Master Techniques in Orthopaedic Surgery

Pediatrics

Master Techniques in Orthopaedic Surgery

Editor-in-Chief
Bernard F. Morrey, MD

Volume Editors

Relevant Surgical Exposures
Bernard F. Morrey, MD
Matthew C. Morrey, MD

The Hand
James Strickland, MD
Thomas Graham, MD

The Wrist
Richard H. Gelberman, MD

The Elbow
Bernard F. Morrey, MD

The Shoulder
Edward V. Craig, MD

The Spine
David S. Bradford, MD
Thomas L. Zdeblick, MD

The Hip
Robert L. Barrack, MD

Reconstructive Knee Surgery
Douglas W. Jackson, MD

Knee Arthroplasty
Paul A. Lotke, MD
Jess H. Lonner, MD

The Foot & Ankle
Harold B. Kitaoka, MD

Fractures
Donald A. Wiss, MD

Pediatrics
Vernon T. Tolo, MD
David L. Skaggs, MD

Soft-Tissue Surgery
Steven L. Moran, MD
William P. Cooney, MD

Peripheral Nerve Surgery
Robert J. Spinner, MD

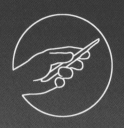

Master Techniques in Orthopaedic Surgery

Pediatrics

Editors

Vernon T. Tolo, MD
John C. Wilson, Jr. Professor of Orthopaedics
Keck School of Medicine
University of Southern California
Director, Childrens Orthopaedic Center
Childrens Hospital Los Angeles
Los Angeles, California

David L. Skaggs, MD
Endowed Chair of Pediatric Spinal Disorders
Associate Professor of Orthopaedic Surgery
Keck School of Medicine
University of Southern California
Associate Director, Childrens Orthopaedic Center
Childrens Hospital Los Angeles
Los Angeles, California

 Wolters Kluwer | Lippincott Williams & Wilkins
Health

Philadelphia • Baltimore • New York • London
Buenos Aires • Hong Kong • Sydney • Tokyo

Acquisitions Editor: Robert Hurley
Senior Managing Editor: David Murphy, Jr.
Developmental Editor: Keith Donnellan, Dovetail Content Solutions
Project Manager: Alicia Jackson
Senior Manufacturing Manager: Benjamin Rivera
Director of Marketing: Sharon Zinner
Creative Director: Doug Smock
Cover Designer: Karen Quigley
Production Service: International Typesetting and Composition

© 2008 by LIPPINCOTT WILLIAMS & WILKINS, a WOLTERS KLUWER business
530 Walnut Street
Philadelphia, PA 19106 USA
LWW.com

Printed in China

Library of Congress Cataloging-in-Publication Data

Pediatrics / editors, Vernon T. Tolo, David L. Skaggs.
    p. ; cm. —(Master techniques in orthopaedic surgery)
  Includes bibliographical references and index.
  ISBN-13: 978-0-7817-9124-3
  ISBN-10: 0-7817-9124-3
 1. Pediatric orthopedics. 2. Orthopedic surgery. I. Tolo, Vernon T.
II. Skaggs, David L. III. Series: Master techniques in orthopaedic
surgery (3rd ed.)
  [DNLM: 1. Orthopedic Procedures—methods. 2. Adolescent. 3. Child.
WS 270 P3719 2008]
  RD732.3.C48P46 2008
  618.92'7—dc22

                                        2007049809

Care has been taken to confirm the accuracy of the information presented and to describe generally accepted practices. However, the authors, editors, and publisher are not responsible for errors or omissions or for any consequences from application of the information in this book and make no warranty, expressed or implied, with respect to the currency, completeness, or accuracy of the contents of the publication. Application of the information in a particular situation remains the professional responsibility of the practitioner.

The authors, editors, and publisher have exerted every effort to ensure that drug selection and dosage set forth in this text are in accordance with current recommendations and practice at the time of publication. However, in view of ongoing research, changes in government regulations, and the constant flow of information relating to drug therapy and drug reactions, the reader is urged to check the package insert for each drug for any change in indications and dosage and for added warnings and precautions. This is particularly important when the recommended agent is a new or infrequently employed drug.

Some drugs and medical devices presented in the publication have Food and Drug Administration (FDA) clearance for limited use in restricted research settings. It is the responsibility of the health care provider to ascertain the FDA status of each drug or device planned for use in their clinical practice.

To purchase additional copies of this book, call our customer service department at (800) 638-3030 or fax orders to (301) 223-2320. International customers should call (301) 223-2300.

Visit Lippincott Williams & Wilkins on the Internet at LWW.com. Lippincott Williams & Wilkins customer service representatives are available from 8:30 am to 6 pm, EST.

10 9 8 7 6 5 4 3 2 1

The editors would like to dedicate this book to our partners, Robert Kay, Jennifer Weiss, Paul Choi, Deirdre Ryan, Alex Arkader, and Nina Lightdale, who help make coming to work each day fun and educational.

I thank Charlene, my wife of 42 years, who has supported me greatly and has encouraged me in so many ways, as she has put up with the time spent on my love of orthopaedics. I also acknowledge the skill and dedication of Phyllis D'Ambra, RN, who has helped my patients and me so often over the past 20 years.

—VTT

I thank my wife, Valerie, and children, Kira, Jamie, and Clay, to whom I can't wait to get home to each night. I am grateful to Janet Jack, RN, my nurse for the past 12 years, both for her expertise in orthopaedics and for her ability to make everyone feel special and cared for.

—DLS

Contents

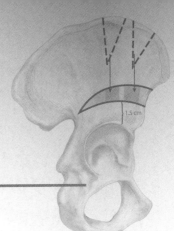

Series Preface

Since its inception in 1994, the *Master Techniques in Orthopaedic Surgery* series has become the gold standard for both physicians in training and experienced surgeons. Its exceptional success may be traced to the leadership of the original series editor, Roby Thompson, whose clarity of thought and focused vision sought "to provide direct, detailed access to techniques preferred by orthopaedic surgeons who are recognized by their colleagues as 'masters' in their specialty," as he stated in his series preface. It is personally very rewarding to hear testimonials from both residents and practicing orthopaedic surgeons on the value of these volumes to their training and practice.

A key element of the success of the series is its format. The effectiveness of the format is reflected by the fact that it is now being replicated by others. An essential feature is the standardized presentation of information replete with tips and pearls shared by experts with years of experience. Abundant color photographs and drawings guide the reader through the procedures step-by-step.

The second key to the success of the *Master Techniques* series rests in the reputation and experience of our volume editors. The editors are truly dedicated "masters" with a commitment to share their rich experience through these texts. We feel a great debt of gratitude to them and a real responsibility to maintain and enhance the reputation of the *Master Techniques* series that has developed over the years. We are proud of the progress made in formulating the third edition volumes and are particularly pleased with the expanded content of this series. Six new volumes will soon be available covering topics that are exciting and relevant to a broad cross-section of our profession. While we are in the process of carefully expanding *Master Techniques* topics and editors, we are committed to the now-classic format.

The first of the new volumes is—*Relevant Surgical Exposures*—which I have had the honor of editing. The second new volume is *Pediatrics*. Subsequent new topics to be introduced are *Soft Tissue Reconstruction*, *Management of Peripheral Nerve Dysfunction*, *Advanced Reconstructive Techniques in the Joint*, and finally *Essential Procedures in Sports Medicine*. The full library thus will consist of 16 useful and relevant titles.

I am pleased to have accepted the position of series editor, feeling so strongly about the value of this series to educate the orthopaedic surgeon in the full array of expert surgical procedures. The true worth of this endeavor will continue to be measured by the ever-increasing success and critical acceptance of the series. I remain indebted to Dr. Thompson for his inaugural vision and leadership, as well as to the *Master Techniques* volume editors and numerous contributors who have been true to the series style and vision. As I indicated in the preface to the second edition of *The Hip* volume, the words of William Mayo are especially relevant to characterize the ultimate goal of this endeavor: "The best interest of the patient is the only interest to be considered." We are confident that the information in the expanded *Master Techniques* offers the surgeon an opportunity to realize the patient-centric view of our surgical practice.

Bernard F. Morrey, MD

Preface

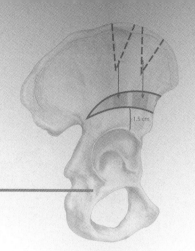

This volume of *Master Techniques in Orthopaedic Surgery* is the first of this excellent series devoted to orthopaedic surgery of children and adolescents. The authors are expert and experienced pediatric orthopaedists who have incorporated lessons learned from their years of clinical experience into each of the 41 chapters. Each chapter either addresses a number of choices of surgical treatment for a distinct clinical condition or concentrates on the technique and nuances of a single surgical procedure that may be used to treat a variety of clinical disorders. An effort has been made to include the most up-to-date surgical techniques that practicing orthopaedic surgeons may not have learned during their training.

Despite the large number of authors and the variety of writing styles, the chapters have been organized in similar fashion throughout, making it easier for readers to quickly find the section or sections they are looking for. Each chapter addresses indications and contraindications, preoperative planning, detailed specifics of the surgical procedure, postoperative management, complications, and "pearls and pitfalls," and includes a short list of references for further reading. All chapters are well illustrated with operative photographs, line drawings, and radiographs.

Several chapters reflect the current approach of treating more pediatric fractures operatively than has been done in years past. As such, they describe up-to-date operative procedures used for these common pediatric fractures. Hip disorders, including congenital hip dislocation, slipped capital femoral epiphysis, and hip dysplasia associated with neuromuscular conditions, are addressed in a number of chapters that provide detailed and easily understood explanations of the osteotomies used to treat these conditions. The treatment of clubfoot has changed quite dramatically in the past decade, and the related chapters highlight the indications and techniques for the recently popular Ponseti treatment and for the extensive surgical release approach. A major section includes chapters on the spine, from the cervical spine to the sacrum, with several chapters focusing on the variety of current surgical approaches being used to treat spinal deformity. Other chapters to attract the reader include those for pediatric sports medicine (discoid meniscus treatment and ACL reconstruction with open physes), pediatric foot deformities requiring osteotomies, leg-length discrepancy, and angular deformity of the lower extremities.

The chapters in this volume will be of value for orthopaedic surgeons specializing in pediatric orthopaedics as well as for orthopaedists who continue to treat children and adolescents as part of a more general orthopaedic practice. In this era of specialization, pediatric orthopaedics is a specialty described by some as general orthopaedics for children and adolescents as defined by age and not by an area of the body, as is the case for much of the specialization in the orthopaedic care of adults. As a result, a very large number of surgical procedures may be considered in the treatment of children and adolescents who have orthopaedic problems, even though each operation may not be done very often. Because of this, it seemed to the editors that the orthopaedic practice community would benefit a great deal from a book such as this that takes a somewhat different approach than is used in other current pediatric orthopaedic textbooks. With the 41 chapters included here, it is hoped that this volume will allow all orthopaedists not only to better understand how to do a specific surgical procedure for their young patients, but also to better understand when and what to do for optimal patient care and outcomes.

Vernon T. Tolo, MD
David L. Skaggs, MD

Contributors

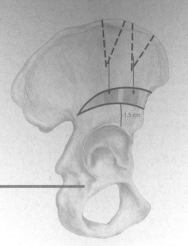

Behrooz A. Akbarnia, MD
San Diego Center for Spinal Disorders
University of California, San Diego
La Jolla, California

Donald S. Bae, MD
Instructor in Orthopaedic Surgery
Harvard Medical School
Department of Orthopaedic Surgery
Children's Hospital Boston
Boston, Massachusetts

Saul M. Bernstein, MD
Southern California Orthopedic Institute
Van Nuys, California

Laurel C. Blakemore, MD
Associate Professor
George Washington University School
of Medicine
Chief, Orthopaedic Surgery and Sports Medicine
Children's National Medical Center
Washington, DC

R. Dale Blasier MD, FRCS(C)
University of Arkansas for Medical Sciences
and Arkansas Children's Hospital
Department of Orthopaedic Surgery
Arkansas Children's Hospital
Little Rock, Arkansas

Jacob M. Buchowski, MD, MS
Assistant Professor of Orthopaedic and Neurological
Surgery
Chief, Degenerative and Minimally Invasive
Spine Surgery
Department of Orthopaedic Surgery
Washington University School of Medicine
St. Louis, Missouri

Robert M. Campbell Jr., MD
Professor of Orthopaedics
The President's Council/Dielmann Chair in Pediatric
Orthopaedics
University of Texas Health Science Center
at San Antonio
Director of The Thoracic Institute
CHRISTUS Santa Rosa Children's Hospital
San Antonio, Texas

Alfred Cook, MD
Department of Orthopaedic Surgery
Northwestern University Feinberg School
of Medicine
Chicago, Illinois

Alvin H. Crawford, MD, FACS
Department of Orthopaedic Surgery
Cincinnati Children's Hospital Medical Center
Cincinnati, Ohio

Michael D. Daubs, MD
Assistant Professor of Orthopaedic Surgery
University of Utah
Salt Lake City, Utah

Richard S. Davidson, MD
Associate Clinical Professor
Children's Hospital of Philadelphia
Hospital of the University of Pennsylvania
Shriners Hospital, Philadelphia
Philadelphia, Pennsylvania

John P. Dormans, MD
Chief of Orthopaedic Surgery
Children's Hospital of Philadelphia
Professor of Orthopaedic Surgery
University of Pennsylvania School of Medicine
Philadelphia, Pennsylvania

John B. Emans, MD
Director
Division of Spine Surgery
Department of Orthopaedic Surgery
Children's Hospital Boston
Harvard Medical School
Boston, Massachusetts

Frances A. Farley, MD
Associate Professor
University of Michigan
Ann Arbor, Michigan

John M. Flynn, MD
Associate Chief of Orthopaedic Surgery
Division of Orthopaedic Surgery
Children's Hospital of Philadelphia
Philadelphia, Pennsylvania

Purushottam A. Gholve, MD, MBMS, MRCS
Research Fellow
Division of Orthopaedic Surgery
Children's Hospital of Philadelphia
Philadelphia, Pennsylvania

Jaime A. Gómez
Columbia University College of Physicians and Surgeons
New York

J. Eric Gordon, MD
St. Louis Shriner's Hospital
Department of Orthopaedic Surgery
St. Louis Children's Hospital and Washington University
 School of Medicine
St. Louis, Missouri

Daniel Hedequist, MD
Division of Spine Surgery
Department of Orthopaedic Surgery
Children's Hospital Boston
Harvard Medical School
Boston, Massachusetts

William L. Hennrikus, MD
Associate Clinical Professor
University of California San Francisco
Children's Hospital Central California
Madera, California

José A. Herrera-Soto, MD
Assistant Director of Pediatric Orthopaedic Fellowship
Orlando Regional Medical Center
Orlando, Florida

Eric W. Hooley, MD
San Diego Center for Spinal Disorders,
University of California, San Diego
La Jolla, California

Charles E. Johnston II, MD
Texas Scottish Rite Hospital for Children
Dallas, Texas

Robert M. Kay, MD
Associate Professor of Orthopaedic Surgery
Keck-University of Southern California
 School of Medicine
Childrens Orthopaedic Center
Childrens Hospital Los Angeles
Los Angeles, California

Najeeb Khan, MD
Department of Orthopaedic Surgery
Northwestern University Feinberg School
 of Medicine
Chicago, Illinois

Yongjung J. Kim, MD
Washington University Medical Center
St. Louis, Missouri

Mininder S. Kocher, MD, MPH
Division of Sports Medicine
Department of Orthopaedic Surgery
Children's Hospital
Harvard Medical School
Boston, Massachusetts

Ken N. Kuo MD
National Health Research Institutes
National Taiwan University Hospital
Taipei, Taiwan

Lawrence G. Lenke, MD
Washington University Medical Center
St. Louis, Missouri

Vincent S. Mosca MD
Associate Professor
Department of Orthopaedics and Sports
 Medicine
University of Washington School of Medicine
Children's Hospital and Regional Medical
 Center
Seattle, Washington

Colin F. Moseley, MD
Chief of Staff
Los Angeles Shriners Hospital
Los Angeles, California

Scott Mubarak, MD
Clinical Professor
University of California San Diego
Children's Hospital
San Diego, California

Peter O. Newton, Jr., MD
Department of Orthopaedics
Children's Hospital San Diego
Department of Orthopaedic Surgery
University of California San Diego
San Diego, California

Kenneth J. Noonan, MD
Associate Professor of Orthopaedics and Rehabilitation
Associate Professor of Pediatrics
University of Wisconsin School of Medicine and Public Health
Madison, Wisconsin

Andrew Perry, MD
Department of Orthopaedic Surgery
University of California San Diego,
San Diego, California

Jonathan H. Phillips, BSc, MB, MS
Orlando Regional Medical Education Faculty
Orlando, Florida

Charles T. Price, MD
Pediatric Orthopaedics
Orlando Regional Healthcare System
Arnold Palmer Hospital for Children
Orlando, Florida

Christopher W. Reilly MD
British Columbia Children's Hospital
Vancouver, British Columbia
Canada

David P. Roye, Jr. MD
St. Giles Professor of Pediatric Orthopaedics
Columbia University College of Physicians and Surgeons
Morgan Stanley Children's Hospital of New York
   Presbyterian
New York

Deidre D. Ryan, MD
Assistant Professor of Orthopaedic Surgery
Keck-University of Southern California School of Medicine
Childrens Orthopaedic Center
Childrens Hospital Los Angeles
Los Angeles, California

Wudbhav N. Sankar, MD
Instructor
Department of Orthopaedic Surgery
University of Pennsylvania Health System
Philadelphia, Pennsylvania

John F. Sarwark, MD
The Children's Memorial Hospital
Chicago, Illinois

Perry L. Schoenecker, MD
St. Louis Shriner's Hospital
Department of Orthopaedic Surgery
St. Louis Children's Hospital and Washington
   University School of Medicine
St. Louis, Missouri

Ernest L. Sink, MD
Assistant Professor
University of Colorado
Department of Orthopaedics
University of Colorado Health Science Center
Denver, Colorado

David L. Skaggs, MD
Endowed Chair of Pediatric Spinal Disorders
Associate Professor of Orthopaedic Surgery
Keck School of Medicine
University of Southern California
Associate Director, Childrens Orthopaedic Center
Childrens Hospital Los Angeles
Los Angeles, California

John T. Smith, MD
Professor
Department of Orthopaedics
University of Utah School of Medicine
Primary Children's Medical Center
Salt Lake City, Utah

Paul D. Sponseller, MD
Riley Professor and Head
Pediatric Orthopaedics
Johns Hopkins Medical Institutions
Baltimore, Maryland

Peter M. Stevens, MD
University of Utah
Department of Orthopaedics
Salt Lake City, Utah

Daniel J. Sucato, MD, MS
Associate Professor
Department of Orthopaedic Surgery
University of Texas at Southwestern
   Medical Center
Texas Scottish Rite Hospital for Children
Dallas, Texas

Vernon T. Tolo, MD
John C. Wilson, Jr. Professor of Orthopaedics
Keck School of Medicine
University of Southern California
Director, Childrens Orthopaedic Center
Childrens Hospital Los Angeles
Los Angeles, California

William Warner, MD
Campbell Clinic
Germantown, Tennessee

Peter M. Waters, MD
Professor of Orthopaedic Surgery
Harvard Medical School
Department of Orthopaedic Surgery
Children's Hospital
Boston, Massachusetts

Jennifer M. Weiss, MD
Childrens Hospital Los Angeles
Children's Orthopaedic Center
Keck-University of Southern California School of Medicine
Los Angeles, California

Bouchaib Yousri, MD
Pediatric Orthopaedics
Orlando Regional Healthcare System
Arnold Palmer Hospital for Children
Orlando, Florida

SECTION I
TRAUMA

1

Closed Reduction and Pinning of Supracondylar Humerus Fractures

David L. Skaggs

INDICATIONS/CONTRAINDICATIONS

Because the operative treatment of supracondylar fractures with reduction and pinning is so effective and safe, the great majority of displaced fractures should be treated operatively. There is little controversy that all closed Gartland type III fractures should have an attempt at closed reduction and pinning. In fractures that are not clearly displaced, three criteria may be helpful in determining whether the fracture should be treated operatively: (a) On a lateral view of the elbow, the anterior humeral line should intersect the capitellum. It does not necessarily need to bisect the capitellum, but it should at least touch it. Initial attempts at a lateral x-ray may be of poor quality and need to be repeated (Fig. 1-1). (b) Baumann's angle should be at least 11 degrees (Fig. 1-2). (c) The medial and lateral column should be intact. Beware of fractures in which the medial column is comminuted, which is usually associated with a loss of Baumann's angle and is an indication for pinning (Fig. 1-3).

Controversy exists as to how much displacement warrants operative reduction. In the past, type II fractures have been treated with closed reduction and casting in hyperflexion to maintain the reduction. Studies have shown that as elbow flexion increases in children with supracondylar fractures, the forearm's compartment pressure increases, and the brachial artery flow decreases, creating an environment ripe for a compartment syndrome. As contemporary case series have such good

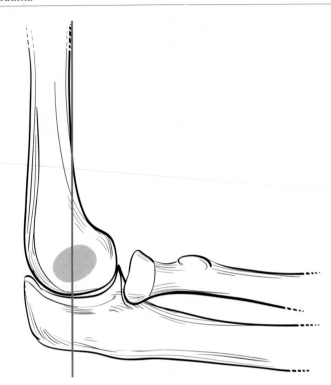

FIGURE 1-1

On a lateral view of the elbow, the anterior humeral line should intersect the capitellum.

outcomes for the closed results and pinning of type II fractures, many believe that it is safer to hold a type II fracture reduced with pins than it is to flex the elbow greater than 90 degrees (Fig. 1-4).

There is little growth and remodeling about the elbow. In most cases, accepting a fracture position in which the capitellum is posterior to the anterior humeral line on the lateral view cannot be reliably predicted to remodel, and the child is likely to permanently end up with less flexion and greater extension of the affected arm. In young children, where the anterior capitellum almost just touches the anterior humeral line, casting in situ may be considered. In general, however, indications for the closed reduction and percutaneous pinning of supracondylar humerus fractures in children are all closed, acute, and displaced (type II and III) fractures.

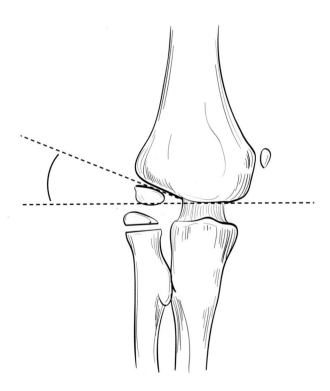

FIGURE 1-2

Baumann's angle is variable, but in general is at least 11 degrees.

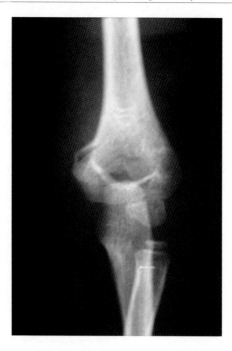

FIGURE 1-3
Look for medial comminution, which is indicative of the fracture being in varus and usually requiring operative reduction and pinning.

PREOPERATIVE PLANNING

The most important part of preoperative planning is assessing the soft tissues. A good rule of thumb is to assume that about 20% of fractures have neurologic or vascular injuries. An examination of the neurovascular status is important, but is often limited by an uncooperative, scared, young child. The ulnar nerve in particular should be assessed if a medial pin is likely. A good way to assess the ulnar nerve's motor portion in young children is to palpate the first dorsal web space for setting of the interosseous muscle as the child attempts to pinch you.

The vascular status consists of two assessments: Is the hand warm and well perfused? and Is the radial pulse present? In a poorly perfused limb, gentle flexion of the elbow to 20 to 40 degrees at presentation is often all that is necessary for perfusion and pulse to return. If the hand remains pulseless and poorly perfused, urgent operative reduction is indicated. Arteriography or other vascular studies are not indicated and only cause a needless delay in treatment.

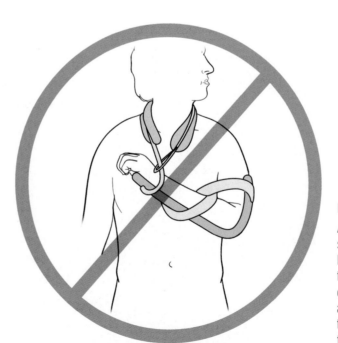

FIGURE 1-4
Avoid casting a supracondylar fracture beyond 90 degrees, as this position increases compartment pressures and decreases perfusion to the hand and forearm.

Although recent studies suggest that a delay in treatment of supracondylar fractures is acceptable, do not confuse a delay in treatment with a delay in assessment. If a fracture shows significant swelling, ecchymosis, puckering of the skin, an ipsilateral forearm fracture, a long delay in treatment, or tense forearm compartments, it is at risk for a compartment syndrome and may require urgent treatment.

At this time, examining the patient's contralateral arm for assessment of the carrying angle may prove helpful when later assessing fracture reduction. Patients are usually consented for possible open reduction.

SURGICAL PROCEDURE

Once in the operating room, the patient receives a general anesthetic and prophylactic antibiotics. It is usually best to place the fluoroscopy monitor opposite the surgeon for ease of viewing (Fig. 1-5).

The patient is positioned supine on the operating table, with the fractured elbow on a radiolucent arm board. Some surgeons use the wide end of the fluoroscopy unit as the table. However, doing so does not allow rotation of the fluoroscopy unit for lateral images of the elbow in cases of unusual instability in which rotation of the arm leads to loss of reduction. It is essential that the arm is far enough onto the arm board that the elbow can be well visualized with fluoroscopy. In very small children, this may mean having the child's shoulder and head on the arm board as well (Fig. 1-6).

The patient's arm is then sterilized and draped. First, traction is applied, with the elbow flexed about 20 degrees to avoid tethering neurovascular structures over an anteriorly displaced proximal fragment. For badly displaced fractures, hold significant traction for 60 seconds to allow soft-tissue realignment, with the surgeon grasping the forearm with both hands and the assistant providing countertraction in the axilla (Fig. 1-7).

If it appears that the proximal fragment has pierced the brachialis, the "milking maneuver" is performed (Fig. 1-8). In this maneuver, the biceps are forcibly "milked" in a proximal-to-distal direction past the proximal fragment, often culminating in a palpable release of the humerus posteriorly through the brachialis.

Next, varus and valgus angular alignment is addressed by moving the forearm. Medial and lateral fracture translation is now corrected by directly moving the distal fragment with one's thumbs, followed by image confirmation. The elbow is then slowly flexed while applying anterior pressure to the olecranon with the surgeon's thumb(s) (Fig. 1-9).

Following a successful reduction (Fig. 1-10), the child's fingers should be able to touch the shoulder. If not, the fracture is still likely in extension (Fig. 1-11). If during the reduction maneuver, the fracture does not stay reduced, and a "rubbery" feeling is encountered instead of the desired "bone on bone" feeling, the median nerve and/or brachial artery may be trapped within the fracture site (Fig. 1-12). If this occurs, an open reduction is generally to remove the neurovascular structures from the fracture site.

Many have described using pronation to assist in reduction, but this should not be automatic. In the most common posterior-medially displaced fracture, the medial periosteum is usually intact. In this

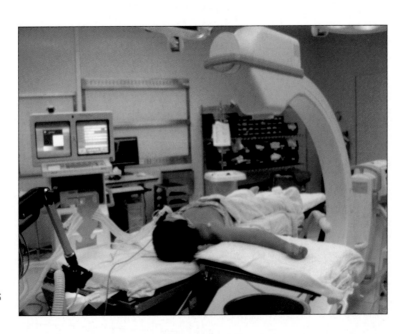

FIGURE 1-5

Positioning the fluoroscopy monitor on the opposite side of the bed allows the surgeon to easily see the images while operating.

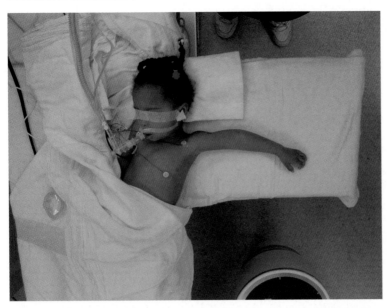

FIGURE 1-6   In small children, imaging of the elbow may be difficult if the arm is not long enough to reach the center of the fluoroscopy unit. By placing the child's head in the crack between the operating room table and the arm board, the elbow is more easily centered for imaging, and the child's head is unlikely to be inadvertently pulled off the side of the bed during the procedure.

instance, pronation may assist in reduction by placing the medial periosteum in tension and closing down the otherwise open lateral column (Fig. 1-13). However, the medial periosteum is often torn in a posterior-laterally displaced fracture, in which case pronation may thus be counterproductive.

The reduction is then checked by fluoroscopic images in anteroposterior, lateral, and oblique planes. The surgeon should verify four points to check for a good reduction: (a) The anterior humeral line intersects the capitellum (Fig. 1-1). (b) Baumann's angle is greater than 10 degrees (Fig. 1-2). (c) The medial and lateral columns are intact on oblique views (Fig. 1-14). If difficulty is encountered maintaining fracture reduction when externally rotating the shoulder for a lateral view of the elbow, consider moving the C-arm instead of the patient's arm (Fig. 1-15).

Some translation (up to perhaps 5 mm) is acceptable, as long as the above other criteria are met (Fig. 1-16). Similarly, a moderate amount of persistent rotational malalignment is also acceptable, as long as the above criteria are met. Because the shoulder joint has so much rotation, it is highly unlikely

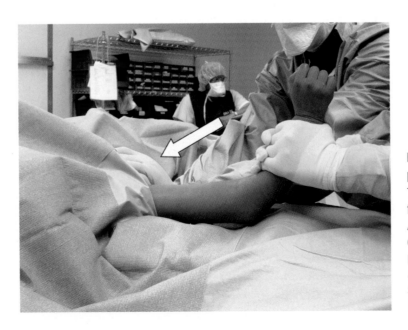

FIGURE 1-7

Reduction maneuver: Traction with elbow flexed 20 to 30 degrees. Assistant provides countertraction against patient's axilla *(white arrow)* to allow for significant traction to be applied.

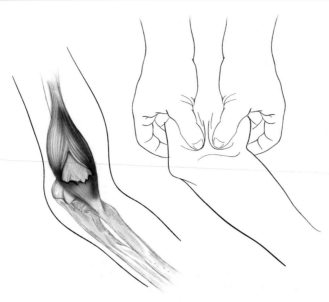

FIGURE 1-8   Brachialis muscle interposition is indicated on the left. The "milking maneuver" frees the brachialis muscle from its location in the fracture, allowing a closed reduction. (Redrawn after Peters C, Scott SM, Stevens P. Closed reduction and percutaneous pinning of displaced supracondylar fractures in children: description of a new closed reduction technique for fractures with brachialis muscle entrapment. *J Orthop Trauma*. 1995;9:430–434, with permission.)

FIGURE 1-9

Reduction maneuver: Flex elbow (*white arrow*) while pushing anteriorly on the olecranon with your thumbs (*red arrow*).

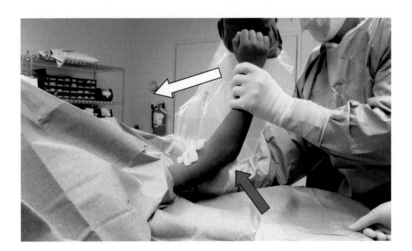

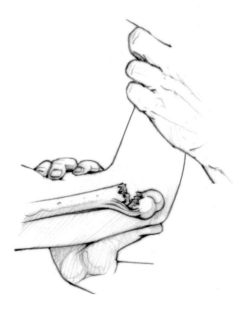

FIGURE 1-10

Reduction maneuver.

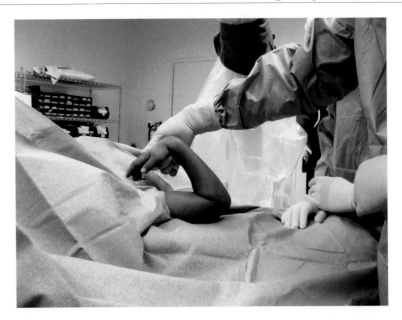

FIGURE 1-11
If fingers cannot touch shoulder, flexion deformity may not be reduced.

to cause a functional problem. Once reduction is satisfactory, use elastic bandage to maintain the elbow in the reduced position of elbow hyperflexion to prevent loss of reduction while pinning (Fig. 1-17)

The elbow is positioned on a folded towel. The surgeon then palpates the lateral humeral condyle. Most commonly, 0.062-in. smooth Kirschner wires (Zimmer, Warsaw, IN) are used, though smaller or larger sizes may be considered if the child is extremely small or large.

The aim of pin placement is to maximally separate the pins at the fracture site to engage both the medial and lateral columns (Fig. 1-18). Whether the pins are divergent or parallel and which pin is placed first are of little importance. Care must be taken to ensure there is sufficient bone engaged in the proximal and distal fragments. It is acceptable to cross the olecranon fossa, which adds two more cortices to improve fixation, but note that this means the elbow cannot fully extend until the pins are removed. In the sagittal plane, to engage the most bone with the K-wire in the distal fragment, the K-wire may go through the capitellum. The reduced capitellum lies slightly anterior to the plane of the fracture; thus, the pin may start a bit anterior to the plane of the fracture and angulate about 10 to 15 degrees posteriorly to maximize osseous purchase. A key element to ensure a correctly placed

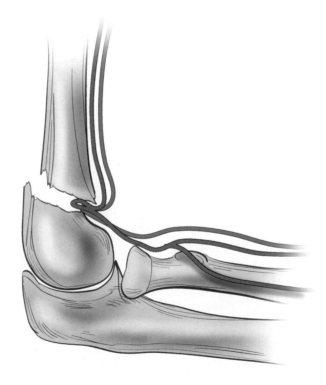

FIGURE 1-12

Brachial artery and median nerve may be trapped at the fracture site. If a reduction feels rubbery and a gap at the fracture site is seen on imaging, entrapment is possible, especially in the setting of vascular compromise or median nerve or anterior interosseus nerve injury.

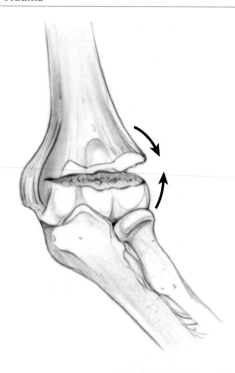

FIGURE 1-13

Pronation closes the hinge as the elbow is flexed, correcting the varus.

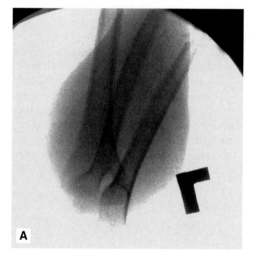
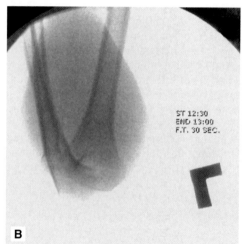

FIGURE 1-14

Oblique views demonstrating intact **(A)** lateral and **(B)** medial columns.

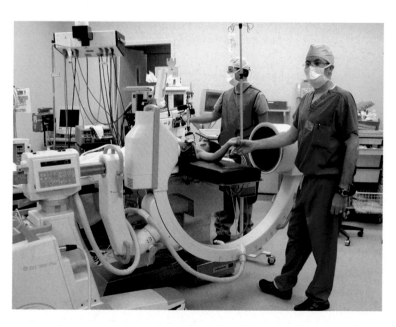

FIGURE 1-15

In very unstable fractures, rotation of the shoulder into external rotation to obtain a lateral image of the elbow may lead to a loss of reduction. In these rare instances, rotating the C-arm, rather than the elbow, is a useful trick.

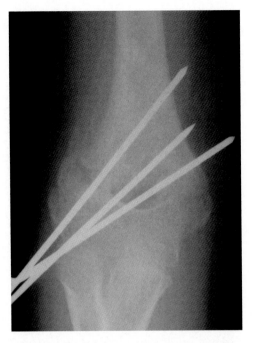

FIGURE 1-16

In this child, about 5 mm of persistent lateral translation was accepted rather than perform an open reduction. There was no noticeable clinical sequelae of this translation.

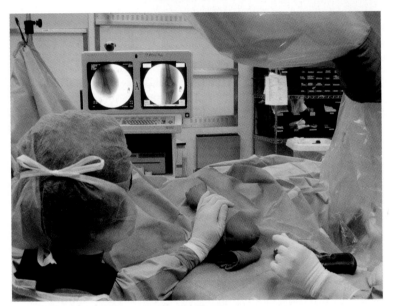

FIGURE 1-17

Holding reduction in hyperflexion with sterile elastic bandage frees the surgeon's hands to concentrate on pin placement. Think of the cartilaginous distal humerus as a pincushion. With the K-wires, not the drill, in your fingers, push them into the cartilage in the exact location and trajectory you want. Verify with imaging, then advance the pin with a drill.

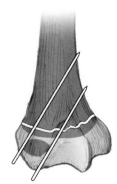
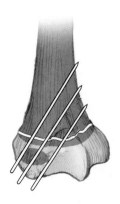
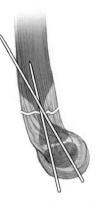

FIGURE 1-18   Separate the pins at the fracture site to engage both the medial and the lateral columns. (Redrawn after Skaggs DL, Cluck MW, Mostofi A, et al. Lateral-entry pin fixation in the management of supracondylar fractures in children. *J Bone Joint Surg.* 2004; 86A:702–707, with permission.)

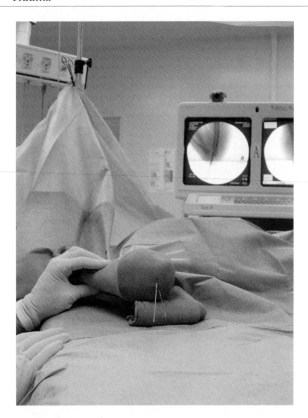

FIGURE 1-19

Assessment of sagittal alignment with lateral view.

pin is to feel the pin go through the proximal cortex. If this feeling is not clearly appreciated, careful fluoroscopic imaging often reveals that the pin did not engage the proximal fragment. As a general rule, it is best to use two pins for Gartland type II fractures and three pins for Gartland type III fractures. Even though two good pins are probably sufficient, placing three pins increases the odds of actually having two good ones.

The K-wire is placed against the lateral condyle without piercing the skin and is checked with anteroposterior fluoroscopic guidance to assess the starting point. The K-wire is held free in the

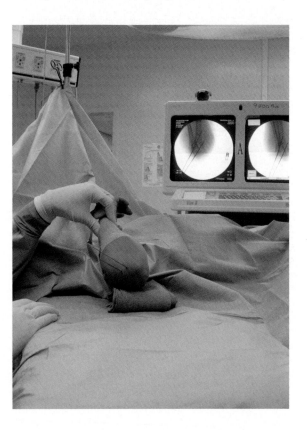

FIGURE 1-20

Check both oblique views to assess reduction of medial and lateral columns.

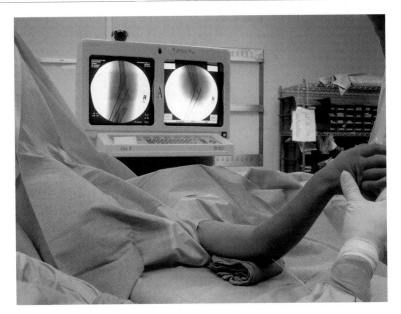

FIGURE 1-21
If the lateral and oblique views show good reduction, remove the tape and check reduction and pin placement in the anteroposterior view with the elbow in relative elbow extension.

surgeon's hand at this point, not in the drill, to allow maximum control. If the starting point and trajectory are correct, the wire may be pushed through the skin and into the cartilage, using the cartilage of the distal lateral condyle as a pincushion that will hold the K-wire in place while you carefully examine the anteroposterior and lateral images. If imaging verifies correct pin placement, advance the pin with a drill (Figs. 1-17 till 1-21). Precise pin placement is an important part of the procedure that should not be rushed, as incorrect pin placement is usually the cause of loss of reduction. The reduction is again checked under fluoroscopy with lateral, oblique, and anteroposterior views.

Stress should be applied in varus and valgus under fluoroscopy to ensure stability (Fig. 1-22). It is important to know about any instability now, rather than a week later. Save the images in which the reduction looks the "worst," particularly if some translational or rotational malreduction is accepted. Keep these images for comparison during postoperative visits to determine whether any movement of the fracture has occurred.

Once the surgeon is satisfied with fracture reduction and pin placement, vascular status is assessed. The wires are bent and cut. The wires are left at least 1 cm to 2 cm off the skin afterward to prevent migration of the wires under the skin. A sterile felt square with a slit cut into it is then placed around the wires to protect the skin (Fig. 1-23).

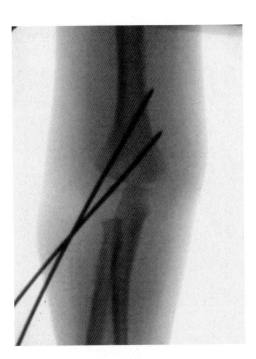

FIGURE 1-22
Stress the elbow. If there is any question about stability, a third pin should be added, or a pin with poor fixation should be replaced.

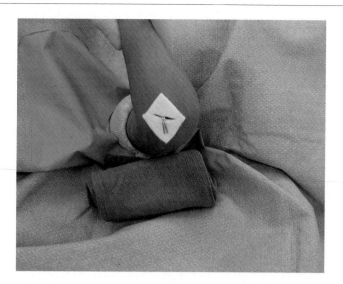

FIGURE 1-23

Skin is protected from pins with felt squares.

Foam is applied to the arm on the anterior and posterior aspects of the elbow (Fig. 1-24). The cast is then applied in 45 to 60 degrees of elbow flexion; flexion to 90 degrees may needlessly increase the risk of compartment pressure (Fig. 1-25). The pins, not the cast, are holding the fracture reduction. Fiberglass casting material is used because of its strength, weight, and radiolucency. When properly applied, fiberglass does not lead to a tight cast.

Alternative Technique: Crossed Pins

Although the majority of supracondylar humerus fractures can be treated with lateral entry pins alone, some good surgeons routinely use crossed pins, entering from the medial and lateral condyles. The danger of placing a medial pin is either direct injury to the ulnar nerve or, more commonly, entrapment of tissue adjacent to the nerve. It has been shown that an incision for medial pin placement cannot be relied on to protect the ulnar nerve, most likely because entrapping tissue adjacent to the nerve may be sufficient to cause constriction of the cubital tunnel. Ulnar nerve instability is present quite often in children. In children under the age of 5, more than half subluxate their ulnar nerve when their elbow is bent more than 90 degrees. If a medial pin is used, the surgeon should insert the lateral pin(s) first and extend the elbow while inserting the medial pin. Remember the principle of not crossing the pins at the fracture site.

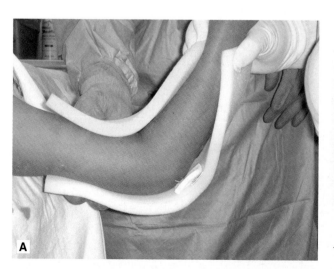
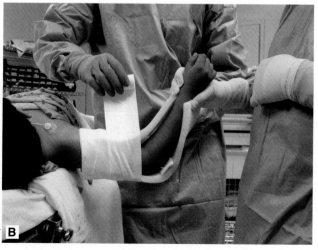

FIGURE 1-24 A, B. Sterile foam is placed directly on the skin. If there is any circumferential dressing placed under the foam, it may be restricting.

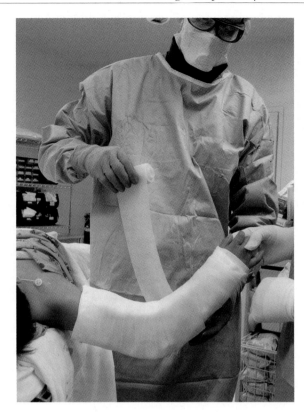

FIGURE 1-25
Cast with elbow flexion no more than 60 degrees, with even less flexion for very swollen elbows.

POSTOPERATIVE CARE

Patients with minimal swelling who are believed to be at little risk for compartment syndrome may be discharged to home with appropriate postoperative instructions. Otherwise children are generally admitted overnight for elevation and observation. The patient customarily returns 5 to 7 days postoperatively, at which time anteroposterior and lateral radiographs are obtained. If the highly unlikely event of a loss of reduction were to occur, this would be noted in sufficient time for re-reduction. This return visit is probably not necessary in most cases. The cast is generally removed 3 weeks postoperatively, at which time radiographs are obtained out of the cast. The pins are removed in the outpatient setting at this time. Range of motion exercises are taught to the family, targeting gentle flexion and extension, to be started a few days after cast removal. The child returns 6 weeks postoperatively for a range-of-motion check, with no radiographs at that time.

COMPLICATIONS TO AVOID

- Vascular: If there is any question of perfusion following fracture reduction in the operating room, the surgical prep may be removed to evaluate the skin color. In addition, a Doppler may be used to assess the pulse. In the case of a poorly perfused hand following reduction, if the hand was well perfused prior to reduction, one must assume that the artery or adjacent tissue is trapped in the fracture site. The pins should immediately be removed to allow the fracture to return to its unreduced position. If there is no pulse postoperatively in an arm that had no pulse preoperatively, but the hand is warm and well perfused, it is probably best to observe the child in the hospital for 48 hours with the arm mildly elevated. The rich collateral circulation about the elbow is generally sufficient.
- Ulnar nerve injury: See above section, "Alternative Technique: Crossed Pins".
- Loss of reduction:
  - Clinical experience of a series of 124 consecutive supracondylar humerus fractures, including completely unstable fractures, has taught us that lateral entry pins, when properly placed, are strong enough to maintain reduction of even the most unstable supracondylar humerus fracture.

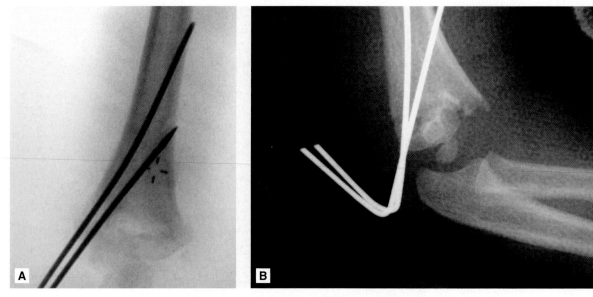

FIGURE 1-26 If the pins are placed too close together, they biomechanically function as one pin, and rotation around the pins is not surprising. **(A)** Intraoperative radiograph. **(B)** Postoperative loss of reduction in the same patient. (From Skaggs DL, Cluck MW, Mostofi A, et al. Lateral-entry pin fixation in the management of supracondylar fractures in children. *J Bone Joint Surg.* 2004;86A:702–707, with permission.)

Improper pin placement, however, jeopardizes stability, whether lateral entry or crossed pins are used (Figs. 1-26–1-28).

○ If a surgeon encounters difficulty placing lateral entry pins in a stable configuration, placement of a medial pin in an extended elbow may be indicated rather than risk loss of reduction.

PEARLS AND PITFALLS

● Aim to separate the pins as far as possible at the fracture site.
● Think of the cartilaginous distal humerus as a pincushion. With the K-wires in your fingers (not the drill), push them into the cartilage in the exact location and trajectory you want. Verify with imaging, then advance the pin with a drill.

FIGURE 1-27

A, B. In accordance with standard fracture principles, pins that cross at the fracture site do not provide stability. (From Skaggs DL, Cluck MW, Mostofi A, et al. Lateral-entry pin fixation in the management of supracondylar fractures in children. *J Bone Joint Surg.* 2004;86A:702–707, with permission.)

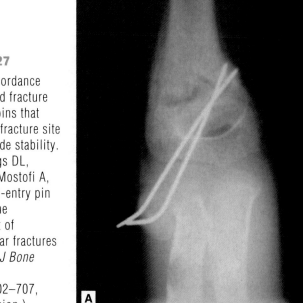
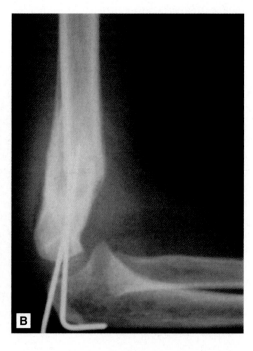

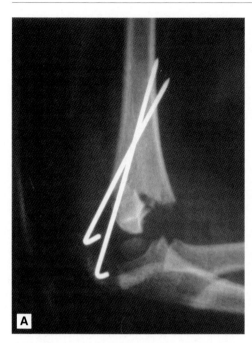
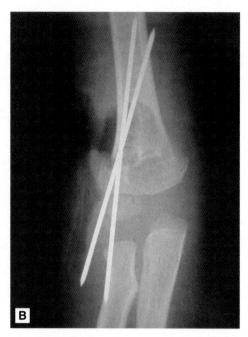

FIGURE 1-28   A, B. Insufficient bone is engaged in the distal fragments, so loss of fixation may be expected. (From Skaggs DL, Cluck MW, Mostofi A, et al. Lateral-entry pin fixation in the management of supracondylar fractures in children. *J Bone Joint Surg.* 2004;86A:702–707, with permission.)

- Do not hesitate to use three pins, especially for most type III fractures.
- If the first pin is in between where you really wanted two pins, just leave it and place one on either side of it, for a total of three pins.
- A small amount of translation or axial rotational malalignment may be accepted rather than doing an open reduction, but accept very little frontal plane or sagittal angular malalignment.
- Following reduction and fixation, stress the fracture under live imaging to the point where you are confident it will not fall apart postoperatively.
- Cast the elbow in significantly less than 90 degrees of flexion to avoid compartment syndrome; the pins are holding the reduction, not the cast.
- If you choose to place a medial pin, extend the elbow when placing the pin to keep the ulnar nerve posteriorly out of harm's way.

REFERENCES

1. Archibeck MJ, Smith JT, Carroll KL, et al. Surgical release of tethered spinal cord: survivorship analysis and orthopedic outcome. *J Pediatr Orthop.* 1997;17:773–776.
2. Battaglia TC, Armstrong DG, Schwend RM. Factors affecting forearm compartment pressures in children with supracondylar fractures of the humerus. *J Pediatr Orthop.* 2002;22:431–439.
3. Lee SS, Mahar AT, Miesen D, et al. Displaced pediatric supracondylar humerus fractures: biomechanical analysis of percutaneous pinning techniques. *J Pediatr Orthop.* 2002;22:440–443.
4. Mapes R, Hennrikus W. The effect of elbow position on the radial pulse measured by Doppler ultrasonography after surgical treatment of supracondylar elbow fractures in children. *J Pediatr Orthop.* 1998;18:441–444.
5. Rasool MN. Ulnar nerve injury after K-wire fixation of supracondylar humerus fractures in children. *J Pediatr Orthop.* 1998;18:686–690.
6. Skaggs DL, Cluck MW, Mostofi A, et al. Lateral-entry pin fixation in the management of supracondylar fractures in children. *J Bone Joint Surg.* 2004;86A:702–707.
7. Zaltz I, Waters PM, Kasser JR. Ulnar nerve instability in children. *J Pediatr Orthop.* 1996;16:567–569.

2 Operative Treatment of Lateral Condyle Fractures

R. Dale Blasier

Lateral condyle fractures are relatively common in children and occur usually as a result of a fall. The extent of displacement depends on the energy of the fall. The fractures usually can be described as either a Salter-Harris type III or a Salter-Harris type IV.

INDICATIONS/CONTRAINDICATIONS

Indications

The need for surgery depends on the type of lateral condyle fracture (Fig. 2-1).

1. An undisplaced fracture generally can be treated by simple immobilization in an above-elbow cast for 4 weeks. An x-ray should be obtained at 1 week to check for late fracture displacement.
2. The relatively unusual hinged-type fracture can be managed by long-arm cast immobilization or by reduction and pinning. The hinged fracture can be proven radiographically by a magnetic resonance image (MRI), an arthrogram, or an ultrasound or by fluoroscopic evaluation under anesthesia. If reduction can be maintained by applying a varus force, the fracture fragment returns to a well-reduced position from the displaced position when the force is released. Reduction can be maintained by direct manual pressure over the lateral condyle while percutaneous pinning is done. If there is any question about the reduction or stability, the fractures should be treated with open reduction and pin fixation.
3. The undisplaced complete fracture can be treated closed. It should, however, be operated on if it displaces later. Therefore close follow-up is required; surgical treatment is needed if lateral displacement of the fracture fragment occurs on the following radiographs.
4. Displaced complete fractures require open reduction and internal fixation to restore alignment of the growth plate and the articular surface.

The Milch classification addresses whether the lateral condyle fracture is confined to the capitellum (type I) thereby leaving the ulna trochlear joint intact and stable or enters the trochlea (type II) and renders the ulnotrochlear joint unstable. This classification is not usually important in terms of treatment, because all significantly displaced intra-articular lateral condyle fractures need to be anatomically reduced and pinned, regardless of whether the fractures affect the ulnotrochlear joint.

In addition to the requirement for surgical treatment of displaced fractures to align the joint surface and align the physis, surgery is required for open fractures and in the very rare case of an irreducible dislocation.

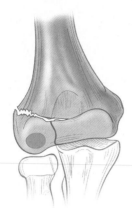
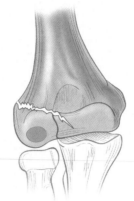

A   Undisplaced fracture   **B**   Hinged fracture

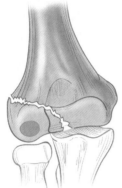
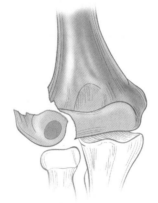

FIGURE 2-1

Lateral condyle
fractures.

    Complete and   Complete and

C   undisplaced fracture   **D**   displaced fracture

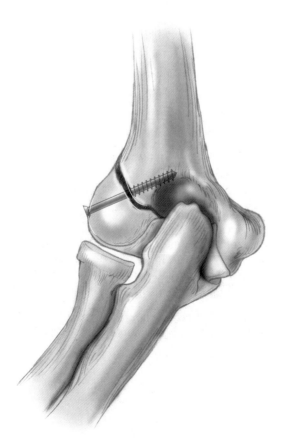

FIGURE 2-2

Screw through
metaphysis.

Contraindications

Surgery should be avoided in patients who present very late, although the exact time following injury at which open reduction should not be attempted remains unclear. In a late case, the surgical landmarks are no longer easily recognized at surgery, and the vascular supply to the fracture fragment may be compromised by dissection.

PREOPERATIVE PLANNING

The surgeon must review the radiographs of the acute fracture to determine the degree of displacement and degree of rotation. If the condylar fragment is not rotated, it can sometimes be treated by closed reduction and pinning under anesthesia. Screws can be used if there is a large enough metaphyseal fragment to accommodate them, as the goal here is to lag the metaphyseal fragment portion of the fracture back to the distal humerus (Fig. 2-2). In some cases, due to the cartilaginous nature of the epiphysis, it will be difficult to tell whether the fragment is hinged into the joint or is complete and somewhat displaced. In this case, one should consider obtaining an MRI or an arthrogram (Fig. 2-3) to determine the extent of the fracture. If fracture reduction is satisfactory after closed manipulation, the fracture should be pinned in this position. If reduction is incomplete or if there is a question about the adequacy of the reduction, the fracture should be opened and reduced anatomically with pin fixation.

In cases where the fracture is old (greater than 6 weeks), it will be necessary to use a computed tomography (CT) scan or MRI of the distal humerus to determine whether the fragments can be reduced.

Surgical Procedure

Some special operating room equipment is necessary. It is useful to have a radiolucent table or arm board to allow easy fluoroscopic access to the distal humerus. Fluoroscopy, of course, is required, and the monitor should be placed in a position easily visible to the surgeon to avoid having to turn away from the operative field. A tourniquet provides a bloodless field. A power drill is required to drill or place pins. Reduction clamps, such as those resembling a towel clip, are often useful. Fixation pins, either stainless steel or resorbable, will be required. After surgery, splint or cast will be required. Preoperative prophylactic antibiotics are used.

For surgery, the patient should be positioned supine on the operating table (Fig. 2-4). It is wise to ask the anesthesiologist to tape the endotracheal tube away from the side of the fracture. The arm should be abducted 90 degrees and internally rotated, giving clear access to the lateral condyle of the humerus. The surgeon should be aware that this position puts tension on the fracture fragment by the attached extensor muscles.

The surgical approach is via a direct lateral incision (Fig. 2-5). This is not the most cosmetic incision after healing. Sometimes it is difficult to feel the landmarks at surgery due to swelling, and it may be worthwhile to consider obtaining a spot fluoroscopic view to ensure the incision is centered over the fracture. It is useful to exsanguinate the limb by means of an elastic wrap or elevation prior to inflation of the tourniquet. Once the incision is made through the subcutaneous tissue, there is no real surgical interval. The surgeon is likely to fall into the fracture site beneath the subcutaneous tissue (Fig. 2-6). The subcutaneous tissue can then be undermined to expose the lateral aspect of the elbow. Washing out the hematoma will assist in visualization.

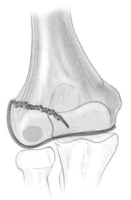
Arthrogram
stops short of
joint surface.

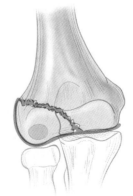
Arthrogram dye
goes through to
joint surface.

FIGURE 2-3

MRI or Arthrogram of gap.

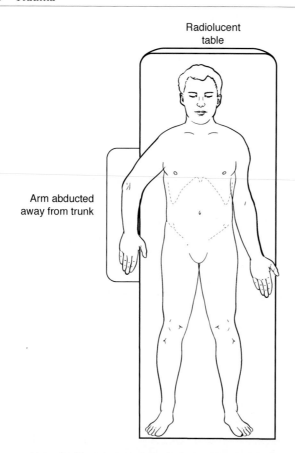

FIGURE 2-4
Supine on table.

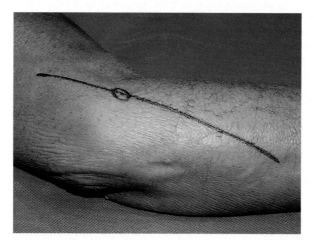

FIGURE 2-5
Lateral incision.

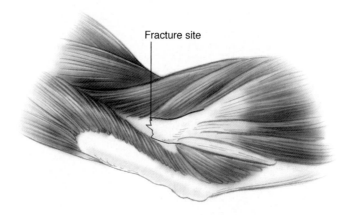

FIGURE 2-6
Falling into the
fracture site.

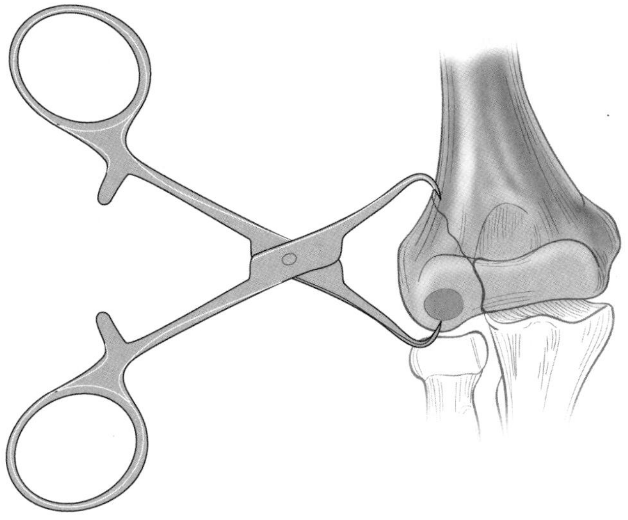

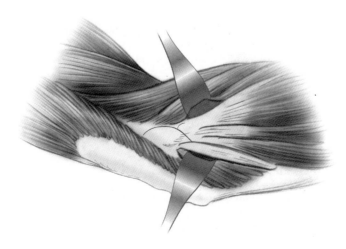

FIGURE 2-7
Clamping the fragment
to the humerus.

The key to obtaining anatomic fracture reduction is the ability to see and feel the reduction at surgery. Some fractures are simply hinged open laterally, and some are completely rotated such that the articular surface of the epiphyseal fragment faces the humerus, and the physeal component faces distally. Once the fragment is rotated back into place, it is helpful to clamp the fragment to the humerus with a towel clip, if possible (Fig. 2-7). It is often necessary to take down the "curtain" of extensor muscles just enough to see into the joint (Fig. 2-8). It is helpful to laterally elevate the torn muscle and periosteum from the distal humerus to better visualize the fracture line. Reduction should be visualized with a retractor in the joint anteriorly to show that the joint's surface is aligned. It is also useful to feel the surface of the distal humerus to make sure that it is relatively smooth. The surgeon should be prepared to accept 1 mm or less of a gap in the articular surface. There should be no appreciable step-off.

Fixation is typically achieved with 0.062-in. (1.5-mm) K-wires. It is best to exclude the K-wires from the surgical wound either by placing the pins through the wound and later placing them through a skin flap or by placing the pins percutaneously from outside the wound.

The pins are typically placed by means of one of two patterns. The pins can be placed parallel diagonally into the metaphysis (Fig. 2-9A). This pin pattern resists rotation in all planes if there is good (greater than 1 cm) spread between the pins. However, it may still be possible for the fragment to separate because the distal fracture fragment can slide along the pins.

The pins can also be placed divergently, such that one pin is parallel to the joint, and the other is parallel to the lateral metaphyseal flare (Fig. 2-9B). Each pin should engage the far (medial) cortex for better fixation. Divergent pin placement resists rotation as well as diastasis at the fragment site. If this pin pattern is used, the more horizontal distal pin should be placed not only through epiphyseal cartilage but also through bone. Spot fluoroscopy in two planes will confirm reduction and pin placement. It is planned that these pins will be temporary. After pin placement, the pins may be cut and left beneath the skin. Though requiring a return trip to the operating room for later removal, this

FIGURE 2-8
Retractor in joint.

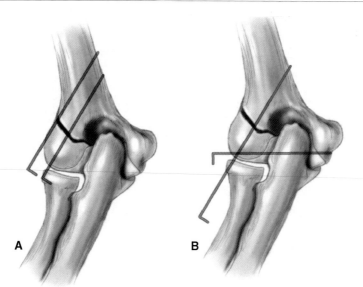

FIGURE 2-9
A, B. Pin patterns.

method offers a low risk of pin tract infection. Another option is to leave the pin bent over and protruding through the skin for later removal in the office without anesthesia; however, there is a small risk of pin tract infection associated with this method.

If there is a sizable metaphyseal fragment that allows screw placement, the fracture may be fixed with small cannulated screws, generally 3.5 mm or smaller. The screw should not cross the growth plate.

The fracture may also be fixed with 1.5-mm resorbable pins, which are made of a plastic polymer that will gradually be resorbed over time. In this method, the fragment is first reduced and then pinned with temporary steel guide wires. Fluoroscopy is issued to confirm anatomic fracture reduction and accurate placement of the guide wires. The guide wires are then sequentially removed and replaced by resorbable pins of a suitable length. Any excess pin is cut and removed.

Regardless of the fixation used, it is wise to test it under fluoroscopy by gently stressing the fracture site prior to closure. If the fracture fragment is clearly mobile in spite of fixation, additional fixation needs to be placed until the fracture is rendered immobile on fluoroscopic examination.

Wound closure is routine. Prior to closure, irrigation is required to remove any debris or contaminants. The extensor muscles need to be tacked back in place with resorbable stitches. Any protruding K-wires should be excluded from the incision if left in a percutaneous position. It is wise to bend the protruding pins to prevent pin migration or to apply pin balls to protect the sharp cut ends. There is generally no fascia to close. The subcutaneous skin and tissue should be reapproximated with resorbable stitches. Steri-Strips and a sterile dressing are applied. The elbow should then be splinted or casted in 90 degrees of flexion.

POSTOPERATIVE MANAGEMENT

Postoperative management includes a wound check at 1 week. Customarily an x-ray will be obtained to make sure that the fragments have not migrated. The elbow should be maintained in above-elbow immobilization for 4 weeks. At the time of cast removal, the pins should be removed in the clinic if they have been left protruding and if elbow range-of-motion exercises have begun. Physical therapy should be reserved only if the child fails to improve the elbow's range of motion within 1 month after cast removal. The surgeon may choose to follow these fractures long term to watch for growth derangement, though this occurrence is very rare.

COMPLICATIONS TO AVOID

True complications can occur as a result of this procedure, including wound infection, pin tract infection, prominence of lateral elbow, nonunion, stiffness, growth derangement, tardy ulnar nerve palsy, derangement of growth (Fig. 2-10), and an ugly scar.

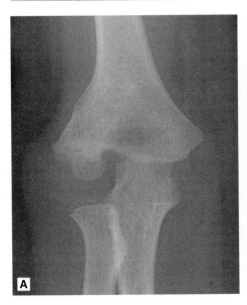
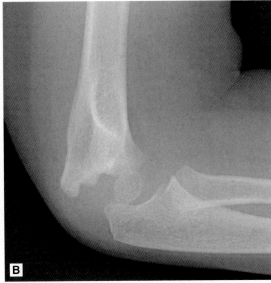

FIGURE 2-10
Anteroposterior **(A)** and lateral **(B)** radiographs of bizarre appearance after healing.

ILLUSTRATIVE CASE

A 7-year-old girl sustained a displaced and rotated fracture of the lateral condyle in a fall (Fig. 2-11). She had open reduction and internal fixation with radiolucent resorbable pins (Fig. 2-12). At 62 months post-op, the architecture and growth are normal (Fig. 2-13).

PEARLS AND PITFALLS

- It is wise to warn the parents of things that can go wrong, so that these become untoward natural history rather than complications.
- If you can't feel the landmarks, it is wise to check the location of the fracture by fluoroscopy to make sure your incision is actually centered over the fracture line.

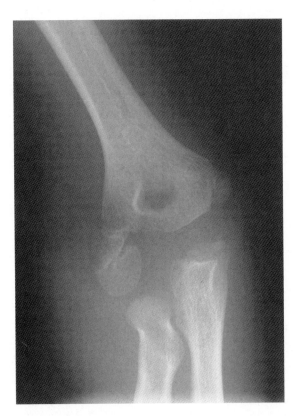

FIGURE 2-11
Displaced, rotated fracture.

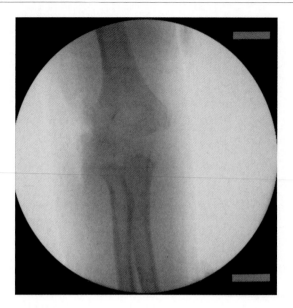

FIGURE 2-12

After open reduction and internal fixation with resorbable pins.

- Don't hesitate to take down some of the common extensor muscle origin off the fracture fragment if you need to see into the joint. Avoid dissection posteriorly, however, which may devascularize the condylar fragment.
- The reduction needs to be nearly perfect, which is why the fracture should be opened in the first place.
- It is wise to stress the fracture under fluoroscopy after fixation. If the fracture wiggles around quite a bit after fixation, then supplemental fixation is required with either additional pins or a tension band suture between the epiphysis and metaphysis.
- Beware of the late-presenting fracture. Up to about 6 weeks after fracture, it is probably best to open, reduce, and pin the fracture. Don't expect an anatomic reduction. After 6 weeks, the fracture should be carefully evaluated by CT or MRI to determine fragment orientation and extent of healing. The decision to proceed with surgery depends on the surgeon's confidence, experience,

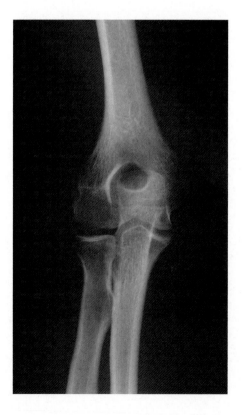

FIGURE 2-13

62 months post-op.

and skill. The challenge is to free the epiphyseal fragment enough to mobilize it back into place without devascularizing it after considerable healing and remodeling have occurred. If the displaced fracture is left alone, the growing body will go a long way to accommodate and remodel the elbow, often resulting in reasonable motion and function. Late surgery may provide an opportunity to make things worse.

REFERENCES

1. Flynn JC, Richards JF Jr, Saltzman RI. Prevention and treatment of non-union of slightly displaced fractures of the lateral humeral condyle in children. An end-result study. *J Bone Joint Surg.* 1975;57:1087–1092.
2. Horn BD, Herman MJ, Crisci K, et al. Fractures of the lateral humeral condyle: role of the cartilage hinge in fracture stability. *J Pediatr Orthop.* 2002;22:8–11.
3. Makela EA, Bostman O, Kekomaki M, et al. Biodegradable fixation of distal humeral physeal fractures. *Clin Orthop Rel Res.* 1992;283:237–243.
4. Morrissy RT, Wilkins KE. Deformity following distal humeral fracture in childhood. *J Bone Joint Surg Am.* 1984;66:557–562.

3 Operative Treatment of Radial Neck Fractures

Saul M. Bernstein

Fractures of the radial neck in which there is significant angulation and/or displacement are relatively rare in children. In a series of 450 patients with radial neck fractures reported by Jeffrey,[3] 80 were younger than 18 years at the time of injury, with 24 children having significant angulation and/or displacement. Gaston et al.[2] reported on 479 radial neck injuries, of which only 100 were in children, with only 13 of these having significant angulation or displacement. Although radial neck fractures with significant angulation are rare in childhood, the treatment can be difficult, and the fractures often result in significant complications.

Radial neck fractures occur equally in boys and girls. The usual mechanism of injury is a fall on the outstretched arm, resulting in a compression impaction injury on the lateral side of the elbow and a traction injury medially.[5,7,8,10] This results in compression angulation with fracture of the radial neck or through the metaphysis. The medial aspect of the elbow may have an avulsion of the distal humeral epicondyle, a fracture of the olecranon, or a medial elbow ligament tear (Fig. 3-1). Jeffrey described these fractures as type I fractures. Complete dislocation of the radial head associated with elbow dislocation with spontaneous reduction is classified as type II fracture.

INDICATIONS/CONTRAINDICATIONS

Indications for treatment vary with the patient's age and the degrees of angulation and/or displacement at the fracture site. In general, angular deformity greater than 30 degrees and displacement greater than 5 mm are appropriate indications for attempted reduction, either closed, semiclosed, or open. It should be noted that the measurement of the angulation at the radial neck fracture site may vary on the radiographs, depending on the amount of rotation on the forearm (Fig. 3-2). The younger the child, the more likely growth will allow some remodeling at the fracture site to help restore alignment, though proximal radial growth is rather slow. However, if a young child sustains a severe radial neck fracture resulting in avascular necrosis or physeal arrest, a poor result is common. Seen primarily in the more severely displaced fractures, avascular necrosis of the radial head and neck may be associated later with hypertrophy of the radial head and shortening of the radius, with resultant increase in elbow valgus as well as loss of forearm rotation.

In general, a radial neck fracture with less than 30 degrees angulation does not need more than a long-arm cast or splint immobilization for 2 or 3 weeks. For those fractures that are angulated more than 30 degrees and/or have more than 5 mm displacement, attempts to obtain fracture reduction are warranted.

In the past, closed reduction under anesthesia was utilized with some success.[6] Closed reduction attempts alone tend to be difficult and are rarely successful. Because this injury is an impaction injury, it can be difficult to gain a reduction. If attempted, closed reduction involves varus stress on the extended elbow, followed by direct manual pressure over the radial neck or head. Doing so theoretically disimpacts the fracture and allows for improvement of the alignment. However, closed reduction should certainly be attempted before open reduction is chosen for treatment of this fracture.

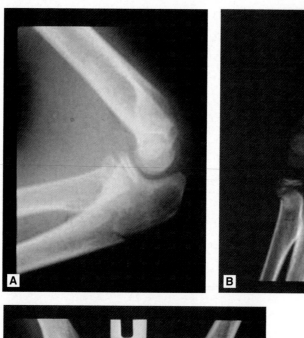

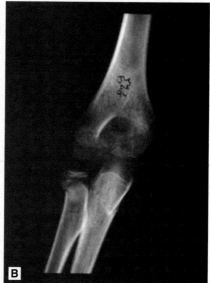

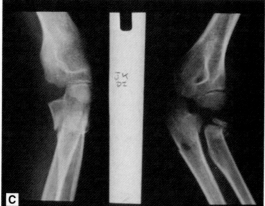

FIGURE 3-1

A–C. Fracture of the radial neck with associated fracture of the olecranon.

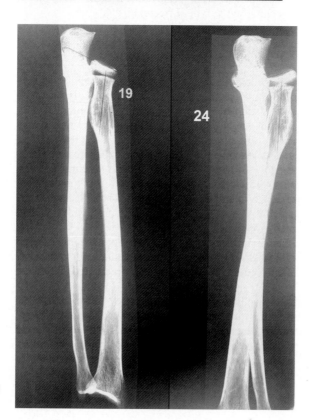

FIGURE 3-2

Note changes in angulation of the radial head with rotation of the forearm.

Open reduction has been associated with significant complications, including infection, synostosis, loss of motion, and nonunion.[1,7,9] Considering the high number of fair or poor results following open reduction of the fracture, other alternative methods should be considered, such as a percutaneous method of reduction (semiclosed) using a small Steinmann pin to disimpact the fracture and gain reduction.

METHOD

Nonoperative Treatment

Patients requiring fracture reduction are treated under general anesthesia. Fractures treated after 4 or 5 days appear to have a higher incidence of avascular necrosis, probably related to rapid healing in the child and the fact that late attempts at reduction may result in more vigorous manipulation and more vascular damage to the radial head and neck. After adequate anesthesia, closed reduction should be attempted. The surgeon should be aware of the position of the posterior interosseous nerve, as it enters through the supinator of the forearm. Repeated trauma to the nerve by manual pressure during closed reduction attempts may cause temporary or possibly permanent paralysis of the nerve. The extended elbow should be placed under varus stress, and the position of maximal deformity should be ascertained with fluoroscopic imaging. Dynamic fluoroscopic examination is the best way to measure the maximum degree of angulation and the amount of displacement. This dynamic imaging also allows the surgeon to determine the best position for application of external manual pressure for attempted reduction. Closed reduction is obtained by pressure of the thumb against the lateral radial head, as visualized on fluoroscopy. If one or two reduction attempts do not result in any improvement, then reduction by (semiclosed) percutaneous methods or by open reduction is needed.

Percutaneous Reduction Technique

If closed reduction does not work, the arm is prepped and sterilely draped in the usual manner. Under fluoroscopic control, the position of maximal angulation and displacement is determined. A small puncture wound is made distally and posterolaterally to the radial head and neck. A firm Kirschner wire or small Steinmann pin is then inserted and directed to the fracture site. The surgeon should be aware of the local anatomy, especially the arcade of Frosch and the posterior interosseous nerve, which courses through this area (Fig. 3-3).

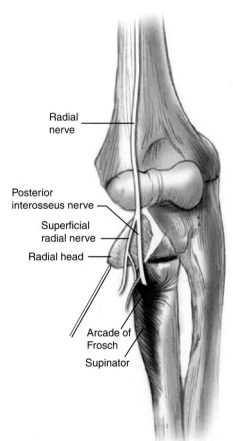

Radial
nerve

Posterior
interosseus nerve

Superficial
radial nerve

Radial head

Arcade of
Frosch

Supinator

FIGURE 3-3

Arcade of Frosch—note proximity of radial nerve to Steinmann pin and fracture.

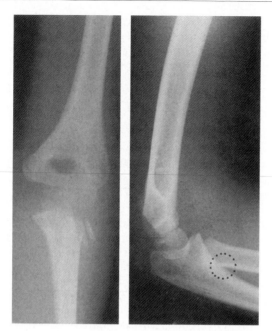

FIGURE 3-4

Markedly displaced fracture of the radial neck.

The pin is directed under fluoroscopic control to the neck or head of the radius. The sharp end of the pin is used, as it gives more stability to the reduction (Figs. 3-4–3-6). The proximal pin end should be padded to prevent physician injury. Pressure is then utilized to disimpact the fracture and reduce the head and neck while partially rotating the forearm. If the reduction is satisfactory, a dressing is applied, followed by a long-arm cast with the elbow flexed to 90 degrees and neutral rotation of the forearm. While a loss of significant reduction is uncommon the literature has noted loss of reduction and recommended pin fixation with flexible nail, leaving the nail in place until healing has occurred.[4] It is advisable not to cross the elbow joint with pins, as pinning the radial head with a Kirschner wire or Steinmann pin through the capitellum into the radial head and neck can result in fracture of the pin and difficulty in pin retrieval.

It is strongly recommended that these fractures not be opened unless reduction cannot be obtained by semiclosed means or unless the radial head and neck fracture fragment is so widely displaced that open reduction is necessary.

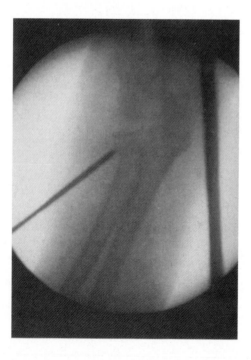

FIGURE 3-5

Reduction by percutaneous Steinmann pin.

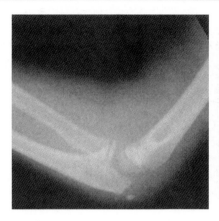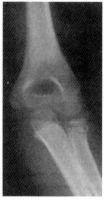

FIGURE 3-6
End result—healed fracture with excellent alignment.

POSTOPERATIVE MANAGEMENT

Postoperative immobilization with a long-arm cast or splint is used for 2 to 3 weeks following fracture reduction. Range-of-motion exercises for the elbow are initiated, as is forearm muscle rotation. Formal physical therapy is reserved for those patients who are slow to regain elbow motion following cast removal. Full activity is resumed after there is adequate elbow motion and pain-free upper extremity function.

COMPLICATIONS TO AVOID

The parents and the injured child should be warned prior to the treatment of the radial neck fracture that this is one of the more difficult pediatric fractures to treat, with approximately 15% to 35% of patients reported to have fair or poor final results. The most common complication is loss of forearm rotation, which may occur from an incompletely reduced fracture or from later radial head hypertrophy, which can occur months after the original fracture has healed. Avascular necrosis, with or without proximal radial physeal arrest, occurs most commonly with radial neck fractures in which there has been wide displacement of the proximal fracture fragment at the time of injury. If open reduction is done on moderately displaced radial neck fractures, care is needed to avoid excessive soft-tissue stripping, which may interfere with the vascular supply to the radial head. If there is a physeal arrest in the proximal radius as a result of this fracture, a valgus deformity of the elbow may occur.

PEARLS AND PITFALLS

- If there is more than 30 degrees angulation and/or 5 mm displacement, fracture reduction is needed.
- Advise the parents *before* the reduction is done that this fracture has a 15% to 35% rate of poor or fair results, even with adequate reduction.
- Attempt to reduce the fracture with percutaneous pin reduction techniques before resorting to open reduction.
- Save open reduction for irreducible fractures or for fractures with wide displacement of the proximal radial neck fracture fragment.
- Avoid placing pins across the capitellar-radial head joint.
- Limit postreduction immobilization for 2 or 3 weeks.

REFERENCES

1. Bernstein SM, McKeever P, Bernstein L. Percutaneous reduction of displaced radial neck fractures in children. *J Pediatr Orthop.* 1993;13:85–88.
2. Gaston SR, Smith FM, Baab O. Epiphyseal injuries of the radial head and neck. *Am J Surg.* 1953;85:266–276.
3. Jeffery CC. Fractures of the head of the radius in children. *J Bone Joint Surg Br.* 1950;32:314–324.
4. Metaizeau JP, Lascombes P, Lemelle JL, et al. Reduction and fixation of displaced radial neck fractures by closed intramedullary pinning. *J Pediatr Orthop.* 1993;13:355–360.
5. Murray RC. Fractures of the head and neck of the radius. *Br J Surg.* 1940;48:106–118.

6. Neher CG, Torch MA. New reduction technique for severely displaced pediatric radial neck fractures. *J Pediatr Orthop.* 2003;23:626–628.
7. Reidy JA, VanGorder GW. Treatment of displacement of the proximal radial epiphysis. *J Bone Joint Surg Am.* 1963;45:1355–1372.
8. Tachdjian MO. *Pediatric Orthopedics.* 2nd ed. Philadelphia: WB Saunders; 1990;3137–3143.
9. Waters PM, Stewart SL. Radial neck fracture nonunion in children. *J Pediatr Orthop.* 2001;21:570–576.
10. Wilkins KE. Fractures and dislocations of the elbow region. In: Rockwood CA, Wilkins KE, King RE, eds. *Fractures in Children.* Philadelphia: JB Lippincott Co; 1984:363–576.

4 Operative Treatment of Forearm Fractures Using Flexible IM Rods

Peter M. Waters and Donald S. Bae

Pediatric diaphyseal fractures of the forearm constitute about 6% of pediatric fractures. Distal metaphyseal and physeal fractures of the radius and ulna are far more common. Diaphyseal radius and ulna fractures are classified as plastic bone deformation injuries, incomplete or greenstick fractures, or complete, displaced fractures. These fractures rarely involve disruption of the distal radio-ulnar joint (Galeazzi fractures) or the proximal radio-ulnar joint (Monteggia fractures). They can coexist with fractures of the humerus, thereby constituting a pediatric floating elbow. Treatment options for displaced radial and ulnar diaphyseal fractures include closed reduction and cast immobilization, closed reduction and intramedullary (IM) fixation, and open reduction with internal fixation. Most plastic deformation and incomplete diaphyseal fractures can be successfully treated with closed manipulation and cast immobilization. Fracture reduction and maintaining postmanipulation alignment in a cast depends on a periosteal tension band. With increasing age and worsening severity of fracture, closed reduction and cast treatment will more often fail to maintain acceptable alignment in complete fractures. In the 1970s, Prevot and Metaizeau introduced elastic intramedullary nail fixation (ESIN) in Nancy, France, to treat unstable fractures with unacceptable alignment.

The goals of closed IM fixation of the forearm are to achieve near-anatomic reduction of the radius and ulna and to maintain fracture alignment throughout the healing process. If fracture stabilization has been carried out with use of percutaneously placed IM rod(s), the periosteum of a child's bone will mechanically resist torsional forces and will aid in healing through its vascularity. Thus, most unstable pediatric forearm fractures can be treated with IM rods instead of the plate-and-screw internal fixation that is required in adult diaphyseal forearm fractures.

Intramedullary fixation offers the advantages of less-invasive surgery and smaller incisions. Restoring the anatomic bow of the radius requires appropriate prebending of the radial elastic nail. Smaller nails (typically 2 to 3 mm in diameter) are chosen to fill approximately one-third of the intramedullary canal. Physeal sparing entry sites are preferred.

In general, fixation of both the radius and the ulna is utilized for fracture alignment and stability. Single-bone fixation, usually with an IM rod in the ulna, has been successfully utilized in unstable fractures in younger children (Fig. 4-1). This technique converts the complete fracture into an incomplete fracture and allows the radius to be rotated to an acceptably reduced position. However, radial stability must be assessed in the operating room under fluoroscopic examination. If there is persistent radial deformity or instability, a radial IM nail needs to be added to the ulnar nail to provide fracture stability. This chapter will address the indications, principles of treatment, techniques, postoperative care, and complications of intramedullary fixation of the forearm in the pediatric patient.

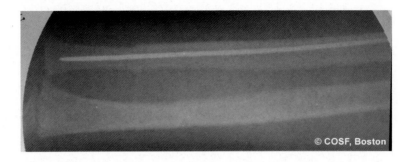

FIGURE 4-1

Single-bone fixation of an unstable forearm fracture with IM rod placement in ulna.

INDICATIONS/CONTRAINDICATIONS

Simplistically, the main indication for internal fixation in a pediatric patient is malalignment of the radial and ulnar fracture(s). However, there is controversy about how much angulation is acceptable in a child's diaphyseal forearm fracture. For acceptable cast treatment, maintenance of the radial bow and angulation of fewer than 10 degrees are desired both acutely and during healing. Failure to achieve or maintain reduction by those standards is an indication for internal fixation. The less stable the fracture is when initially reduced, particularly in an older child, the clearer are the indications for internal fixation. A floating elbow is also an indication for internal fixation to obviate the need for circumferential cast immobilization, thereby lessening the risk of the development of a compartment syndrome. Open fractures, pathologic fractures, or refractures are also considered indications for internal fixation in the forearm. (Table 4-1 provides a summary of the indications for internal fixation of pediatric forearm fractures.)

Possible contraindications for the use of IM nails for radius and ulna diaphyseal fractures include an older patient or a severely contaminated open fracture. If all growth plates in the forearm are closed, it may be better to use plate-and-screw internal fixation, as the rate of delayed union of the radius and ulna in older teens and adults appears to be higher with IM nail treatment than if some growth is remaining. If there is a type III open fracture with marked soft-tissue injury and wound contamination, use of an external fixator to facilitate soft-tissue care would be preferred.

PREOPERATIVE PLANNING

Preoperative anteroposterior (AP) and lateral radiographs of the radius and ulna need to include views of the elbow and wrist. This is particularly important at the elbow to prevent the orthopaedist from not recognizing a possible coexisting Monteggia-type injury at the radial head. Entry sites for the nail are planned and are to some degree based on the diaphyseal level of the fracture, particularly in the case of the radial fracture. The entire instrument set for inserting flexible IM nails must be available, and all IM nail sizes from 2 mm to 4 mm need to be sterile and ready for use. Fluoroscopy needs to be set up in the operating room. A radiolucent arm operating table is used.

SURGICAL PROCEDURE

Closed reduction IM fixation of the pediatric forearm is performed in the operating room under general anesthesia. The affected arm is draped to the side on a radiolucent arm table, with the child supine and the shoulder abducted 90 degrees. Antibiotic prophylaxis against infection is given prior to the incision. Usually the bone easiest to reduce is stabilized first. For the ulna, apophyseal and metaphyseal proximal entry sites have both been utilized (Fig. 4-2). Because the olecranon

TABLE 4-1   Indications for Internal Fixation of Pediatric Forearm Fractures
Open fracture
Loss of reduction with closed treatment
Irreducible fracture with >10 degrees of angulation
Older child with unstable fracture
Floating elbow injury
Pathologic fracture
Refracture

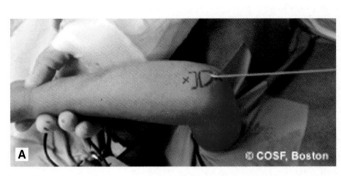 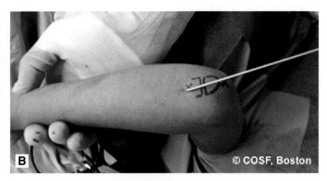

FIGURE 4-2   Intraoperative proximal ulna entry sites for intramedullary fixation: Apophyseal **(A)** and metaphyseal **(B)**.

apophysis does not contribute significantly to the growth of the ulna, most pediatric orthopaedists will pass a small-diameter, smooth rod across the proximal ulnar apophysis, thereby allowing a straight passage of the nail down the ulnar medullary canal. Alternatively, a split is made in the anconeus muscle on the subcutaneous border of the ulna, and an appropriate bend is made in the nail for passing the rod from the proximal to the distal end of the ulna. Distal entry between the flexor carpi ulnaris tendon and the extension carpi ulnaris tendon has also been used. The size of the nail used depends on the size of the medullary canal on radiograph. The thinnest diameter of the ulna is located at its distal end; the ulna nail is usually 2 to 3 mm in diameter.

If a proximal apophyseal entry point is used, a small incision is made in the skin crease overlying the midportion of the olecranon. The proximal ulnar cortex is entered with fluoroscopic guidance using a power drill to insert a Steinmann pin into the intramedullary canal. Care must be taken not to penetrate beyond the cortex with this sharp pin, as a false passage may be created. The Steinmann pin is removed, and the straight elastic nail is then tapped with a mallet down to the fracture site (Fig. 4-3). Closed manipulation of the ulna fracture site is performed, and the nail is passed across the ulna fracture. On rare occasions, if interposed tissue prevents anatomic reduction, an open reduction is necessary through a small incision (Fig. 4-4). Passage of the pin to a point just proximal to the distal ulnar physis completes the ulnar fixation.

As mentioned previously, in children between the ages of approximately 8 and 12 years, single-bone fixation may be sufficient to align both bones in an acceptable, stable position. More often, however, dual-bone fixation is necessary. Radial IM fixation is performed using a distal nail entry site. Anatomical options include (a) proximal to the Lister tubercle between the third and fourth extensor compartments (Fig. 4-5), (b) the radial-side metaphysis proximal to the physis (Fig. 4-6), and (c) the ulnar-side metaphysis between the fourth and fifth extensor compartments. For each of these entry sites, the extensor pollicis longus tendon, the radial sensory nerve, and the digital extensor tendons need to be protected. A small incision is usually made at the entry site to avoid iatrogenic tendon or sensory nerve damage during nail placement.

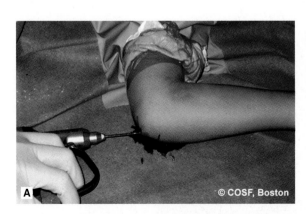 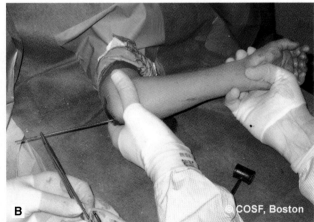

FIGURE 4-3   Intraoperative passage of the ulna rod through the apophysis. **A.** Power drilling is used for cortical entry only. **B.** A mallet is then used to pass the IM nail down the medullary canal.

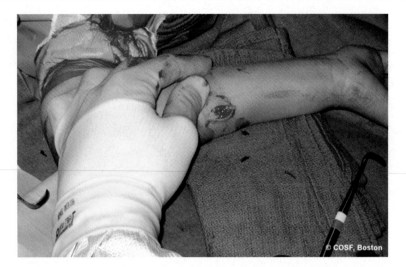

FIGURE 4-4

Incision for open reduction and rod passage is used in difficult reductions to lessen the risk of compartment syndrome.

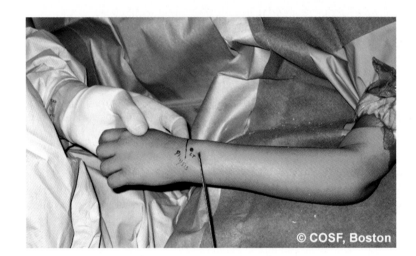

FIGURE 4-5

Intraoperative radial entry site proximal to Lister tubercle.

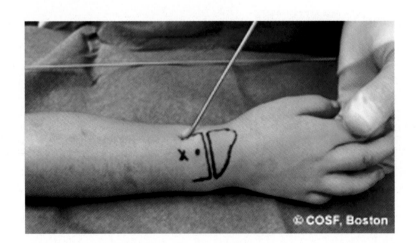

FIGURE 4-6

Intraoperative radial entry site proximal to physis on the radial side.

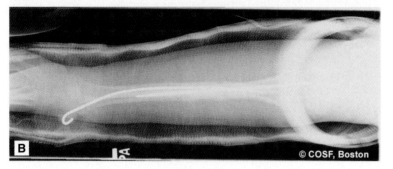

FIGURE 4-7

(A, B) Intramedullary fixation of radius and ulna fractures with elastic titanium nails that were precontoured prior to placement.

With the radial elastic nail, three-point bending is necessary to maintain the radial bow and radial fracture alignment (Fig. 4-7). The degree of bend should lead to overall filling of the intramedullary canal at the thinnest portion of the radius, which is in the mid-diaphyseal region. The bend in either an elastic or a stainless pin should be sufficient to avoid impaling the opposite cortex during insertion. The cortical entry site should be widened to allow for better control of nail passage during insertion. Again, insertion with a power drill should be used only at the entry site and not beyond to prevent creating a troublesome false passage. The nail is inserted from distal to proximal with a mallet, all the time controlling the nail's rotational position. Passage across the fracture site can usually be performed by twisting the rod tip. Confirmation of successful placement of the nail across the fracture is made with fluoroscopy. The nail is then tamped into the proximal radial neck region.

Approximately 5% to 10% of radius and/or ulna fractures require an open reduction. This is usually because the surgeon is unable to obtain an anatomic reduction to allow for nail passage percutaneously across the fracture site; rarely is it because the surgeon selected a nail of too large a diameter. With repeated attempts at closed manipulation, the risk of compartment syndrome increases. Therefore, excessive or overzealous attempts at achieving percutaneous reduction and fixation should be avoided. Difficulty in attaining radial reduction is most often due to interposed periosteum or extensor muscle in the fracture site. With open reduction, the surgeon should not only be mindful of the posterior interosseous nerve location when exposing the midproximal radius but also be prepared for the possibility of a displaced neurovascular bundle when exposing the ulna. All open fractures require irrigation and debridement of the fracture site and, thus, open reduction. Intramedullary nail fixation can be used to stabilize open radial and/or ulna fractures, unless marked wound contamination exists.

POSTOPERATIVE MANAGEMENT

The decision of whether to bury the tips or leave the end of the IM nail exposed depends on the length of time the surgeon plans to leave the IM fixation in place. Surgeon preference also influences the chosen site of nail insertion. Intramedullary forearm fixation has been removed as early as 4 to 6 weeks and as late as 1 year following fracture. Surgeons who prefer to remove the IM nails after approximately 6 weeks of healing will usually leave the tips exposed (Fig. 4-8), avoiding skin breakdown over buried pins and possible infection, especially with proximal ulnar apophyseal pins. Early nail removal may require additional cast or brace treatment until there is full fracture healing. Surgeons who worry about early refracture or a loss of fracture alignment usually leave the IM fixation in place for approximately 6 months or until there is clearly complete healing. These buried pins can cause problems with irritation of the extensor tendon, sensory nerves, or the skin.

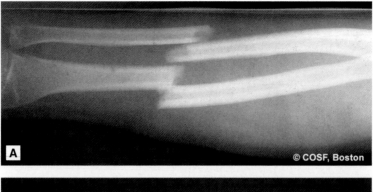

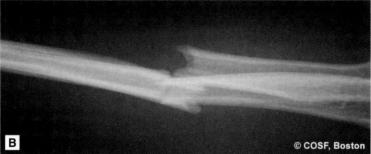

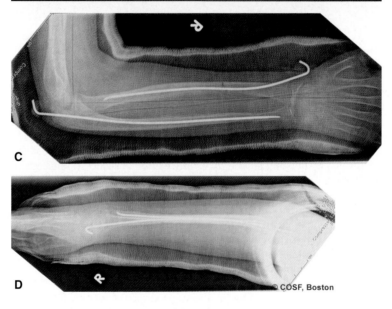

FIGURE 4-8

A, B: Displaced, unstable radius and ulna diaphyseal fractures treated with intramedullary fixation (can be either elastic titanium nails or Kirschner smooth wires), with pins left external for early removal **(C, D).**

The use of postoperative cast, splint, or brace immobilization also varies widely among surgeons. There is no clear evidence for the superiority of one technique over another. The less conservative surgeon will splint the forearm only temporarily for soft-tissue injury, excessive pain, or a comminuted fracture pattern at higher risk for loss of fracture alignment. The more conservative surgeon will use a cast or splint until sufficient healing is seen radiographically in order to prevent nail migration, nail bending, fracture malalignment, or delayed bone healing.

A summary of the treatment principles using forearm IM nails is presented in Table 4-2.

TABLE 4-2   Principles of Treatment
Fracture stability and alignment
Minimal incisions, as compared with plating
Periosteum resists torsional forces
First fix the bone easiest to reduce
Small-diameter nails, typically 2–3 mm in diameter (not canal filling; ~1/3 canal fill)
Maintenance of anatomic radial bow
Physeal sparing entry sites, if possible

TABLE 4-3   Complications of Intramedullary Fixation of Pediatric Forearm Fractures

Nonunion of the ulna
- Open fracture
- Distraction from too large a pin
- Early motion
- Comminuted fracture

Extensor pollicis longus (EPL) rupture
- Sharp edge of pin at Lister tubercle
- Attritional rupture

Extensor tendon or radial sensory nerve irritation

Compartment syndrome
- Prolonged attempts at closed reduction or passage of nail

Refracture
- Inadequate healing before rod removal (4%–8%)

Forearm stiffness
- Minor loss of <20 degrees (<2%)
- Major loss of >40 degrees (unlikely)

Reangulation of fracture due to early removal in older patient
Malangulation of the radius with single-bone ulna fixation
Hypertrophic scar/keloid formation
Hardware irritation

COMPLICATIONS TO AVOID

There is a low incidence of complications related to IM fixation of the radius and ulna (Table 4-3). Irritation of the radial sensory nerve, extensor tendons, and skin occur with long or prominent buried nail tips and usually resolves with nail removal. More worrisome extensor pollicis longus and extensor digitorum communis tendon ruptures have occurred with buried implants; these tendon ruptures require reconstructive surgery. Refracture has occurred in 4% to 8% of fractures, with a higher incidence after early nail removal in older patients. Malangulation of the radius with only single-bone ulnar fixation and reangulation with early rod removal have also been described; both tend to occur in older children. Loss of forearm rotation is rare, with approximately 2% of patients having fewer than 20 degrees loss and none having more than 40 degrees loss in one series. Nonunion has been described in cases of open fractures, distraction at the fracture site, and initiation of early motion in older patients. The nonunions may have been avoided with smaller-diameter pins, to avoid distraction at the fracture site; longer protection before mobilization; or plate-and-screw fixation in selected instances, particularly in older patients.

PEARLS AND PITFALLS

- Use of IM flexible nails for radius and ulna fractures provides satisfactory fracture stabilization and alignment in a less-invasive manner than would be achieved with plates and screws.
- Fracture reduction is usually accomplished closed, but mini open reduction should be used if fracture reduction is difficult.
- Usually 2 to 3 mm flexible nails are used for fracture fixation.
- The ulna nail is usually inserted first.
- Although sometimes the placement of a nail in only the radius or ulna will suffice to provide fracture reduction and stability, usually a nail is placed in both bones.
- The radial nail needs to be contoured to maintain the anatomic radial bow.
- Multiple unsuccessful attempts at IM nail passage are associated with a higher incidence of forearm compartment syndrome.

REFERENCES

1. Blaiser RD, Salamon PB. Closed intramedullary rodding of pediatric adolescent forearm fractures. *Operat Tech Orthop.* 1996;3:128–133.
2. Flynn J, Waters PM. Single bone fixation of both bone forearm fractures. *J Pediatr Orthop.* 1996;16:655–659.
3. Lee S, Nicol RO, Stott NS. Intramedullary fixation for pediatric unstable forearm fractures. *Clin Orthop.* 2002;402:245–250.
4. Metaizeau JP, Ligier JN. Surgical treatment of fractures of long bones in children. *J Chir (Paris).* 1984;121:527–537.
5. Prevot J, Guichet M. Elastic stable intramedullary nailing for forearm fractures in children and adolescents. *J Bone Joint Surg.* 1996;20:305.

5 Operative Treatment of Femur Fractures Using Flexible IM Nails

Wudbhav N. Sankar and John M. Flynn

Until the early 1990s, most children who sustained a femoral diaphyseal fracture were treated with spica casting or traction followed by delayed casting. In recent years, however, there has been an increasing trend among pediatric orthopaedic traumatologists to perform operative fixation to mobilize the child, minimize the psychosocial impact of prolonged casting, and accelerate return to function. In older children and adolescents, surgeons have also recognized that operative management has yielded less shortening and angular deformity than did traction and casting. Through the 1970s and 1980s, treatment preferences evolved from traction and casting to external fixation, standard plating, and adult-style reamed intramedullary nailing. However, complications from external fixation (refracture and pin-site complications), open plating (morbidity of open surgery), and reamed nailing (avascular necrosis of femoral head and risk of physeal closure) limit the widespread use of these techniques to treat the skeletally immature child. Although the French have used titanium elastic nails (TENs) with great success for a number of decades, it was not until the mid-1990s that elastic nailing gained acceptance in the United States. Since then, several studies have shown flexible nailing to have a very favorable risk-benefit profile as a treatment for femoral shaft fractures in children. The rapid nationwide adoption of flexible nailing as a standard of care at many pediatric trauma centers attests to the relatively short learning curve for surgeons and the effectiveness and safety for patients.

INDICATIONS/CONTRAINDICATIONS

Currently, in most centers, TENs are the most popular choice for stabilizing a typical pediatric femur fracture in the school-aged child. For children age 5 and younger who have an isolated femoral shaft fracture, early spica casting remains the most common treatment. In young children with multitrauma, TENs are being used with increasing frequency. In adolescents older than 11 years and/or heavier than 50 kg, TENs have been used successfully, although a higher rate of complications has been reported. Because TENs do not involve a "rigid" fixation like a plate or locked nail, they are more suited for length-stable fractures, such as transverse or short oblique patterns. Long spiral and comminuted femur fractures can be treated with TENs, though the risk of shortening is increased. TENs are best suited for midshaft femur fractures, as a higher rate of malunion has been reported in distal and proximal fracture locations.

PREOPERATIVE PLANNING

All children with femoral shaft fractures should undergo a full trauma evaluation in search of other injuries. Full-length anteroposterior (AP) and lateral radiographs of the femur should be obtained to evaluate the fracture; in addition, radiographs of the hips and pelvis are standard for high energy trauma. The nail size can be estimated by measuring the narrowest diameter of the femoral canal. In general, the appropriate nail is 40% of the smallest medullary diameter. For example, if the narrowest diameter were 1 cm, two 4-mm nails would be used. The largest possible nail diameter should always be used. Most pediatric femoral canals are wide enough to accommodate either a 3.5-mm or 4.0-mm nail.

SURGICAL PROCEDURE

Patient Positioning

Titanium elastic nailing can be performed on either a fracture table or a radiolucent table. The fracture table is often preferred as it allows the surgeon to get the fracture out to length and optimally reduced before prepping and draping. Others report good results without the use of a fracture table. When the radiolucent table is used (as may be necessary for children with a femur fracture and other lower-extremity fractures or severe short-tissue injuries), an assistant pulls traction, which complicates the process of getting AP and lateral images in fractures where it is difficult to pass the nail across the fracture site.

On the fracture table, both feet are padded with Webril and placed into the foot holders. The uninjured leg is abducted widely out of the way so that the image intensifier can be positioned between the legs, with sufficient room remaining for an assisting surgeon (Fig. 5-1). The C-arm monitor is positioned next to the patient's contralateral shoulder, so that the monitor is in the direct line of sight for both the surgeon and the assistant. Prior to preparing and draping the injured leg, the surgeon uses the C-arm image to visualize the fracture site. Traction is used to get the fracture out to length. This is a good time for the surgeon to rehearse the maneuver that aligns the fracture for nail passage and to note the position of the image intensifier that will yield good AP and lateral images of the fracture. Proper rotation can be ensured by noting the position of the patella and compensating for any external rotation of the hip, especially in the more proximal fracture. The entire injured extremity is then prepped from the upper thigh down to the foot holder. Circumferential drapes are used so that the entire leg is accessible from both the medial and the lateral sides.

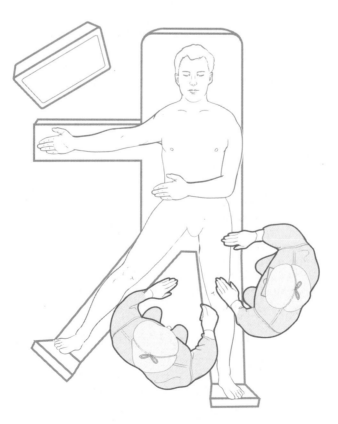

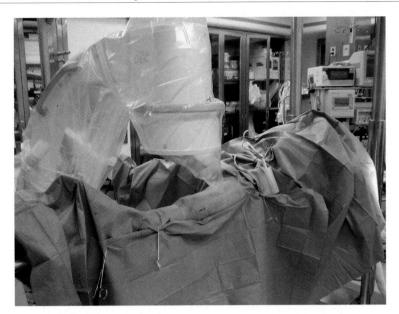

FIGURE 5-2
The extremity is circumferentially draped to allow access to both sides of the leg. A 2-cm skin incision is marked from the site of bony insertion extending distally.

Nail Entry

The first step in the surgical procedure is selecting the proper nail entry sites. The C-arm image intensifier is used to obtain an AP image of the knee. The distal femoral physis is visualized, and its position is marked on the skin to warn the surgeon to avoid deep dissection in this area. The proper nail entry point for the standard retrograde technique is 2 to 3 cm proximal to the distal femoral physis, just below the metaphyseal-diaphyseal junction. A longitudinal skin incision is made on both the medial and lateral leg extending from the site of bony insertion distally 1 to 2 cm to minimize soft-tissue damage during nail insertion (Fig. 5-2). The incisions are deepened with electrocautery, and a hemostat is used to spread down to the bone. The same hemostat may be used to palpate the femur to get a sense of the anteroposterior dimension. Ideally, the starting points should be in the center of the femur in the sagittal plane. A drill (with a soft-tissue protector) is used to open the femoral cortex at the medial and lateral insertion sites. Although an awl is available, a drill offers better control and can give the exact hole size needed. The size of the drill bit should be larger than the size of the nail; thus, a 4.5-mm drill would be used to place a 4.0-mm nail. The drill is first directed perpendicular to the cortex; once the cortex is breached, the drill (still running) is slowly angled sharply up the shaft of the femur (Fig. 5-3). This creates a track that greatly facilitates nail insertion. The cancellous bone of the distal femur can be very dense in young, active children. If the surgeon drills too transversely across the femur, the nail will follow that track, and it will be quite difficult to turn the nail up the femur. An oblique track, aiming up the shaft, will allow the surgeon to quickly pass the nail up to the fracture site.

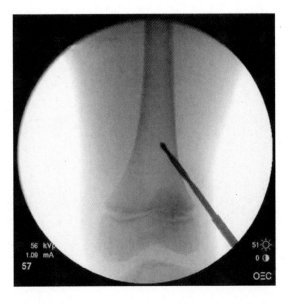

FIGURE 5-3
While running, the drill is angled sharply up the shaft of the femur to create a tract for nail passage.

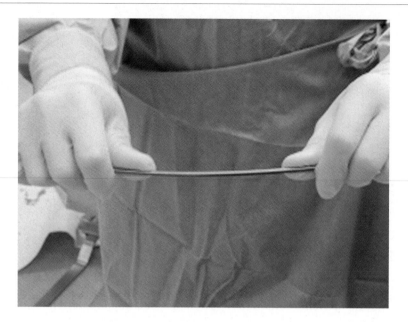

FIGURE 5-4

Elastic nails are prebent by hand so that the apex of the bend will be at the fracture site.

Prior to insertion, the elastic nails are bent by hand into a gentle C shape, such that the apex of the bend will be at the fracture site (Fig. 5-4). It is often easier to use the T-handle chuck rather than doing this by hand.

After prebending, the first nail is introduced through the lateral drill hole. Sometimes it is easier to find the hole and enter the femur if the hooked tip is turned caudal. Under image-intensifier control, the tip is then turned cranial and tapped up the femur toward the fracture site (Fig. 5-5). The same technique is used to insert and advance the second nail through the medial femoral cortex (Fig. 5-6). Some surgeons prefer to pass one nail across the fracture site before introducing the second nail. If there is any question as to the position of the nails, a lateral view should be consulted. The nail tips are sharp enough to penetrate the cortex (Fig. 5-7).

Fracture Reduction and Nail Passage

Under fluoroscopic imaging, the fracture should be reduced before the nails are passed across the fracture site. The F tool can be extremely helpful in correcting flexion of the proximal fragment or medial/lateral displacement (Fig. 5-8). Alternatively, a mallet can be used to direct either the proximal or the distal fragment to improve fracture alignment. Once reduction is achieved on both the AP and lateral views, the surgeon should try to advance the nail that appears more difficult to pass across the fracture site (Fig. 5-9). Although this may seem counterintuitive, if the easiest nail is passed across first, it may hold the fracture in a displaced position, making passage of the second nail quite

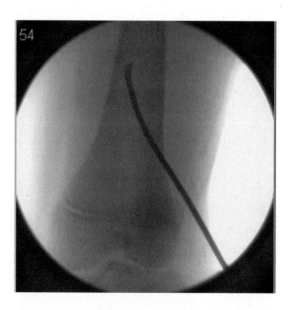

FIGURE 5-5

The first nail is advanced up the femoral shaft.

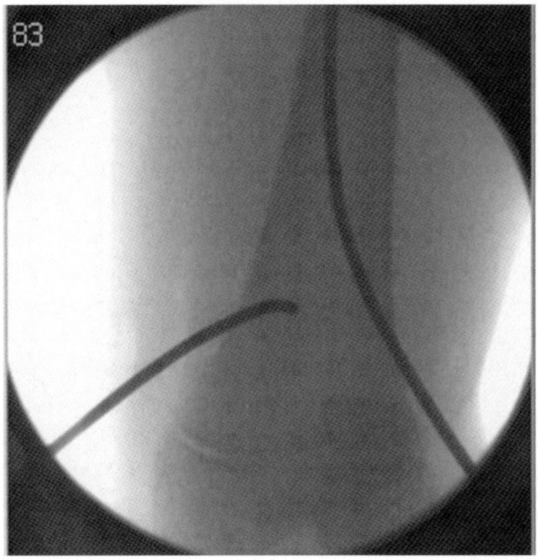

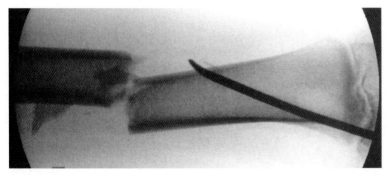

FIGURE 5-6

The second elastic nail is first inserted with the hooked tip pointing caudad; the hook is then rotated cephalad, and the nail is tapped up to the fracture site.

FIGURE 5-7   Nail tips are sharp enough to penetrate the cortex. (Courtesy Skaggs DL, Flynn JM. *Staying Out of Trouble in Pediatric Orthopaedics.* Philadephia: Lippincott Williams & Wilkins, 2005.)

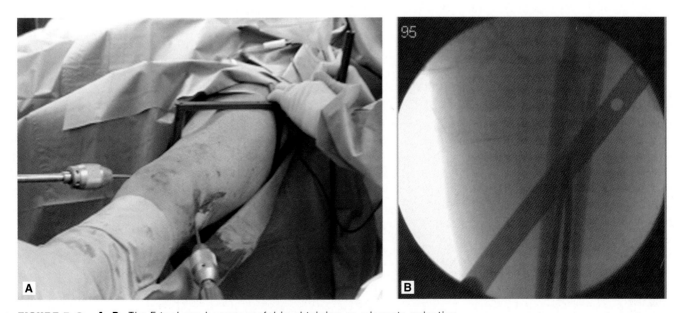

FIGURE 5-8   **A–B.** The F tool can be very useful in obtaining an adequate reduction.

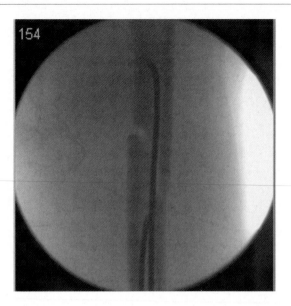

FIGURE 5-9

The more difficult nail is first passed beyond the fracture site.

difficult. Rotation of the nail is sometimes very helpful to thread the nail into the canal of the proximal fragment. It is sometimes helpful to temporarily turn the hooked tip of the nail 180 degrees so that it can "catch" the opposite cortex and facilitate passage across the fracture site (Fig. 5-10). The intramedullary position of the first nail should be confirmed on a lateral view before the second nail is advanced. Once both nails are across the fracture site, they should be tapped forward a few centimeters, and proper position of the nails should again be confirmed on both the AP and lateral fluoroscopic views (Fig. 5-11). Once the intramedullary status in the proximal fragment is confirmed, both nails are advanced to their final proximal position. The nail inserted through the lateral femoral cortex should end laterally near the apophysis of the greater trochanter. The nail inserted through the medial distal femur should end medially at the lesser trochanter or femoral neck in proximal fractures

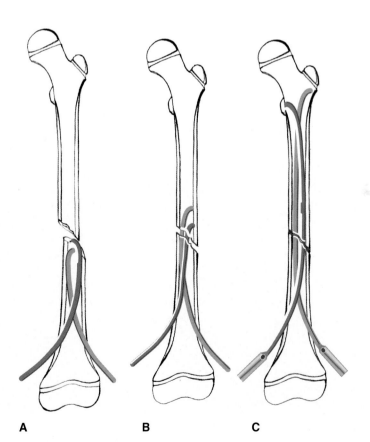

FIGURE 5-10

A–C. Reduction can often be aided by turning the hooked tip 180 degrees to "catch" the opposite cortex.

A   B   C

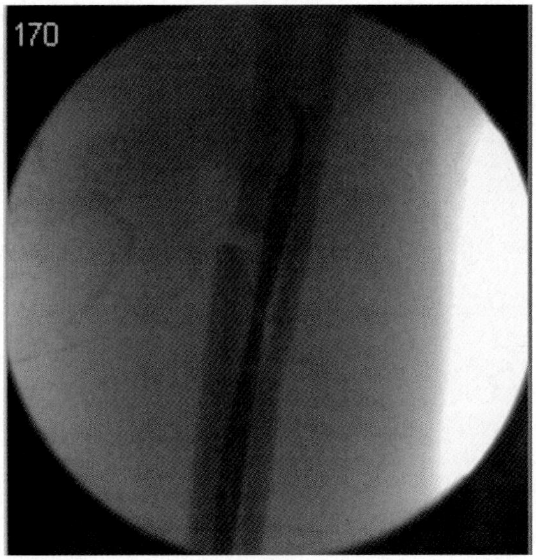

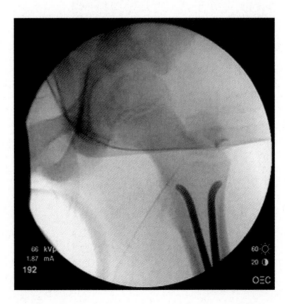

FIGURE 5-11

After confirmation of intramedullary position using a lateral image, the second nail is advanced past the fracture site.

(Fig. 5-12). The final position of the nails should form a divergent C configuration. As first designed by the French, TENs achieve biomechanical stability from this symmetric arrangement, which creates six points of fixation and allows the construct to act as an internal splint.

Final Steps

The fracture site is again visualized with the image intensifier on both the AP and lateral views to confirm reduction. If the fracture site is distracted, traction can be removed, and the surgeon can gently impact the leg to close the fracture gap. It is also important to confirm proper rotational alignment of the injured extremity at this time by making sure there is a true AP of the proximal and distal femur in the same plane. The nails are then backed out a few centimeters, cut at the skin surface, and tapped back in with a tamp. At their final position, the nail ends should lie along the metaphyseal flare, ending proximal to the physis with only 1 to 2 cm of the nail outside the cortex (Fig. 5-13) if future removal is planned.

Most surgeons plan to remove nails in 6 to 9 months DLS. In this case, nails may be left flush with the metaphysis. It is extremely important when performing this last step to avoid bending the nails away from the skin. Although this facilitates nail cutting, as well as later hardware removal, the cut end becomes more prominent and increases the risk of soft-tissue irritation. A hemostat is then used to sweep any remaining soft tissue out from under the nail tip, again to minimize soft-tissue irritation at the entry site. After irrigation, the medial and lateral wounds are closed in a layered fashion using 2.0 Vicryl sutures, and subcuticular 4.0 Monocryl for skin.

FIGURE 5-12

Final proximal position of the nails.

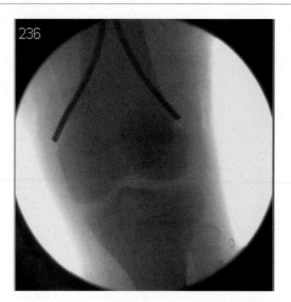

FIGURE 5-13

TENs should be backed out, cut, and advanced so that the nail ends proximal to the physis.

SPECIAL CASES

For more proximal femoral shaft fractures, an alternative technique using one retrograde nail and one antegrade nail is suggested. The antegrade nail is inserted laterally through the apophysis of the greater trochanter and ends at the distal lateral femoral cortex. The retrograde nail is inserted through the medial distal femur and ends medially by the lesser trochanter (as described above; Fig. 5-14). Just as in the more conventional retrograde technique, the more difficult of the two elastic nails is first passed across the fracture site. Although this nailing technique provides increased stability for proximal femoral shaft fractures, it does introduce the theoretical possibility of trochanteric apophyseal damage, although this has never been reported with the use of TENs.

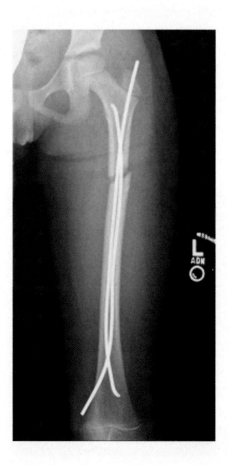

FIGURE 5-14

Proximal femur fracture treated with one retrograde nail and one antegrade nail inserted through the greater trochanter apophysis. Ideally, the retrograde nail could be advanced further up femoral neck.

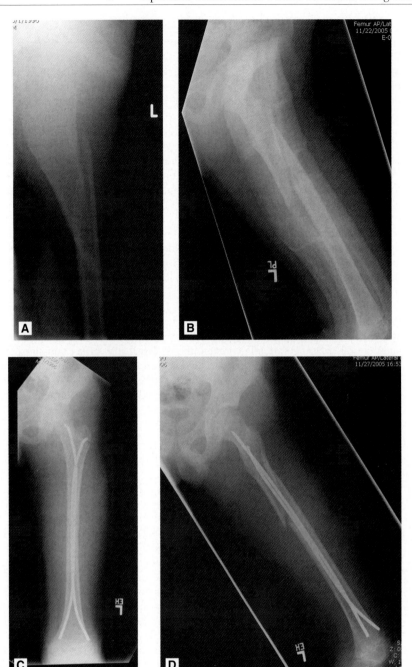

FIGURE 5-15

Anteroposterior **(A)** and lateral **(B)** radiographs of a proximal femur fracture in a 8-year-old boy. AP **(C)** and lateral **(D)** radiograph 3 weeks after surgery. Note the very proximal placement of the nails and the separation of the nails proximally to maximize stability.

EDITOR'S NOTE: PROXIMAL FEMUR FRACTURES

An alternative technique for treating proximal femoral fractures, such as subtrochanteric fractures, with TENs is to place both nails in the standard retrograde fashion (Fig. 5-15). With this technique, the nail entering medially goes up the femoral neck, and the nail entering laterally goes into the greater trochanter, ideally engaging the cartilaginous apophysis. Note on Figure 5-15C that the nails are left flush with the metaphysis, as no future removal is planned.

POSTOPERATIVE MANAGEMENT

Patients are usually placed in a knee immobilizer to minimize knee motion and to keep the children more comfortable during the early postoperative period. Although the immobilizer certainly does not truly protect the fracture site, it does help stabilize the knee, which can buckle due to quadriceps injury and reflex inhibition. Patients may be managed with patient-controlled analgesia (PCA) for the first postoperative day before being converted to oral narcotics such as oxycodone. Unlike plating, locked nailing, and external fixation, TENs is not "rigid fixation." Therefore, expect children to have more pain and muscle spasm than you would see with other fixation methods. For stable fracture patterns (e.g., transverse, short oblique), early weight bearing may begin the day after surgery. For more unstable fracture patterns (e.g., comminuted), toe-touch weight-bearing status should be maintained until early callus is seen on postoperative radiographs. In rare cases in which the fracture is judged to be particularly length unstable, a "one-leg walking spica" may be used for 3 to 4 weeks until there is enough callus that shortening is unlikely. Healing of femoral shaft fractures typically occurs between 2 and 4 months. Typically, young children (<10 years old) will be active and relatively pain free in 2 or 3 months. Older children may take 3 to 6 months. A limp is very common, and parents should be warned in advance. Sometimes, late after surgery, the primary cause of the limp is soft-tissue irritation by the nail tips; this limp will resolve within a couple weeks after nail removal.

After a fracture is completely healed, the hardware may be removed about 6 to 9 months after injury. Although some surgeons leave the elastic nails in permanently, nail removal may decrease soft-tissue irritation at the entry site, may provide psychologic closure of the injury for the family, and may (at least theoretically) prevent the risk of a stress riser and subsequent fracture at the insertion site after the child has grown for a few years and the nail is more proximal in the femur. However, nail removal does carry the risk of a second anesthetic; as such, the final decision on this controversial topic should be left to the family and the treating surgeon.

COMPLICATIONS TO AVOID

The most common complication associated with the use of TENs is soft-tissue irritation at the nail entry site, reported to be between 7% and 33%, depending on the series. This complication can be minimized by leaving the nails flush against the distal femur and by leaving no more than 1 to 2 cm of the nail ends out of the cortex. Some children have developed a knee effusion due to nail-tip irritation. Nonunions are extremely rare with the use of TENs. Malunion is also uncommon but is more likely to occur in heavy children (>50 kg) with either proximal or distal fractures or in length-instable fractures. TENs can certainly be used with great success in bigger, older children, but there is now clear evidence that the risk of malunion and shortening is greater in this population. Therefore, the surgeon should have a thorough discussion with the family before surgery regarding the risks and benefits of TENs for this population. In these higher-risk patients/fractures, there are important considerations in choosing the treatment method, and the surgeon is essentially helping the family decide which set of risks and complications they are willing to tolerate. For instance, in some cases, a locked nail can be used, though with a small risk of avascular necrosis and tougher removal. Submuscular plating is ideal for some of these fractures, though with the downsides of more incisions; a more difficult, lengthy, radiation-intensive procedure; and a much more difficult and potentially bloody implant removal. External fixation may also be better than TENs, especially in very proximal and distal fractures, with the downsides of pin problems, knee stiffness, and refracture risk. By considering all these issues, the surgeon and family can come to a satisfactory decision.

ILLUSTRATIVE CASE

An 8-year-old boy was seen after being struck by a motor vehicle while crossing the street. A full trauma evaluation revealed a left midshaft femur fracture as the patient's only injury (Fig. 5-16). On the morning after admission, the patient was taken to the operating room, where his femur was stabilized with titanium elastic nails. The patient was discharged from the hospital uneventfully on the second day after surgery. At his first postoperative visit, one week after surgery, the patient demonstrated excellent fracture alignment (Fig. 5-17). His knee immobilizer was discontinued, and his weight-bearing status was advanced to weight bearing as tolerated. Four months after surgery, the patient showed near-complete healing of his fracture; his only complaint was minor irritation at the lateral nail insertion site (Fig. 5-18). The elastic nails were removed 8 months after the index operation. One year after his injury, the patient demonstrated complete healing with no clinical deficits (Fig. 5-19).

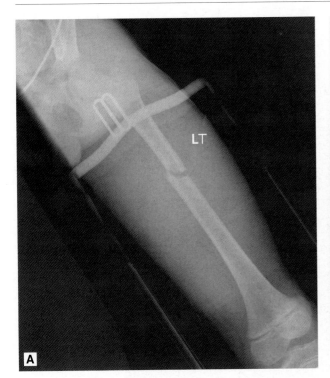

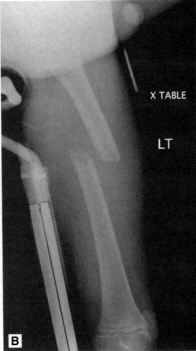

FIGURE 5-16

AP **(A)** and cross-table lateral **(B)** demonstrate a short oblique left femur fracture.

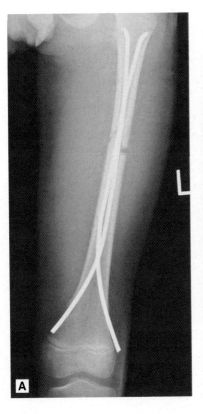

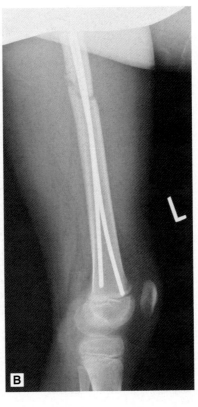

FIGURE 5-17

AP **(A)** and lateral **(B)** radiographs taken 1 week after fracture stabilization with titanium elastic nails.

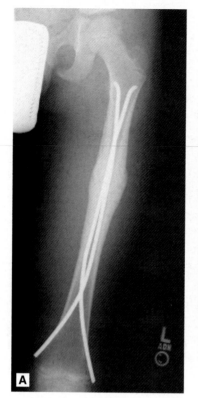
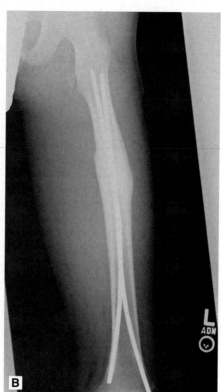

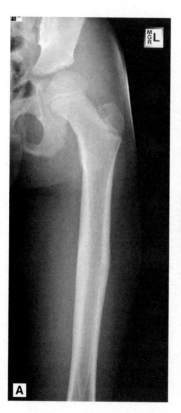
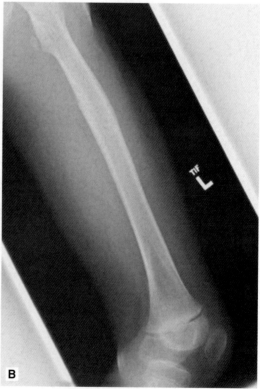

FIGURE 5-19
AP **(A)** and lateral **(B)** radiographs 1 year after injury and 4 months after nail removal.

REFERENCES

1. Flynn JM, Hresko T, Reynolds RA, et al. Titanium elastic nails for pediatric femur fractures: a multicenter study of early results with analysis of complications. *J Pediatr Orhthop.* 2001;21:4–8.
2. Flynn JM, Launay F, Moroz L, et al. Titanium elastic nailing of pediatric femur fractures: predictors of complications and poor outcomes. JBJS, Oct 2006.
3. Heinrich SD, Drvaric DM, Darr K, et al. The operative stabilization of pediatric diaphyseal femur fractures with flexible intramedullary nails: a prospective analysis. *J Pediatr Orthop.* 1994;14:501–507.
4. Ho CA, Skaggs DL, Tang CW, et al. Use of flexible intramedullary nails in pediatric femur fractures. *J Pediatr Orthop.* 2006;26:497–504.
5. Ligier JN, Metaizeau JP, Prevot J, et al. Elastic stable intramedullary pinning of long bone shaft fractures in children. *Z Kinderchir.* 1985;40:209–212.
6. Luhmann SJ, Schootman M, Schoenecker PL, et al. Complications of titanium elastic nails for pediatric femoral shaft fractures. *J Pediatr Orthop.* 2003;23:443–447.
7. Sink EL, Gralla J, Repine M. Complications of pediatric femur fractures treated with titanium elastic nails: a comparison of fracture types. *J Pediatr Orthop.* 2005;25:577–580.

6 Early Spica Cast Treatment of Femur Fractures

William L. Hennrikus and Scott Mubarak

INDICATIONS/CONTRAINDICATIONS

Early spica casting is indicated for the otherwise healthy child age 1 to 6 years old with an isolated femoral shaft fracture stemming from a low-energy injury with intact soft tissue, no evidence of compartment syndrome, and a reliable home environment. There has been a trend to place IM flexible nails in younger children with isolated femoral shaft fractures, and at times, one may consider IM flexible nails in children ≤6 years of age, depending on the family's wishes and other factors. Femoral fractures in children younger than 1 year of age are best treated with another method, such as a Pavlik harness. In addition, femoral fractures in children older than 6 years of age and in children younger than 6 years of age with an open fracture or multi trauma are not routinely treated with a spica cast; instead, surgical treatment is usually preferred.

Spica cast treatment for the child up to 6 years of age minimizes hospitalization and allows the child to return to the home environment in 1 to 2 days. Attention to detail during cast application and adherence to the indications for the use of spica casting are necessary to achieve a good result.

PREOPERATIVE PLANNING

All the necessary materials and assistants needed for application of the cast should be in the room at the start of the procedure. Three assistants are needed to hold the child on the spica table during application of the cast. A radiology technician and fluoroscopic or permanent radiographic imaging are also required. Materials needed include a spica table, an arm rest bar (such as a 60 in. × 4 in. × 1/8 in. sheet of stainless steel), and a 2 in. × 2 in. × 3 ft. wood block to elevate the proximal legs of the spica table (Fig. 6-1). The wood elevator tilts the spica 10 degrees so that the patient's perineum fits snugly onto the perineal post on the spica table. If the procedure is performed in the operating room, a wood elevator is not needed; instead, the operating room table can be tilted 10 degrees for the same effect. Necessary casting and padding materials include stockinette in multiple sizes (2 in., 3 in., and 4 in.) to cover the legs and abdomen, a folded towel to pad the abdomen, Webril cotton in multiple sizes (2 in., 3 in., and 4 in.), one-quarter self-sticking foam padding to pad bony prominences such as the sacrum and spine, fiberglass in multiple sizes (2 in., 3 in., and 4 in.), fiberglass splints for reinforcing the cast junction between the torso and the leg, towels to provide space for the abdomen, and a bucket of water (Fig. 6-2). Materials needed to trim the cast include a cast saw, an industrial-sized staple gun, and moleskin. A one-fourth-inch diameter wood dowel bar should also be available to connect the legs in the cast for added stability, though this is usually not needed when fiberglass is used (Fig. 6-3). In addition, an instructional handout for the family about spica cast care is very helpful. Finally, special seat belt straps are required in some states to secure the child in a spica cast during transportation in an automobile.

Application of the spica does not need to be done as an emergency procedure. In general, if the child arrives at the emergency department during normal working hours, the cast can be applied

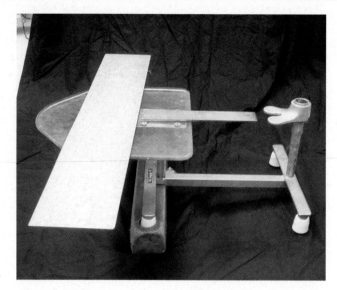

FIGURE 6-1

Spica table with arm board and wood elevator.

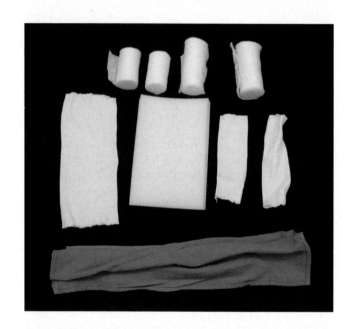

FIGURE 6-2

Materials to pad the spica cast.

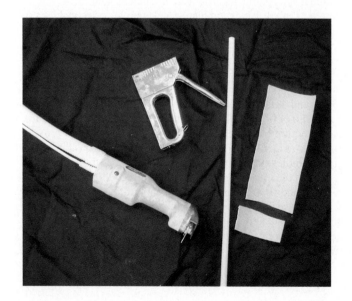

FIGURE 6-3

Additional materials to trim the cast and stabilize the legs.

in an immediate fashion. Although the procedure can be done in the emergency department or procedure room with conscious sedation, fracture reduction and molding may be best accomplished in the operating room with live imaging, a dedicated anesthesiologist, and a great deal of assistance. If the child arrives at the emergency department in the evening or on a weekend, the child can be admitted, and the injured leg can be placed in Buck skin traction with a small amount of weight (e.g., 5 lb.) until assistants and an operating room are available. Surgeons should be wary of the possibility of compartment syndrome with tightly wrapped skin traction or ipsilateral leg or foot trauma.

Parents are informed of the risks and benefits of the procedure prior to application of the cast. (See "Complications to Avoid.") The most important risk to inform the parents of is the potential need to change treatment and remove the spica cast due to unacceptable shortening or angulation. About one in five children placed in an early spica cast will require a change in treatment. This is also the time to set the parents' expectations that the child will limp for 6 months following a femur fracture; if the child stops limping early, it will just increase the parents' overall satisfaction with the care. In addition, parents should be informed that overgrowth is not completely predictable. Despite the surgeons' best efforts, there is a small risk that a child treated with a spica cast for a femoral fracture will have a permanent 2-cm or greater leg length difference and may need an epiphyseodesis at an older age.

SURGICAL PROCEDURE

Spica casts can be applied in the emergency room setting, in the clinic setting, or on the ward under sedation for small children age 3 years or younger. In general, the spica cast is more easily applied in the operating room under general anesthesia for older or uncooperative children. The one-and-a-half spica cast is preferred, with the cast extending from the nipple level to the mid- to distal tibia level on the injured side and to the mid- to distal femur level on the uninjured side. The child is placed supine on the spica table, with the child's arms secured to the arm board with Webril cotton or held across the child's chest by an assistant. Securing the arms in this fashion simplifies holding the child. The spica table is tilted 10 degrees downward by placing the wood elevator under the proximal legs of the spica table or by tilting the operating room bed.

One assistant holds each leg at the ankle and applies gentle traction to the affected side. The goal of positioning the leg is to match the position of the distal fragment to the proximal fragment. For the typical midshaft femoral fracture, the legs are positioned with the hip and knee in mild flexion and with the hip in 20 degrees of abduction and 15 degrees of external rotation, allowing for the effects of the abductor and psoas muscles on the proximal fragment. Proximal one-third fractures should be positioned with more hip flexion. A folded towel at least 2 in. thick is placed on the child's chest and abdomen beneath the stockinette to prevent the cast from being too tight and to allow full respiratory excursion while in the cast. If in doubt, make the abdomen padding larger. If the child starts to have decreased oxygen saturation during casting, this is most likely an indication of tight wrapping; removal of the towels is usually curative.

Next, stockinette is applied to all areas to be casted, followed by three layers of Webril cotton. Some surgeons use a Gore-Tex cast underliner on the skin as the first layer of the cast, which has the theoretical advantage of being breathable and waterproof; this is not a requirement, however. Extra Webril is applied to bony prominences, such as the fibula head, iliac crest, greater trochanters, and patella. Additional Webril is applied at the top and bottom of the cast so that a soft edge results when the stockinette is folded over. Some surgeons place a self-sticking one-fourth-inch foam pad on the back of the child over the cotton to prevent pressure areas on the sacrum and spine that could result from supine positioning while in the cast.

Just before placing the casting material, AP and lateral imaging may be practiced to make certain the images can be obtained in an expedient fashion while the casting material is hardening, allowing for real-time manipulation of the fracture. Fiberglass rather than plaster is utilized, because fiberglass is lighter, stronger, easier to x-ray through, easier to wedge, and water resistant. Typically four layers of fiberglass are rolled. The fiberglass is rolled over the Webril, taking care to leave a half-inch area of uncovered Webril at the superior torso and inferior leg area of the cast. The extra Webril in these areas ensures a soft edge when the stockinette is folded over. In addition, fiberglass splints are applied to the groin, buttock, and knee to strengthen the cast and, in most cases, to obviate the need for a connecting bar between the legs. Not using a connecting bar between the legs makes carrying the child on a parent's hip easier and simplifies peroneal care.

In particular, a splint should be incorporated at the resident's triangle section of the cast at the inferior lateral buttock area bilaterally. This area typically does not get enough fiberglass coverage from rolling the fiberglass. Splints can be made from a roll of 3-in. fiberglass. Typically splints are about 6 to 20 in. long and six layers thick.

Most fractures tend to angulate into varus; therefore, a valgus mold is applied to the fracture site while the cast is still wet (Fig. 6-4). Aiming for 5 to 10 degrees of valgus at the initial cast application is a reasonable goal, as the fractures often drift into varus over the oncoming weeks.

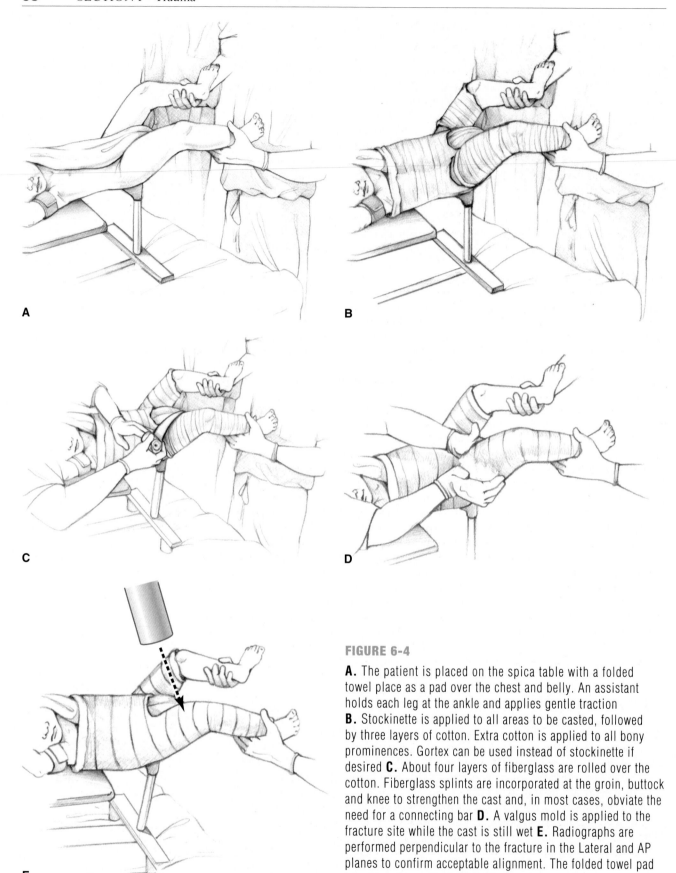

A

B

C

D

E

FIGURE 6-4

A. The patient is placed on the spica table with a folded towel place as a pad over the chest and belly. An assistant holds each leg at the ankle and applies gentle traction **B.** Stockinette is applied to all areas to be casted, followed by three layers of cotton. Extra cotton is applied to all bony prominences. Gortex can be used instead of stockinette if desired **C.** About four layers of fiberglass are rolled over the cotton. Fiberglass splints are incorporated at the groin, buttock and knee to strengthen the cast and, in most cases, obviate the need for a connecting bar **D.** A valgus mold is applied to the fracture site while the cast is still wet **E.** Radiographs are performed perpendicular to the fracture in the Lateral and AP planes to confirm acceptable alignment. The folded towel pad is removed once the cast is hardened.

Next, the stockinette edges are folded back at the torso and legs and are wrapped with fiberglass to eliminate any rough edges. The perineal area is trimmed with the cast saw superior to the gluteal fold, and the stockinette is folded back and may be held in place with staples or an assistant's fingers. Moleskin is applied to any remaining rough edges of the cast. Biplane radiographs are obtained in the operating room to assess fracture alignment.

One may accept up to 2 cm of shortening at the extreme, but 1 cm is preferable, as further shortening may occur over time. Magnification on the images may be estimated by taping a metal marker of known length (a paper clip) to the cast at the level of the fracture. Up to 10 degrees of angulation in the frontal plane (with a strong preference of valgus over varus), 20 degrees of anterior bow, and 10 degrees of posterior bow are acceptable. In the under 6-year-old age group, fractures aligned within these limits will usually remodel and overgrow to near normal alignment over a 1- to 2-year interval.

Unacceptable angulation can usually be corrected by wedging the cast. Wedging the cast to correct angular deformity is performed by making a 300 degree out of 360 degree circular cut in the cast at the level of the deformity. The cast spreader is used to open the wedge, which levers the cast to correct the angulation. The wedge is held open with plastic spacers, and radiographs are performed to document the improvement in fracture alignment. The cast is then overwrapped with fiberglass at the wedge site. The proximal and distal fragments should be checked for rotational alignment; AP and lateral imaging can be used to evaluate that both fragments are in the same plane. Rotational malalignment may be corrected by a circumferential circular cut of the cast and rotation of the distal fragment relative to the proximal fragment, followed by image verification of correct alignment.

Unacceptable angulation, despite wedging or shortening of greater than 2 cm in the spica cast, can be corrected by changing the cast, by removing the cast and applying traction, or by using an external fixator or IM nails.

POSTOPERATIVE MANAGEMENT

Parents are instructed about cast care, positioning in the cast, perineal skin care, diapering in the cast, methods for carrying and transferring the child, car seat regulations, and so forth. Remember, there are no hypochondriacs in a cast. In addition, the parents are provided with a handout about spica cast care. In general, the child in the spica cast can be turned from side to side or onto his or her stomach as tolerated. Larger children are provided with a reclining wheelchair; smaller children can be transported at home with a wagon padded with pillows and blankets. Parents may be provided with special straps to secure the child to the car seat for transportation home.

The child with a femur fracture in a spica will usually have pain and muscle spasms for about a week. A 10-day prescription for liquid acetaminophen (Tylenol) with codeine for pain and liquid diazepam for muscle spasms may be prescribed.

Weekly biplane radiographic follow-up is indicated for the first 2 to 3 weeks to ensure that fracture alignment and length are maintained in the cast. Shortening is best measured on the lateral film by the overlap of the bony projections. Measurement of shortening on the AP film can be distorted and less accurate due to the flexion of the cast at the hip and knee and a resultant lack of a true AP radiograph. Angulation is measured on both the lateral and AP radiographs by drawing a line down the long axis of both fragments and measuring the angle. At weekly follow-up visits, unacceptable angulation can usually be corrected by wedging the cast.

After 2 weeks, the patient is seen on an outpatient basis as deemed necessary until the fracture is united. In general, duration of casting can be estimated as the child's age in years plus 3 additional weeks; however, the radiographs must be examined to confirm callus formation. For example, a 5-year-old would be in the spica cast for 5 plus 3 weeks, or 8 weeks total. Parents should be informed that if the child is having increasing pain or agitation, they should visit the doctor immediately, as it may be a sign of skin or other problems. At the time of cast removal in the office, the parents are informed that the child may not be able to walk for about 3 weeks and will limp for about 3 to 6 months. Subsequent follow-up visits are scheduled for 3 months, and then at 1 year for clinical and radiologic examinations. Additional follow-up may be needed on a case-by-case basis for such concerns as angulation or shortening. Physical therapy is usually not needed.

COMPLICATIONS TO AVOID

The most common complications of femoral fractures treated with a spica cast are shortening, angulation, and skin rashes. During treatment in the spica cast, one may accept up to 2 cm of shortening, up to 10 degrees of varus angulation to 20 degrees of valgus, 20 degrees of anterior bow, and 10 degrees of posterior bow, with more angulation acceptable in very young children. Fractures healing within these parameters will predictably remodel and overgrow nicely during the 2 years following cast removal. The alignment of the normal uninjured femur is 8 degrees of anterior bowing and 0 angulation in the frontal plane. Wedging of the cast within the first 2 weeks of spica application can usually correct angular deformity to within acceptable limits. Unacceptable angulation despite wedging or shortening of greater than 2 cm in the spica cast can be corrected by changing the cast, by removing the cast and placing the child's leg in traction, or by applying an external fixator or flexible IM rods. About one in five patients will require a cast change or change of treatment due to unacceptable angulation or shortening in the spica. Parents should be informed of this risk prior to spica cast application.

Compartment syndrome can result from applying the cast in pieces with a short-leg cast applied first, traction applied via the short-leg cast, and positioning of the leg in the sitting position with the hip and knee flexed to 90 degrees. In the past, such "90-90" spica casts were advocated to enable traction to be applied across the femur. This position is no longer recommended, as it may lead to severe soft-tissue problems over the anterior ankle and/or proximal posterior calf (Fig. 6-5). Careful application of the cast in one piece with the hip and leg in more extension and with the foot out of the cast can minimize the risk of compartment syndrome and soft-tissue problems. If there is unacceptable shortening with the spica cast technique, the next step is to move to an alternative treatment method.

Severe skin rashes under the cast may be an additional reason for changing the cast. This is most common in children under the age of 2 who are not yet toilet trained. Typically the rash stems from urine and feces getting on the skin at the perineal area. Clear cast care instructions and handouts for the parents about cast care can help minimize the skin rash problem. Using a Gore-Tex cast underliner may also minimize skin problems in this age group.

Less common complications include superior mesenteric artery syndrome, compartment syndrome, decubitus ulcers, and skin burns from the cast saw. Superior mesenteric artery syndrome is rare but can result from excessive lordosis in the cast. Decubitus ulcers can be minimized by placing one-fourth-inch foam padding on the back side of the cast over the cotton Webril and under the fiberglass. Encouraging parents to turn the child in the spica cast from side to side and onto his or her stomach as tolerated also helps minimize prolonged pressure on the lumbar and sacral areas. Cast burns can be minimized by meticulous use of the cast saw and protecting the skin at the time of cast removal by placing a plastic protective cutting stick under the cast in line with the planned cast saw cut.

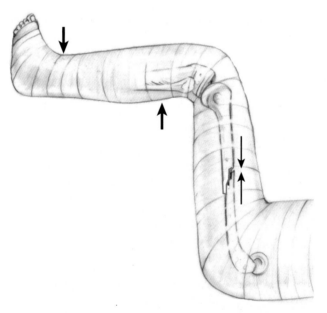

FIGURE 6-5   After the child awakens from general anesthesia, there is a shortening of the femur from muscular contraction, which causes the thigh and leg to slip somewhat back into the spica. This causes pressure to occur at the corners of the cast (see arrows; i.e., proximal posterior calf and anterior ankle). (Redrawn after Mubarak SJ, Frick S, Sink E, et al. Volkmann contracture and compartment syndromes after femur fractures in children treated with 90/90 spica casts. *J Pediatr Orthop.* 2006;26:567–572, with permission.)

Finally, femoral fractures in children are usually the result of normal trauma, such as falling from a bicycle or from a porch. However, be certain to consider and rule out child abuse in a case of a femoral fracture in any young child, especially in children who are not yet walking. Abuse is suggested by an unreasonable history, inappropriate delay in coming to the hospital, a history of previous abuse, multiple acute fractures, and evidence of any additional fractures in various stages of healing. In general, the fracture pattern of the femur alone, such as a spiral fracture pattern, does not rule in or rule out abuse.

ILLUSTRATIVE CASE

A 3-year-old boy presented to the emergency department in the early evening with a fracture of the femur after having fallen from a slide (Fig. 6-6). The fracture was an isolated, closed injury, and the child was otherwise healthy with a good home environment. The patient was admitted and placed into 3-lb Buck skin traction overnight. The next morning, after administering morphine analgesia, a spica cast was applied in the clinic by the method described. Portable fluoroscopic imaging demonstrated satisfactory alignment in the cast (Fig. 6-7). Follow-up radiographs at 1 week demonstrated satisfactory alignment. Follow-up radiographs at 2 weeks demonstrated that the fracture had drifted into varus; the cast was wedged. Radiographs after wedging demonstrated satisfactory alignment. The cast was removed after 6 weeks; the patient returned for a visit at 3 months and demonstrated a minimal limp and no functional problems. At the 1-year visit, the child's gait was normal, and the hip and knee motion and rotation were symmetrical. The leg lengths measured clinically by tape measure from the anterior iliac spine to the medial malleolus demonstrated a 3-mm shortening on the injured limb. The thigh circumference measured with a tape measure 5 cm above the superior pole of the patella demonstrated a 4-mm difference. The patient and the parents were unaware of the mild limb length or circumference differences. Radiographs at this time demonstrated near complete remodeling (Fig. 6-8). The patient did not return for any additional follow-ups.

PEARLS AND PITFALLS

- The injury radiographs of the fractured femur must include the hip and knee to avoid missing a concomitant hip dislocation, femoral neck fracture, or occult knee injury.
- Malreduction from femur fractures often occur with the fracture fragments drifting into a varus position. Therefore, a valgus mold should be applied over the femur at the time of cast application.

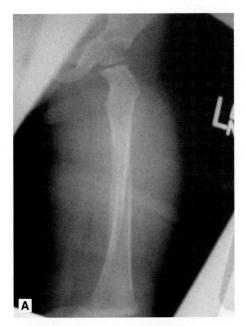
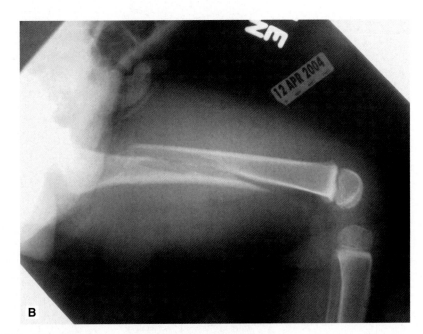

FIGURE 6-6   Anteroposterior **(A)** and lateral **(B)** radiographs of fractured femur.

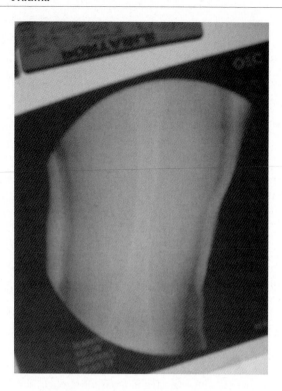

FIGURE 6-7

Fluoroscopic image of well-aligned fracture in cast.

- It is easy to forget to check for correct rotational alignment. Make certain to verify that both the proximal and distal fragments show an AP and lateral view in the respective x-rays. If an AP view is noted on one fragment and a lateral view on the other fragment, rotation may be off by 90 degrees.
- Always consider child abuse in the differential diagnosis of a young child with a femur fracture. If child abuse is strongly suspected, one option is to delay application of the spica cast and, place the child's limb into temporary skin traction until the nonaccidental trauma workup is completed.

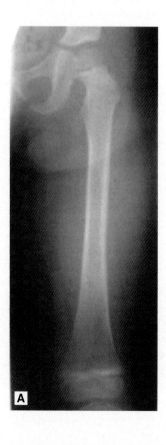
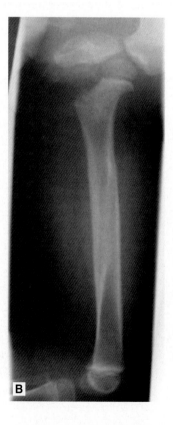

FIGURE 6-8

AP **(A)** and lateral **(B)** radiographs of healed fracture 1 year later.

- About one in five patients treated with a spica cast will demonstrate unacceptable shortening or angulation, necessitating a change of the cast or a change in treatment. Inform the parents of this risk prior to spica cast application.

RECOMMENDED READING

1. Beals RK, Tufts E. Fractured femur in infancy: the role of child abuse. *J Pediatr Orthop.* 1983;3:583–586.
2. Illgen R, Rodgers WB, Kasser JR, et al. Femur fractures in children: treatment with early spica casting. *J Pediatr Orthop.* 1998;11:481–487.
3. Irani RN, Nicholson JT, Chung SMK. Long term results in the treatment of femoral shaft fractures in young children by immediate spica immobilization. *J Bone Joint Surg.* 1976;58A:945–951.
4. Kasser JR. Femur fractures in children. In: *Instructional Course Lectures;* vol. 41. American Academy of Orthopaedic Surgeons; 1992:403–408.
5. Martinez AG, Carroll NC, Sarwark JF, et al. Femoral fractures in children treated with early spica cast. *J Pediatr Orthop.* 1991;11:712–716.
6. Mubarak SJ, Frick S, Sink E, et al. Volkmann contracture and compartment syndromes after femur fractures in children treated with 90/90 spica casts. *J Pediatr Orthop.* 2006;26:567–572.
7. Schwend RM, Werth C, Johnston A. Femur shaft fractures in toddlers and young children: rarely from child abuse. *J Pediatr Orthop.* 2000;20:475–481.
8. Staheli LT, Sheridan GW. Early spica cast management of femoral shaft fractures in young children. *Clin Orthop Relat Res.* 1977;126:162–166.
9. Wiess AP, Schenck RC, Sponseller PD, et al. Peroneal palsy after early cast application for femoral fractures in children. *J Pediatr Orthop.* 1992;12:25–28.

7 Operative Treatment of Femur Fractures Using Submuscular Plating

Ernest L. Sink

Operative stabilization is the treatment of choice for pediatric femur fractures in most children older than 5 years. Flexible elastic nailing is successful for the majority of diaphyseal femur fractures (the middle 60% of the femur). Reports show that the complication rate was greater when titanium elastic nails were used to stabilize comminuted and long oblique length-unstable fractures and that there is an increased risk of complications in children over 10 years old. Therefore, in length-unstable fractures, different methods of stabilization, such as external fixation, trochanteric-entry rigid nails, and submuscular bridge plating, have been implemented to achieve greater stability.

Plate osteosynthesis is a proven method for stabilizing pediatric fractures. The use of submuscular bridge plating for comminuted femur fractures allows for rigid stabilization, minimally invasive techniques, avoidance of avascular necrosis (AVN) of the femoral head, and stabilization of the diasphyseal/metaphyseal junction.

INDICATION/CONTRAINDICATIONS

The procedure is indicated for patients from ≥5 years to skeletal maturity. The fracture patterns most amenable to bridge plating are comminuted or long oblique length-unstable fractures in which methods such as intramedullary elastic nails are less appealing. Submuscular plating is also a reliable option for proximal or distal one-third femur fractures. For these fractures, there needs to be room for two to three screws in the proximal or distal diaphyseal region. Because this method has a relative contraindication in patients with transverse fractures, flexible IM nails may be used instead of bridge plating for transverse or short oblique mid-diaphyseal fractures.

PREOPERATIVE PLANNING

All patients should be carefully evaluated for other injuries, including knee or hip injuries. The operating room should have a traction bed and a C-arm (fluoroscope). No preoperative templating is required, as the plate length and contour are chosen under sterile conditions. It is important to have the long plates and the appropriate screw set available. Finally, it may be necessary to evaluate the natural rotation of the contralateral leg before draping.

SURGICAL PROCEDURE

Patients are positioned supine on a fracture table. The well leg is extended and slightly abducted to allow a true lateral fluoroscopic image of the fractured femur. Alternatively, a "well leg" holder may be used. Provisional reduction to restore femoral length and rotation is obtained with boot traction and verified fluoroscopically (Fig. 7-1). Final alignment is performed with plate fixation, as described later.

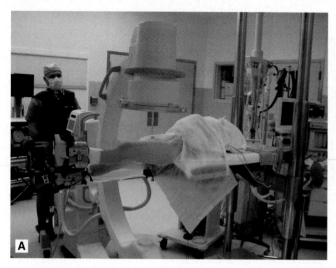
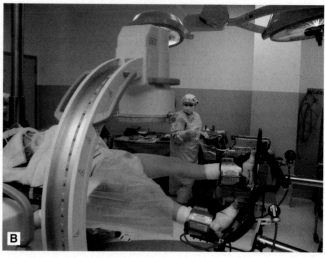

FIGURE 7-1 **A.** Patient position on the fracture table. **B.** The well leg is slightly extended to allow good anterior–posterior and lateral views of the femur.

A narrow 4.5-mm plate is most often used, as it is readily available, is easy to contour, and has percutaneous screw placement that is forgiving. A locked plate may also be used in osteopenic patients or in very proximal or distal fractures that have little available room for screws. A nonlocking plate achieves enough stability in this age group and allows easier percutaneous screw placement as compared with a locking plate. If a locking plate is used, a combination of locking and nonlocking screws is needed to reduce the femur to the plate. In addition, it may be easier to place the locking screws with direct plate exposure rather than percutaneous exposure. Self-tapping screws are essential for easier percutaneous insertion. In smaller children, a long, narrow, 3.5-mm plate may be used, though a 4.5-mm plate will fit most femurs, even in younger children.

The plate length chosen is usually 10 to 16 holes, depending on fracture location and patient size. The plate commonly spans from just below the greater trochanteric apophysis to the metaphysis of the distal femur. If possible, the plate length should allow six screw holes proximal and distal to the fracture. A table plate bender contours the plate similar to the lateral femur, with a slight bend proximally and distally to accommodate the proximal and distal metaphysis. The final femoral varus/valgus alignment is the same as the plate, so it is important to contour the plate as close to anatomic as possible. The usual practice is to place the precontoured plate on the anterior thigh and then use the anterior-posterior view on the C-arm to shadow the plate with the lateral femur cortex checking the contour (Fig. 7-2). Usually, there is no significant (greater than 5 degrees) misalignment as a result of incorrect contouring.

FIGURE 7-2

A. A narrow, 4.5-mm contoured plate is placed on the anterior thigh to shadow the lateral cortex of the femur to evaluate the length and contour of the plate. **B.** The fluoroscopic image confirming adequate plate contouring.

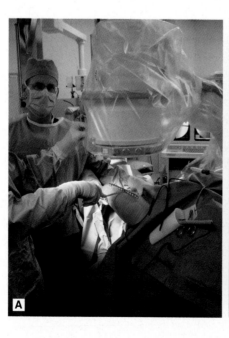
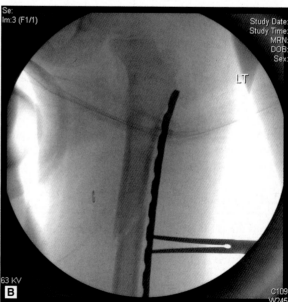

A small (4 to 7 mm) incision is performed at the distal lateral thigh. The exposure is advanced through the tensor fascia to expose the distal oblique fibers of the vastus lateralis muscle. Blunt dissection is performed deep to the distal muscle fibers to enter the plane between the vastus lateralis and the lateral femur periosteum. This plane is easily entered and allows proximal plate advancement with minimal force (Fig. 7-3). The plate is then slowly tunneled proximally in this plane. A Kocher clamp may be used to grasp the distal aspect of the plate for guidance. Care is taken to keep the plate on the lateral femur as it is advanced proximally past the fracture to the region of the greater trochanteric apophysis. The plate may be more difficult to pass along the lateral femur past the fracture; the surgeon may correct this by pulling the plate back and redirecting it. The C-arm may also aid the surgeon in plate advancement (Fig. 7-4).

Once the plate is fully advanced, it should sit comfortably on the lateral femur. Anterior-posterior and lateral images are then obtained to ensure that the plate is in a good position in both planes and that the femoral length is restored. The plate is provisionally fixed to the femur with a Kirschner wire (K-wire) placed in the most proximal and distal screw holes (Fig. 7-5). If the fracture is "sagging" posterior, the femur can be lifted in an anterior direction while a K-wire is placed through the plate to engage the femur in this region.

A long plate and correct screw placement are important for construct stability. A screw should be placed in close proximity to the proximal and distal extent of the fracture (Fig. 7-6). The remaining screws are placed as far apart as possible. Obtaining maximal screw spread with a long plate will improve construct stability due to the long working length of the plate. Three screws

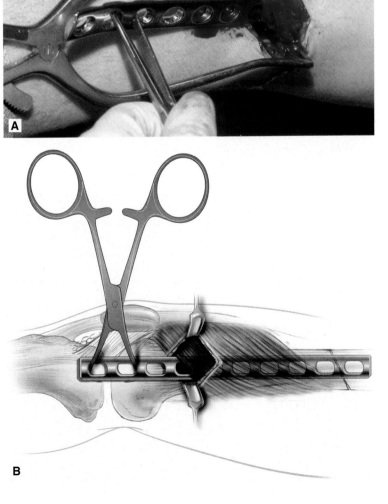

FIGURE 7-3

A. The plate being advanced proximally deep to the distal oblique fibers of the vastus lateralis. **B.** Artist's drawing of the plate advancement.

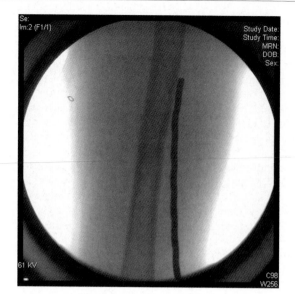

FIGURE 7-4

Fluoroscopic image of the plate gliding past and proximal to the fracture along the lateral periosteum.

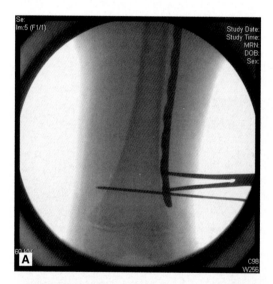

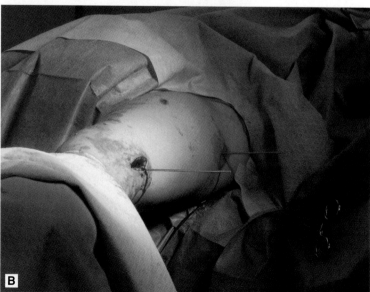

FIGURE 7-5

A–B. The plate is temporarily secured to the femur with a Kirschner wire placed in the most proximal and distal screw holes. The fluoroscopic image **(A)** confirms that the plate is in a good position to start screw fixation.

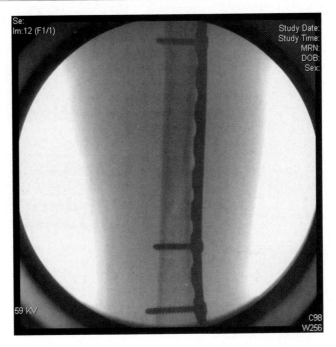

FIGURE 7-6

Intraoperative fluoroscopic image illustrating the plate bridging the fracture, with two screws placed in proximity to the proximal and distal margins of the fracture.

proximal and three screws distal to the fracture are optimal. The first screw placed should be near the proximal or distal extent of the fracture, where the femur is farthest from the plate. A screw in this area will reduce the femur to the plate and act as a "reduction screw." As the screw engages the far cortex, the femur will be reduced to the precontoured plate (Fig. 7-7). The fracture is thus "bridged," and no attempt is made to place a screw to lag the fracture fragments.

The technical aspects of percutaneous screw placement are as follows (Fig. 7-8): Screws are placed using a "perfect circles" technique. With the fluoroscopic image in the lateral plane, a #15 blade scalpel is placed on the skin over the hole and is then rotated horizontal to the beam through the skin, tensor fascia, and vastus fascia. A 3.2-mm drill is placed in this small incision using a free-hand technique, and its location in the desired hole is confirmed with fluoroscopy. The hole is then drilled through both cortices. The length of the screw is approximated by placing the depth gauge on the anterior thigh as the image is rotated to the anterior-posterior view. A 0 Vicryl suture is tied around the 4.5-mm, fully threaded, cortical screw head so the screw will not be lost in the soft tissue if it inadvertently disengages from the screwdriver. The screw is then placed through the plate and across the femur. The suture ties are cut, and the incisions are closed with absorbable subcuticular sutures after all screws are placed.

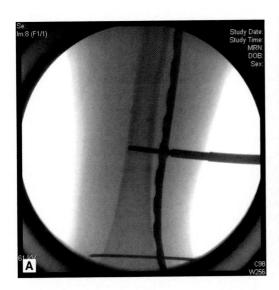
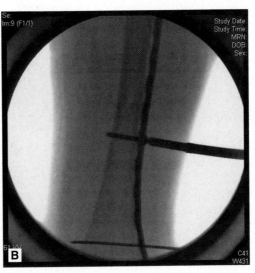

FIGURE 7-7

A. Intraoperative fluoroscopic image illustrating the first screw being placed just distal to the fracture, where the femur is farthest from the plate. **B.** As the screw engages the opposite cortex, the femur is reduced to the plate.

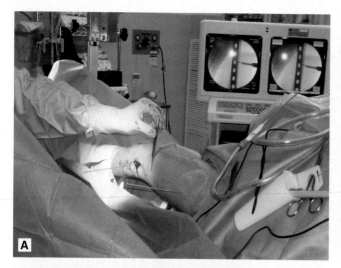

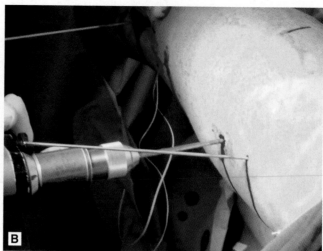

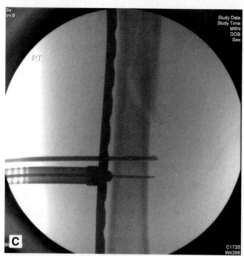

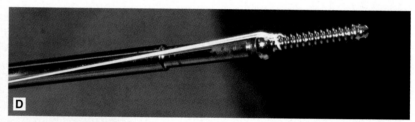

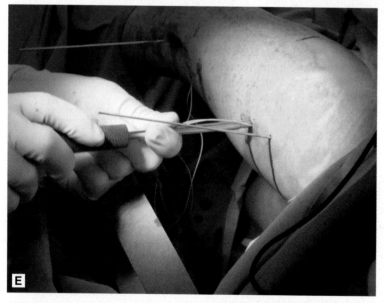

FIGURE 7-8 **A.** Method used to localize the appropriate screw hole and then make the percutaneous incision for the screw placement. Using the lateral floroscopic image the tip of a #15 blade knife is placed over the desired screw hole. The blade of the knife is then rotated 90 degrees along the beam of the C-arm, and the knife is directed to the desired plate hole. (Note: The K-wires temporarily secure the plate to the femur.) **B.** Drilling with freehand technique. **C.** Fluoroscopic image of the depth gauge on the anterior thigh to approximate screw length. **D.** The screw with a Vicryl suture tied around the screw head so it will not be lost in the soft tissue. **E.** A screw being placed percutaneous.

POSTOPERATIVE MANAGEMENT

A soft dressing is applied after surgery. Patients may be placed in a knee immobilizer for early comfort with mobilization. No casting is required in the early postoperative period. Active knee range of motion is encouraged, as comfort allows. Patients are kept non–weight bearing or touch-down weight bearing until bridging callous is seen (usually at 6 to 10 weeks). Progressive weight bearing is then encouraged. Once bridging callus is apparent on three or four cortices, activity as tolerated and sports are allowed in a graded manner. This is usually between 10 and 14 weeks post-op.

The plate is removed in most patients at around 6 months. If the plate is removed closer to or past a year, it may be too difficult to remove percutaneously due to tissue and bone ingrowth. There are no clear indications for plate removal. Most parents, when offered the option of plate removal, will elect for removal. Surgeons may want to be more aggressive in offering plate removal for younger children, as they have more bony overgrowth and leg growth potential. In the adolescent ages, removal may be approached on an individual basis; family and surgeon preferences are factors for removal. In either case, the plate can be removed through the same percutaneous incisions. The screws are removed using image guidance. A dull Cobb elevator is slid along the outer part of the plate to free up surrounding tissue. Then the Cobb, with the sharp end directed away from the bone, is advanced between the plate and the bone, thus freeing up the plate. Once the plate is completely freed, it can be removed from the distal incision where it was advanced. Patients are then allowed weight bearing as tolerated and should be kept from running or sports for 6 weeks.

COMPLICATIONS TO AVOID

Reported complications are rare. There is one reported case of plate failure in a patient with a 3.5-mm titanium plate. This complication has not been reported with stainless steel plates or with larger 4.5-mm plates. A 3.5-mm plate would be more acceptable in smaller or younger children. There is also one reported complication of refracture in a patient; the author believed the plate was removed too early. This can be avoided by ensuring complete fracture union before plate removal. Malunion is possible and can be potentially avoided with appropriate plate contouring. Nonunion has not been reported, as this technique is best applied in closed, comminuted fractures where the fracture region is "bridged." A rotational malunion is more likely to occur. Attention to rotation is important before screw placement. Using the opposite extremity and fracture geometry appearance with fluoroscopy with initial traction setup is recommended.

ILLUSTRATIVE CASE

An 8-year-old girl sustained a proximal one-third oblique femur fracture with a nondisplaced butterfly segment (Fig. 7-9). A submuscular plate technique was chosen. The plate was placed from distal to proximal. Good screw purchase was obtained on the proximal three screws, although the fracture line extended to the second proximal screw. The distal screws were widely spaced along a long plate. At 6 weeks, bridging callous was easily seen, and the patient started to bear weight as tolerated.

DISCUSSION

The submuscular bridge plating technique has simplified management of the complex, length-unstable comminuted or long oblique pediatric femur fracture. Plating may also be considered as an option in treating proximal or distal third fractures where elastic nails may have poor stability. A better understanding of plate mechanics has improved femoral shaft plating techniques. The long plate working length in submuscular plating results in less strain on the plate and screws. In addition, callous formation occurs rapidly, as the soft tissues around the fracture are left relatively undisturbed. Earlier callous formation results in earlier load sharing, which means decreased cumulative strain on the plate and screws. Thus plate failure has not been a complication with this technique. Finally the technique has a relatively straightforward learning curve for the orthopaedic surgeon already familiar with standard plating techniques.

PEARLS AND PITFALLS

- Submuscular bridge plating is indicated for length-unstab long oblique or comminuted femur fractures.

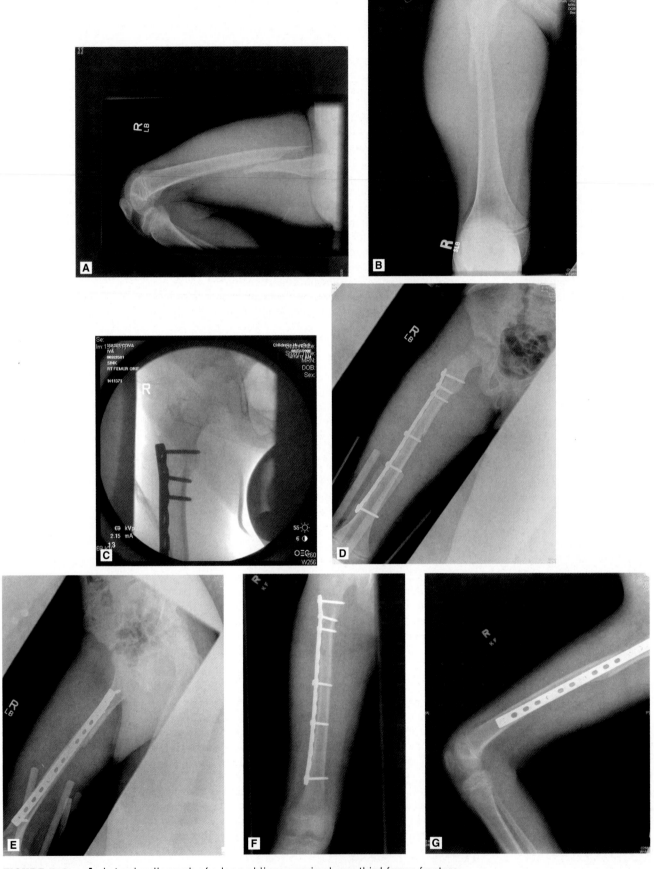

FIGURE 7-9 **A.** Lateral radiograph of a long oblique proximal one-third femur fracture. **B.** Anterior-posterior radiograph of a same fracture. **C.** Fluoroscopic image of stable proximal fixation. **D.** Postoperative anterior-posterior radiograph after bridge plating. **E.** Postoperative lateral radiograph after bridge plating. **F.** Anterior-posterior radiograph 6 weeks post-op. **G.** Lateral radiograph at 6 weeks, indicating bridging callus.

- For rigid stabilization, a long, narrow, 4.5-mm plate is used, spanning from the greater trochanteric apophysis to the distal metaphysis.
- Precontour the plate to conform to the lateral femur, as the final alignment of the fracture is that of the plate.
- Obtain as much screw spread as possible for three screws proximal and three screws distal to the fracture.
- Tie a #1 or O-Vicryl suture around the head of the screw prior to insertion so the screw will not be lost in the soft tissue.
- Place screws in close proximity to the proximal and distal extent of the fracture, but avoid the temptation to lag the fracture (bridge the fracture).
- The first screw should be in the screw hole closest to the proximal or distal aspect of the fracture, where the femur is farthest from the plate. As the screw in this region engages the femur, it will reduce the fracture to the plate.

REFERENCES

1. Agus H, Kalenderer O, Eranilmaz G, et al. Biological internal fixation of comminuted femur shaft fractures by bridge plating in children. *J Pediatr Orthop.* 2003;23:184–189.
2. Caird MS, Mueller KA, Puryear A, et al. Compression plating of pediatric femoral shaft fractures. *J Pediatr Orthop.* 2003;23:448–452.
3. Eren OT, Kucukkaya M, Kockesen C. Open reduction and plate fixation of femoral shaft fractures in children aged 4 to 10. *J Pediatr Orthop.* 2003;23:190–193.
4. Flynn, JM, Hresko T, Reynolds RAK, et al. Titanium elastic nails for pediatric femur fractures: multicenter study of early results with analysis of complications. *J Pediatr Orthop.* 2001;21:4–8.
5. Fyodrov I, Sturm PF, Robertson WW. Compression-plate fixation of femoral shaft fractures in children aged 8 to 12 years. *J Pediatr Orthop.* 1999;19:578–581.
6. Hedequist DJ, Sink EL. Technical aspects of bridge plating for pediatric femur fractures. *J Orthop Trauma.* 2004;19:276–279.
7. Heinrich SD, Drvaric DM, Darr K, et al. The operative stabilization of pediatric diaphyseal femur fractures with flexible intramedullary nails: a prospective analysis. *J Pediatr Orthop.* 1994;14:501–507.
8. Kanlic EM, Anglen JO, Smith DG, et al. Advantages of submuscular bridge plating for complex femur fractures. *Clin Orthop.* 2004;426:244–251.
9. Kregor PJ, Song KM, Routt ML, et al. Plate fixation of femoral shaft fractures in multiple injured children. *J Bone Joint Surg.* 1993;75:1774–1780.
10. Luhmann SJ, Schootman M, Schoenecker PL, et al. Complications of titanium elastic nails for pediatric femoral shaft fractures. *J Pediatr Orthop.* 2003;23:443–447.
11. Moroz LA, Launay F, Kocher MS, et al. Titanium elastic nailing of fractures of the femur in children. Predictors of complications and poor outcome. *J Bone Joint Surg.* 2006;88:1361–1366.
12. Rozbruch SR, Muller U, Gautier E, et al. The evolution of femoral shaft plating technique. *Clinic Orthop.* 1998;354:195–208.
13. Sink EL, Gralla J, Repine M. Complications of pediatric femur fractures treated with titanium elastic nails: a comparison of fracture types. *J Pediatr Orthop* (in press).
14. Sink EL, Hedequist DJ, Morgan SJ, et al. Results and technique of pediatric femur fractures treated with submuscular bridge plating. *J Pediatric Orthop.* 2006;26:177–181.
15. Ward WT, Levy J, Kayne A. Compression plating for child and adolescent femur fractures. *J Pediatr Orthop.* 1992;12:626–632.

8 Operative Treatment of Femur Fractures Using a Greater Trochanteric Entry IM Nail

Jonathan H. Phillips

Fractures of the shaft of the femur are among the most common causes for admission of children to hospitals. Treatment of these fractures accounts for a significant percentage of surgical procedures that are performed to treat pediatric fractures. The incidence of pediatric femur fracture in the United States is approximately 27 per 10,000 population. Management of this injury has undergone a significant evolution in the past decade, with more emphasis given to operative management than was previously the case. This chapter describes a new device developed by the author for the intramedullary fixation of femoral shaft fractures in children with open physes. The implant has been in use for approximately 9 years at the author's institution and is the subject of ongoing study.

INDICATIONS/CONTRAINDICATIONS

In general, the Pediatric Locking Nail (PLN, BIOMET, Parsippany, NJ) is indicated for treatment of femoral shaft fractures in patients over the age of 8 with a fracture below the lesser trochanter but above the supracondylar area. Comminution and instability are not contraindications because proximal and distal interlocking screws achieve considerable stability of the fracture when treated with this technique. The nail's controlling diameter is 8.5 mm, so the minimal femoral canal diameter is 9 mm. Attempting to insert this nail in canals smaller than 9 mm can lead to comminution. Open fractures, after appropriate debridement, can be stabilized with this nail.

As yet, an upper age limit has not been defined. Though the nail is ideally suited for patients with open physes, it can also be used in the skeletally mature individual. In a heavy, older adolescent with closed physes, however, consideration should be given to the use of available intramedullary devices used to treat adults with a femoral shaft fracture.

PREOPERATIVE PLANNING

As in all trauma situations, the child with a femur fracture for whom the use of this nail is being considered should be thoroughly evaluated clinically. Particular emphasis is placed on the diagnosis of any concomitant knee or hip injuries. Preoperative orthogonal radiographs of the injured femur are necessary, and an anteroposterior pelvis radiograph, along with radiographs of the ipsilateral knee, is advisable.

Careful evaluation of the limiting diameter of the intramedullary (IM) canal is mandatory. Because the minimum diameter of this nail is 8.5 mm, a 9-mm canal is the smallest that can accommodate this device without IM reaming. The nail is usually inserted unreamed, though the IM canal can be reamed if necessary. In the indicated age group (older than 8 years), however, this technique is seldom needed.

Preoperative evaluation of the radiographs for occult fracture comminution will avoid surprises during the operation. It is common to have undisplaced facture lines around the radiographically obvious fracture, particularly with a spiral fracture pattern. Often a fracture extension distally toward the supracondylar region or proximally to the trochanters can be diagnosed before becoming clinically evident during nail insertion. As long as these fracture line extensions are recognized, allowance for them can be achieved by modifying the surgical technique. For instance, if there is concern about comminution of the fracture by the nail in a very complex fracture pattern, a mini open technique with temporary bone clamp stabilization of the fracture during nail insertion may be useful.

Certain fracture patterns, in and of themselves, are more troublesome for nail insertion. The proximal subtrochanteric fracture typically leads to an underestimation of the degree of displacement in both the axial and the sagittal planes. The deforming force of the psoas muscle pulls the proximal fragment into external rotation and sometimes into marked flexion. With a more "parallel to the ground" approach using reamers and awls, the thin posterior cortex of the intertrochanteric area can be easily breached, causing unnecessary delay and intraoperative revision of the nail's entry pathway. Thorough preoperative evaluation will usually allow the surgeon to anticipate this potential problem, which can be minimized by placing the patient on the fracture table with flexion of the hip. In addition, starting the entry point for the nail more posteriorly and aiming the guide pin anteriorly (toward the ceiling) will be helpful in these proximal femur structures.

For the more distal femoral shaft fracture, the preoperative planning must be especially thorough. Depending on the fracture configuration (transverse, oblique, or spiral), this nail in its present iteration is not suitable for fractures more distal than 4 cm proximal to the distal femoral physis, particularly in a large femur with a capacious distal IM canal in which little stability of the fracture will be achieved, even with a firm distal interlocking screw.

SURGICAL PROCEDURE

After an appropriate preoperative evaluation of any comorbid factors, the patient is taken to the operating room, where a fracture table has been set up and fluoroscopy is available. Preoperative prophylactic antibiotics are given. General anesthesia and complete muscle paralysis are preferable for ease of fracture reduction. A closed reduction of a widely displaced fracture is advisable, as this will greatly simplify instrumenting the femur and passing the nail. During this maneuver, any buttonholing of fracture fragments through the quadriceps may be diminished or actually eliminated. By looking at the fluoroscopic images at this stage, one can get a sense of how much persistent soft-tissue interposition is present and whether a small open-reduction incision is likely to be needed. The patient's foot on the injured side is then placed in the traction boot. Under fluoroscopic control, traction is applied to align the fracture linearly. Care must be taken not to overdistract the fracture or apply too much tension; in smaller children, it is especially easy to distract the hip joint significantly, which may increase the risk of avascular necrosis of the femoral head; imaging the hip joint at this point will help avoid this problem. In addition, excessive pressure of the perineum against the fracture table's perineal post is well recognized as a cause of possible pudendal nerve palsy. The incidence of this complication is minimized by wrapping the post with cotton padding and by not overdistracting with traction.

Assuming the fracture is adequately aligned and the well leg is appropriately positioned for unobstructed fluoroscopic access (Fig. 8-1), the injured thigh and adjoining areas are prepped and draped according to the surgeon's preferences. Any open wounds of the thigh should then be debrided and irrigated.

The approach to the entry point in the greater trochanter should be made so that the guide pin for the trochanteric reamer enters the middle of the intertrochanteric portion of the canal (Fig. 8-2).

On the anteroposterior fluoroscopic image, the guide pin should pierce the lateral aspect of the greater trochanter at least 5 mm below the tip. The guide pin should not be placed centrally in the apex of the greater trochanter, as this brings the reamer too close to the femoral head vascular supply that is coursing through the piriformis fossa. In addition, the angle of the guide pin to the long axis of the femur should be 30 degrees or more to ensure that the shaft of the nail, when inserted, is medialized in the capacious upper end of the femur. This allows full seating of the threads of the proximal interlocking screw.

A small open incision is advisable the first few times a surgeon uses this device so that direct palpation of the trochanter can be made. After familiarity is achieved with this local anatomy, a percutaneous technique is easily achieved (Fig. 8-3) after appropriate positioning of the guide pin the 9 mm reamer is used to open the lateral cortex of the trochanter, avoiding the calcar as pedestal formation here will block passage of the nail. (Fig 8-4). The appropriate sized nail is then mounted on the proximal targeting device and bends fashioned: thirty degrees proximally and 15 to 20 degrees distally.

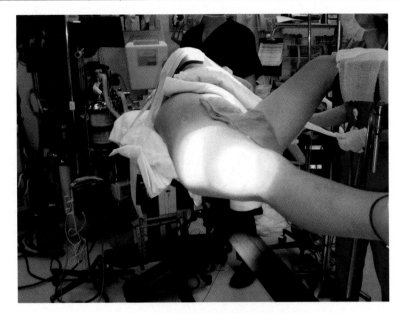

FIGURE 8-1

Typical position on the fracture table.

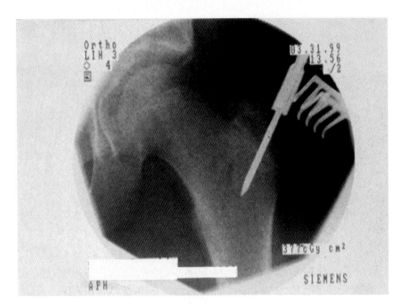

FIGURE 8-2

The guide pin is inserted into the center of the intertrochanteric area of the femur on the anteroposterior radiographic projection.

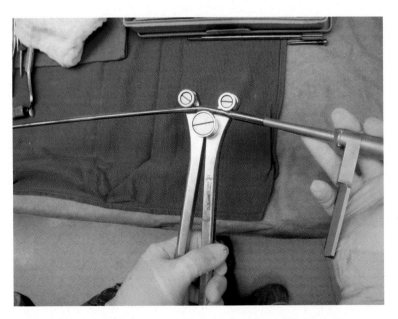

FIGURE 8-3

Proximal nail contouring. A similar smaller bend is made in the distal end of the nail. Left and right femurs are instrumented with left and right bends appropriately.

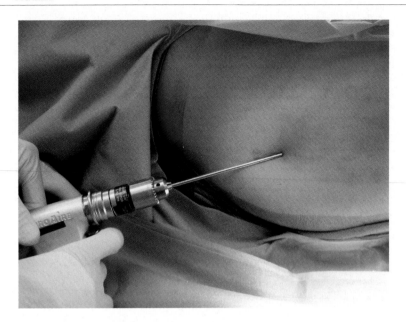

FIGURE 8-4

Percutaneous positioning of the guide pin in the appropriate planes at the greater trochanter.

With the correct-length nail mounted and contoured, the nail is introduced through the greater trochanter and around the curves of the intertrochanteric area. Impaction with a mallet may be necessary (Fig. 8-5).

If the nail does not pass this area easily, it should be removed, and a greater bend in the tip of the nail should be made. (However, the bigger the bend in the tip, the larger the effective diameter of the nail when it crosses the femoral isthmus.) Rotation of the nail in the axial plane is another useful maneuver for easing nail passage through the intertrochanteric area. The nail is then driven, often by hand but perhaps with a mallet, across the fracture site. Again, because the tip has a bend in it, the nail can be steered appropriately to access the canal of the distal fracture fragment. The nail is then seated such that its tip is short of the distal femoral physis (Figs. 8-6 and 8-8). The fracture site is checked with the image intensifier to ensure that it is not distracted. The nail is then interlocked as follows. The targeting arm is attached to the proximal targeting device, and a stab incision is made appropriate to the position of the drill guide assembly. The drill is then tapped down to the lateral cortex of the proximal femur. A 3.5-mm drill is used to interlock the proximal end of the nail (Figs. 8-7 and 8-8).

Note that the tip of the screw is slightly smaller than 4 mm and has a pilot thread. The screw's subcapital thread achieves fixation in the lateral cortex of the femur. For this reason, because the locking screws are usually unicortical, care must be taken not to enlarge the drill hole in the lateral cortex; otherwise, adequate hold of the screw will not be achieved. If there is doubt about the bone quality,

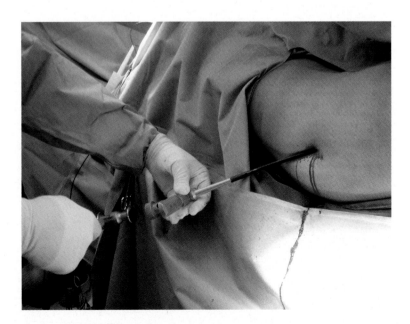

FIGURE 8-5

Impaction of the nail through the intertrochanteric area.

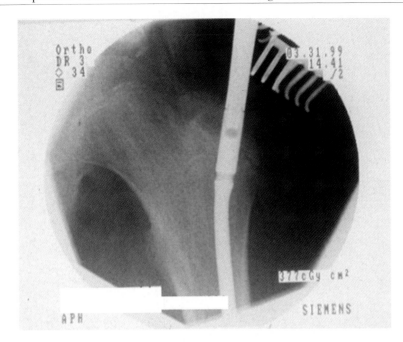

a bicortical technique should be used for this screw. The depth gauge fits inside the drill guide tube once the drill bushing is removed. A fluoroscopic image can help check accurate screw length measurement.

Once satisfactory rotation at the fracture site is confirmed, distal interlocking is performed using the perfect circles technique on the image intensifier (Fig. 8-9). Once again, it is important not to excessively enlarge the lateral cortical drill hole or else screw purchase will be compromised. A high-quality lateral fluoroscopic image of the distal screw is important to ensure that the screw has passed through the interlocking hole and is not in front of or behind the nail. Confirmatory fluoroscopic images of the proximal construct and the fracture site will confirm accurate implant placement and fracture reduction at these levels.

The procedure is completed with closure of the wounds.

POSTOPERATIVE MANAGEMENT

Crutch walking is instituted immediately postoperatively, with the patient bearing partial weight on the injured limb for about 6 weeks or until three bridging cortices are seen on radiographs of the femoral fracture (Fig. 8-10).

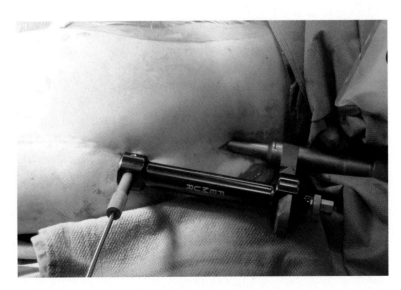

FIGURE 8-7
The proximal interlocking hole is drilled through the drill bushing (different case from previous figures).

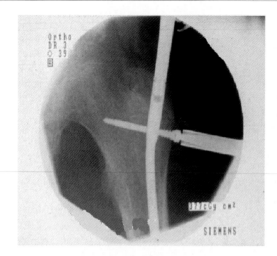

FIGURE 8-8
Proximal interlocking
screw placement.

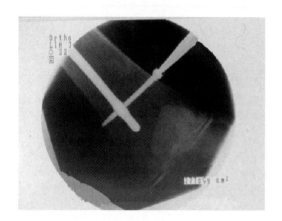

FIGURE 8-9
Distal interlocking
screw.

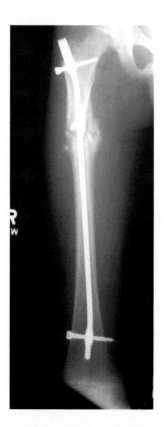

FIGURE 8-10
Healed subtrochanteric
fracture at about seven
weeks.

Routine nail removal is usually performed at about 9 months after injury, as long as complete healing is evident on radiographs. Removal of the nail is done as the reverse of insertion. The distal interlocking screws are located by fluoroscopy and are readily removed. The proximal end of the nail is accessed with a guide pin, and the reamer is used to remove the fibrous tissue at the interface with the locking bolt. Once the extraction device is firmly engaged in the nail, the locking screws can be removed. The nail is extracted with a slap hammer.

COMPLICATIONS

Possible complications include those that can be associated with any surgical procedure involving the treatment of fractures, especially the possibility of wound infection and the possibility of malunion, delayed union, or nonunion at the fracture site. Because malunion would most commonly involve rotational malalignment, it is important to align the rotational position of the distal fracture fragment appropriately during fracture reduction and adjustment of the fracture table. The risk of delayed or nonunion at the fracture site is minimized by ensuring that overdistraction at the fracture site does not occur when the IM nail is placed.

Aside from the general risks associated with the operative treatment of fractures, most of the potential complications with this procedure are related to technical errors. If there is inadequate preoperative assessment of the radiographs, occult fracture comminution may not be recognized, leading to fracture propagation during IM nail insertion, often leading to the need for open reduction. The guide pin can be placed inaccurately, particularly in subtrochanteric fractures, leading to penetration of the posterior femoral cortex in the intertrochanteric area. This situation can be avoided in proximal fractures by placing the guide pin at about a 45-degree angle to the operating table. Overreaming the entry point will lead to increased difficulty in passing the nail. Overbending of the nail tip will increase the effective diameter of the nail, making passage of the nail through the isthmus difficult. Underbending of the nail's proximal end makes interlocking screw placement more difficult and may lead to a varus deformity at the fracture site. Inaccurate drilling of the distal interlocking screw hole will lead to the screw backing out postoperatively.

PEARLS AND PITFALLS

- Use of this IM nail is primarily for those children over age 8 and adolescents.
- The minimal femoral IM canal diameter to allow use of this nail is 9 mm.
- Careful assessment of the preoperative x-rays is needed to identify occult areas of fracture comminution, which will affect IM nail placement.
- The entry point for this IM nail is at the lateral aspect of the greater trochanter.
- The nail allows more or less contouring of the proximal and distal ends to facilitate insertion.
- The feature of interlocking proximal and distal screws allows for use of this flexible nail in essentially all femoral shaft fractures in this age group.
- IM nail removal is carried out 1 year or less after insertion.

SUGGESTED READINGS

Little has been written on this specific subject. To the author's knowledge, no other interlocked flexible femoral nail specifically designed for pediatric applications has been described. However, the following articles provide excellent background for developments over the past 20 years in this area.

1. Carey TP, Galpin RD. Flexible intramedullary nail fixation of pediatric femoral fractures. *Clin Orthop.* 1996;332:110–118.
2. Cramer KE, Tornetta P, Spero CR, et al. Ender rod fixation of femoral shaft fractures in children. *J Pediatr Orthop.* 2000;376:119–123.
3. Fein LH, Pankovich AM, Spero CM, et al. Closed flexible intramedullary nailing of adolescent femoral shaft fractures. *J Orthop Trauma.* 1989;3:133–141.
4. Gordon EJ, Swenning TA, Burd TA, et al. Proximal femoral radiographic changes after lateral transtrochanteric intramedullary nail placement in children. *J Bone and Joint Surg Am.* 2003;85:1295–1301.
5. Letts M, Jarvis J, Lawton L, et al. Complications of rigid intramedullary rodding of femoral shaft fractures in children. *J Trauma.* 2002;52:504–516.
6. Luhmann SJ, Schootman M, Shoeneker PL, et al. Complications of titianium elastic nails for pediatric femoral shaft fractures. *J Pediatr Orthop.* 2003;23:443–447.
7. Mann DC, Weddington J, Davenport K. Closed ender nailing of femoral shaft fractures in adolescents. *J Pediatr Orthop.* 1986;6:651–654.

CEREBRAL PALSY

9 Lower Extremity Surgery in Children with Cerebral Palsy

Robert M. Kay

The manifestations of cerebral palsy, though due to a central nervous system (CNS) lesion, are often first evident in the musculoskeletal system. As a result, the initial diagnosis of cerebral palsy is often made by the orthopaedist, especially in children with mild cerebral palsy. Cerebral palsy occurs in approximately 1 in 500 children, a rate that has not changed significantly despite medical advances of the past several decades.

Children with cerebral palsy often have associated medical problems, including CNS maladies (seizures), pulmonary complications (including bronchopulmonary dysplasia, chronic pulmonary insufficiency, and frequent pneumonias), gastrointestinal problems (including gastroesophageal reflux, malabsorption, and ulcers), aspiration, and genitourinary problems (including incontinence and infection).

PATHOLOGY

Cerebral palsy is a static encephalopathy due to hypoxic or anoxic brain injury. The hypoxic or anoxic event may occur during pregnancy, at the time of delivery, or following delivery. The diagnosis of cerebral palsy resulting from a postnatal insult is common, though the temporal cutoff for a diagnosis of cerebral palsy is arbitrary. Most physicians use the diagnosis of cerebral palsy to include a static encephalopathy due to an event that occurs before the child reaches 2 years of age.

In all of these instances, damage to the brain, including the motor cortex, occurs. This commonly results in spasticity and hyperreflexia in the affected extremities. Hypotonia is less common in the extremities but is not uncommon in the trunk. Some children have mixed tone. In other instances, the result is choreoathetoid cerebral palsy with increased, nonvoluntary movements of the extremities.

PRESENTATION

Children with cerebral palsy first present to the orthopaedist for myriad reasons. Common reasons for referral include limping, leg-length discrepancy, foot problems, toe walking, tight muscles, and/or poor use of the hands.

The diagnosis of cerebral palsy is often easily made when the appropriate history has been elicited from the parents, even before the child is examined. A detailed birth history should include problems during the pregnancy and/or delivery, possible hypoxic events, and duration of hospitalization.

On average, children should sit at 6 months, stand at 8 months, and walk at 12 months. If a child does not reach these milestones by 1.5 times these ages (i.e., sit by 9 months, stand by 12 months, and walk by 18 months), an investigation into the developmental delay is warranted. Another helpful question is whether the child demonstrates handedness before 1 year of age. If a child shows a preference for a hand before 1 year of age, a diagnosis of hemiplegia is common.

On physical examination, range of motion is checked along with muscle tone, selective motor control, and upper and lower extremity reflexes. Typically tone and reflexes are increased in the affected extremities, whereas selective motor control is decreased.

THE DECISION FOR SURGERY

Many children with spastic cerebral palsy ultimately benefit from surgical intervention. However, the results of surgery are less reproducible in children with choreoathetoid cerebral palsy.

In general, the goals for intervention in children with cerebral palsy include improving function and/or preventing deformity and/or pain. Many children undergo reconstruction of the hips to prevent or treat dislocation and potential pain, even if those children are nonambulatory. Though hip dislocations occur in ambulatory children, they are much less common than in children who are nonambulatory.

In ambulatory children who require surgery for gait abnormalities, surgery is most commonly undertaken when the child is between the ages of 5 and 10 years. One of the most important concepts in appropriate surgical treatment of these children is to postpone surgery until the child has fulfilled the following criteria:

- The gait disturbances are interfering with function.
- Nonsurgical interventions will no longer suffice to address the gait disturbances.
- The child has failed to make significant functional progress over the preceding 6 months (i.e., the child has plateaued).

If surgery is undertaken while the child is making rapid functional progress, the child will miss out on the rapid functional gains during the recuperative period and may never be able to recoup the lost opportunity of such a rapid gain. A more prudent approach is to wait until the child plateaus, at which point surgical intervention can facilitate and expedite additional functional progress.

An important concept is the fact that the different levels of the lower extremities are interconnected and that a deviation at one level often impacts the alignment and function at other levels. A classic pitfall of not appreciating this interconnectedness is the child in marked equinus with unrecognized hamstring tightness who undergoes isolated heel-cord lengthening and ends up in significant crouch gait.

PREOPERATIVE PLANNING

Children with cerebral palsy generally have complex walking patterns, often involving multiple-level abnormalities involving one or both lower extremities. Evaluation should include both static and dynamic parameters. Previous authors have demonstrated poor correlation of static and dynamic measures in children with cerebral palsy.[9]

Three-dimensional computerized motion analysis, when available, provides objective information regarding dynamic joint deviations in multiple joints simultaneously and often impacts surgical decision making.[5,6]

The surgical plan is based on the functional gait limitations put in the context of the individual's bony and soft-tissue deformities. Contractures and/or deviations at any level in the lower extremity affect the biomechanical alignment and function at other levels. Failure to address the various problems simultaneously results in suboptimal treatment outcomes. Single-event multilevel surgery (SEMLS) of the lower extremities is the preferred treatment because it allows simultaneous correction of multiple deformities, thus providing for optimal alignment of the lower extremities while limiting the child to a single recuperative period. In contrast, correcting such problems subsequently would require additional recuperative periods, with their attendant psychosocial implications, as well as the standard risks of surgeries and hospitalizations.

SOFT-TISSUE SURGERY

Hip

Hip Adductor Lengthening   Tightness of the hip adductors and flexors are common in both ambulatory and nonambulatory children with CP. Hip adductor tightness is more common and manifests with both static and dynamic tightness. During gait, these children often strike their knees against one another or their legs may actually cross (scissor) during gait.

INDICATIONS/CONTRAINDICATIONS.   When available, computerized motion analysis aids in assessment prior to planned hip adductor lengthening. Studies have demonstrated poor correlation between static and dynamic measures in children with cerebral palsy.[9] Visually, excessive femoral anteversion, especially when combined with excessive knee flexion, may be confused with hip adduction deformity. Gait analysis can help determine whether there is true hip adduction during gait.

The indication for hip adductor lengthening is the presence of dynamic hip adduction in combination with static tightness of the hip adductors. In general, adductor lengthenings are indicated when children have 20 degrees or less of hip abduction with the hip extended.

SURGICAL PROCEDURE.   A 3- to 4-cm transverse incision is made in the proximal groin crease. Tenotomy scissors are used to incise the fascia in line with the skin incision. The adductor longus (the tightest tendon, which is palpable anteriorly) is identified and isolated from surrounding tissue with a clamp and/or finger. A right-angle clamp is placed around the adductor longus and slid as far proximally as possible. Electrocautery is then used to transect the musculotendinous unit (Fig. 9-1A).

The gracilis is then identified and isolated. The gracilis is easily separated from the remainder of the adductors by abducting the hip and extending the knee, thus placing the gracilis on tension (Fig. 9-1B). Electrocautery is used to transect the muscle as proximal as possible.

Further adductor lengthening is rarely needed after the adductor longus and gracilis are addressed. If further lengthening is needed (usually if hip abduction is less than 45 degrees in extension after the aforementioned lengthenings), then a portion of the adductor brevis is transected until 45 degrees of abduction in extension is possible. The anterior branches of the obturator nerve are protected during the lengthening (Fig. 9-1C). When feasible, the deep fascia is closed to minimize the risk of drainage and infection. Although these wounds rarely become infected, closure with surgical glue may provide some protection from soiling.

POSTOPERATIVE MANAGEMENT.   After hip adductor lengthening surgery, the child is placed in an A-frame cast with each leg abducted at least 25 to 30 degrees for 3 to 4 weeks. If only a mild lengthening is performed in an adolescent, a hip abduction pillow or orthosis may be considered to facilitate postoperative care.

Following cast removal, a hip abduction orthosis is used at night for at least the first 6 to 12 months postoperatively to minimize the risk of recurrence. Physical therapy, focusing on range of motion, gait, and strengthening, is begun at the time of cast removal.

COMPLICATIONS TO AVOID.   Acute complications following adductor lengthening are unusual. However, obturator neurectomy and/or excessive lengthening of the adductors can result in excessive weakness of the adductors, with resultant hip abduction and pelvic instability during standing and gait. Recurrent deformity is seen with some regularity, though the frequency and severity can be minimized by postoperative use of a hip abduction orthosis.

PEARLS AND PITFALLS.
- Obturator neurectomies should not be performed because of the frequent occurrence of overcorrection and fixed abduction following such surgery.
- Excessive hip adductor lengthening must be avoided. Regardless of etiology, fixed hip abduction makes standing extremely difficult and can even preclude sitting in standard wheelchairs.
- Make sure to differentiate between apparent excessive hip adduction (as may be seen with femoral anteversion and knee flexion) and true hip adduction.

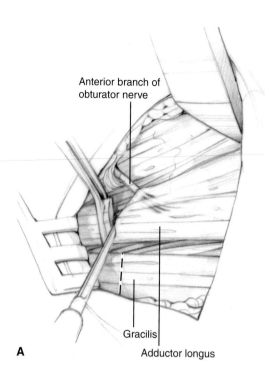

Anterior branch of
obturator nerve

Gracilis

Adductor longus

A

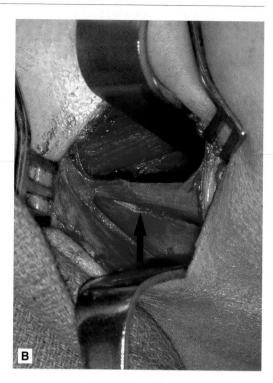

B

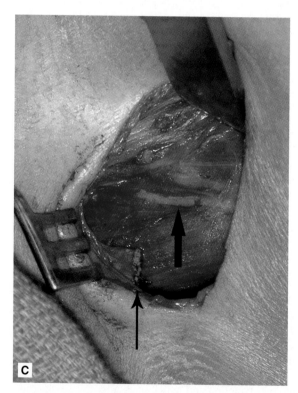

C

FIGURE 9-1 **A.** The adductor longus is first isolated and transected. Next, the gracilis is isolated and transected. The anterior branch of the obturator must be preserved. **B.** Isolation of the gracilis during hip adductor lengthening. The arrow points to the gracilis. The gracilis is brought under tension by a combination of hip abduction and knee extension. **C.** Branches of the anterior obturator nerve as they run across the adductor brevis. These branches should be preserved in order to preserve adductor strength and prevent excessive hip abduction postoperatively. The small arrow points to the transected gracilis muscle and the large arrow to anterior branches of the obturator nerve.

Psoas Recession

INDICATIONS/CONTRAINDICATIONS.   Psoas tightness manifests with the inability to get the affected limb into a trailing position. It is important to remember that this and other gait abnormalities can be due either to a problem at the apparently involved level or to abnormalities at other levels. For example, excessive hip flexion seen in crouched gait may be due to excessive ankle dorsiflexion and/or excessive knee flexion, even in the absence of a true hip flexion contracture.

The main indication for psoas recession is excessive hip flexion in terminal stance in patients with at least a 10-degree flexion contracture on static examination.

Computerized motion analysis is helpful in assessing these children preoperatively, as there is a tendency to overestimate the presence of excessive hip flexion with visual observation of gait.[15]

SURGICAL PROCEDURE.   Hip flexor power is best preserved when the psoas is lengthened fractionally rather than via a simple tenotomy. Such a recession is performed well proximal to the musculotendinous junction by cutting the tendon and leaving the adjacent muscle intact.

Before cutting the psoas tendon, it is important to be certain that this is the psoas and not the adjacent neurovascular structures. Skaggs et al.[13] described three tests that should be performed before cutting the tendon: (a) identifying muscle fibers leading into the tendon, (b) noting that the musculotendinous unit tightens with internal rotation of the hip, and (c) checking that the leg does not "jump" with a brief stimulation of the "tendon" via electrocautery.

This surgery is usually described as being performed through a separate 5-cm anterior bikini incision, using a standard anterior approach to the hip. The tensor-sartorius interval is identified as the soft spot just distal to the anterior superior iliac spine (ASIS). Tenotomy scissors or a small hemostat are used to pierce the deep fascia and open the interval. A strip of fat should be seen between the tensor fascia lata and sartorius. The lateral femoral cutaneous nerve should be identified in this interval and protected. The rectus femoris is deep in this interval (just anterior to the hip capsule). Dissection is carried out medial to this, and the pelvic brim can be palpated. The hip is flexed to relax the psoas, and a right-angle retractor, such as a Sofield retractor, is used to retract the psoas while exposing the tendon on its undersurface (Fig. 9-2A). The three tests described by Skaggs

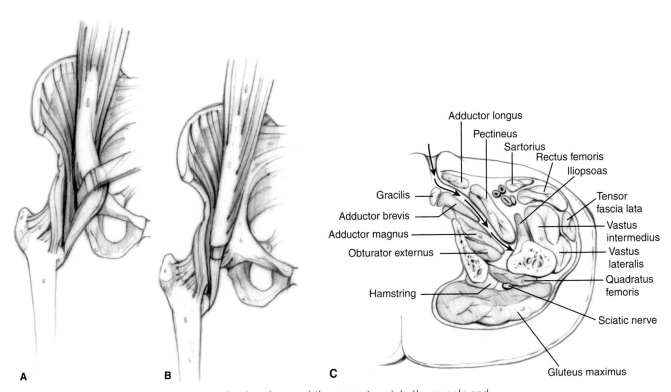

FIGURE 9-2   A. A right-angle retractor is placed around the psoas to rotate the muscle and expose the tendon on its undersurface. **B.** After recession, the cut ends of the tendon separate, revealing underlying muscle. There is continuity of the musculotendinous unit. **C.** If the psoas recession is to be performed through the adductor lengthening incision, the plane of dissection is posterior to the pectineus. Once the iliopsoas tendon is identified, it is traced as far proximal as possible (adjacent to the pelvic brim), and a recession is performed, as illustrated in **A** and **B.**

et al.[5] are checked prior to transecting the tendinous portion of the psoas. A fractional lengthening is performed by cutting the tendon well proximal to the musculotendinous junction, thereby preserving hip flexor strength (Fig. 9-2B).

In thin children undergoing simultaneous hip adductor tendon lengthening, the incision described above can be used for psoas lengthening. By dissecting posterior to the pectineus, the psoas tendon can be easily palpated (Fig. 9-2C). Dissecting scissors are used to incise the sheath around the psoas, and the musculotendinous unit is identified. The psoas is traced as proximal as possible (generally to near its exit from the pelvis). A right-angle retractor (preferably a Sofield retractor) is placed around the psoas in order to expose the tendon. (As noted above, the tendon lies on the underside of the muscle.) The three tests noted above for confirming the appropriate localization are performed. Once the musculotendinous unit is identified, a right-angle clamp is placed around the tendinous portion of the psoas, which is then transected while the adjacent muscle fibers are left intact.

POSTOPERATIVE MANAGEMENT. Psoas recessions are almost universally combined with other lower-extremity surgeries. As a result, the postoperative care is affected by these other surgeries. Regardless of the other procedures, following psoas recession, the child is placed into a prone position for 6 hours daily, beginning on postoperative day 1. The proning is usually broken into three sessions daily, each lasting 2 hours. The child is allowed to weight bear and ambulate as tolerated immediately postoperatively if these activities are not contraindicated by the other procedures.

COMPLICATIONS TO AVOID. Damage to the femoral neurovascular structures is a rare, though potentially devastating, complication of hip flexor lengthening. The risk of femoral nerve injury in particular is minimized by the aforementioned surgical technique.

A much more common complication is hip flexor weakness. Excessive weakness is minimized by performing a fractional lengthening of the psoas rather than a psoas tenotomy.

PEARLS AND PITFALLS.

- The psoas musculotendinous unit will tighten with internal hip rotation. This is a useful test for intraoperatively differentiating the tendon from the femoral nerve.
- Because of better preservation of hip flexor power, fractional lengthening of the psoas is preferred to psoas tenotomy.

Knee

Hamstring Lengthenings

INDICATIONS/CONTRAINDICATIONS. Hamstring lengthening is indicated for children with excessive knee flexion in terminal swing and stance and with popliteal angles greater than 40 degees. In general, various nonoperative options will have been tried prior to surgery, such as knee immobilizers at night, a home stretching program, and/or botulinus toxin A injections into the hamstrings.

SURGICAL PROCEDURE. A single midline incision (usually 4–5 cm) is made at the junction of the middle and distal thirds of the posterior thigh. The medial hamstrings are almost universally tight in those with hamstring contractures and are approached first. It is extremely rare to find a child with isolated lateral hamstring tightness in the absence of previous hamstring surgery.

The dissection is carried medially and the semitendinosus is isolated. (The semitendinosus is the most superficial posteromedial structure and is tendinous in nature.) Isolation of the semitendinosus is most easily accomplished by dissecting directly toward the tendon with tenotomy scissors or electrocautery. The deep fascia is incised with dissecting (tenotomy) scissors. Once the tendon is isolated, a right-angle clamp is placed around the semitendinosus tendon from lateral to medial to minimize the risk of neurovascular damage (Fig. 9-3A). In most cases, the semitendinosus is transected with electrocautery at approximately the level of the musculotendinous junction. If a concomitant distal rectus femoris transfer (DRFT) is to be performed, the semitendinosus is transected proximal to the musculotendinous junction to allow for sufficient length for the DRFT.

The fascia over the semimembranosus is incised with tenotomy scissors, and the muscle is isolated. The discrete aponeurosis is then cut with a knife. A #15 blade provides finer control and feel than does electrocautery (Figs. 9-3B and 9-3C). The aponeurosis is cut transversely at two levels, with the underlying muscle left undisturbed. The proximal cut should be made first so that the tissue is still on tension when the distal cut is made. It is not necessary to lengthen the gracilis; it does not appear to be a significant cause of medial hamstring tightness, and routine lengthening will cause excessive knee flexor and hip extensor weakness.

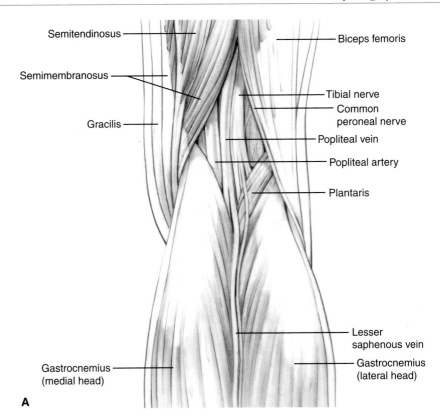

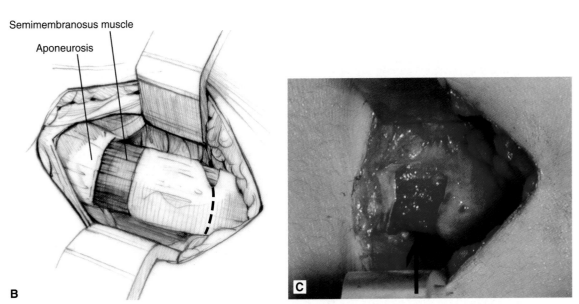

FIGURE 9-3   A. Anatomy of the posterior distal thigh and knee. The semitendinosus is the most superficial medial hamstring. Because the neurovascular structures are relatively close during the surgery, the right-angle clamp should be placed from lateral to medial when isolating the semitendinosus to minimize the potential risk of neurovascular injury. These structures are at highest risk during posterior capsulotomy. **B.** Aponeurotic lengthening of the semimembranosus is typically performed at two levels. When the biceps femoris requires lengthening, a comparable aponeurotic lengthening is performed, also typically at two levels. **C.** Typical appearance following aponeurotic lengthening of the semimembranosus. This photograph demonstrates the lengthening at one of the two levels typically performed. The arrow points to the underlying muscle, which is left intact. Note the white aponeurosis, which has separated, allowing additional knee extension despite preservation of the underlying muscle.

In the past, rechecking a popliteal angle with each sequential hamstring lengthening was thought to be necessary. However, it now appears that rechecking a popliteal angle may put undue tension on the nerve (with a theoretical increase in the risk of peroneal nerve palsy), so it is no longer necessary to check the popliteal angle intraoperatively (Fig. 9-4). Instead, the knee is brought into full extension, with the ipsilateral hip extended. If the knee easily falls into extension following the medial hamstring lengthening, the lateral hamstrings are not lengthened.

If the lateral hamstrings are quite tight following medial hamstring lengthening, the biceps femoris should be lengthened. The biceps femoris can be accessed easily through the midline incision that was used for the medial hamstring lengthening. Dissection is aimed directly toward the tight biceps femoris with dissecting scissors or electrocautery. The fascia over the biceps is incised, and the discrete aponeurotic band, located laterally in the biceps, is identified and isolated. This band should be transected at two levels using a #15 blade (as with the semimembranosus), leaving the underlying muscle intact.

Posterior knee capsulotomy is only very rarely indicated in children with CP, though it has been advocated by previous authors. In almost all children who are potential candidates for posterior capsulotomy, the capsule itself is not as tight as the neurovascular bundle following hamstring lengthening. Therefore, the posterior capsulotomy is rarely of significant benefit in children with CP (unlike those with significant knee contractures associated with other maladies, such as arthrogryposis).

When necessary, posterior knee capsulotomy may be performed with the patient supine or prone. Although it is certainly easier to perform concomitant surgeries at other levels with the child supine, posterior capsulotomy is more difficult with the child supine if the knee flexion contractures exceed 20 degrees. If knee capsulotomy is requisite, it may be worth positioning the child prone, even if other surgeries may require reprepping the child supine. The posterior capsulotomy may be performed through a midline incision (usually 6–8 cm in the distal third of the thigh). The dissection is deepened between the semimembranosus medially and the biceps femoris laterally. The peroneal and tibial nerves, as well as the popliteal artery and vein, are identified, isolated, and protected in this direct, posterior approach (Fig. 9-3A). Vessel loops may be placed around these important structures if desired. With the neurovascular structures protected, dissection is carried directly toward the femur until the medial and lateral heads of the gastrocnemius are identified. An elevator is then used to sweep these off the posterior knee capsule, which is then divided with either a #15 blade or electrocautery. When the knee is extended, the capsule is seen to spread.

In children with marked crouch and patella alta, some physicians advocate patellar tendon shortening and extension osteotomy of the femur in conjunction with hamstring lengthening. When performed, this operation should be reserved for children with severe crouch in adolescence. However, these procedures are often not requisite, as severe crouch can often be attained without the addition of patellar tendon shortening and femoral extension osteotomy.

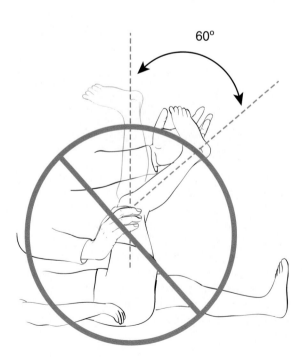

FIGURE 9-4

The popliteal angle test should *not* be performed intraoperatively, as this can cause undue tension on the sciatic nerve, with potential deleterious effects on the nerve (particularly the peroneal branch) postoperatively.

POSTOPERATIVE MANAGEMENT.   Hamstring lengthening is often combined with other procedures. In general, a long-leg walking cast can be used for 3 to 4 weeks following hamstring lengthening. Most children with CP will stand, but not walk, with the cast(s), due to the children's limited balance, strength, and motor control. Following cast removal, knee immobilizers are used at night for at least 6 to 12 months.

For children with significant knee flexion contractures (≥20 degrees) and marked crouch (usually ≥45 degrees) preoperatively, a knee-ankle-foot orthotic (KAFO) is often helpful to enhance gait for at least the first 3 to 6 months following cast removal. In such children, the initial postoperative casts may be changed at 3 weeks and measurement for KAFOs may be done. The long-leg casts are continued until the KAFOs are ready for delivery.

COMPLICATIONS TO AVOID.   Though rarely discussed, genu recurvatum is relatively common following hamstring lengthening. The risk is significantly greater following combined medial and lateral hamstring lengthening than is that following isolated medial hamstring lengthening.[8] Because of this risk of recurvatum, as well as risks of increased anterior pelvic tilt and weak hip extension, lateral hamstring lengthening should not routinely be performed in all cases.

Unfortunately, numerous cases of extreme recurvatum also occur after some isolated medial hamstring surgeries. In almost every one of these cases, the medial hamstring surgery consists of a simple transection of each medial hamstring (semitendonosus, semimembranosus, and gracilis). Such routine transection of all the medial hamstrings should never be performed in ambulatory children with CP, because it leads to significant hip extensor weakness, genu recurvatum, anterior pelvic tilt, and the inability to achieve adequate knee flexion in swing phase.

Neuropraxia is well known following hamstring lengthening surgery. The risk appears to be less if the popliteal angle is not checked intraoperatively.

Recurrent hamstring contracture is possible as well. Postoperative casting followed by the use of knee immobilizers for at least 6 months postoperatively seems to decrease this risk.

PEARLS AND PITFALLS.
- Lateral hamstring lengthening is not needed in many cases. Medial hamstring lengthening suffices in most cases to allow sufficient knee extension.
- Combined medial and lateral hamstring lengthening increases the risk of genu recurvatum postoperatively.
- Posterior knee capsulotomy is rarely indicated in children with cerebral palsy. The neurovascular bundle is often under sufficient tension following combined medial and lateral hamstring lengthening that knee capsulotomy will usually not safely allow additional knee extension.
- Avoid extending the knee (to assess or lengthen hamstrings) with the hip flexed 90 degrees intraoperatively, as this is associated with stretch injury of the peroneal nerve.

Distal Rectus Femoris Transfer

INDICATIONS/CONTRAINDICATIONS.   Distal rectus femoris transfer is a relatively new operation, first described in 1987 by Gage et al.[3] The indications for surgery are a stiff knee in swing phase in conjunction with overactivity of the rectus femoris in swing phase. The stiff knee may cause difficulty with foot clearance due to decreased magnitude and/or delayed timing of peak knee flexion in swing phase.

SURGICAL PROCEDURE.   A 4 to 5 cm longitudinal incision is made over the distal anterior thigh. The distal tip of the incision is over the proximal pole of the patella. The deep fascia over the quadriceps tendon is incised with dissecting scissors. It is easiest to separate the rectus from the remainder of the quadriceps mechanism proximally (usually starting 4–5 cm proximal to the patella). This is often easiest to do by incising longitudinally (for a length of 1–2 cm) from to deep along the medial or lateral border of the quadriceps tendon 4 to 5 cm proximal to the Freer. This makes it easier to find the plane between the rectus femoris and the vastus intermedius. The plane is smooth and should separate easily. The interval is first developed with a septum elevator and then blunt dissection with the index finger. If developing this plane is difficult, the surgeon is likely within the rectus tendon rather than in the plane between the two aforementioned tendons. The Freer elevator is used to penetrate the extensor mechanism immediately adjacent to the lateral border of the rectus femoris. Blunt dissection frees the lateral border of the rectus, which is separated from the vastus intermedius as distally as possible using blunt dissection. The rectus is transected about 1 cm proximal to the patella (Fig. 9-5A). The tendon is freed from all underlying attachments after placement of a whip stitch using a size 1 or 2-0 nonabsorbable braided suture, depending on tendon size (Fig. 9-5B). The tendon is then pulled distally, and care is taken to free the tendon from any soft-tissue attachments proximally as far as the finger

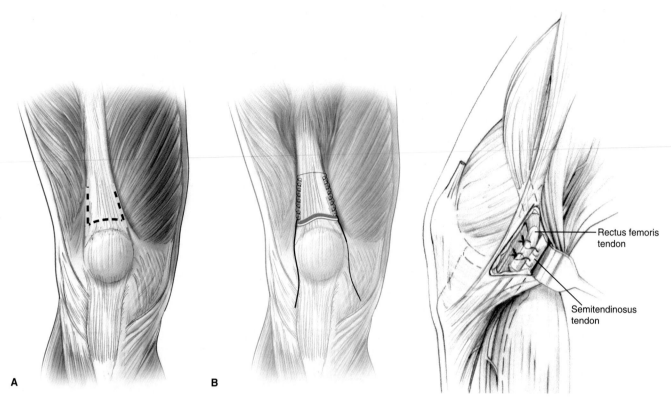

A   **B**

FIGURE 9-5   Technique for distal rectus femoris transfer (DRFT). Care must be taken to separate the rectus from the remainder of the quadriceps. The DRFT is best found about 4 to 5 cm proximal to the patella after incising longitudinally adjacent to the quadriceps tendon. **A.** The rectus is transected approximately 1 cm proximal to the patella. **B.** A whip stitch is then placed in the rectus stump. **C.** When available, the semitendinosus is the preferred recipient tendon. Because Pulvertaft-type anastamosis does not appear to confer significant advantage and increases the risk of damage to the recipient tendon, it is not usually performed.

can reach. This allows for a direct line of pull toward its future distal attachment. When such soft-tissue attachments are released, the rectus should have an excursion of at least 1.5 to 2 cm when manual traction is applied (Fig. 9-5).

When possible, it is a good idea to transfer the rectus to the semitendinosus (Fig. 9-5C), as this has a longer lever arm than do the other two common transfers (to the gracilis or the sartorius). Lateral transfer to the iliotibial band can also be performed, though this is done less frequently than are the medial transfers.

Small rakes are then used to retract the medial skin flap, and dissection is made deep to the fascia overlying the vastus medialis. Other authors advocate making this tunnel outside the fascia; however, there is often so little subcutaneous tissue that such a technique would result in the rectus transfer being immediately subcutaneous. The vastus medialis is retracted, and the intermuscular septum is incised using electrocautery. A large window (at least 3–4 cm in length) is made in the septum to keep the DRFT from being tethered, particularly proximally. If the semitendinosus or gracilis is to be used as the recipient tendon, the tendon stump can be brought into the anterior compartment. This procedure is facilitated by placing a whip stitch in the distal tendon stump before bringing the recipient tendon anteriorly. The transfer is completed under some tension, with the knee flexed about 20 degrees. As an alternative, the knee can be placed in 10 to 20 degrees of flexion, and both tendons can be placed under tension to determine the appropriate amount of tendon overlap, if any, for the DRFT. Once the determination is made regarding the appropriate degree of tendon overlap, the knee can be flexed and the DRFT completed with the predetermined amount of overlap obtained.

With the knee flexed 10 to 20 degrees, there should be a palpable rebound to the tendon when palpated following transfer. Depending on the tension of the transfer, the DRFT may be side to side or end to end. When there is sufficient length, some surgeons prefer a Pulvertaft repair, in which the smaller tendon is weaved through the larger, though this does not appear to confer any significant advantages when nonabsorbable sutures are used. In fact, in some children with small tendons, a Pulvertaft repair may be associated with a significant risk of compromising the integrity of the recipient tendon and with resultant postoperative tendon rupture.

If the sartorius is the recipient, the rectus is wrapped around approximately 50% of the sartorius in napkin-ring fashion and sutured to itself. The rectus is then also sutured to the sartorius in at least one site to prevent proximal migration of the DRFT.

POSTOPERATIVE MANAGEMENT.   Postoperatively, care is generally dictated by associated surgeries. Some surgeons recommend immediate mobilization of the knee following DRFT to prevent scarring of the tendon. However, immediate motion is not necessary for three primary reasons: (a) patients routinely gain significant knee flexion in swing even when immobilized postoperatively, (b) immediate mobilization is not used for the vast majority of tendon transfers in the upper and lower extremities without apparent deleterious results, and (c) higher rates of wound complications and scar widening have been encountered when immediate postoperative mobilization following DRFT was allowed.

COMPLICATIONS TO AVOID.   Because of its anterior knee location, the scar often spreads, so perform the closure with this in mind. Dehiscence is also possible, but less common.

Functional complications include failure to improve knee flexion in swing. This could potentially be due to suture pullout, an indirect pull of the DRFT, surgical scarring, or insufficient tension of the transfer.

Because excessive crouch may be seen after DRFT, this procedure is not recommended in children who are gross motor function classification system (GMFCS) level IV patients or in those without good knee extensor strength and/or with marked crouch (usually ≥40 degrees) preoperatively.

PEARLS AND PITFALLS.
- The rectus needs to be freed along its medial and lateral borders proximally to allow for a direct line of pull.
- Do not perform this transfer in those who are GMFCS level IV ambulators or those with weak knee extensors and/or marked crouch preoperatively.

Triceps Surae Lengthening   Traditionally, triceps surae lengthening has been via lengthening of the Achilles tendon. With or without heel-cord lengthening, crouch is a common problem as children who have CP age, especially those with diplegia and quadriplegia.

INDICATIONS/CONTRAINDICATIONS.   Surgical lengthening is indicated in those children with an equinus contracture evident on static and dynamic examination. Nonsurgical management, including night splints, range-of-motion exercises, and/or serial casting, often delay or obviate the need for surgical lengthening of the triceps surae. Previous authors have shown that observational gait analysis tends to overestimate ankle equinus (and thus the need for triceps surae lengthening).[15]

Most children with equinus contracture who need triceps surae lengthening can be treated with gastrocnemius recession. If triceps surae lengthening is indicated, the Silfverskiöld test may be used, as described below, to determine whether to perform Achilles tendon lengthening or gastrocnemius recession. If the ankle can be dorsiflexed to at least neutral with the knee flexed and the hind foot inverted, then gastrocnemius recession is indicated. If the ankle remains in equinus, the Achilles tendon is lengthened.

SURGICAL PROCEDURE.
Gastrocnemius Recession.   Traditionally, gastrocnemius recession has been performed through a straight posterior incision; however, a medial approach is often quicker and easier, while also leaving a more cosmetic scar.

The medial longitudinal incision is approximately 2 to 3 cm anterior to the posterior aspect of the calf. A 2.5- to 3.0-cm incision is made in the middle third of the calf. The location is best determined by palpating the gastrocnemius while dorsiflexing the ankle; tightening of the aponeurosis can generally be easily palpated at the appropriate level for the incision (Fig. 9-6A).

The incision is deepened in line with the skin incision, and the deep fascia is incised. The plane posterior to the gastrocnemius (and anterior to the deep fascia) is developed by blunt dissection. Two right-angle (Sofield) retractors are used—one is posterior to the gastrocnemius, which exposes the gastrocnemius and protects the sural nerve and lesser saphenous vein, while the second progressively advances medial to lateral to expose the entire width of the gastrocnemius aponeurosis (Fig. 9-6B and 9-6C).

In a single, transverse recession of the gastrocnemius, the ankle is dorsiflexed with the knee extended and the hind foot inverted until 10 degrees of dorsiflexion is obtained. Failure to invert the

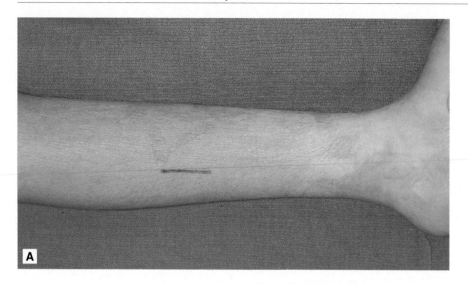

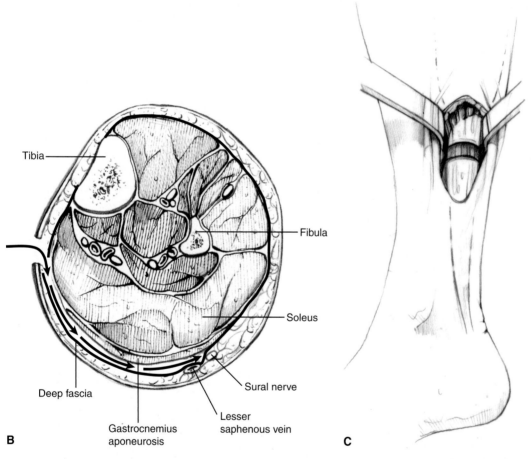

FIGURE 9-6   The technique for gastrocnemius recession is easily performed through a medial incision in the middle third of the calf. **A.** The deep fascia is incised, and dissection is carried out posterior to the gastrocnemius. **B.** The lesser saphenous vein and sural nerve are protected in the posterior flap. (The author prefers a single-level recession of the gastrocnemius.) **C.** To preserve calf strength and minimize the risk of overlengthening, the intraoperative goal should be 10 degrees of dorsiflexion with the knee extended and the hind foot inverted.

hind foot will result in dorsiflexion through the foot (rather than through the ankle) and in insufficient correction of the equinus. The cut ends of the aponeurosis should spread so that the cut ends remain parallel. If they converge laterally, then the recession has not been completed.

Achilles Tendon Lengthening.   Achilles tendon lengthening can be performed in many ways—open versus percutaneous, sliding versus Z-lengthening. Open Achilles tendon lengthening is recommended in children with CP, especially those with diplegia or quadriplegia. The risk of overlengthening appears greater with percutaneous lengthening.[1]

For mild to moderate lengthenings (usually in children with static dorsiflexion preoperatively to within 20–25 degrees of neutral), an open sliding lengthening may be performed, as described by White.[14] A longitudinal incision (usually 6–8 cm) is made over the medial lower leg, approximately 2 cm anterior to the posterior border of the Achilles. Sharp dissection is carried down through the tendon sheath of the Achilles. Two cuts are made, each through slightly more than 50% of the tendon substance. The first cut is through the anterior portion of the tendon distally, and the second is through the medial portion of the tendon proximally. Once the cuts are completed, the ankle is dorsiflexed to 10 degrees with the knee extended and the hind foot inverted. The portions of the tendon will be noted to slide over one another, though the tendon will remain intact (Fig. 9-7).

For more severe deformities (usually at least 30 degrees of fixed equinus preoperatively), an open Z-lengthening of the Achilles is preferred. The tendon is cut longitudinally in its midline for essentially the entire length of the incision; the distal cut comes out through the medial half of the tendon (unless there is hind-foot valgus preoperatively, in which case the distal cut is lateral). The proximal cut is in the opposite direction from the medial cut and is therefore usually lateral (Fig. 9-8).

One of the basic principles of tendon surgeries, including Achilles tendon lengthening, is that when cutting halfway across a tendon, it is best to start in the middle of the tendon and cut to the side of the tendon. This will prevent accidentally transecting the entire tendon, which can easily occur when cutting from the border of the tendon proceeding toward the tendon's center.

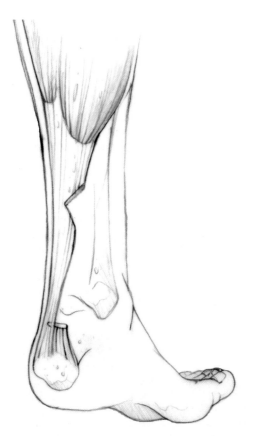

FIGURE 9-7   Sliding lengthening of the Achilles tendon. The distal cut (just proximal to the tendon insertion into the calcaneus) should be made first; this cuts through slightly more than 50% of the tendon width anteriorly. The proximal cut is made through slightly more than 50% of the medial side of the tendon. The goal of dorsiflexion intraoperatively is 10 degrees with the knee extended and the hind foot inverted (as noted for the gastrocnemius recession).

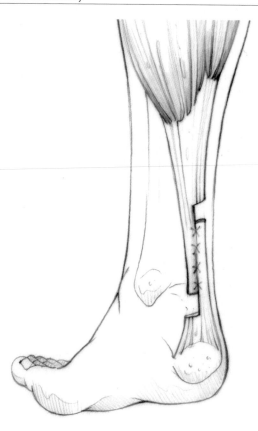

FIGURE 9-8

Z-lengthening of the Achilles tendon. The distal cut usually exits medially (except in valgus feet). Z-lengthening is often required in severe contractures or in repeat Achilles tendon lengthenings.

The tendon is repaired in a side-to-side fashion with size 1 nonabsorbable suture with multiple figure-eight sutures. There should be palpable rebound to the tendon when the ankle is held in neutral position. If not, the tendon needs to be repaired with more overlap of the tendon ends to minimize the risk of overlengthening and crouch.

In addition, for severe deformities (usually at least 30 degrees of equinus), the tightness of the toe flexors must be checked following Achilles tendon lengthening. This is done by bringing the ankle to neutral dorsiflexion and checking the toes for toe flexor tightness and clawing. If these are present with the ankle in neutral and absent with the ankle in equinus, then there is tightness of the extrinsic toe flexors. Such extrinsic tightness is well treated by fractional lengthening of the toe flexors (flexor digitorum longus and flexor hallucis longus) in the distal third of the calf. These lengthenings are performed through the same medial incision in the posteromedial distal calf that is used for lengthening the Achilles tendon. (A zigzag incision is often used for equinus contractures of at least 50 degrees to enhance surgical exposure.) The fascia over the posteromedial compartment is opened in the distal third of the lower leg. The flexor digitorum longus (FDL) is the second-most-anterior tendon (Fig. 9-9) and can generally be differentiated easily from the posterior tibial tendon because of its location and smaller caliber. The surgeon can confirm correct tendon identification by noting that the musculotendinous unit moves as the second through fifth toes are passively flexed and extended. The posterior tibial neurovascular bundle is directly posterior to the FDL and should be identified and protected. An intramuscular fractional lengthening of the FDL is performed via an intramuscular tenotomy several centimeters proximal to the musculotendinous junction. This is done by placing a right-angle clamp around only the tendinous portion of the FDL well proximal to the musculotendinous junction, using electrocautery to transect the isolated tendon. The second through fifth toes are then brought into extension with the ankle dorsiflexed to neutral. This results in a fractional lengthening with preservation of continuity of the FDL's musculotendinous unit. Dissection is then carried out posterior to the neurovascular bundle, and the flexor hallucis longus (FHL) is identified. The FHL has a larger muscle belly than the FDL at this level, and its identity may be confirmed by noting its excursion upon extending and flexing the great toe. A comparable intramuscular tenotomy (as described for the FDL) is used to fractionally lengthen the FHL, and the hallux is brought into extension with the ankle in neutral dorsiflexion.

POSTOPERATIVE MANAGEMENT.   Following triceps surae lengthening, casting is typically used for 6 weeks postoperatively. Weight bearing is allowed immediately unless contraindicated because of other concomitant surgery, such as osteotomies of the femur, tibia, and/or foot. The initial casts are

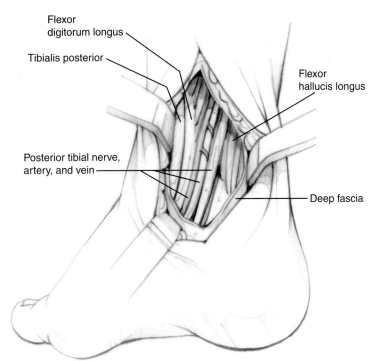

Flexor
digitorum longus

Tibialis posterior

Flexor
hallucis longus

Posterior tibial nerve,
artery, and vein

Deep fascia

FIGURE 9-9

Anatomy of the posteromedial lower leg. The posterior tibial tendon is directly posterior to the tibia and anterior to the flexor digitorum longus (FDL). Like the flexor hallucis longus (FHL), the FDL's muscle belly extends quite distally. The posterior tibial neurovascular bundle lies between the FDL and the FHL.

generally changed at 3 to 4 weeks postoperatively so that new braces may be measured and readied for delivery when casting is discontinued 6 weeks postoperatively.

COMPLICATIONS TO AVOID.   The most serious complication is overlengthening of the tendon with a calcaneal gait postoperatively. It is important to realize that a calcaneal gait is also seen in many children who have never undergone triceps surae lengthening. Because this complication has such a poor long-term prognosis, it is imperative to do everything possible to avoid it. Gait analysis is very helpful in confirming equinus. Observational gait analysis overestimates ankle equinus and can result in the performance of unnecessary heel-cord lengthening surgery.[15]

In children with mild contractures (dorsiflexion within a few degrees of neutral), the contracture will generally respond well to serial casting without the need for surgery. If other surgery is being performed, many of these mild contractures will stretch out in the postoperative casts used for the other procedures, even if the triceps surae is not lengthened surgically. When surgery is performed, the goal should be to obtain only about 10 degrees of dorsiflexion intraoperatively, whether a gastrocnemius recession or Achilles tendon lengthening is performed. Percutaneous Achilles lengthenings appear to increase the risk of calcaneus in bilaterally involved children.

Recurrent contracture is most common in hemiplegics. Recurrence is minimized by the use of AFOs postoperatively.

PEARLS AND PITFALLS.
- Observational gait analysis overestimates ankle equinus, thus overestimating the need for heel-cord lengthening.
- When a child toe walks while wearing AFOs, the toe walking is due to excessive flexion at the knee and/or hip.
- Minimize triceps surae lengthening, as excessive dorsiflexion is a very difficult problem to overcome.
- In most cases do not perform percutaneous Achilles lengthenings in bilaterally involved children with CP.

SURGERIES FOR VARUS FEET

Varus foot deformities are common in children with CP. Varus deformities have been reported in approximately 10% of diplegic and quadriplegic children sent for gait analysis and in 30% of hemiplegic children so referred.[16] The varus may be seen in conjunction with equinus deformities (i.e., equinovarus feet) or may be isolated. Varus is typically due to soft-tissue imbalance or may be due to overpull of the anterior tibialis, posterior tibialis, triceps surae, or a combination thereof.

Traditional teaching is that the posterior tibialis is responsible for the vast majority of varus feet in children with CP. Unfortunately, this teaching is wrong.

When the varus foot deformity is due to the anterior and/or posterior tibialis, the two muscles are responsible for an equal number of cases. The anterior tibialis is caused in approximately one-third of cases, the posterior tibialis in one-third, and both the anterior and posterior tibialis in the remaining third.[10]

Initially, the varus deformity is flexible. As time passes, the deformity may become fixed. The Coleman block test, though quite useful in able-bodied patients, often cannot be performed in children with CP due to their problems with balance, coordination, and/or mentation. The foot can, however, be manipulated by the examiner, with the patient sitting or lying prone, in order to assess the stiffness of the varus deformity. For fixed deformities, bone surgery is necessary in conjunction with soft-tissue surgery to afford sufficient correction. One of the most important concepts when performing bone surgery is to address the underlying soft-tissue imbalance. If the underlying soft-tissue balance is not corrected, recurrent deformity due to ongoing soft-tissue imbalance is nearly unavoidable.

Soft-Tissue Surgeries for Varus Feet

Indications/Contraindications   Surgery is indicated when nonsurgical management does not suffice to control the foot position. Typically, the greatest functional problem is that the varus compromises stability in stance phase (though it also interferes with swing phase prepositioning of the foot for stance phase). Nonoperative treatment with braces, stretching casts, passive stretches, and/or botulinus toxin injections is indicated before considering surgery. Braces that have a wraparound hind-foot component are typically required to control significant varus (and to minimize pressure sores).

Traditional teaching has been that the posterior tibial tendon is responsible for the vast majority of varus deformities in children with CP. However, dynamic electromyography and computerized motion analysis reveal that the anterior and posterior tibial muscles are responsible for the varus with comparable frequencies, and both are often contributory in the same patient.[10]

Surgical Procedure

ANTERIOR TIBIAL TENDON TRANSFER.   When the anterior tibial tendon is causative, either split or whole transfer is recommended to balance the foot. The author prefers split transfers, having seen significant numbers of cases of both over- and undercorrection following whole tendon transfers of the anterior tibial tendon.

With a split transfer, three incisions are typically used: (a) a 2- to 3-cm incision in the dorsomedial hind foot over the anterior tibial tendon insertion, (b) a 3- to 4-cm incision over the distal lower leg, and (c) a 2-cm incision over the dorsolateral hind foot just lateral to the toe extensors (Fig. 9-10A).

The author rarely transfers the tendon to the cuboid. Because the cuboid is relatively small in many children with CP, bringing the tendon through it and tying sutures over a button is often necessary for such transfers. Skin callus, necrosis, and/or hypersensitivity of the plantar foot are common sequelae when buttons are used.

The author usually connects the split transfer to the peroneus tertius or brevis. The author's preferred recipient tendon is the peroneus tertius, as it has an excellent line of pull to receive the anterior tibial tendon transfer. It is important to remember that the tendon is absent in approximately 10% of people. In the vast majority of children with CP, this tendon is of good caliber to receive the anterior tibialis (Fig. 9-10B). If this is not the case, however, the anterior half of the peroneus brevis is split from the remainder of the peroneus brevis tendon and is brought dorsally to receive the split anterior tibial tendon transfer.

A longitudinal 3- to 4-cm incision is made over the distal lower leg to access the anterior tibial tendon. The distal end of this incision is 2 to 3 cm proximal to the ankle. The incision is deepened and the extensor retinaculum is entered with dissecting scissors or a #15 blade.

Next, the distal portion of the anterior tibial tendon (ATT) is exposed and harvested through the aforementioned 2- to 3-cm oblique incision over the dorsomedial hind foot. This incision is directly over the distal portion of the ATT, which can be identified by manual palpation. If difficulty is encountered when trying to identify the tendon, a right-angle clamp is placed around the ATT in the lower leg wound, and the tendon is placed under tension so its distal portion is easily palpable. Alternatively, the foot may be plantarflexed to place the ATT under tension. The incision is deepened with dissecting scissors, and the ATT sheath is incised. A right-angle clamp is placed around the ATT and advanced distally until the bony insertion of the ATT is encountered. Two tests to confirm that this is the ATT and not the extensor hallucis longus (EHL) tendon are (a) advancing the clamp distally until bone is encountered at the medial cuneiform and

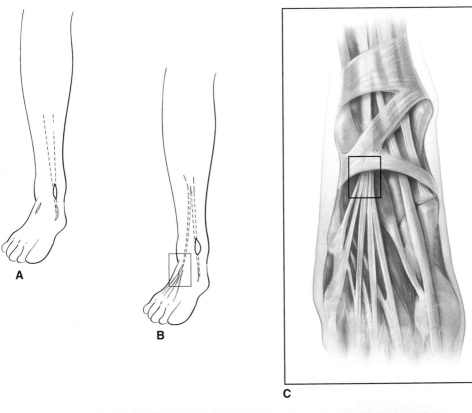

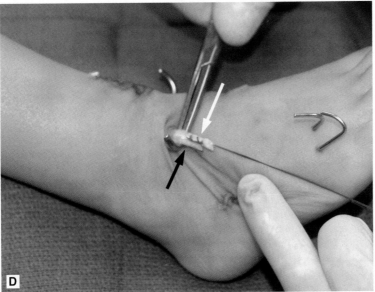

FIGURE 9-10   Split anterior tibial transfer to the peroneus tertius. **A.** Site for the three incisions. **B.** Location of the transfer and the balance of the pull of the anterior tibialis following transfer. The split transfer should be outside the retinaculum to the dorsal hind foot to allow a direct line of pull. **C.** Enlargement of the outlined portion of **B** showing relevant anatomy. The peroneus tertius, which provides an excellent recipient tendon in the majority of children with cerebral palsy, is located just lateral to the toe extensors. **D.** Clinical photograph demonstrating a typical overlap of the anterior tibial tendon (with whip stitch) and the peroneus tertius, which provides a large amount of tissue for healing. The child had also undergone simultaneous tibial and midfoot osteotomies.

first metatarsal base and (b) putting the tendon under tension (by lifting the clamp) and noting that the first ray is supinated and the great toe does not extend. A wooden tongue blade is placed under the distal portion of the ATT. The tendon is split in its midsubstance for a distance of approximately 2.5 cm; then the plantar half of the tendon is cut distally. The medial/plantar half of the ATT is harvested to minimize the lever arm of the remaining portion of the tendon. A 2-0 whip stitch of nonabsorbable suture is placed through the tendon stump, and the tendon is passed into the lower leg deep to the extensor retinaculum. A curved (Ober) tendon passer is placed antegrade from the lower leg incision under the retinaculum, emerging from the dorsomedial hind-foot incision. The starting location proximally is just anterior and medial to the ATT and should pass easily into the distal incision. The tendon passer is used to bring the medial/plantar half of the ATT under the retinaculum into the lower leg wound. In the process, the ATT naturally splits longitudinally in its midportion.

The peroneus tertius or peroneus brevis will have been exposed by this point in the surgery. A 1- to 1.5-cm incision is made in the dorsolateral hind foot, directly lateral to the toe extensors. Tenotomy scissors are used to dissect down to the peroneus tertius. The peroneus tertius is directly lateral to the long extensor to the fifth toe (Fig. 9-10C). This is confirmed by placing tension on the peroneus tertius and noting that the hind foot everts and the fifth toe does not extend. If the tendon has a caliber comparable to that of the split ATT, then the peroneus tertius is used to receive the transfer. If not, then the peroneus brevis is used.

The peroneus brevis requires a 4 to 5 cm incision over the distal course of the tendon before it inserts into the fifth metatarsal base. If the brevis is used, it is split similarly to the method described for the ATT, with one important exception: Whereas the peroneus brevis is split longitudinally in its midsubstance with a #15 blade, the proximal cut in the brevis is dorsal and at least 5 to 6 cm proximal to the tendon insertion into the fifth metatarsal base. As with the split ATT, a 2-0 nonabsorbable whip stitch is placed in the portion of the peroneus brevis to be used for transfer.

Regardless of which tendon is used to receive the transfer, the split portion of the ATT is passed superficial to the retinaculum to the dorsolateral hind foot. This is accomplished by using dissecting scissors to create a tunnel outside the extensor retinaculum connecting the lateral hind-foot incision with the lower leg incision and using a tendon passer (from distal to proximal) to retrieve the split ATT. There are two reasons for transferring outside the retinaculum: (a) it allows the tendon to have a direct line of pull, and (b) it maximizes the preservation of dorsiflexion strength. The tendon should pass easily through this tunnel.

The tendon is sutured to the peroneus tertius in a side-to-side fashion with figure-eight sutures of nonabsorbable 2-0 sutures. The peroneus tertius is not cut in order to receive the transfer. The foot is held in neutral dorsiflexion and mild eversion, with the tendons overlapped significantly to maximize tension in the transferred tendon. This also allows for a large surface area of tendon overlap for tendon-to-tendon healing (Fig. 9-10D). Completion of the transfer to the peroneus brevis is similar, though care must be taken to bring the brevis to the dorsolateral hind foot so that the transferred tendon has a direct line of pull and makes an angle of at least 45 degrees to the foot.

POSTERIOR TIBIAL TENDON TRANSFER. When the posterior tibial tendon is causative, whole or split transfer is indicated. As noted earlier, the author prefers split transfers as there have been many cases of overcorrection of whole posterior tibial tendon transfers.

A four-incision technique may be used. This technique includes (a) a 2- to 3-cm incision over the medial hind foot (posterior tibialis insertion), (b) a 4-cm incision over the medial lower leg, (c) a 1-cm incision just posterior to the fibula in the distal third of the lower leg, and (d) a 3- to 4-cm incision over the peroneal sheath just distal to the lateral malleolus in the hind foot.

The procedure begins by making the four incisions noted above. The lateral incision over the peroneal sheath is deepened, and the peroneal tendon sheath is incised with a #15 blade or scissors. The peroneus brevis is identified (just dorsal to the peroneus longus). To confirm that the tendon is the brevis and not the longus, the tendon is placed under tension: Both will evert the hind foot, but only the peroneus longus plantarflexes the first ray.

The lateral lower leg wound is deepened, and the retinaculum is incised just posterior to the fibula. Attention is turned medially, and the medial lower leg incision is made. This incision is deepened, and the retinaculum over the posterior tibial tendon is incised just posterior to the posteromedial tibial border. The posterior tibial tendon (PTT) is directly posterior to the tibia and is the largest tendon present. The FDL is immediately posterior to the PTT, and tension on the FDL will plantarflex the toes if confusion arises about the relevant anatomy.

The final incision is made over the medial hind foot directly over the PTT. The tendon is generally readily palpable just inferior and distal to the medial malleolus. If this is not evident, hind-foot eversion places the PTT on tension and often facilitates identification. The tendon sheath is incised with scissors or a #15 blade, and the tendon is traced to its insertion into the navicular. The plantar half of the PTT is harvested using a #15 blade after a wooden tongue blade is placed under the PTT

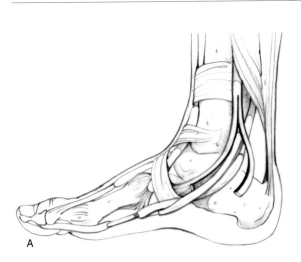
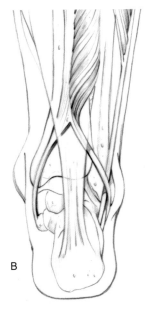

FIGURE 9-11   Split posterior tibial tendon transfer to the peroneus brevis. **A.** Posterior tibial tendon after the plantar half has been harvested distally and the tendon split proximal to the medial malleolus. **B.** Appearance of the two limbs after completion of the split transfer, thus balancing the previous varus pull of the PTT.

(as for the split ATT transfer), and a 2-0 nonabsorbable whip stitch is placed in the harvested plantar half of the PTT.

A tendon passer is passed antegrade from the medial lower leg wound, distal to the medial malleolus and into the medial hind-foot incision to retrieve the split portion of the PTT. As the split portion is drawn into the lower leg wound, the tendon naturally splits longitudinally along the PTT cut made in the medial hind foot. This split is extended as proximal as possible (Fig. 9-11A).

The split PTT is then passed directly posterior to the tibia and into the lateral lower leg wound. The following help accomplish this: (a) All posterior soft tissue is retracted using a right-angle retractor (such as a Sofield); (b) a tendon passer is passed just posterior to the tibia and the posterior border of the fibula until the tip emerges from the lateral lower leg incision; (c) a 0 or 2-0 suture is folded over on itself and passed through the lateral incision, and the looped end is retrieved with the tendon passer; (d) the ends of the PTT whip stitch are passed through the loop in the suture; and (e) the suture (with the split PTT) is brought out through the lateral wound.

Next a tendon passer is brought retrograde from the lateral hind-foot wound, through the peroneal tendon sheath, and into the lateral lower leg wound to retrieve the PTT. The split PTT is then sutured in either a Pulvertaft or a side-to-side fashion with figure-eight sutures of a 2-0 nonabsorbable suture (Fig. 9-11B).

Postoperative Management   Postoperative care is the same following either anterior or posterior tibial tendon surgery. A short leg cast is worn for 6 weeks postoperatively and immediate weight bearing is allowed. Bracing (foot orthoses [FOs], supramalleolar orthosis [SMOs], ankle foot orthoses [AFOs]) is used for at least 6 months postoperatively to help protect the transfer. The cast is usually changed once, at 3 to 4 weeks postoperatively, to measure for braces that will be placed at the time of cast removal at 6 weeks.

Complications to Avoid   The most common complication is recurrent or residual deformity. The risk of this complication should decrease, however, as there is increasing recognition of the frequent contribution of the anterior tibialis to varus foot deformity in children with CP. Residual deformity may also occur if a rigid (bony) deformity is not recognized and treated at the time of surgery.

Overcorrection is rare. The risk of this appears higher if whole tendon transfers are performed in children with CP. In addition, overcorrection may be seen if surgery for a varus foot is performed in the absence of significant varus. Unfortunately, many physicians attribute intoeing in children with CP to a varus foot and posterior tibial dysfunction, even if no varus is actually present preoperatively.

Vascular complications have been reported following whole PTT transfer through the interosseous membrane.

Pearls and Pitfalls

- Dysfunction of the anterior tibialis, the posterior tibialis, and combined dysfunction of the two muscles are each responsible for approximately one-third of varus feet in children with CP.
- Soft-tissue surgery will not suffice if the deformity is rigid. Bone surgery will be needed in such cases.
- Bone surgery should not be performed in isolation. Soft-tissue balancing is requisite to maximize the long-term prognosis following osseous surgery.

Bone Surgery for Varus Feet

Indications/Contraindications   If there is fixed hindfoot varus, calcaneal osteotomy is necessary to afford sufficient correction. Though the Coleman block test is often used in able-bodied children, such a test is usually not feasible in children with CP. The foot can be manipulated to check for fixed hind-foot varus.

Surgical Procedure   A preferred osteotomy for varus feet is a Dwyer lateral-closing wedge osteotomy. This osteotomy is carried out through an oblique incision that begins over the dorsal aspect of the calcaneus just anterior to the Achilles tendon and ends plantar to the calcaneus 1 to 2 cm proximal to the calcaneocuboid joint. To minimize the risk of wound slough, it is important to incise perpendicular to the skin and calcaneus and to minimize undermining of the skin flaps.

The concept of the osteotomy is that a lateral-closing wedge is removed to shorten the lateral column of the calcaneus and to correct the varus (Fig. 9-12A). The sural nerve is identified and protected, and the peroneal tendon sheath is incised so that the peroneal tendons can be retracted in a plantar direction. The calcaneus is osteotomized parallel to the posterior facet, with the cut exiting the superior aspect of the calcaneus anterior to the Achilles insertion. It is usually easiest to place a Crego elevator over the superior aspect of the calcaneus anterior to the Achilles both to direct the cuts and to protect the soft tissues. A critical step in performing such an osteotomy is to direct both cuts so that they converge at the medial cortex; this allows for excellent bony contact of the cut edges of the calcaneus along the entire width of the osteotomy. Sometimes it may be helpful, especially as experience is being gained with this osteotomy, to leave an osteotome in one limb of the osteotomy while performing the second cut; this ensures appropriate convergence of the two cuts

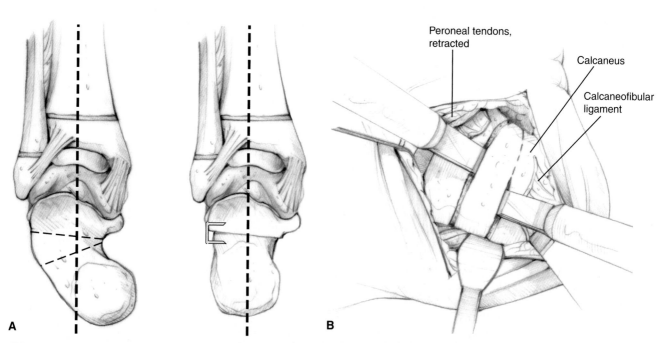

Peroneal tendons, retracted

Calcaneus

Calcaneofibular ligament

A   **B**

FIGURE 9-12   Dwyer osteotomy of the calcaneus for rigid hind-foot varus. **A.** A lateral-closing wedge of bone is removed to correct the varus and bring the calcaneus in line with the long (weight-bearing) axis of the tibia. **B.** The two osteotomy cuts converge to meet at the medial cortex. While gaining experience with the osteotomy, it is often helpful to leave an osteotome in the first cut while making the second cut.

(Fig. 9-12B). Staples can be used for osteotomy fixation, though smooth Kirschner wires (usually 2.0 mm) may be used in children with poor bone stock. Closure of the incision with nonabsorbable mattress sutures has been found to lead to fewer wound complications than does closure with absorbable sutures.

Postoperative Management   Postoperatively, the child is placed into a short-leg nonwalking cast. This cast is changed to a walking cast at 3 to 4 weeks postoperatively. If K-wires are used, they are removed in the office at the time of cast change. The short-leg walking cast is removed at 6 to 8 weeks postoperatively.

Complications to Avoid   Recurrent or residual deformity can occur if an insufficient wedge of bone is resected laterally or if soft-tissue balance is not obtained at the time of surgery. Common causes of inadequate soft-tissue balancing are insufficient tension on the tendon transfer or not surgically addressing the offending muscle(s) causing the varus.

Wound complications are relatively common following any lateral approach to the calcaneus. However, the frequency of this complication can be minimized by developing full thickness flaps during surgical dissection and by using nonabsorbable skin sutures during wound closure.

Pearls and Pitfalls   Bone and soft-tissue surgery must be combined when there is fixed bony deformity in conjunction with soft-tissue causes of varus. Failure to address both will result in residual and/or recurrent deformity.

SURGERY FOR VALGUS FEET

Valgus feet are very common in patients with diplegia and quadriplegia. Approximately 30% of all children with CP sent to the gait lab have been noted to have pes valgus.[16] This deformity is less common in children with hemiplegia. The deforming soft-tissue forces are opposite those found in varus feet, with overpull of the evertors (the peroneals) relative to the invertors (posterior and anterior tibialis). As with varus deformities, correction of valgus deformities requires appropriate soft-tissue balancing. Unlike surgery for varus deformities, however, bone surgery is almost universally needed when surgery is indicated to correct a valgus foot deformity.

Commonly described osteotomies include a medial calcaneal slide and a lateral column (calcaneal) lengthening as described by Evans[2] and popularized more recently by Mosca.[11] The author prefers a calcaneal lengthening osteotomy when possible, because it can correct the underlying deformity rather than create a second, compensatory deformity. Though unusual, both of these osteotomies (calcaneal lengthening and calcaneal slide) may be used in the same foot with a severe deformity.

Indications/Contraindications

The prime indications for surgery for valgus feet are (a) valgus feet that cannot be braced effectively and (b) lever arm dysfunction interfering with function. Occasionally, foot pain may also be significant.

Preoperative examination should include an assessment of the ankle because ankle valgus can be confused with hind-foot valgus. Clinical examination and/or radiologic assessment aid in this evaluation. On an AP ankle radiograph, the distal fibular physis should be at the level of the ankle mortise. If the distal fibular physis is located more proximally, then ankle valgus is contributing to at least some of the apparent pes valgus.

Because a calcaneal lengthening osteotomy corrects the underlying deformity, it is the preferred osteotomy in the majority of cases in which a calcaneal osteotomy is indicated for pes valgus. However, a calcaneal slide may be preferred in the following instances: (a) a stiff deformity that is not passively correctable, (b) fixed valgus following previous subtalar fusion, and (c) children with marked ligamentous laxity.

Calcaneal Lengthening Osteotomy

Indications/Contraindications   A calcaneal lengthening osteotomy is the most common procedure because it corrects the underlying deformity. The indications are as noted above.

Surgical Procedure   An approximately 5-cm straight lateral incision is made parallel to the foot's plantar aspect. The distal tip of the incision is at the level of the calcaneocuboid joint. (The joint can be localized by palpation of the distal calcaneus while abducting and adducting the foot.) The sural nerve and its branches are sought and protected.

Lengthening of the peroneus brevis in conjunction with a calcaneal lengthening osteotomy is necessary for two important reasons: (a) to allow greater opening of the osteotomy and greater correction of the deformity and (b) to enhance soft-tissue balance between the hind-foot invertors and evertors. A Z-lengthening of the peroneus brevis is performed, and its ends are tagged for ease of identification and repair. The peroneus longus is only lengthened in the more severe cases. Lengthening the peroneus longus should be avoided when possible because it plantarflexes the first metatarsal and, therefore, resists the tendency toward forefoot supination, which is common with hind-foot valgus. When the peroneus longus is lengthened, its ends are tagged with a different color suture than was used on the peroneus brevis to distinguish one from the other when the tendons are subsequently repaired.

A separate 4-cm incision is made medially over the distal portion of the course of the PTT. The tendon is retracted, and a full-thickness ellipse of the talonavicular joint capsule is removed.

Subperiosteal dissection is performed 2 to 2.5 cm proximal to the calcaneocuboid joint. A septum elevator is placed over the dorsum of the calcaneus. It should easily slide into the gap between the anterior and middle calcaneal facets. Fluoroscopic imaging confirms this as the site for the osteotomy. The lateral third of the plantar fascia is incised off the calcaneus to facilitate opening of the osteotomy. A Homan retractor is placed over the dorsum of the calcaneus between the anterior and middle facets and is used to direct the osteotomy (Fig. 9-13A). A lamina spreader (with broad blades) is inserted into the calcaneus to open the osteotomy site. As the osteotomy is opened, deformity correction is evident, and the arch will become apparent.

The bone graft is a trapezoidal-shaped wedge that is twice as wide laterally as medially (Fig. 9-13B–13C). Typically, the lateral edge is 14 to 16 mm, with the medial edge measuring 7 to 8 mm; the exact size is determined by how much the lamina spreader can open the osteotomy. It is important to check that the osteotomy is truly opening and that the calcaneal bone is not simply being compressed by the lamina spreader. It is also important to check that the plantar fascia is not preventing the osteotomy from opening while the lamina spreader is being used.

The trapezoidal bone graft is then created with a power saw. Either an allograft bone block or a tricortical autogenous iliac crest bone graft may be used. Allograft and autograft both incorporate rapidly (Fig. 9-14).

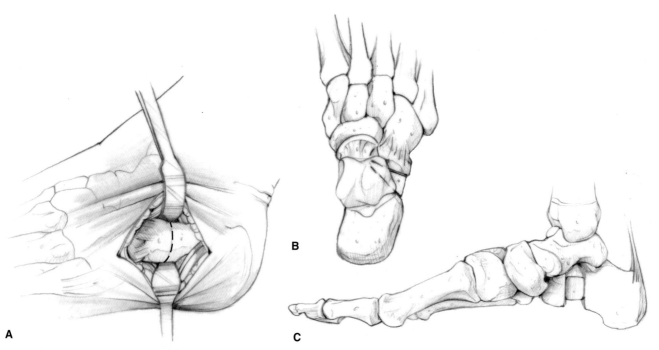

FIGURE 9-13   Calcaneal lengthening osteotomy. **A.** The calcaneus is cut 2 to 2.5 cm proximal to the calcaneocuboid joint, between the anterior and middle facets. Exposure is facilitated with a Homan retractor or septum elevator dorsally and a Chandler retractor plantarly at the osteotomy site. **B–C.** A trapezoidal bone graft (approximately twice as wide laterally as medially) is inserted to enhance talar head coverage by the navicular and to correct the talar sag. No fixation is needed, though a 2.0-mm K-wire can be inserted across the calcaneocuboid joint prior to opening the osteotomy if the surgeon is concerned about calcaneocuboid joint subluxation as the foot is corrected.

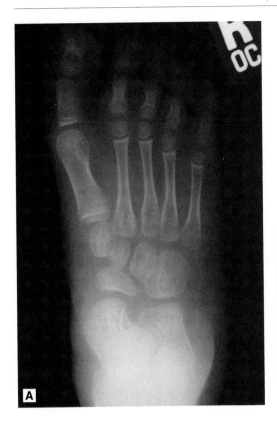

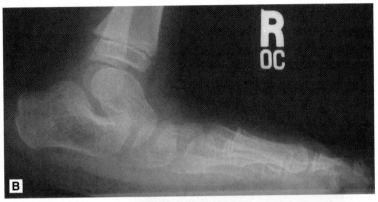

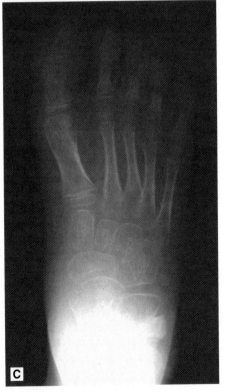

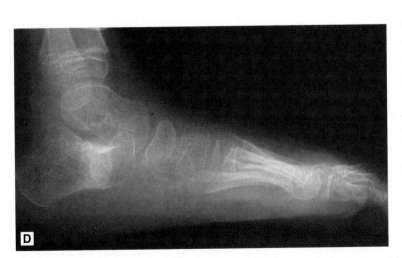

FIGURE 9-14   AP **(A)** and lateral **(B)** preoperative x-rays of a 7-year-old boy with CP and pes valgus. The AP view demonstrates significant lateral displacement of the navicular relative to the talar head. The lateral view demonstrates talar sag and a midfoot break. Postoperative AP **(C)** and lateral x-rays **(D)** show appropriate correction. On the AP, the navicular covers the talar head well. On the lateral, the talar sag and midfoot break are corrected.

Following insertion of the bone graft into the calcaneal osteotomy, the talonavicular joint capsule is plicated with figure-eight sutures of a slowly absorbable (e.g., PDS) size 0 suture. This medial plication often enhances correction of the foot. However, plication of the PTT has not been found to add significantly to correction.

The peroneal tendons are repaired independently in a side-to-side fashion with figure-eight nonabsorbable size 2-0 sutures.

If the associated forefoot supination is not flexible, then isolated correction of the hind-foot valgus will result in a foot with a corrected hind foot, persistent forefoot supination, and no floor contact by the medial forefoot. Such a foot is at high risk of recurrent hind-foot deformity if the forefoot supination is not corrected. This correction is generally accomplished with a plantarflexion osteotomy of the medial column (such as a dorsal opening wedge or plantar closing wedge at the level of the medial cuneiform or first metatarsal base). If the osteotomy is at the level of the first metatarsal base and if the physis is open at the time of surgery, care must be taken to avoid the physis with the dissection, osteotomy, and fixation.

Postoperative Management   A short-leg nonwalking cast is used postoperatively. This cast is changed to a short-leg walking cast 3 to 4 weeks postoperatively. The short-leg walking cast is removed at 6 to 8 weeks postoperatively.

Complications to Avoid   Although wound complications are relatively common following any lateral approach to the calcaneus, they are less common when using nonabsorbable mattress sutures to close the incision.

Recurrent deformity can be minimized by appropriate soft-tissue balancing with lengthening of the peroneus brevis (and sometimes longus), as well as the medial plication. Recurrence is more common in severe ligamentous laxity.

Pearls and Pitfalls

- The ankle should be checked for valgus preoperatively. Surgery for pes valgus will fail if the apparent pes valgus is actually due to ankle valgus.
- Calcaneal lengthening osteotomy is best able to correct the pes valgus deformity in children with CP while maintaining subtalar range of motion.
- Soft-tissue balancing is crucial for correcting this deformity and maintaining the correction.
- Results of this surgery are poor in those with marked ligamentous laxity.

Calcaneal Medial Sliding Osteotomy

Indications/Contraindications   A medial sliding calcaneal osteotomy is preferred for (a) rigid hind-foot deformities that are not passively correctable, (b) fixed valgus following previous subtalar fusion, and (c) children with marked ligamentous laxity.

Surgical Procedure   An oblique incision is made from the dorsal-posterior aspect of the calcaneus to the plantar-anterior surface, as described above for a Dwyer osteotomy. Care is taken to create thick soft-tissue flaps to maintain soft-tissue integrity. One-half- and three-quarter-inch straight osteotomes are used for the osteotomy. The osteotomy is parallel to the posterior facet and should be straight across or angled slightly cephalad when proceeding from lateral to medial; this will prevent binding of the two fragments when the distal fragment is displaced medially. The medial cortex needs to be osteotomized and the posterior (distal) fragment mobilized. The distal fragment is generally displaced one-third to one-half the width of the calcaneus (Fig. 9-15). Fixation of the calcaneus is with K-wires or screws. When K-wires are used, smooth wires, generally 2.0 to 2.4 mm in diameter, are generally preferred for fixation. Smooth K-wires provide sufficient fixation and are easily removed in the office. When screws are used, large cancellous or cannulated screws (generally 4.5–6.5 mm in diameter) are preferred. A washer can enhance fixation and prevent the screw head from migrating into the calcaneus.

Postoperative Management   As with a calcaneal lengthening osteotomy, a short-leg nonwalking cast is used postoperatively for 3 to 4 weeks, followed by a short-leg walking cast for an additional 3 to 4 weeks.

Complications to Avoid   Wound complications are common following calcaneal osteotomies, though the risk is less when nonabsorbable sutures are used for wound closure.

Recurrent deformity is not uncommon, especially if soft-tissue balancing (particularly with peroneal tendon lengthening) is not performed.

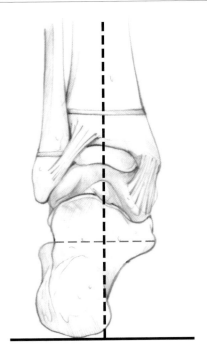 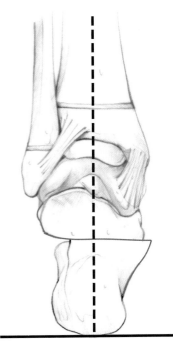

FIGURE 9-15

Medial calcaneal sliding osteotomy for pes valgus. The calcaneus is cut obliquely (parallel to the posterior facet). The plantar fragment is translated medially one-half to one-third the diameter of the calcaneus before fixation. After this translation, the calcaneus is in line with the long (weight-bearing) axis of the tibia.

Pearls and Pitfalls

- A sliding osteotomy is a good option in cases where calcaneal lengthening may not be helpful, including in rigid valgus deformities or in children with marked ligamentous laxity.
- The osteotomy should be angled cephalad as directed from lateral to medial to prevent binding of the distal fragment as it is displaced medially.
- Avoid injury of the posterior medial neurovascular bundle and toe flexors by avoiding overpenetration of the osteotome medially. A lamina spreader may be placed in an incomplete osteotomy. Cutting of the medial cortex is completed under direct visualization with a pituitary or Kerrison rongeur.
- After completing the osteotomy, a blunt instrument, such as a Chandler elevator, may be placed across medially to loosen the periosteum and to allow medial translation.

Subtalar Fusion

Indications/Contraindications   Subtalar fusion is rarely necessary, despite its previously widespread use. This procedure places undue stress on adjacent joints and does not guarantee a good long-term result. The author has inherited many patients who ended up with severe deformities in the hind foot and midfoot following previous subtalar fusions. Thus the subtalar fusion should be reserved for the following groups of patients: (a) patients who have significant recurrence after calcaneal lengthening osteotomies, (b) adolescents with very severe pes valgus deformities, and (c) children or adolescents with severe valgus and marked ligamentous laxity.

Surgical Procedure   The approach is through an oblique (Ollier) incision in a skin crease from the lateral aspect of the toe extensor tendons (at the level of the calcaneocuboid joint distally) to the plantar aspect of the calcaneus proximally. The incision is deepened to and through the deep fascia, and the extensor digitorum brevis (EDB) origin is incised with a U-shaped incision along its medial, proximal, and lateral borders. The distal portion of the EDB is left intact, and the EDB is reflected distally. The extra-articular portions of the subtalar joint are exposed using a combination of curettes and rongeurs to remove the soft tissues. A one-fourth-inch straight osteotome is used to remove the extra-articular cortical bone from the dorsal aspect of the calcaneus and the plantar aspect of the talus, thus exposing cancellous bone (Fig. 9-16A). To maintain appropriate alignment, the subtalar fusion can be fixed with a 4.5-mm cannulated screw from the dorsal talar neck, through the subtalar joint, and exiting the lateral calcaneus (Dennyson-Fulford technique). The subtalar joint is held in the corrected position as the guide wire and then the screw is passed. A washer is often helpful to enhance screw purchase. If the bone is of poor quality, a second cannulated screw may be passed

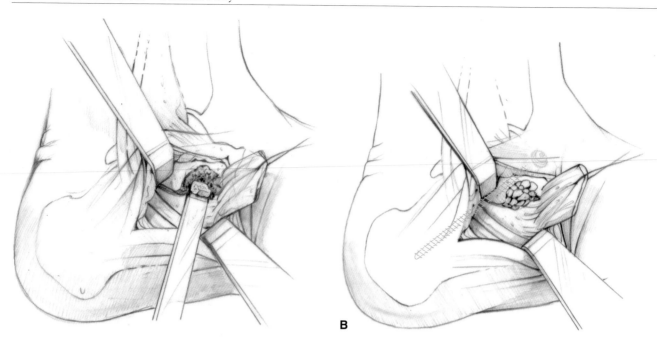

FIGURE 9-16 Subtalar fusion with Dennyson-Fulford technique. Initially, the extensor digitorum brevis is reflected distally, and the subtalar joint is prepared. **A.** After soft tissue has been removed, the bone on the dorsum of the calcaneus and plantar aspect of the talus are decorticated using osteotomes. **B.** The screw is inserted from the dorsomedial talus and exits the lateral calcaneus. Bone graft is placed in the subtalar joint.

from the heel through the posterior aspect of the calcaneus and up into the talus. Cancellous allograft or autograft bone is used to pack the significant extra-articular gap that results from the correction of severe deformities (Fig. 9-16B).

Postoperative Management As with a calcaneal osteotomy, a non-weight-bearing cast is used for 3 to 4 weeks, followed by a short-leg walking cast for 3 to 4 weeks. When smooth K-wires are used, they are removed in the office at the cast change 3 to 4 weeks postoperatively.

Complications to Avoid Recurrent deformity and hardware failure may be seen following subtalar fusion. Recurrent deformity is most common if soft-tissue balancing is not achieved at the time of subtalar fusion. Hardware failure may be seen when there is a marked gap laterally following correction of severe valgus. The risk of hardware failure is decreased when a structural block of bone is inserted into this lateral gap or when two screws are used for fixation.

The author has seen several cases of "failed" subtalar fusions with residual deformity due to failure of the surgeon to recognize that the valgus deformity was due to ankle valgus rather than pes valgus.

Pearls and Pitfalls
- In the vast majority of patients with CP undergoing osseous foot surgery, a joint-preserving osteotomy is preferable to subtalar fusion.
- Care must be taken to be certain that the valgus deformity is from the foot and not the ankle.

Surgery for Dorsal Bunions

Dorsal bunion is a common deformity seen in children with CP and is due to overpull of the anterior tibialis. The first metatarsal is elevated and the first metatarsophalangeal (MTP) joint is flexed, with resulting pressure over the dorsum of the foot over the first metatarsal head (Fig. 9-17).

Indications/Contraindications In general, shoes with a wide, deep toe box are sufficient to alleviate symptomatology. However, in the face of progressive deformity, surgery may be considered if the child is symptomatic despite appropriate brace and/or footwear.

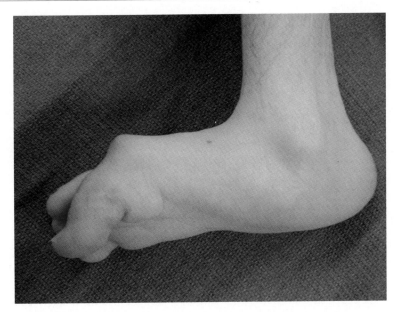

FIGURE 9-17

Clinical photograph of an 18-year-old boy with a fixed dorsal bunion. Overpull of the anterior tibialis, elevation of the first metatarsal, and flexion of the first metatarsophalangeal joint are evident.

Surgical Procedure   It is important to distinguish between flexible and rigid deformities because the treatments are different. For flexible deformities, soft-tissue balancing is sufficient. Part of the correction requires weakening the overpull of the anterior tibialis, through either a lengthening or a transfer. A split anterior tibial tendon transfer (as described earlier) is often preferred in ambulatory children, because this helps maintain dorsiflexion and minimizes the risk of a subsequent hind-foot deformity.

The flexor hallucis longus (FHL) is transferred to the first metatarsal head to correct the hyperflexion of the first MTP joint. This is accomplished through an approximately 3- to 4-cm incision over the medial aspect of the forefoot. The FHL is identified and isolated and a distal tenotomy is performed by the FHL's insertion. The FHL is then passed through an appropriately sized drill hole in the plantar aspect of the first metatarsal head, looped back, and sutured to itself with nonabsorbable sutures (generally 2-0) to prevent the metatarsal head from drifting dorsally.

For residual deformity after such soft-tissue correction, an osteotomy of the medial column is indicated. This osteotomy may be performed through the medial cuneiform; an alternative site is through the first metatarsal base. In either case, an opening dorsal or closing plantar osteotomy is performed. A dorsal opening wedge osteotomy of the medial cuneiform may be preferred, as this is often stable without internal fixation (Fig. 9-18). If the osteotomy is at the base of the first metatarsal, care must be taken to avoid the physis if it is open at the time of surgery. To avoid this physis in growing children, this generally results in an osteotomy that is diaphyseal and is located far from the site of deformity, which is another reason to use the medial cuneiform instead.

Rigid deformities are rare in ambulatory children, usually occurring in more severely involved children. Surgical reconstruction is usually indicated for children with rigid deformities who are having marked difficulties with footwear. If such children continue to have pain, pressure sores, or breakdown despite the use of accommodative shoes, surgery should be considered. For these rigid deformities, the first MTP joint usually has marked degenerative changes, with full thickness cartilage loss; thus, fusion of the first MTP joint is indicated. The surfaces of the joint are removed with a small sagittal saw or osteotomes to create flat bony surfaces that result in mild (usually 10–15 degrees) dorsiflexion at the MTP joint when the bone surfaces are opposed. Fixation is usually done with smooth, 1.6-mm (0.062-in.) K-wires. Two crossed K-wires supplemented by a longitudinal K-wire placed retrograde through the tip of the great toe can be used. The anterior tibialis should also be weakened (as noted above) to allow the first metatarsal head to be brought in a plantar direction. For nonambulatory children, however, a Z-lengthening of the anterior tibialis is often preferred, because dorsal bunions are most commonly seen associated with calcaneal deformities in nonambulators. An osteotomy of the medial cuneiform or first metatarsal base may be used to bring the first metatarsal head more plantar.

Postoperative Management   A short-leg walking cast is used for 6 to 8 weeks postoperatively. If pins are used, they are removed at 4 to 6 weeks postoperatively.

Complications to Avoid   Recurrent deformity may be seen. This is minimized by weakening the anterior tibialis via tendon lengthening or transfer. Wound complications are rare.

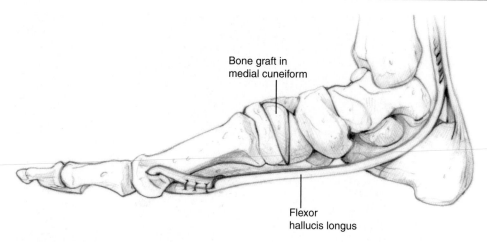

Bone graft in
medial cuneiform

Flexor
hallucis longus

FIGURE 9-18 Surgical reconstruction for flexible dorsal bunion deformity. For all dorsal bunion surgeries, the anterior tibial pull on the first metatarsal must be decreased (via tendon lengthening or transfer). In addition, for a deformity that is flexible at the first MTP joint (MTPJ) level, the FHL tendon is cut distally and brought through a drill hole in the plantar aspect of the first metatarsal head to pull down the head and prevent excessive flexion at the first MTPJ. If there is a fixed dorsiflexion deformity of the first ray in the midfoot, then a dorsal opening wedge osteotomy is also performed. Both the FHL transfer and the medial cuneiform osteotomy are depicted.

Pearls and Pitfalls
- Treatment of either flexible or rigid deformity requires soft-tissue balancing, including weakening of the anterior tibialis via tendon lengthening or transfer.
- Rigid deformities are generally associated with significant degenerative changes of the first metatarsophalangeal joint and require fusion of this joint.

ROTATIONAL OSTEOTOMIES OF THE LOWER EXTREMITIES

Rotational malalignment of the lower extremities is common in children with CP. Such rotational malalignment causes significant lever arm dysfunction,[4] which interferes with gait mechanics and ambulatory ability. In comparison to their able-bodied peers, children with CP lack balance, strength, and muscle selectivity. Because of these differences, rotational malalignment often necessitates surgical correction in children with CP.

Indications for operation include lower extremity long-bone torsion with resultant lever arm dysfunction interfering with walking and/or running.

Femoral Rotational Osteotomies

Indications Traditional teaching has been that femoral rotational osteotomies should be performed proximally. More recent studies have demonstrated comparable results for proximal and distal femoral osteotomies.[7]

Distal femoral osteotomies are preferred in the majority of cases for children with CP. The benefits of distal femoral osteotomy include (a) a smaller incision, (b) less soft-tissue dissection, (c) minimal blood loss, and (d) no remaining hardware once the pins are removed in the office 4 weeks postoperatively.

Proximal osteotomies are indicated in coxa valga and hip subluxation and in skeletal maturity. Skeletal maturity is an indication for proximal surgery for two reasons: (a) to avoid casting and allow immediate mobilization in older, larger children, and (b) to avoid potentially prolonged casting and/or malunion due to delayed healing.

Correction with proximal and distal osteotomies appears comparable. With either location of osteotomy, the amount of correction measured at surgery should be 1.5 to 2 times the amount deemed necessary based on preoperative static examination and dynamic gait data. For example, if the surgeon is aiming for a final correction of 20 degrees of hip rotation, intraoperative correction of 30 to 40 degrees is necessary.[7] Optimal correction results in neutral hip rotation during stance phase postoperatively; thus, if hip rotation during gait were 20 degrees internal preoperatively, then intraoperative correction of 30 to 40 degrees would be recommended to normalize postoperative hip rotation.

Distal Femoral Osteotomy

SURGICAL PROCEDURE. Some surgeons prefer to perform this surgery using a pneumatic thigh tourniquet, though this is not necessary. When not using the tourniquet, the distal femoral physis is located with the aid of fluoroscopy. In general, the physis is at the junction of the mid and proximal thirds of the patella.

A 4- to 5-cm longitudinal incision is made laterally, with the distal end of the incision at the level of the physis. A subvastus approach is made to the distal femur after incising the iliotibial band. This is most easily accomplished in a distal-to-proximal direction using electrocautery to mobilize the vastus off the intermuscular septum. Care must be taken to cauterize any perforating vessels encountered. Fluoroscopic imaging is used to localize the osteotomy site (generally 2–2.5 cm proximal to the distal femoral physis). The increased healing capacity and increased cross-sectional area in the metaphysis relative to the diaphysis make it very important to perform a metaphyseal osteotomy.

Subperiosteal dissection is carried out at the level of the osteotomy. Two derotation pins are placed through the surgical incision parallel to one another and parallel to the physis, with one proximal and the other distal to the planned osteotomy site to judge the amount of rotation through the osteotomy. After placement of the pins, an oscillating saw is used to osteotomize the femur perpendicular to its long axis and parallel to the physis. A large elevator (such as a large Crego or large Chandler) may be used to protect the posterior structures during the osteotomy. It is also important to make sure that the saw does not have a large excursion through the posterior femur to avoid the neurovascular structures. Osteotomes can be used as needed to complete the osteotomy. A bone-holding clamp is placed on the proximal fragment, and the distal fragment is rotated. Rotation of the distal fragment is most easily accomplished by flexing the knee to 90 degrees and grasping the lower tibia to attain a sufficient lever arm for rotation (Fig. 9-19). The osteotomy should be checked to ensure that there has not been significant translation in the coronal and sagittal planes. A sterile goniometer is used to measure the angle of derotation by measuring the angle between the derotation pins, which were parallel prior to the osteotomy.

Fixation is with smooth K-wires in a crossed configuration. Three pins are usually all that is needed for most children, though two pins are likely to be biomechanically sufficient in many children. In the majority of children, 2.4-mm K-wires can be used, though 2.8-mm wires may be considered in children who weigh more than 30 to 35 kg (Fig. 9-20). The pins are inserted retrograde from the metaphysis and exiting in the diaphysis or metadiaphyseal junction. Whether two of the three pins are inserted from medial or lateral is based on surgeon preference and ease of insertion.

POSTOPERATIVE MANAGEMENT. A long-leg cast is placed at the time of surgery. The child is allowed to begin weight bearing, as tolerated, at 3 to 4 weeks postoperatively. The cast is changed

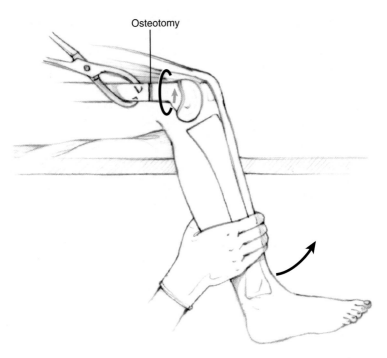

Osteotomy

FIGURE 9-19

For a distal femoral osteotomy, rotation of the distal fragment is most easily performed as follows: (a) placing a bone-holding clamp (such as a small lobster-claw clamp) on the femur just proximal to the osteotomy, (b) flexing the knee to 90 degrees, and (c) rotating the leg by grasping near the ankle.

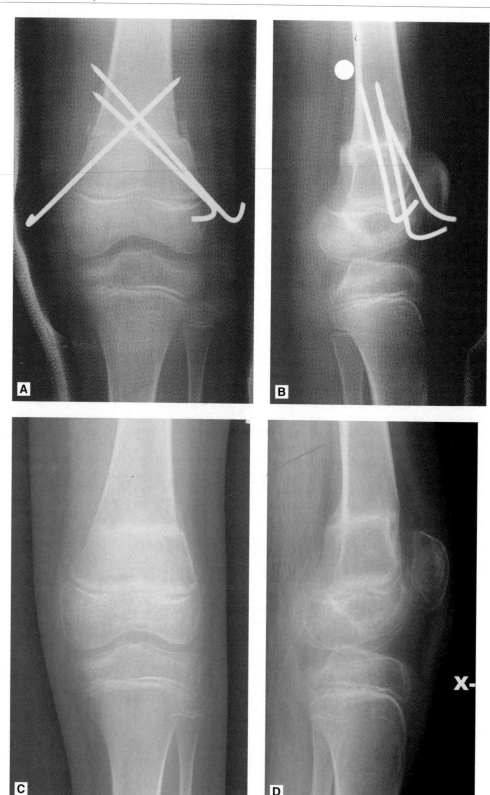

FIGURE 9-20

Radiographs 1 month **(A, B)** and 2 months **(C, D)** postoperatively following distal femoral rotational osteotomies in a 12 year old with cerebral palsy who underwent single-event multilevel surgery (SEMLS). One-month post-op AP **(A)** and lateral radiographs **(B)** of the left knee demonstrate appropriate location of the osteotomy in the metaphysis, appropriate bony contact, early healing, and fixation with three 2.4-mm smooth pins. The osteotomy should be parallel to the joint and perpendicular to the long axis of the femur. Because the bone is not cylindrical in the metaphysis, it is typical to see a step-off on the AP and/or lateral views. Pins were removed in the office on the date of these x-rays, and weight bearing was initiated. Two months post-op AP **(C)** and lateral **(D)** radiographs of the left knee demonstrate appropriate healing and alignment.

and the pins removed in the office 4 weeks postoperatively. Casting is continued until bone healing is complete, which is almost universally by 2 months postoperatively.

COMPLICATIONS TO AVOID. The most common complication following distal femoral osteotomy is loss of fixation. This complication was reported in 6% of one series of distal femoral osteotomies, with a rate of 8% (3/37) in femurs fixed with staples and in none of the 14 osteotomies fixed with K-wires. Fixation loss appears to be very rare in children with open physes whose osteotomies are fixed with K-wires.

Knee stiffness is very common after 2 months of casting but should resolve within 1 to 2 months following cast removal.

PEARLS AND PITFALLS.

- Distal femoral osteotomy has comparable results and complication rates to proximal femoral osteotomy but requires less soft-tissue dissection and prevents the need for reoperation for retained hardware.
- A distal femoral osteotomy should be performed in the metaphysis to allow for increased surface area for bony healing and more rapid healing.
- Fixation with K-wires appears superior to fixation with staples, with lower rates of loss of fixation.
- With either proximal or distal femoral osteotomy, the amount of correction noted on both static and dynamic examinations (i.e., static examination and instrumented gait analysis) measured at least 1 year postoperatively will generally be 50% to 65% of that measured at the time of surgery. As a result, if 20 degrees of correction are desired, the intraoperative correction should be 30 to 40 degrees.

Proximal Femoral Osteotomy

SURGICAL PROCEDURE.   Because most of the children undergoing proximal femoral rotational osteotomies are undergoing multiple-level surgery due to other concomitant gait deviations, the osteotomies should be performed with the child supine.

A standard lateral approach is made to the proximal femur. The incision is straight lateral, and the proximal-most extent is at the vastus ridge. The fascia lata is incised in line with the skin incision, and the vastus lateralis is elevated off the vastus ridge. A 1.6- to 2.0-mm guide wire is placed into the proximal femur, beginning laterally approximately 1.5 cm distal to the trochanteric apophysis. The guide pin is placed so that the neck-shaft angle postoperatively will be 120 to 125 degrees in ambulatory children. (This contrasts with the more typical neck-shaft angle of approximately 100–110 degrees in nonambulators.)

The K-wire is inserted to a depth corresponding to the blade length of the blade plate to be inserted. (For example, for a Toddler blade plate with a 38-mm blade length, the pin is inserted to a depth of 38 mm.) The length of K-wire in the femur is checked by placing the same-size guide wire adjacent to the first wire (with the tip at the site where the guide wire enters the femur) and measuring how much of the second wire protrudes relative to the inserted wire (Fig. 9-21).

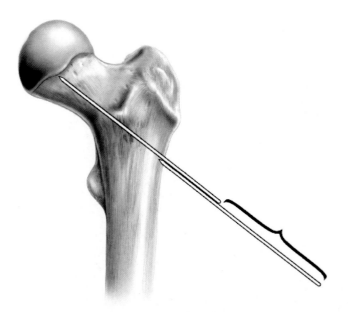

FIGURE 9-21   Method for determining the needed depth for the blade plate. A guide wire is placed into the femoral neck. A second wire, which must be the same length as the guide wire, is placed adjacent to the guide wire and advanced until it abuts the lateral femoral cortex. The amount the second pin protrudes beyond the guide wire equals the depth of the guide wire in the femur. The guide wire should be advanced until its length in the proximal femur equals the blade length of the blade plate to be inserted. The blade plate chisel is then advanced to the tip of the guide wire, with no need to read the depth off the chisel.

Based on preoperative templating, the appropriate-size chisel is inserted into the proximal femur immediately cephalad to the guide wire. The position of the chisel must be checked in the AP and lateral views to confirm appropriate position in all planes. The chisel is inserted until its tip is at the tip of the guide wire. (This is much easier than trying to read the depth off the underside of the blade plate chisel.)

The femur is then marked for the osteotomy. Depending on the blade plate to be used, the distance from the chisel insertion site to the osteotomy site varies. For AO 90-degree blade plates, these distances should be 10, 12, and 15 mm for the infant, toddler, and child blade plates, respectively.

After the osteotomy site is marked, derotation wires are placed parallel to one another through the surgical incision. Care must be taken to insert the proximal wire very near the chisel so that the wire will not interfere with the final osteotomy cut. The distal wire is distal to the distal osteotomy cut.

The femoral osteotomy is made perpendicular to the femoral shaft. If a shortening osteotomy is to be performed, the second cut is also perpendicular to the femoral shaft (and thus parallel to the first cut). To minimize limb length discrepancy, the femur should not be shortened when performing a unilateral osteotomy. Shortening of the femur helps decrease overall tone of the muscles spanning the femur—most notably the hamstrings—to relieve excessive knee flexion. The final cut is made in the proximal fragment, with the cut parallel to the chisel in all planes if a 90-degree plate is used (Fig. 9-22). If a different angle plate is used, then the cut is not parallel to the chisel in the coronal plane. For every degree above 90 degrees of the plate angle, the cut should be angled an equal number of degrees away from the chisel. For plates with less than a 90-degree angle, the cut should be angled toward the chisel by the number of degrees that the angle differs from 90 degrees. As an example, if a 100-degree plate is used, the cut is angled 10 degrees away from the chisel in the coronal plane. For an 80-degree plate, the cut should be angled 10 degrees toward the chisel.

A standard plate can be bent with plate benders prior to insertion in order to fine-tune the desired neck-shaft angle postosteotomy and to increase the length of the blade that can be accommodated in the proximal fragment. When this is done, the angle of the final cut is as noted in the preceding paragraph.

For children in whom an infant plate is used, the screw hole in the shoulder of the plate can be used to enhance fixation in the proximal fragment. This screw is generally angled posterior so that purchase of the posterior cortex can be obtained.

The amount of derotation is ascertained by using a goniometer to measure the angle between the derotation pins. After fixation is obtained, hip internal and external rotations are checked and compared with the preosteotomy values as a second check of the amount of derotation performed.

POSTOPERATIVE MANAGEMENT.   Postoperatively, the child is placed in an A-frame cast, spica cast, or hip abduction pillow for 4 weeks. An A-frame cast or abduction pillow may be used if fixation

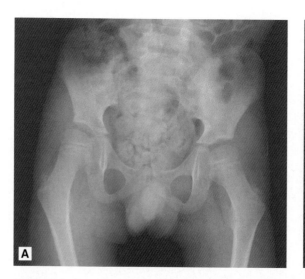 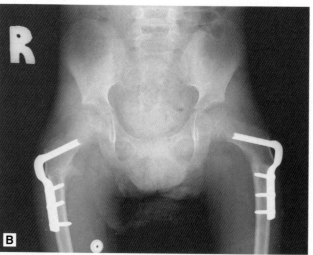

FIGURE 9-22   Radiographs demonstrating bilateral proximal femoral osteotomies. This child underwent bilateral varus derotational osteotomies (VDROs) as part of SEMLS. Bilateral femoral osteotomies were indicated because of gait deviations, including internal hip rotation and foot progression angles more than 50 degrees internal. Because of relative coxa valga and migration percentages approximating 30% bilaterally, the rotational osteotomies were done proximally, and a mild varus was performed concomitantly. Preoperative AP pelvis radiograph **(A)** and 2-month postoperative x-ray **(B)** demonstrate healed osteotomies in satisfactory alignment.

and bone quality are both good; a spica cast is used in other children. With either type of cast, the child begins physical therapy with weight bearing, as tolerated, at the time of cast removal 4 weeks postoperatively. If no cast is used, weight bearing, as tolerated, is allowed 3 to 4 weeks postoperatively. Because many children with CP may develop significant spasm at the time of cast removal, benzodiazepines, such as diazepam, may be indicated on an as-needed basis for the first week or two following cast removal.

COMPLICATIONS TO AVOID.   Common complications include significant blood loss and need for blood transfusion. Undercorrection and/or recurrent deformity may occur. A second surgery is often necessary for removal of hardware, though this is not a complication.

PEARLS AND PITFALLS.
- Proximal femoral derotational osteotomies are generally preferable to distal osteotomies in children with significant coxa valga and/or hip subluxation or in skeletally mature individuals.
- As with distal femoral osteotomy, postoperative correction measured at least 1 year postoperatively will generally be 50% to 65% of that measured at surgery.
- Excessive varus (neck-shaft angle less than 120 degrees) should be avoided in children who walk extensively.
- Pins marking rotation are placed distally and proximally before making the osteotomy; otherwise, measurement of correction will not be possible.
- Lateral imaging should be checked to ensure that sagittal alignment has not been inadvertently changed.

Tibial Rotational Osteotomies

Indications   Tibial torsion with resultant lever arm dysfunction is common in children with CP. When this is of functional consequence, tibial rotational osteotomy is indicated. Distal tibial osteotomies are easier and much safer to perform than are proximal osteotomies. Proximal osteotomies result in significant risks of neurologic damage and compartment syndrome.

In the majority of cases of distal tibial osteotomy, the fibula does not require osteotomy. The inherent stability of this construct results in excellent alignment without significant loss of alignment. The author has performed rotational osteotomies of 45 degrees and more without needing to osteotomize the fibula.

Isolated distal tibial osteotomy in children with CP has reliable outcomes with low rates of complications.[12]

Surgical Procedure   A sterile tourniquet is recommended for this procedure, as this allows the surgeon to check the thigh-foot angle intraoperatively preceding and following derotation of the tibia.

The physis is located via fluoroscopic imaging. An approximately 2.5- to 3-cm longitudinal incision is made over the anteromedial subcutaneous border of the tibia. The distal end of the incision is at the level of the physis. The saphenous vein is identified and protected, and full thickness flaps are developed. The periosteum is incised longitudinally, beginning 1.5 cm proximal to the physis and proceeding as far proximal as possible (based on the length of the incision). At the distal end of the incision (1.5 cm proximal to the physis), the periosteum is cut anteriorly and posteriorly in a T fashion; subperiosteal dissection is carried out using Crego elevators.

Derotation pins are placed proximal and distal to the proposed osteotomy, and a metaphyseal osteotomy is performed 2 to 2.5 cm proximal to the physis. A wide (14-mm) Crego elevator is placed to protect the soft tissues during osteotomy. Osteotomes may be preferred for this osteotomy because they facilitate early healing and allow a smaller incision to be used than would be needed if a power saw were used. The osteotomy should be perfectly parallel to the physis and perpendicular to the long axis of the tibia; otherwise, derotation will lead to angular deformity (Fig. 9-23). The osteotomy is easily completed without the need for drill holes (Fig. 9-24). After completing the osteotomy, the distal fragment is rotated until the desired correction is obtained. The amount of correction can be ascertained by using a sterile goniometer to measure the angle between the previously parallel pins.

Thigh-foot angle in able-bodied subjects is usually 10 to 15 degrees external. When derotation is performed, the desired thigh-foot angle is generally less than 10 to 15 degrees external, because correction to a thigh-foot angle of greater than 10 to 15 degrees can cause lever arm dysfunction and because of the tendency toward external tibial torsion in children with CP as they get older.[16]

As a result, when internally rotating the tibia to correct excessive external torsion, the surgeon should aim for a thigh-foot angle of 0 to 5 degrees external postoperatively. When correcting internal tibial torsion, the surgeon should aim for a thigh-foot angle of approximately 5 degrees external (Fig. 9-24).

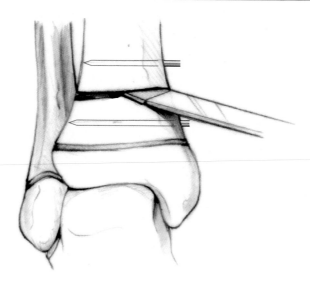

FIGURE 9-23 Technique for distal tibial osteotomy. After placement of derotation pins proximal and distal to the planned osteotomy, an osteotome is used to cut the distal tibial metaphysis perpendicular to the long axis of the tibia and parallel to the physis. Osteotomy of the fibula is not necessary, even when rotating the distal fragment 40 degrees or more.

If osteotomy of the tibia is performed in conjunction with correction of a significant foot deformity (i.e., metatarsus adductus, pes varus, or pes valgus), the foot deformity should be corrected prior to the tibial osteotomy. The reason for this sequence is that a significant foot deformity will result in an abnormal thigh-foot angle, and correction of the tibial torsion before correcting the foot deformity will more likely result in over- or undercorrection of the tibial deformity. In contrast, with initial correction of the foot deformity, the residual abnormality in thigh-foot angle is known and can be precisely corrected (Fig. 9-25).

Postoperative Management Postoperatively, a long-leg nonwalking cast is used for 3 to 4 weeks. At the 3- to 4-week post-op visit, the K-wires are removed in the office, new AFOs (if indicated) are measured, and the child is placed into a short-leg walking cast for an additional 3 to 4 weeks. The cast is generally removed at 6 to 8 weeks postoperatively once bone healing is sufficient.

Complications to Avoid Serious complications are rare with distal tibial osteotomies. Unlike with proximal tibial osteotomies, neurovascular complications appear to be extremely rare, and compartment syndromes have not been reported. Wound complications occur in approximately 5% of children, and deep infections in approximately 1%.

Pearls and Pitfalls

- Rotational osteotomies of the distal tibia are much safer and easier to perform than proximal tibial osteotomies.
- Osteotomy of the fibula is not required, even for correction of at least 45 degrees.

SUMMARY

Optimal treatment of children with CP requires a thorough understanding of normal and abnormal gait. Essential to this is the recognition that abnormalities at the hip, knee, or ankle impact the biomechanical alignment and function at the other levels of the lower extremities. Important examples include the importance of correcting lever arm dysfunction in conjunction with hamstring lengthening to maximize the chance of improving knee extension during stance phase.

The timing of surgery is also of paramount importance. Although many children have ongoing gait deviations, the decision for surgery should be postponed until the child has reached a functional plateau for at least 6 months prior to surgery. Both before and after surgery, spasticity management and appropriate use of physical therapy, home programs, and orthotics are requisite.

Once the decision for surgery has been made, the child's gait must be carefully evaluated. Computerized motion analysis, when available, allows the most in-depth assessment of pathologic gait. Even when computerized motion analysis is not available, however, a thorough examination of static

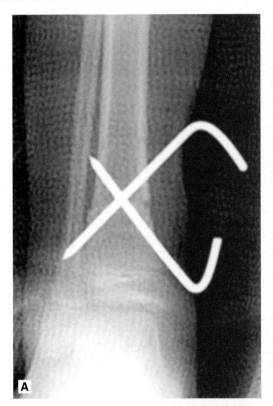

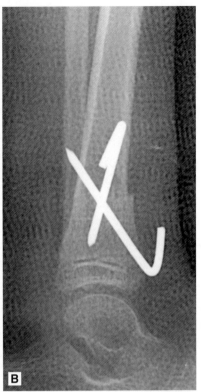

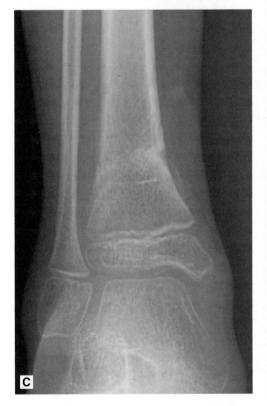

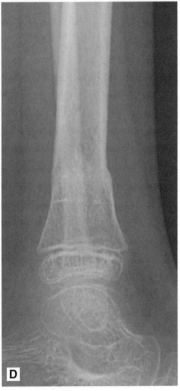

FIGURE 9-24

Radiographs demonstrating tibial rotational osteotomy 4 weeks **(A, B)** and 8 weeks **(C, D)** postoperatively. The radiographs at 4 weeks show appropriate healing and alignment. Hardware was removed at this time, and the child was placed in a short-leg walking cast. The radiographs at 8 weeks demonstrate a healed osteotomy. Casting was discontinued at this time.

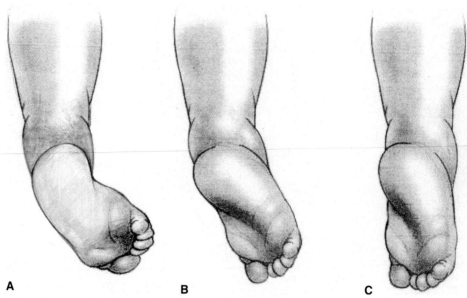

A **B** **C**

FIGURE 9-25 When correcting both a foot deformity as well as tibial torsion, the foot deformity should be corrected first. **A.** Markedly abnormal thigh-foot angle before surgical correction. **B.** Once the foot deformity is corrected, the amount of tibial rotation necessary is evident. **C.** Alignment following tibial rotation.

and dynamic parameters is requisite. Slow-motion videotape analysis of a child's gait may provide useful additional information when a gait lab is not readily accessible.

Single-event multilevel surgery, optimally in conjunction with computerized gait data, has been shown to be safe and effective in children with CP, with consideration given to the impact of surgical intervention at one level on other levels of the lower extremities. Such surgery allows simultaneous correction of multiple deformities, thus optimizing biomechanical alignment. This surgery also results in the need for fewer operations during childhood—with fewer general anesthetics (and its attendant risks), less risk of other iatrogenic adverse events (including adverse drug events), less time off school, fewer recuperative periods, and less psychologic trauma.

REFERENCES

1. Borton DC, Walker K, Pirpiris M, et al. Isolated calf lengthening in cerebral palsy: outcome analysis of risk factors. *J Bone Joint Surg Br.* 2001;83(3):364–370.
2. Evans D. Calcaneo-valgus deformity. *J Bone Joint Surg Br.* 1975;57(3):270–278.
3. Gage JR, Perry J, Hicks RR, et al. Rectus femoris transfer to improve knee function of children with cerebral palsy. *Dev Med Child Neurol.* 1987;29(2):159–166.
4. Gage JR, Schwartz M. Pathological gait and lever-arm dysfunction. In: Gage JR, ed. *The Treatment of Gait Problems in Cerebral Palsy.* Cambridge: Cambridge University Press; 2004:180–204.
5. Kay RM, Dennis S, Rethlefsen S, et al. The effect of preoperative gait analysis on orthopaedic decision making. *Clin Orthop Relat Res.* 2000;372:217–222.
6. Kay RM, Dennis S, Rethlefsen S, et al. Impact of postoperative gait analysis on orthopaedic care. *Clin Orthop Relat Res.* 2000;374:259–264.
7. Kay RM, Rethlefsen SA, Hale JM, et al. Comparison of proximal and distal rotational femoral osteotomy in children with cerebral palsy. *J Pediatr Orthop.* 2003;23(2):150–154.
8. Kay RM, Rethlefsen SA, Skaggs D, et al. Outcome of medial versus combined medial and lateral hamstring lengthening surgery in cerebral palsy. *J Pediatr Orthop.* 2002;22(2):169–172.
9. McMulkin ML, Gulliford JJ, Williamson RV, et al. Correlation of static to dynamic measures of lower extremity range of motion in cerebral palsy and control populations. *J Pediatr Orthop.* 2000;20(3):366–369.
10. Michlitsch MG, Rethlefsen SA, Kay RM. The contributions of anterior and posterior tibialis dysfunction to varus foot deformity in patients with cerebral palsy. *J Bone Joint Surg Am.* 2006;88(8):1764–1768.
11. Mosca VS. Calcaneal lengthening for valgus deformity of the hindfoot: results in children who had severe, symptomatic flatfoot and skewfoot. *J Bone Joint Surg Am.* 1995;77(4):500–512.
12. Ryan DD, Rethlefsen SA, Skaggs DL, et al. Results of tibial rotational osteotomy without concomitant fibular osteotomy in children with cerebral palsy. *J Pediatr Orthop.* 2005;25(1):84–88.
13. Skaggs DL, Kaminsky CK, Eskander-Rickards E, et al. Psoas over the brim lengthenings: anatomic investigation and surgical technique. *Clin Orthop Relat Res.* 1997;339:174–179.
14. White WJ. Torsion of the Achilles tendon: its surgical significance. *Arch Surg Am.* 1943;46:784.
15. Wren TA, Rethlefsen SA, Healy BS, et al. Reliability and validity of visual assessments of gait using a modified physician rating scale for crouch and foot contact. *J Pediatr Orthop.* 2005;25(5):646–650.
16. Wren TA, Rethlefsen S, Kay RM. Prevalence of specific gait abnormalities in children with cerebral palsy: influence of cerebral palsy subtype, age, and previous surgery. *J Pediatr Orthop.* 2005;25(1):79–83.

RECOMMENDED READING

1. Gage JR. Surgical treatment of knee dysfunction in cerebral palsy. *Clin Orthop Relat Res.* 1990;253:45–54.
2. Gage JR. Gait analysis: an essential tool in the treatment of cerebral palsy. *Clin Orthop Relat Res.* 1993;288:126–134.
3. Gage JR, ed. *The Treatment of Gait Problems in Cerebral Palsy.* Cambridge: Cambridge University Press; 2004.
4. Kay RM, Rethlefsen SA, Dennis SW, et al. Prediction of postoperative gait velocity in cerebral palsy. *J Pediatr Orthop Br.* 2001;10:275–278.
5. Kay RM, Rethlefsen SA, Fern-Buneo A, et al. Botulinum toxin as an adjunct to serial casting treatment in children with cerebral palsy. *J Bone Joint Surg Am.* 2004;86:2377–2384.
6. Kay RM, Rethlefsen SA, Kelly JP, et al. Predictive value of the Duncan-Ely test in distal rectus femoris transfer. *J Pediatr Orthop.* 2004;24:59–62.
7. Kay RM, Rethlefsen S, Reed M, et al. Changes in pelvic rotation after soft tissue and bony surgery in ambulatory children with cerebral palsy. *J Pediatr Orthop.* 2004;24:278–282.
8. Kay RM, Rethlefsen SA, Ryan JA, et al. Outcome of gastrocnemius recession and tendo-Achilles lengthening in ambulatory children with cerebral palsy. *J Pediatr Orthop Br.* 2004;13:92–98.
9. Ounpuu S, Muik E, Davis RB, et al. Rectus femoris surgery in children with cerebral palsy. Part II: a comparison between the effect of transfer and release of the distal rectus femoris on knee motion. *J Pediatr Orthop.* 1993;13:331–335.
10. Perry J, ed. *Gait Analysis: Normal and Pathologic Function.* Thorofare, NJ: SLACK Incorporated; 1992.
11. Rethlefsen S, Kay R, Dennis S, et al. The effects of fixed and articulated ankle-foot orthoses on gait patterns in subjects with cerebral palsy. *J Pediatr Orthop.* 1999;19:470–474.
12. Rethlefsen S, Tolo VT, Reynolds RA, et al. Outcome of hamstring lengthening and distal rectus femoris transfer surgery. *J Pediatr Orthop Br.* 1999;8:75–79.
13. Skaggs DL, Rethlefsen SA, Kay RM, et al. Variability in gait analysis interpretation. *J Pediatr Orthop.* 2000;20:759–764.

10 Open Reduction of a Congenital Dislocated Hip and Salter Innominate Osteotomy

Colin F. Moseley

INDICATIONS/CONTRAINDICATIONS

Open reduction is the treatment of choice for congenital hip dislocation after the age of 18 months. Because it is better to leave a hip dislocated than to produce a reduced but dysplastic hip, the surgeon must conclude that there is an age after which the operation is not indicated, probably around 4 or 5 years for bilateral hip dislocation and 8 years for unilateral hip dislocation. The Salter innominate osteotomy should be a routine component of open reduction of congenital hip dislocation, because it redistributes forces and promotes modeling of the acetabulum.

PREOPERATIVE PLANNING

After induction of anesthesia, examination under fluoroscopy is performed to determine the amount of femoral anteversion. The femur is rotated until the femoral neck and the femoral head ossific nucleus line up with the femoral shaft. Femoral anteversion is calculated by subtracting the amount of external rotation required from 90 degrees to obtain this fluoroscope view. Arthrogram prior to open reduction is useless. The acetabulum cannot be visualized because it is filled with pulvinar, and the femoral head is always somewhat out of round. The need for femoral shortening cannot be determined in advance and is not related to the x-ray appearance. Derotation osteotomy is performed when there is more than 50 degrees of femoral anteversion or when the stability of the hip reduction demands it.

SURGICAL PROCEDURE

Setup

The patient is positioned supine on a radiolucent table, with the hip elevated on a bump. The bump should be placed under the iliac crest but not under the buttock to avoid pushing the gluteal muscles up against the hip and limiting exposure of the sciatic notch. The radiolucent table is used to permit examination before surgery and for a later x-ray to check the lengths of the pins used for the Salter osteotomy.

Technique

The surgical procedure will be described as if being performed as the first procedure on the hip of a 2 year old. It should be recognized that secondary procedures are substantially more difficult, because few of the anatomical landmarks are easily identified. The dimensions mentioned must be increased for larger children.

The incision is made 1 cm below the iliac crest and inguinal ligament and should extend about 5 cm (Fig. 10-1) posterior to the anterior superior iliac spine (ASIS) and 3 cm medially to this. The best approach is to think of the superficial exposure in three stages: First, the iliac crest; second, the interval between sartorius and tensor fascia femoris muscles; and third, the middle portion and the lateral femoral cutaneous nerve.

The incision is extended to the iliac crest, retracting the overhanging external oblique muscle if necessary. Some fibers may have to be released from the iliac crest to expose its cartilaginous center. Using the thumb and forefinger as guides, the surgeon incises the iliac apophysis exactly in the middle (Fig. 10-2). Each half of the iliac apophysis can be popped off cleanly with pressure of the thumb in a sponge. The ilium is exposed subperiosteally, and a sponge is packed back into the sciatic notch on each side.

The interval between the sartorius and the tensor fascia lath muscles lies on a straight line between the ASIS and the patella. The deep fascia is incised on that line, starting 15 mm distal to the ASIS (Fig. 10-3). The interval can be recognized by fat around the lateral femoral cutaneous nerve. The nerve passes distally and laterally beneath the still intact part of the deep fascia. The fascia is then incised carefully and the nerve identified, mobilized, and retracted medially (Fig. 10-4).

The bony ridge between the ASIS and anterior inferior iliac spine (AIIS) is now exposed. Unlike the iliac crest, this ridge is sharp and narrow and does not provide an easy target. The experienced surgeon can accomplish this exposure by palpating the AIIS and making one cut from

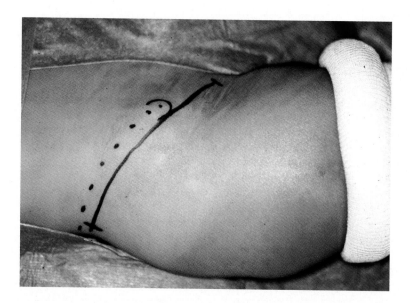

FIGURE 10-1

The incision.

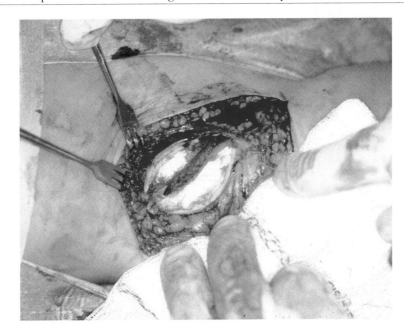

FIGURE 10-2
Exposure of the ilium.

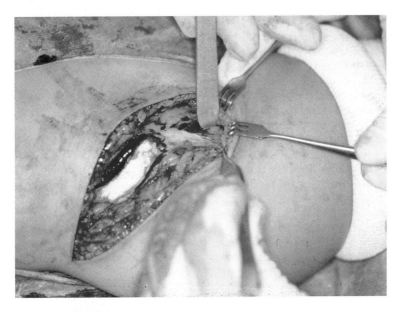

FIGURE 10-3
Developing the distal interval.

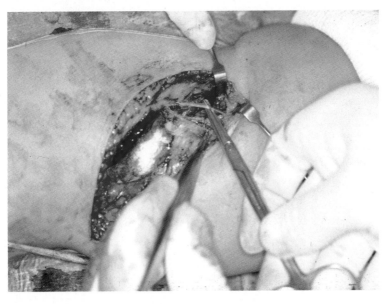

FIGURE 10-4
Exposure of the lateral femoral cutaneous nerve.

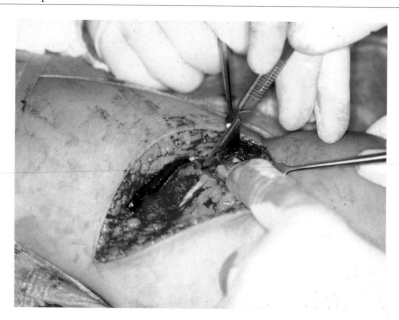

FIGURE 10-5

Exposure of the interspinous ridge.

the AIIS to the ASIS, but most will prefer to make small 2- to 3-mm cuts along the ridge, starting superiorly and elevating the periosteum progressively until the AIIS is reached. The AIIS is recognized as the cartilaginous apophysis of origin of the straight or direct head of the rectus femoris muscle (Fig. 10-5).

The tendon of the straight head of the rectus femoris is immediately obvious in the depth of the interval extending distally from the AIIS. Its medial and lateral borders are identified and the tendon transected as far proximally as possible, preferably at the takeoff of the rectus femoris reflected head, which may not be easily identified because it is incorporated into the false acetabulum. The straight head of the rectus femoris tendon does not need to be tagged, because it does not retract out of the wound.

The iliopsoas muscle comprises the medial wall of the surgical interval, emerging from behind the medial periosteum of the iliac crest. Its tendon lies on the posterior aspect; however, it only begins at the level of the pubis, so the surgeon must look for it rather distally at the pelvic rim. It is identified by rolling the muscle medially on itself to identify the posterior aspect of the muscle and the tendon. When the tendon is visualized, a right-angle clamp can be inserted into the muscle just anterior to the tendon (Fig. 10-6), separating the tendon from the muscle, and can be used to deliver the tendon into the wound, where it can be transected.

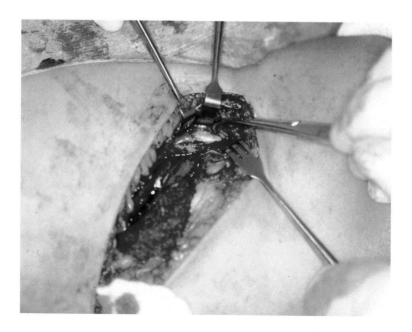

FIGURE 10-6

Releasing the psoas tendon.

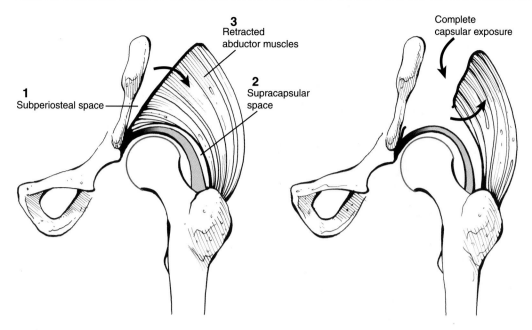

FIGURE 10-7

Exposing the hip capsule.

The hip capsule now constitutes the base of the exposed interval and can be cleaned with an elevator. The goal is to develop two intervals that almost meet medially (Fig. 10-7).

The hip capsule is visible as a smooth, shiny, white layer (Fig. 10-8). Frequently some fibers of the iliopsoas originate from the anterior capsule (the capsulopsoas muscle) and can be cleared off the hip capsule with the elevator.

It is important to develop the superior pericapsular interval and to extend that exposure as far medially as possible, right to the bone at the superior aspect of the false acetabulum. This interval is not easily visualized, particularly with very high-riding femoral heads; therefore, the exposure is done largely by palpation. This layer can be joined to the lateral iliac subperiosteal layer by cutting the intervening tissue with heavy scissors from anterior to posterior (Fig. 10-9).

Attention can then be turned to the anterior and inferior capsule. Exposure is extended as far medially as possible along the pubic ramus, thereby exposing the anterior origin of the hip capsule. This step is extremely important to allow the initial release and later repair of the capsule.

The capsule incision is begun with a scalpel. Once entered, heavy scissors are used to avoid damaging the articular cartilage of the head. The incision is T-shaped, with the stem of the T horizontal (not in line with the neck) and extending from the margin of the acetabulum to a point laterally that will lie at the acetabulum margin once the hip is reduced. The umbrella of the T is immediately along the margin of the acetabulum, extending posteriorly and as far distally as possible.

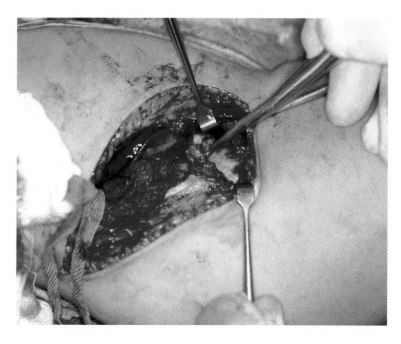

FIGURE 10-8

Developing the pericapsular interval.

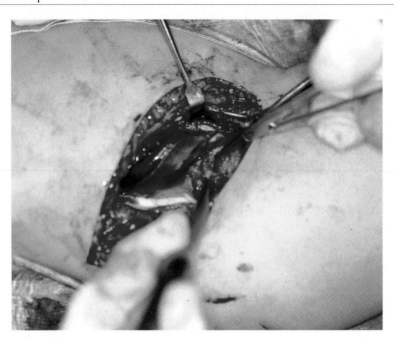

FIGURE 10-9

Exposing the capsule.

In making the superior limb of the incision, the surgeon should inspect the cut edge to be sure that the labrum has not been splayed out beneath the capsule instead of being in its usual location within the acetabulum.

The distal extension of this incision medially is important, as that part of the capsule can constitute a barrier to reduction. It is exposed by balancing the tip of a right-angle retractor on the pubic ramus as far medially as possible (Fig. 10-10), without letting it slip superiorly or inferiorly.

The ligamentum teres ligament is usually the first anatomized structure seen upon opening the hip capsule. It can be hooked with a right-angle clamp and is transected at its insertion on the femoral head, producing a relatively spherical femoral head surface without a prominence (Fig. 10-11). This ligament should then be cleared of peripheral attachments, transected at its origin in the depth of the acetabulum, and removed.

The transverse acetabular ligament is palpated and then transected with scissors while palpating this area. This ligament must be completely released to allow the labrum, to which it is attached at each end, to retract, thereby allowing the acetabulum's entrance to widen for full reduction of the femoral.

Once the transverse acetabular ligament has been released, the labrum needs no further attention. It is a very soft structure and will be extruded out of the way by the reduced femoral head. Some have suggested making radial cuts, but this is not only unnecessary but also ineffective, because the labrum usually has a very wide base and cannot be "folded" out.

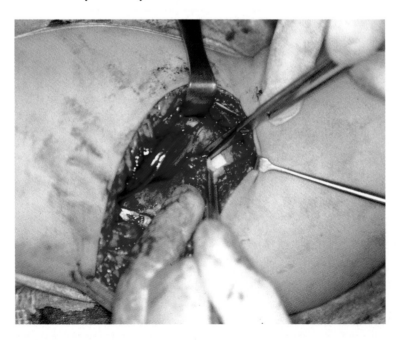

FIGURE 10-10

Opening the capsule.

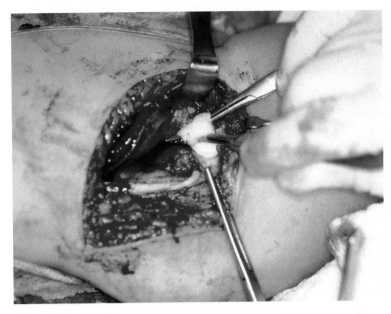

FIGURE 10-11
Excising the ligamentum teres.

The pulvinar is not considered a real obstruction by those who say that it will simply extrude out of the acetabulum when the head is reduced. Others prefer to remove the pulvinar tissue with a rongeur in order to expose the acetabulum's articular cartilage.

Redundant portions of the hip capsule can be trimmed. First the triangular superior flap formed by the T incision can be excised. Second, now that the extent of the false acetabulum can be visualized, the capsule can be elevated from the lateral iliac wing down to the superior margin of the true acetabulum, where the capsule is excised, taking care to avoid the labrum.

The femoral head can now be reduced, usually with a satisfying clunk. The reduction can then be assessed for stability by adducting and extending the hip. The surgeon must take note of the muscular tension generated by the reduction. Because the Salter osteotomy will further increase the tension across the hip joint, a decision must be made about the need for a shortening osteotomy of the femur. Although this will almost never be necessary in the 2-year-old child, the likelihood does increase with older children. The adductor longus tendon can be palpated at this point and, if too tight, can be released percutaneously.

Reference should also be made to the preoperative assessment of femoral anteversion. If this is more than 50 degrees, a derotation femoral osteotomy should be performed, whether or not femoral shortening is required.

In anticipation of the capsulorrhaphy, three heavy, nonabsorbable sutures are placed but not tied (Fig. 10-12A). On the femoral side, they are inserted 2 to 3 mm apart along the superior cut edge of the inferior capsular, with the most lateral suture placed right at the apex, at the most lateral part of the cut edge. On the acetabular side, the sutures are placed a few millimeters apart, with the medial

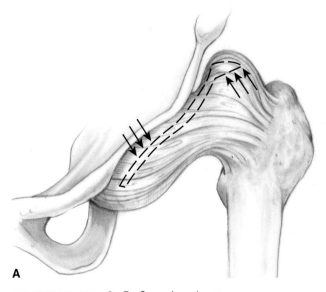

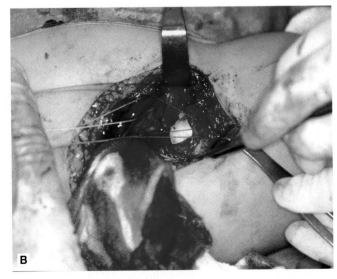

FIGURE 10-12   A, B. Capsule sutures.

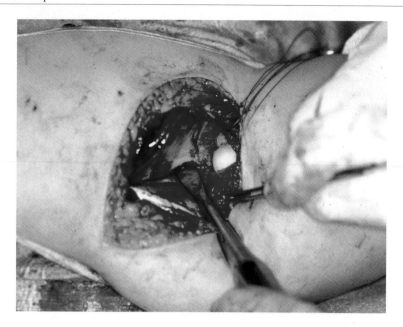

FIGURE 10-13

Preparing for the Salter osteotomy.

one being placed as far medially as possible (Fig. 10-12B). Placement of this medial suture requires superior retraction along the pubic ramus.

To prepare for the Salter innominate osteotomy, a channel for passing a Gigli saw is developed, using a periosteal elevator into the sciatic notch from both the medial and lateral aspects (Fig. 10-13).

Chandler retractors are placed in the sciatic notch. To the surgeon, the notch appears farther away on the lateral aspect than on the medial (Fig. 10-14). This is because on the medial side, the surgeon is looking at the pelvic brim and not at the actual notch. Remembering this will facilitate passage of the saw.

Twisting the Chandler retractors provides a space for the Gigli saw (Fig. 10-15). The best strategy is to start on the medial aspect and aim the tip of the saw at the lateral retractor so that it strikes and then rides up its blade. Alternatively, one can use special channeled retractors designed by Mercer Rang that, when placed in the notch, facilitate passage of the saw. When the Gigli saw appears laterally, it can be grasped and pulled through (Fig. 10-16).

Before beginning the cut, the limbs of the saw should be oriented transversely so that the plane between the limbs intersects the pelvis at the desired point of anterior exit of the cut, just at the top of the AIIS (Fig. 10-17). This should be a straight cut to facilitate fitting the bone wedge.

A wedge of bone is cut from the anterior part of the iliac crest that includes the ASIS and the interspinous ridge (Fig. 10-18). A triangular wedge of about 30 degrees with straight sides is fashioned from this bone (Fig. 10-19).

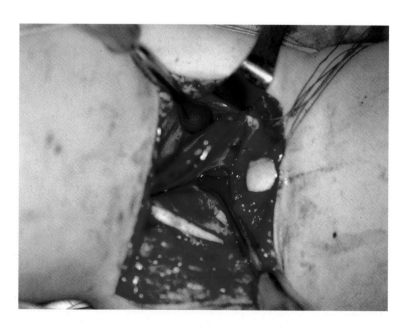

FIGURE 10-14

Providing access to the sciatic notch.

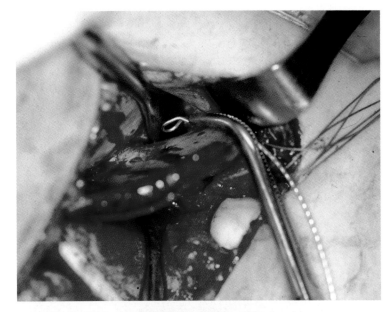

FIGURE 10-15
Passing the Gigli saw.

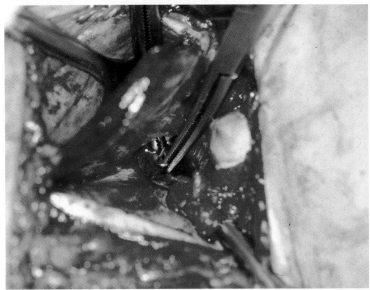

FIGURE 10-16
Delivering the Gigli saw.

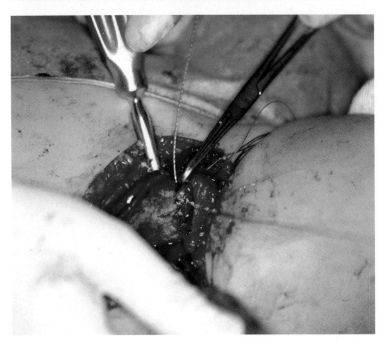

FIGURE 10-17
Making the pelvic cut.

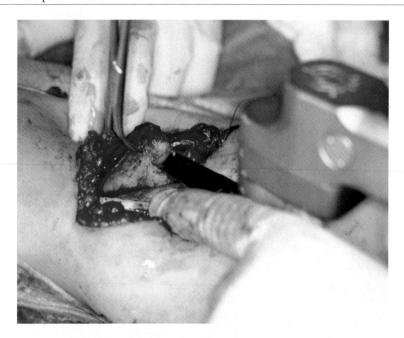

FIGURE 10-18
Cutting the wedge.

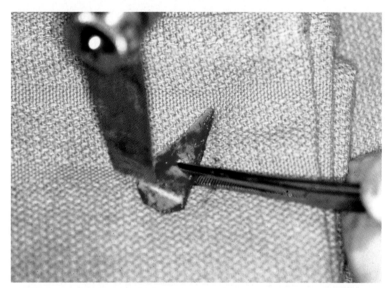

FIGURE 10-19
Shaping the wedge.

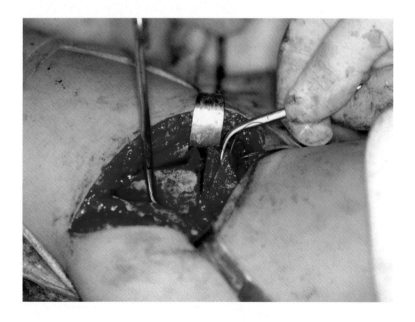

FIGURE 10-20
Opening the pelvic
osteotomy.

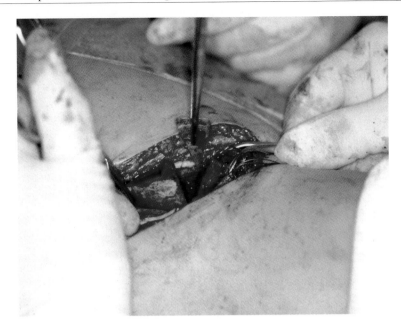

FIGURE 10-21
Inserting the wedge.

Two sharp towel clips are applied to the pelvis. The upper clip can be applied so that its crotch impinges on the crest, allowing it to function as a lever. The lower clip is placed deep to the AIIS on the inferior hemipelvis (Fig. 10-20). Care should be taken to place the inferior towel clip through bone and not just through the apophysis to avoid separation from the underlying bone when traction is applied. The wedge is opened by exerting traction on the lower clip and leverage on the upper one. Forward displacement of the lower segment improves the axis of rotation and thereby the coverage achieved by the redirection.

The bone wedge should be gently placed into the gap (Fig. 10-21). Forcing it in only serves to separate the fragments without gaining the necessary rotational correction. The cut surface of the pelvis is much broader than the graft. Therefore, the graft should be placed as far medially as possible to minimize the chance that the pins used for fixation will intrude into the acetabulum. Lengthening at the medial margin of the osteotomy should be avoided.

The graft is fixed in place by two threaded pins. The first pin engages only the very tip of the superior pelvic segment but passes through the middle of the graft. The second, more superior pin achieves better purchase of the pelvic segment but passes near the tip of the wedge (Fig. 10-22). Both pins pass into the distal pelvis medially and posteriorly to the acetabulum.

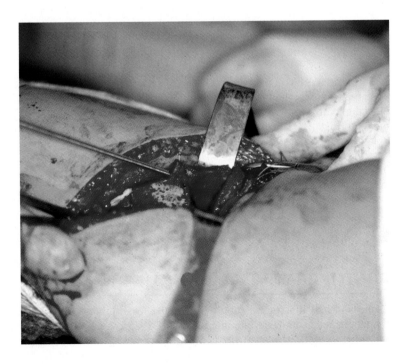

FIGURE 10-22
Pin fixation.

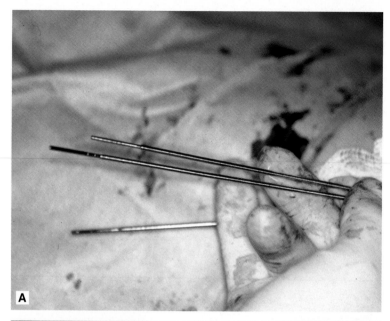

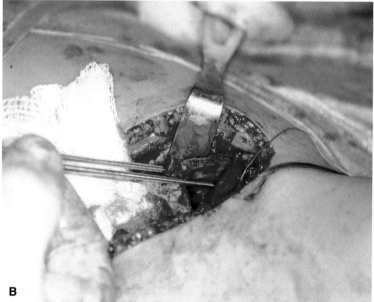

FIGURE 10-23

A, B. Ensuring correct pin depth.

The desired depth of pin penetration is to, but not through, the triradiate cartilage. In the 2-year-old child, this depth is about 12 to 13 mm into the distal segment. Determining how far the pin has penetrated into the distal segment is a simple, quick procedure: Use pins that have a smooth, unthreaded butt end (Fig. 10-23A). Mount the pin so that the shoulder (the transition between the threaded and nonthreaded portions) is visible. After insertion of the first pin, place a similar pin alongside the first, with the tip at the level of the cut surface of the distal segment (Fig. 10-23B). The relative displacement of the shoulders of the two pins shows the depth of penetration into the distal segment. An x-ray is taken to assess depth of penetration, and the pins are adjusted accordingly. The pins are then cut off at the bone. The capsulorrhaphy is then completed by tying the previously placed capsule sutures.

The iliac crest is closed using a vertical double throw stitch to ensure good apposition of the cut surfaces. The deep fascia is closed with care to avoid entrapping any fibers of the lateral femoral cutaneous nerve.

POSTOPERATIVE MANAGEMENT

A one-and-half hip spica is applied with the leg in about 20 degrees of flexion, 30 degrees of abduction, and neutral or slight internal rotation. Care is taken to produce a good cast mold posterior and superior to the greater trochanter. The spica is worn for 3 months.

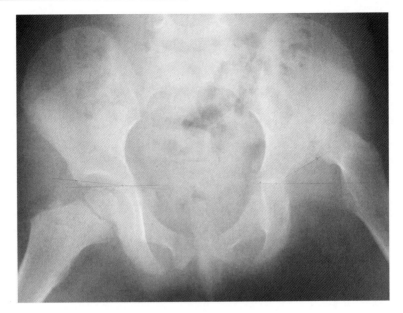

FIGURE 10-24

The x-ray shows a shallow acetabulum, an absent teardrop, a blunt acetabular lip, and a small femoral ossific nucleus.

COMPLICATIONS TO AVOID

The most serious complication is redislocation of the femoral head. This risk can be minimized by careful application of the spica cast, achieving the mold with plaster instead of fiberglass. The patient is maintained in a supine position and never in a prone, sitting, or vertical position. This prevents the child's weight from being born by the thighs on the legs of the cast, which can push the hips up and out, risking dislocation. For younger patients who are not toilet trained, parents must make a supreme effort to keep the cast clean and dry. Not doing so can lead to severe skin problems and could necessitate anesthesia to replace the cast.

ILLUSTRATIVE CASE

A girl presented at the age of $3^1/_2$ years with a dislocated left hip (Fig. 10-24). It was evident when she first began to walk that her gait was abnormal, but she had received no prior treatment.

She underwent an open reduction, Salter osteotomy, and shortening osteotomy of the femur (Figs. 10-25 and 10-26).

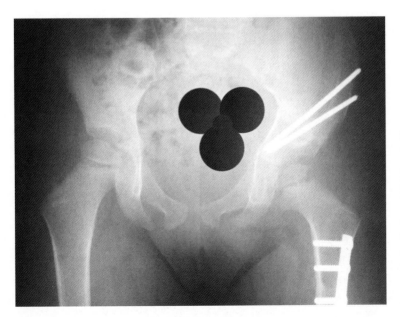

FIGURE 10-25

This x-ray was taken 1 year after the procedure, at the age of $4^1/_2$ years. The femoral head is deeply reduced and well covered. In the usual course of events, the femoral plate would have been removed at about this time.

FIGURE 10-26

This is the follow-up x-ray at the age of 6 years, 2¹/₂ years after the open reduction. Note that the femoral head, although deeply reduced in the acetabulum, is somewhat lateralized with respect to the pelvis due to the widened teardrop, which represents the thickened medial wall of the acetabulum.

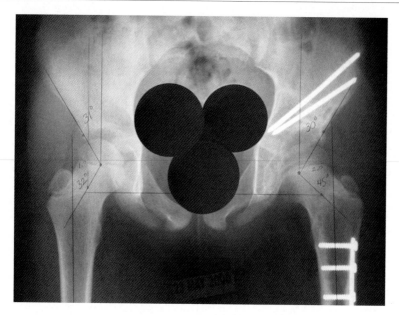

At the age of 11 years, she was functioning normally with no limp, pain, or disability. The hip looks excellent radiologically (Fig. 10-27).

PEARLS AND PITFALLS

- The lateral femoral cutaneous nerve must be retracted medially. Because it exits the pelvis beneath the inguinal ligament and the origin of that ligament has been moved medially, the nerve should also be retracted medially.
- The stem of the T-shaped incision into the capsule must be superior enough, because the inferior flap is used in the repair.
- Careful attention should be paid to the release of the anteroinferior capsule. Although this can be difficult to access, failure to adequately release the capsule can leave an obstruction to reduction.

FIGURE 10-27

The ossific nucleus has formed well, with no evidence of avascular necrosis, and the head appears spherical and congruent. The center edge angle measures 30 degrees.

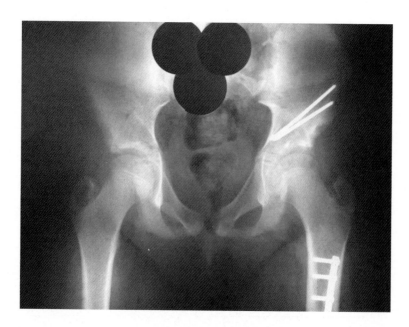

- At the time of the trial reduction, the surgeon must assess the need for femoral shortening. Some tension is required to maintain the reduction, but excessive tension can lead to avascular necrosis.
- Because the Salter osteotomy moves the capsular origin from the pubic ramus more distal and makes it harder to access, the sutures for the capsulorrhaphy should be placed before the innominate osteotomy is done.

REFERENCES

1. Akagi S, Tanabe T, Ogawa R, et al. Acetabular development after open reduction for developmental dislocation of the hip. 15-year follow-up of 22 hips without additional surgery. *Acta Orthop Scand.* 1998;69(1):17–20.
2. Albinana J, Dolan LA, Spratt KF, et al. Acetabular dysplasia after treatment for developmental dysplasia of the hip: implications for secondary procedures. *J Bone Joint Surg Br.* 2004;86(6):876–886.
3. Crawford AH, Mehlman CT, Slover RW, et al. The fate of untreated developmental dislocation of the hip: long-term follow-up of eleven patients. *J Pediatr Orthop.* 1999;19(5):641–644.
4. Galpin RD, Roach JW, Wenger DR, et al. One-stage treatment of congenital dislocation of the hip in older children, including femoral shortening. *J Bone Joint Surg Am.* 1989;71(5):734–741.
5. Haidar RK, Jones RS, Vergroesen DA, et al. Simultaneous open reduction and Salter innominate osteotomy for developmental dysplasia of the hip. *J Bone Joint Surg Br.* 1996;78(3):471–476.
6. Salter RB. Role of innominate osteotomy in the treatment of congenital dislocation and subluxation of the hip in the older child. *J Bone Joint Surg.* 1966;48A:1413.
7. Zionts LE, MacEwen GD. Treatment of congenital dislocation of the hip in children between the ages of one and three years. *J Bone Joint Surg Am.* 1986;68(6):829–846.

11 Dega Acetabuloplasty

Paul D. Sponseller

Professor W. Dega, working in Poznan, Poland, described an incomplete iliac osteotomy in 1969.[2,3] Reported just a few years after Pemberton's osteotomy, the Dega osteotomy was part of a continuum of incomplete osteotomies that also include the Pembersal and the San Diego osteotomy.[1,2,3] These osteotomies correct the acetabulum while hinging on portions of the symphysis pubis and the triradiate cartilage (Fig. 11-1). Because of this second point of hinging, these osteotomies have the potential to not only reorient the acetabulum but also to reshape it. They differ in the extent of the bone cut on the inner and outer tables of the acetabulum—the extent of the remaining hinge. The Pemberton cuts both the inner and the outer tables of the ilium, and hinges on the ischial limb of the triradiate cartilage. The Pembersal extends past the ischial limb of the triradiate cartilage, freeing the acetabulum to rotate more. The San Diego osteotomy preserves the entire medial cortex and cuts through the cortical bone of the sciatic notch in an attempt to produce equal anterior and posterior coverage.[3]

The Dega osteotomy, the subject of this chapter, preserves the inner table of the pelvis posterior to the iliopectineal line. It also preserves the entire cortex of the sciatic notch. The amount of intact medial cortex determines the direction of rotation of the acetabulum.

INDICATIONS

The Dega has been described primarily for use in developmental dysplasia of the hip, a condition in which the posterior portion of the acetabulum is far better developed than the anterior portion. However, some patients with neuromuscular dysplasia or skeletal dysplasia (such as spondyloepiphyseal dysplasia or Morquio syndrome) may also be candidates for this procedure if the coverage needed is primarily anterolateral.[1,2,3,4] The lower age limit for the osteotomy is primarily determined by bone quality, which must be strong enough (on the younger end) to support the hinge process yet not too stiff (on the older end) to hinge plastically. For the bone to be adequately plastic, the triradiate cartilage should ideally be open. Therefore, the ideal age range is approximately between 2 and 12 years. Dega is also ideal for bilateral procedures, because the stress on the symphysis pubis is probably less than that from a complete iliac osteotomy.

CONTRAINDICATIONS

Patients with an acetabulum that is too small to adequately contain the femoral head, even after reorientation, should be treated by another procedure, such as a shelf arthroplasty or Chiari Osteotomy. Patients with extreme osteopenia may not tolerate the reorientation without settling and loosening the interference fixation.

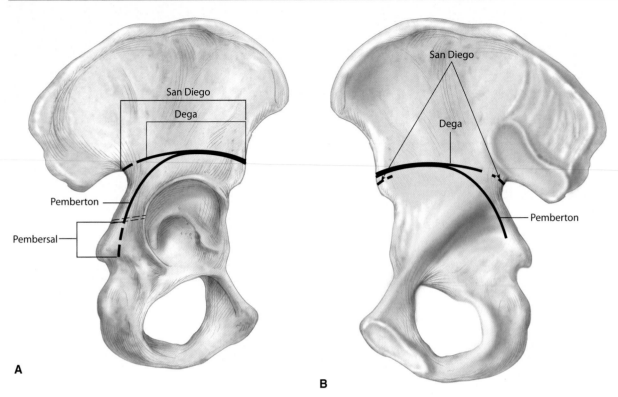

FIGURE 11-1 Comparison of Dega, Pemberton, Pembersal, and San Diego. **A.** View from lateral aspect of pelvis. **B.** View from medial aspect of pelvis.

PREOPERATIVE PLANNING

The range of hip flexion should be assessed. If flexion is less than 90 degrees preoperatively, it will only worsen after surgery and may limit the patient's ability to sit. The rotation and resting position of the hip should also be assessed. The acetabuloplasty tends to produce some apparent external rotation (10–20 degrees), which can be compensated for by additional internal rotation of the femur if an osteotomy of this bone is also being performed.

Imaging consists of an anteroposterior radiograph of the pelvis. An abduction–internal rotation radiograph, taken with the hip in extension, will also give an idea of the degree of potential coverage and possibly the need to perform an open reduction.

Some surgeons like to obtain a preoperative three-dimensional computed tomogram to assess the acetabular pathology. Others feel that this information can be gained intraoperatively by fluoroscopy, inspection, and noting the response of the acetabulum to redirection.

SURGICAL PROCEDURE

The patient is placed supine, with the pelvis on a fluorolucent table. Slight elevation of the involved hemipelvis may be produced by placing a "bump" under the iliosacral region. If both sides are to be operated on at one session, a square towel under the sacrum will elevate them both. The fluoroscope should be positioned over the patient from the opposite side.

The incision described by Dega extends from a point inferior to the anterior superior iliac spine (ASIS) and proceeds posteriorly and inferiorly.[2] Alternatively, the straight "bikini" incision described by Salter can be used in the skin tension lines that run obliquely from posterosuperior to anteroinferior to the ASIS. This incision produces a cosmetically superior result, with no sacrifice in operative exposure. The lateral femoral cutaneous nerve, which is identified under the fascia lata, is freed and retracted medially. The tensor-sartorius interval is developed up to the ASIS. The iliac apophysis is split as far along the iliac crest as possible, allowing exposure for eventual bone graft if autograft is desired.

In the depths of the tensor-sartorius interval, the lateral femoral circumflex vessels should be sought and coagulated. The lateral surface of the ilium should be exposed. Bleeding from bony nutrient foramen should be stopped. Some surgeons prefer subperiosteal exposure of the inner table of the ilium as well to prevent inadvertent harm to structures during cutting of the medial wall with

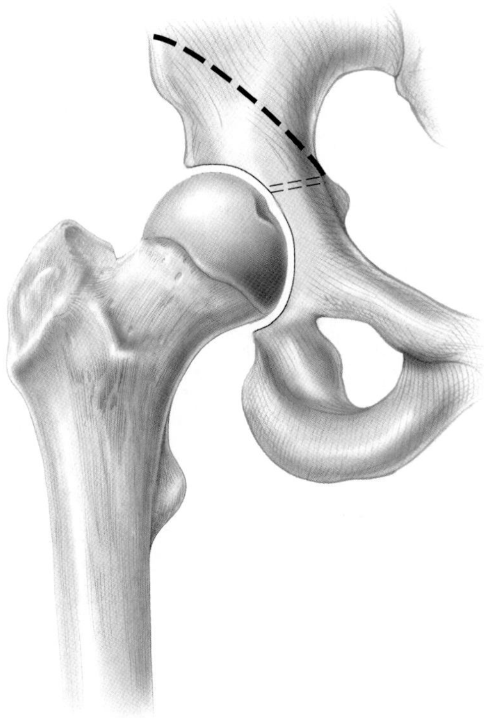

FIGURE 11-2
Outline of fluoroscopic view of cut for Dega osteotomy.

the osteotome. If a capsulorrhaphy is indicated, the tendon of the rectus femoris muscle should be tagged and detached. If a capsulorrhaphy is not needed, the tendon may be left intact. The exposure on the medial surface of the ilium should extend at least to the iliopectineal line so that the extent of the osteotomy may be visualized.

The level and direction of the osteotomy is then marked by a Steinmann pin. The pin should be just cephalad to the anterior inferior iliac spine (AIIS) and directed caudally to the medial end of the triradiate cartilage (Fig. 11-2). Enough cortex (at least 1–1.5 cm in a 4 year old) must be left above the acetabulum to prevent the supra-acetabular bone from deforming when the segment is levered down. The osteotomy is initiated with a 1/4-in. osteotome. After one complete pass of the osteotome, additional cuts are continued anteriorly and posteriorly to the initial pass. On the lateral surface of the ilium, these cuts, which preserve the cortex of the sciatic notch, outline a semicircular path. These cuts can be controlled by using a curved osteotome from anterior to posterior with a downward orientation of the handle as viewed from the front. As the osteotomy becomes complete, the surgeon should test the malleability of the acetabulum by levering downward with a 1/2-in. osteotome.

When the acetabulum is sufficiently mobile, the correction is imaged with an osteotome levering down on the acetabulum. If the correction is adequate, the size of the desired bone graft is estimated. It is a scalene triangle with an obtuse angle between the base and the caudal surface. Usually the base is between 1 and 2 cm (Fig. 11-3). The bone graft must be large enough and properly sized to be intrinsically stable when wedged into the ilium. The source of the bone graft is typically one or more of the following, depending on the surgeon's preference: A set of tricortical wedges from the ipsilateral iliac crest, a wedge of bone resulting from concomitant shortening osteotomy of the ipsilateral femur, or a single structural allograft. If autologous iliac grafts are used, there must be more than one to maintain intrinsic stability, and they should be placed next to each other to prevent tilting.

If an open reduction of the hip with capsulorrhaphy is performed as part of the procedure, it is easier to close the capsule before inserting the graft in the osteotomy. Once the osteotomy is opened, the capsule is pushed inferiorly out of direct view. Thus, it is easier to judge the position of the femoral head and the approximation of the capsule before graft insertion.

One challenge during graft insertion is to lever open the osteotomy site while maintaining an open space for the graft. It may be preferable to place two small threaded Steinmann pins before opening the osteotomy (Fig. 11-4), with one pin perpendicular to the outer cortex and the other anterior to it and inferior to the osteotomy. The pins should form a 20- to 25-degree angle. The osteotomy is levered open using a broad osteotome. It is held open with a toothed laminar spreader while the osteotome is removed. This opens up the entire area to access for inserting the bone graft(s). The graft(s) are wedged into place and gently tamped so that the cortical surface of the wedge is aligned with that of the lower osteotomy segment. If it is too far inside the osteotomy site, the bone will subside into the cancellous surface. If it is outside, extrusion is possible. Once the graft is in place, the Steinmann pins should be approximately parallel. The graft is then tested for stability. It should not

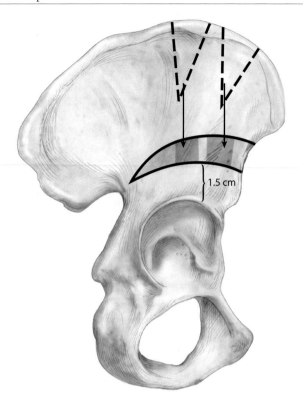

1.5 cm

FIGURE 11-3

Dega osteotomy with grafts wedged in place.

be able to be pulled out or tilted. The pins may then be removed. Any additional loose cancellous graft is packed in the available open osteotomy surface. The iliac apophyseal cartilage is reapproximated, restoring a normal contour to the ilium. The incision is closed in the usual fashion.

After all portions of the procedure are complete, it is a good idea to take an anteroposterior pelvic radiograph with the surgical drapes removed. A spica cast is then applied. Flexing the hips in the cast facilitates care.

POSTOPERATIVE MANAGEMENT

The patient is kept non–weight bearing on the operated side for 6 weeks. The cast is then removed and range of movement is allowed. Depending on the incorporation of the graft, weight bearing is allowed at the surgeon's discretion.

COMPLICATIONS

Serious complications are rare with this osteotomy. Overzealous opening of the osteotomy may lead to loss of the medial hinge and loss of angular correction. Harvesting of an iliac crest graft too close to the osteotomy may result in cracking of the ilium. A graft that is not strong enough may deform. If several grafts are inserted, they should all be under compression so that one does not back out. If the graft is inserted too far medially, it may collapse into the surrounding cancellous bone. Cortical contact is important.

Insufficient correction of the underlying acetabular pathology is a possibility. Options include using a larger wedge, correction via femoral osteotomy, or addition of an acetabular shelf augmentation at the time of surgery.

Finally, there is a suggestion that excessive pressure on the femoral head from an iliac osteotomy may result in avascular necrosis (AVN) of the femoral head.[3,5] It is difficult to separate the influence of reducing dislocation from the pressure of the osteotomy itself. In addition, the triradiate cartilage may be affected by the osteotomy, either through leverage forces or crack propagation. The incidence of functionally significant alteration in growth seems to be very low.

ILLUSTRATIVE CASE

This 5$\frac{1}{2}$-year-old girl presented with bilateral untreated developmental dysplasia of the hip after being recently adopted from abroad (Fig. 11-5A). She had a significant Trendelenburg gait. Bilateral one-stage open reduction of the dislocated hips was performed. The femora osteotomies

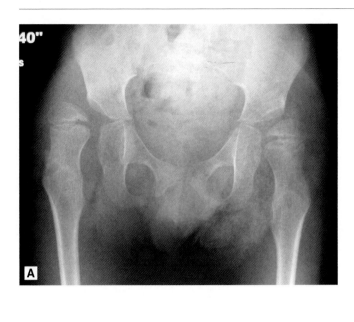

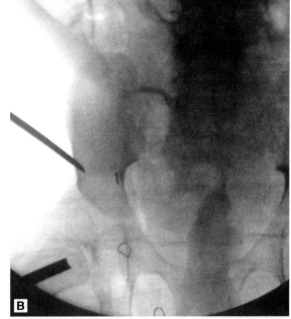

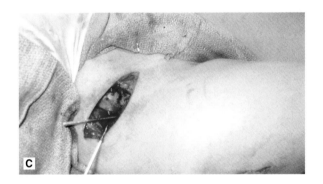

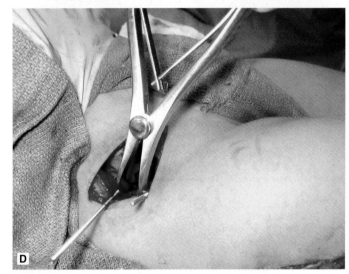

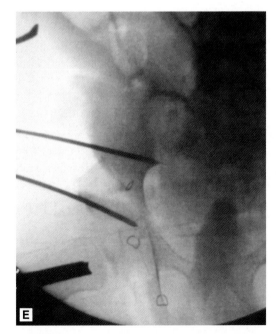

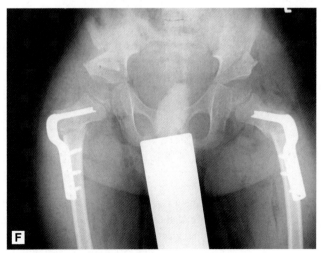

FIGURE 11-4   Dega osteotomy in child with cerebral palsy. **A.** Preoperative radiograph. **B.** Initial location and direction for osteotomy. **C.** Threaded Steinmann pins in place to facilitate graft insertion. **D.** Laminar spreader maintaining osteotomy for graft insertion after it has been opened. **E.** Graft in place. **F.** Postoperative radiograph.

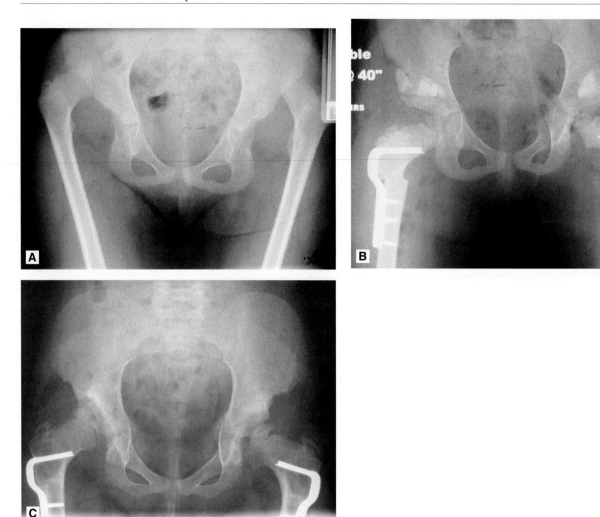

FIGURE 11-5   Dega osteotomy in $5^1/_2$-year-old girl with developmental dysplasia of the hips.
A. Preoperative radiograph illustrating upsloping acetabular sourcil. **B.** Immediate postoperative
reduction with graft from femoral osteotomies. **C.** One-year post-op. Note some graft subsidence
on right.

involved 1.5 cm of shortening. The bone graft was used for the Dega osteotomies. Satisfactory
reduction was achieved, and the acetabulum was corrected to a stable shelf with a horizontal sourcil
with the Dega (Fig. 11-5B). One year later (Fig. 11-5C), proximal femoral growth was preserved.
Some subsidence of the osteotomy was seen on the right.

PEARLS AND PITFALLS

- Have allograft bone in reserve.
- Complete a capsulorrhaphy before final graft insertion.
- Use threaded Steinmann pins to hold the osteotomy once it is opened.
- The bone graft must be structurally stable.
- The outer graft cortex should line up with the cortex of the surrounding bone.
- Preserve an adequate medial hinge to maintain compression across the osteotomy.
- Do not overcorrect the acetabulum.
- Do not allow the osteotome to pass too far through the medial cortex of the ilium to avoid injury
  to surrounding structures, such as the deep femoral artery.

EDITOR'S NOTE

One of the most appealing aspects of the Dega osteotomy is that the direction of increased acetabular coverage may be chosen intraoperatively by choosing where to leave intact ilium to act as a hinge. As Dr. Sponseller describes in this chapter, by leaving intact the sciatic notch, as well as the posterior half of the medial table, anterior and lateral coverage may be obtained. If one desires more posterior coverage, the osteotomy may extend through the sciatic notch, leaving the midportion of the medial iliac table intact to act as a hinge. In this instance, the sciatic notch should be subperiosteally dissected and protected the inner and outer tables with Chandler retractors. Although this may technically be considered a San Diego osteotomy, these two osteotomies are along a continuum in my mind. DLS

REFERENCES

1. Coleman SS. The subluxating or wandering femoral head in developmental dislocation of the hip. *J Pediatr Orthop.* 1995;15(6):785–788.
2. Grudziak JS, Ward WT. Dega osteotomy for the treatment of congenital dysplasia of the hip. *J Bone Joint Surg Am.* 2001;83A(6):845–854.
3. McNerney NP, Mubarak SJ, Wenger DS. One-stage correction of the dysplastic hip in cerebral palsy with the San Diego acetabuloplasty: results and complications in 104 hips. *J Pediatr Orthop.* 2000;20(1):93–103.
4. Ozgur AF, Aksoy MC, Kandemir U, et al. Does Dega osteotomy increase acetabular volume in developmental dysplasia of the hip? *J Pediatr Orthop Br.* 2006;15(2):83–86.
5. Ruszkowski K, Pucher A. Simultaneous open reduction and Dega transiliac osteotomy for developmental dislocation of the hip in children under 24 months of age. *J Pediatr Orthop.* 2005;25(5):695–701.

12 Varus Derotation Osteotomy of Proximal Femur

Vernon T. Tolo

A proximal femoral osteotomy is commonly used to treat a variety of abnormal conditions of the hip by realigning the femoral head within the acetabulum. This procedure can be used at any age but is seldom performed before 1 year of age. Although proximal femoral osteotomy may be done alone, it is commonly combined with other surgical procedures under the same anesthesia. Intraoperative dynamic arthrography of the hip is usually used to help determine the optimal position of the femoral head within the acetabulum, particularly if there is incomplete ossification of the proximal femoral epiphysis. The need for casting after proximal femoral osteotomy is determined by the stability of proximal femoral fixation, cooperativeness of the child, age of the child, or the need to stretch soft tissues that have been lengthened as an adjunctive procedure to the femoral osteotomy.

INDICATIONS/CONTRAINDICATIONS

The most common indications for a proximal femoral varus derotation osteotomy (VDO) occur in children with developmental dysplasia of the hip (DDH), hip subluxation, or dislocation associated with spastic cerebral palsy (CP). VDO is also used for the surgical treatment of Legg-Perthes disease and of hip subluxation or dislocation related to many genetic and neuromuscular disorders too numerous to individually mention. In all of these conditions, the proximal femoral varus osteotomy is customized to address the specific hip problem present. Although the exact manner in which the VDO is performed for a specific patient may vary, the principles are constant in each operative procedure. The goals of proximal femoral osteotomy include improvement of hip motion, improvement in the distribution of forces across the hip to allow more normal hip development and growth, and prevention of premature degenerative articular cartilage changes.

Proximal femoral varus osteotomy is contraindicated in CP patients with long-standing hip dislocation, which is commonly associated with extensive articular cartilage erosion and flattening of the femoral head. This malformation of the femoral head is secondary to many years of contact between the femoral head and the lateral iliac wing. The coincident articular cartilage erosions seem to be a major source of hip pain in these spastic individuals. If a malformed femoral head with articular cartilage erosions to subchondral bone is placed into the acetabulum, hip pain and motion worsen, and further hip surgery is nearly always needed soon thereafter. In these patients, surgical procedures that are better than a VDO would include a femoral head and neck resection with muscle or implant interposition or a Schanz proximal femoral valgus osteotomy with or without femoral head resection.

There may be a relative contraindication for VDO in patients with Legg-Perthes disease. In ambulatory children and adolescents, it is preferable not to create a proximal femoral neck-shaft angle of less than 115 to 120 degrees, as this may weaken the hip abductors sufficiently to cause a persistent Trendelenburg gait. In patients with Legg-Perthes disease, when the femoral head is flattened somewhat, the neck-shaft angle tends to be about 130 to 135 degrees. If more than 20 degrees of varus is needed to contain or cover the lateral femoral head, a VDO alone may result in a femoral neck-shaft angle of less than 110 degrees. In such cases, therefore, consideration should be given to use of a shelf arthroplasty or a combination of a limited VDO and shelf arthroplasty. Remodeling the femoral neck-shaft angle into more valgus will occur in younger individuals who have a normal proximal femoral phsis, including young patients with spastic CP. This remodeling into valgus is not present in most patients with Legg-Perthes disease due to the proximal femoral physeal involvement and the age at which surgical treatment is usually performed.

PREOPERATIVE PLANNING

The majority of patients in whom a VDO is used either present to the orthopaedist with a limp (with or without pain) when walking or are nonambulatory children and teenagers with neuromuscular disorders, mainly spastic CP. A delay in the diagnosis of hip dislocation until walking age still occurs more often than would be hoped and is often the reason for a painless limp in a young child who has been walking only a short time. Birth history factors that increase the chance of a hip dislocation at birth include breech presentation, a family history of DDH in the mother or siblings, and being firstborn.

Whereas children with DDH often have few or no coexisting medical conditions that may have an impact on surgical treatment with a VDO, those with hip dysplasia associated with CP and other neuromuscular disorders always have coexisting medical conditions. As a part of the medical history, therefore, it is important to determine whether the child has been, and is being, treated for seizures, gastroesophageal reflux, pulmonary compromise, or a cardiac disorder, all of which are common in children and teenagers with spastic quadriplegia CP. Prior to a VDO, the preanesthesia evaluation will commonly include consultation with a pulmonologist; evaluation by a cardiologist, including an echocardiogram; and discussion with the neurologist supervising the seizure treatment. Seizure medications are continued up to the time just before surgery and are reinstituted as soon as possible postoperatively.

Physical examination is important to help determine the planes of correction needed at the time of the VDO. The gait is observed in those children who walk. If pain is present, the painful leg will have a shorter stance phase as part of the antalgic gait. Look for a Trendelenburg gait, in which the child leans over the affected hip when standing on that leg; this finding indicates hip abductor weakness associated with nearly all chronic hip disorders. Leg length discrepancy is checked with the child standing and by observing the superior iliac wing level on each side. A Trendelenburg test is done in the same position by having the child stand on one leg at a time while the orthopaedist observes the pelvic movement. Hip motion in three planes, six directions should be measured and recorded. With DDH, if the hip is fully dislocated, motion of the affected hip will be limited in abduction, but other planes of motion are often normal. If there is hip pain or Legg-Perthes disease, hip internal rotation with the patient in the prone position is the first plane of motion lost and is the most useful examination to detect early hip problems. Flexion and extension of the hip is usually preserved relatively well even when there is a moderate to severe hip disorder present.

Careful notation prior to surgery of hip range of motion is needed when planning the VDO. Because the proximal femoral osteotomy can correct abnormalities in three planes (varus/valgus, rotation, and flexion/extension) through a single bone cut, the final goal of the surgery is to realign the femoral head congruently with the acetabulum, as well as to align the limb distal to the osteotomy in the same plane as the opposite side so that the foot progression angle is the same bilaterally when the ambulatory child is walking after surgery.

In patients with neuromuscular disorders, the physical examination differs somewhat from that used with DDH patients. Most neuromuscular disease patients for whom a VDO is used have spastic quadriplegia or diplegia forms of CP, but a smaller number have disorders with low muscle tone. With spastic quadriplegia patients, associated scoliosis and pelvic obliquity are common, require ongoing assessment, and need to be treated often, as does the hip dysplasia. Patients with CP are nearly always born with their hips well located. However, the hips may gradually subluxate or dislocate during growth due to excessive muscle tone and contractures in the hip adductor and flexor muscles. If a unilateral hip subluxation or dislocation occurs, the legs drift into a "windswept" position, with one hip adducted and the other abducted. If this windswept position is treated relatively early (before the age of 5 or so) with hip adductor and psoas tenotomies to allow for the restitution of hip symmetry, progressive hip subluxation or dislocation can often be prevented, thereby avoiding the need for a VDO as part of the surgical treatment. If hip subluxation or dislocation is present past the age of 5, it is usually necessary to perform a VDO, in addition to the adductor and psoas tenotomies, to keep the femoral head located in the acetabulum. If hip subluxation or dislocation is bilateral, both hips should be treated at the same operative session.

In older children and teenagers with a windswept position, x-rays may show subluxation on one side (the adducted hip) and a well-located hip on the other side (abducted hip). The subluxated hip will require at least adductor and psoas tenotomies with a VDO to relocate the femoral head. Although the x-ray demonstrates that the abducted hip has a well-located femoral head, it is common for this hip to have an abduction contracture, which prevents the hip from being brought to a neutral position or into an adducted position. If this physical finding is present, a VDO is needed on the abducted hip as well as on the adducted hip to allow both legs and hips to be brought to a neutral position for wheelchair sitting. If there is a fixed abduction hip contracture present that is not treated with a VDO, the patient will quickly redevelop a windswept position after the contralateral VDO and tenotomies have been performed, which can lead to a consequent risk of redislocation of the adducted hip.

Low muscle tone can lead to hip subluxation in some children with muscle disorders or in CP patients who have had selective dorsal rhizotomy. Hip motion is usually not limited in this group of children, with abduction common to 90 degrees, normal internal and external rotation, and full flexion. If the child is not walking and spends the whole day in the wheelchair, there may be some flexion contractures. On examination, the hips can often be subluxated and relocated with minimal effort, a maneuver that is usually painless. If hip subluxation or dislocation worsens, VDO may be indicated. If a VDO is done in nonambulatory patients with low muscle tone, the varus correction needed to maintain reduction is often greater than with other conditions, and the final femoral neck-shaft angle necessary to stabilize the hips is usually about 100 degrees. In this situation, an additional acetabular osteotomy is often used at the same time to increase joint stability.

The initial imaging studies for patients who may require a VDO are anteroposterior (AP) radiographs of the pelvis, with the hips first in a neutral position and then in an abducted, flexed position (frog-leg lateral view). The AP radiograph in the neutral position shows the femoral head position when sitting or standing and demonstrates the degree of subluxation or dislocation present, as well as the status of acetabular development. The AP radiograph with the legs in the frog-leg position demonstrates whether the femoral heads can and will reduce into the acetabulum when the hip is abducted. If the femoral heads reduce into the acetabulum on this radiograph, open reduction of the hip is usually not necessary, and the hip can usually be treated successfully with tenotomies and a VDO. If the femoral head does not reduce into the acetabulum on the abducted view, open reduction of the femoral head, in addition to the tenotomies and VDO, is planned. If there is acetabular dysplasia on the AP radiographs, an additional pelvic osteotomy is planned in addition to the tenotomy and VDO. These pelvis and hip radiographs are the primary imaging studies necessary to determine the need for surgery and for a VDO. A dynamic hip arthrogram, done as the first stage of the VDO operative procedure, is used to determine the exact position in which the femoral head will be placed surgically.

Advanced imaging studies that can be useful in some patients who require a VDO include computed axial tomography (CT) and magnetic resonance imaging (MRI). The latter is useful in patients with a hip disorder or hip subluxation who have pain with walking. Although hip subluxation itself can cause groin pain with activity, this pain may also be present from an injury to the labrum or adjacent soft tissue, which is demonstrated on the MRI and which would require repair or debridement. CT is useful mainly to develop three-dimensional (3D) reconstructions, which can clearly show the bony anatomy of the femoral head and acetabulum and can be evaluated from 360 degrees. Three-dimensional CT reconstructions can be used to measure the acetabular version and can assist in deciding where acetabular coverage may be needed as a part of the hip reconstruction procedure. CT can also be used to measure the degree of femoral anteversion present preoperatively to guide the amount of rotational correction needed through the VDO to normalize the femoral version.

Prior to surgery, the parents of patients should be informed that blood transfusion may be needed during or after the VDO, particularly if the child is small or if bilateral VDO is planned. Usually blood transfusion is not needed, but parents should be given the opportunity to provide donor-designated blood. Transfusion needs rarely exceed one unit of packed red blood cells, if that. The need for blood transfusion is increased if bilateral VDO and pelvic osteotomies are done at the same surgical session. If the patient is taking nonsteroidal anti-inflammatory medication for control of hip pain, this should be stopped about 1 week before surgery to prevent additional perioperative blood loss.

Just prior to surgery, in the preoperative holding area, the operating surgeon answers any questions the parents have regarding the surgery, and informed consent is reaffirmed. The correct site of the planned hip surgery is confirmed with the parents (and patient, if alert and old enough), and the surgeon marks the surgical site.

SURGICAL PROCEDURE

The patient is positioned supine on a radiolucent operating table to allow periodic fluoroscopic evaluation throughout the surgical procedure. General anesthesia with endotracheal intubation is carried out in routine fashion. In patients with spastic CP, placement of an epidural catheter after general anesthesia is induced can help diminish the need for intraoperative anesthetic medications and allows for localized pain control for 2 to 3 days postoperatively. A Foley urinary catheter is used if the operative procedure is planned for 3 hours or more or if epidural anesthesia is used.

If surgery is planned for only one hip, a roll is placed under the thoracolumbar spine on the operative side to elevate that side of the pelvis about 20 degrees. This position is particularly helpful if a pelvic osteotomy is planned in addition to the VDO. The entire leg and hemipelvis are prepped to the midthoracic level, and sterile drapes are placed. Preoperative prophylactic antibiotics are given intravenously prior to the incision. Also prior to any incision, a "time-out" is used to confirm the patient's identity, the operative procedure planned, and the site of the surgical procedure.

A dynamic examination of the hip is performed under live fluoroscopy to see if the femoral head reduces fully into the acetabulum or if the femoral head remains dislocated or subluxated with hip abduction maneuvers. If the femoral head reduces into the acetabulum, a hip arthrogram is performed. A 22-gauge spinal needle is inserted under fluoroscopic control into the hip joint. The author prefers an anterolateral approach, aiming the needle at the base of the femoral head directly onto the proximal femoral neck and attempting to insert the needle tip into the sulcus formed as the hip capsule is elevated off the femoral neck in this location due to the size of the femoral head. A medial approach can also be used effectively (Fig. 12-1). The trocar is left in the spinal needle during needle insertion. Once the desired position is reached, the hip is rotated gently. If the needle is in the bone of the femoral neck, the needle will rotate in the same direction as the hip. If the needle is through the capsule but not in the bone, the needle will rotate in the direction *opposite* the hip rotation—the desired needle position. Radio-opaque dye is then injected through IV tubing into the hip joint, with live fluoroscopic examination used throughout the dye insertion. It is important to avoid extravasation of the radio-opaque dye, particularly in the superior-lateral aspect of the hip joint, so that the arthrogram study yields the most and best information to form a final surgical plan for the VDO. Once confirmation of an intra-articular injection is obtained, about 3 cc of dye is inserted into the hip joint. The needle is removed, and the hip is placed through a full range of motion to allow for dispersal of the dye over the entire femoral head.

Examination of the hip is again performed under live fluoroscopy. Of particular interest are the presence of a medial or superior dye pool with different hip positions and the appearance of the cartilaginous lateral acetabulum (Fig. 12-2). If there is a medial dye pool in the neutral position of adduction/abduction, yet the femoral head reduces into the acetabulum with abduction, the amount of hip abduction necessary to allow full reduction and disappearance of the medial dye pool is carefully noted. The amount of abduction required to lead to full reduction and a congruent position of the femoral head in the acetabulum is the amount of varus correction that will be needed when the VDO is done. If there is limited abduction due to contracture of the hip adductors, tenotomy of the adductor longus is performed in children with DDH. In patients with spastic CP, more extensive hip adductor lengthening is done, usually including the adductor longus, adductor brevis, and gracilis muscles. After adductor release has been completed, repeat hip examination under fluoroscopy is performed, and plans are finalized for the amount of varus and rotational correction to be achieved with the VDO for optimal final hip position.

In younger children, the hip arthrogram will also help determine the need for a pelvic osteotomy in addition to the VDO. Children with hip subluxation will show an increased acetabular angle on an AP radiograph of the hip. However, this may be either bony acetabular dysplasia or unossified

FIGURE 12-1

Dynamic hip arthrography is important to determine the position of the femoral head within the acetabulum, as well as to assess the lateral edge of the acetabulum. The 22-gauge spinal needle can be inserted either through a medial approach (shown here) or through an anterolateral approach.

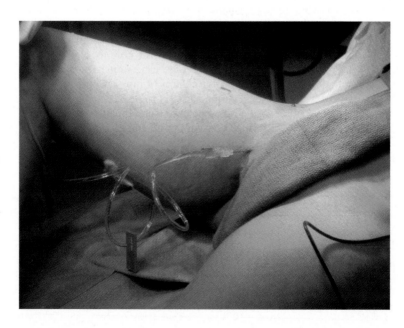

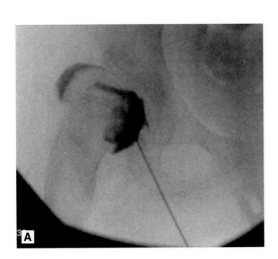
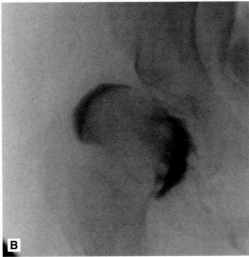

FIGURE 12-2

A. Medial needle insertion for dynamic hip arthrogram with injection of 3 cc radio-opaque dye. **B.** Medial dye pool is present with hip in neutral or slightly adducted position. Medial dye pool improved with hip abduction so that open reduction not needed.

lateral acetabular cartilage. Once the femoral head is reduced, the arthrogram will show how much acetabular coverage is present. If there is cartilaginous acetabular coverage present, reduction of the femoral head will usually allow a return to normal ossification of this lateral acetabular cartilage, and there is often no need for an additional pelvic osteotomy. However, if there is insufficient lateral acetabular coverage once the femoral head is reduced, an acetabular surgical procedure should be done after the VDO has been completed.

In patients with DDH in which the hip is not reducible, even under general anesthesia, an arthrogram with the hip dislocated will demonstrate the elongated hip capsule and perhaps some flattening of the femoral head. However, the arthrogram is less useful in this situation than when the femoral head can be reduced into the acetabulum. If the hip is irreducible and the hip adductor muscles are contracted, tenotomy of the adductor longus is done, and the hip is then reexamined. If the femoral head is still irreducible, open reduction is needed, with or without femoral osteotomy (see Chapter 10).

The incision for the VDO begins at the tip of the greater trochanter, which is palpable on the proximal lateral thigh, and extends along the lateral thigh parallel to the femoral shaft. The length of the incision should be sufficient enough to allow for easy placement of the blade plate fixation device. The fascia lata is split in line with the skin incision. The vastus lateralis muscle is retracted anteriorly with a self-retaining retractor, and the posterolateral portion of the vastus lateralis is identified. Using electrocautery, this fascia and periosteum are incised with electrocautery posteriorly, just anterior to the level of the gluteus maximus tendon, and down to bone; very little muscle is cut. Care needs to be taken not to migrate posterior to the femoral shaft, as the sciatic nerve is close by, and cutting the adjacent perforating vessels in this posterior location will cause more blood loss. Incision of the vastus lateralis fascia is carried cephalad to the base of the greater trochanter. Fluoroscopy is used to identify the level of the greater trochanter apophysis. A transverse incision is made to the bone, just distal to this apophysis, and is carried medially to the base of the femoral neck. Subperiosteal dissection is used to reflect the vastus lateralis anteriorly so that the anterior surface at the base of the femoral neck is visualized, as are the anterior and lateral proximal femoral shaft. Visualization of the base of the femoral neck helps to avoid making the osteotomy cut into the medial base of the femoral neck. It also allows the surgeon to directly visualize the degree of femoral anteversion or retroversion that is present, which helps in placing the guide pin and blade plate in the correct plane.

Fluoroscopy is used to locate the appropriate starting point on the proximal lateral femoral metaphysis for the guide pin. A Steinmann pin is inserted up the femoral neck to a point just short of the physis (Fig. 12-3). The starting point for this pin needs to be high enough to just allow the pin to pass up the inferior femoral neck and low enough to avoid having the osteotomy come across the medial base of the femoral neck. The pin is inserted at an angle that will allow for the amount of varus correction that was determined from the hip arthrogram data. If a 90-degree blade plate is to be used for fixation of the osteotomy and 40 degrees of varus correction is desired, the pin should be inserted at a 50-degree angle relative to the femoral shaft (Fig. 12-3B).

As the pin is being inserted, the visualized anterior surface of the base of the femoral neck is held parallel to the operating room tabletop, so that the pin does not have to be angulated either anteriorly or posteriorly during pin insertion. A stout Steinmann pin is preferred to prevent some bending when

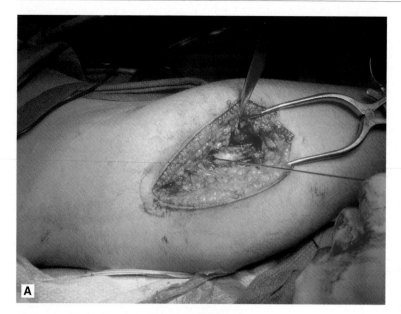

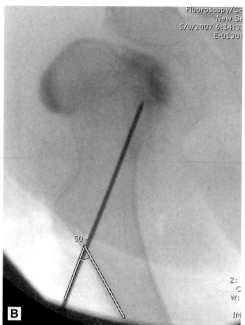

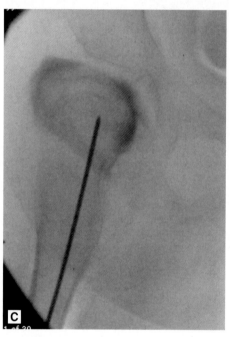

FIGURE 12-3 **A.** A Steinmann pin is inserted into the femoral neck as a guide pin for insertion of the chisel for the blade plate. **B.** AP fluoroscopic view demonstrates position of Steinmann pin to obtain 40 degrees varus correction when using a 90-degree blade plate for fixation. **C.** Frog-leg lateral view of femoral neck demonstrates satisfactory position of the Steinmann pin to serve as guide to allow for safe chisel and blade plate insertion.

the pin position is checked on the frog-leg lateral view after insertion. Once the pin has been inserted and appears satisfactory on the AP fluoroscopic view, the hip is placed in a flexed, abducted position to obtain a lateral fluoroscopic image (Fig. 12-3C). The goal is for the pin to be in the center of the femoral neck on the lateral view and in the inferior half of the femoral neck on the AP view. The necessary length of blade plate is measured by placing another identical Steinmann pin next to the inserted pin and using a ruler to determine the length of the pin inside the bone (Fig. 12-4).

Once the guide pin is confirmed as being in the appropriate position to provide the planned correction, the blade plate's chisel is inserted under fluoroscopic control (Fig. 12-5). Two or three small drill holes are made in the lateral cortex, about 1 mm cephalad to the entry point of the guide pin. If the guide pin has been placed in a central location on the lateral fluoroscopic view, the chisel should

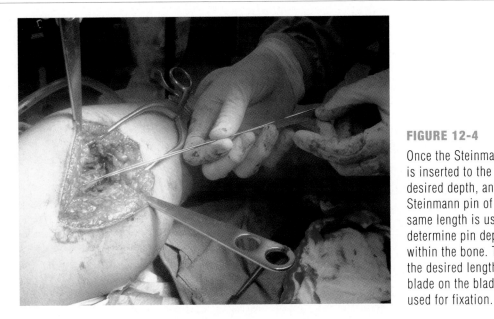

FIGURE 12-4

Once the Steinmann pin is inserted to the desired depth, another Steinmann pin of the same length is used to determine pin depth within the bone. This is the desired length of the blade on the blade plate used for fixation.

be placed at the level of these drill holes and centered on the guide pin. The chisel is then hammered into the femoral neck while being held centered on the guide pin, as shown via periodic fluoroscopic checks. Care needs to be taken to avoid tilting the chisel during this insertion to avoid leading to a flexed or extended position of the blade plate. If flexion or extension correction at the VDO is desired (usually it is not), however, tilting of the chisel during insertion is appropriate. The depth of the chisel insertion is to about 5 to 10 mm less than the tip of the guide pin. Fluoroscopic examination at this point is required to confirm that the chisel is inside the femoral neck in all views (Fig. 12-6).

The next step is to perform the femoral osteotomy. The 90-degree blade plate to be used should be carefully examined. Most blade plates have an offset of 15 to 20 mm distal to the blade, which allows the proximal fragment to tuck into this offset, thus avoiding lateralization of the proximal femur (Fig. 12-7). The osteotomy needs to be cut distal to the chisel at a distance that is a few millimeters less than the measured offset in the blade plate being used. Prior to making the transverse osteotomy, the saw is used to make marks on the anterior femoral shaft a few centimeters above and below the planned osteotomy site; these marks will become the guide for the amount of rotational correction desired. (If these rotational guide marks are made on the lateral femoral shaft, the blade plate will cover them so that they will not be visible.)

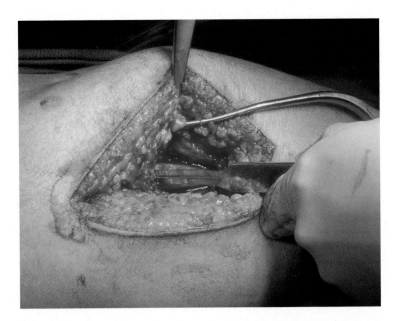

FIGURE 12-5

The chisel is inserted just superior to the Steinmann pin, using the pin as the guide to centralize the chisel.

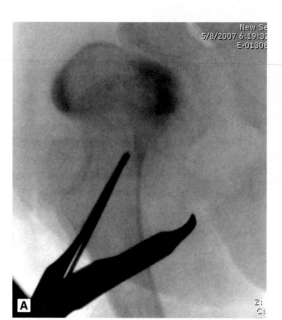
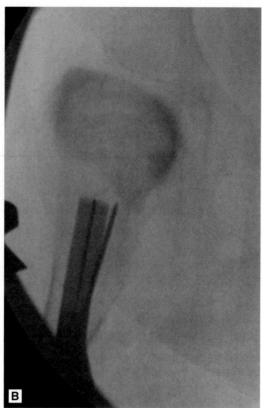

FIGURE 12-6   **A.** AP fluoroscopic view demonstrates satisfactory position of the chisel.
B. Lateral fluoroscopic view demonstrates central position of the chisel in the femoral neck.

An alternate method for determining the amount of rotational correction involves the insertion of two K-wires (one above and one below the planned osteotomy site) prior to the osteotomy (Fig. 12-8A). These K-wires act as a goniometer to let the surgeon know the amount of rotational correction that is being achieved at final plate placement. The proximal femoral osteotomy should be made perpendicular to the long axis of the femoral shaft. To obtain more bone contact at the osteotomy surfaces, a medial wedge of bone is removed from the proximal fragment, with care being taken not to cut into the femoral neck. This osteotomy saw cut should start about halfway across the proximal cut surface to avoid excessive leg shortening and should be made in a direction parallel to the chisel that is still in the femoral neck (Fig. 12-8B).

FIGURE 12-7

A commonly used blade plate. The osteotomy needs to be made so that it lies within the proximal plate's 15–20 mm offset to prevent lateralization of the femur.

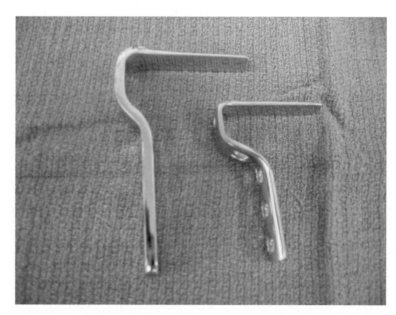

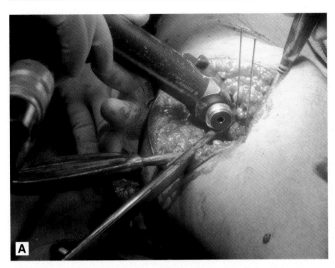
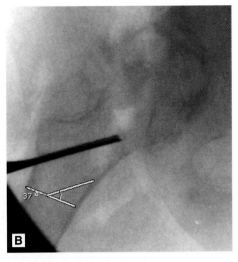

FIGURE 12-8   A. The osteotomy is completed with a power saw, excising a medially based wedge of bone. The K-wires shown in this patient are being used to assess the amount of rotational correction achieved. **B.** To obtain the planned correction when using a 90-degree blade plate for fixation, a medially based wedge of bone is removed, as demonstrated on this AP fluoroscopic view.

Once the medial wedge is cut, it is usually necessary to free this piece of bone from the psoas tendon, because this wedge usually includes at least a part of the lesser trochanter. The tendon can be cauterized directly off the bone surface of the wedge that is to be removed. This maneuver allows at least partial release of the psoas tendon to prevent it from blocking full femoral head reduction. If necessary to stabilize the proximal fragment, this tendon can be firmly held with a tenaculum with the femoral head reduced. To prevent the blade plate from deviating away from the path cut by the chisel, it is helpful to keep this proximal osteotomy fragment stabilized when the chisel is removed and the blade plate is inserted. The blade plate should be mounted on the insertion device prior to chisel removal. The chisel is then removed and the blade plate pushed into the chisel channel up the femoral neck (Fig. 12-9). Once the blade plate is nearly all the way in place, a mallet can be used to complete the insertion. Prior to complete insertion, fluoroscopic evaluation of the blade plate position is necessary to confirm that the position is satisfactory on both the AP and the lateral views (Fig. 12-10). Once the satisfactory position has been confirmed, the blade plate is fully inserted. A tamp is used for final insertion (Fig. 12-11).

The distal femoral fragment is then brought to the proximal osteotomy site and is held to the side plate with Verbrugge clamps. The distal fragment is placed in the desired position of rotation prior to being clamped to the side plate. Cortical screws are then placed to anchor the distal fragment to

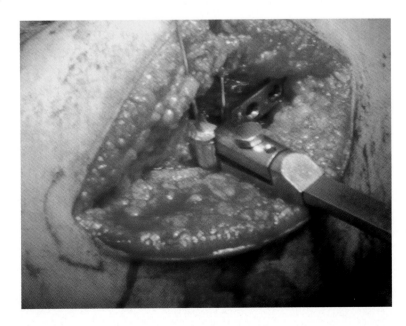

FIGURE 12-9

The blade plate is inserted into the channel cut by the chisel.

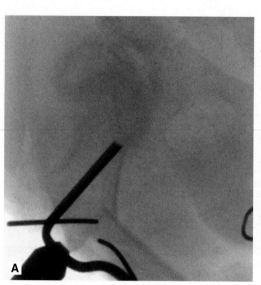
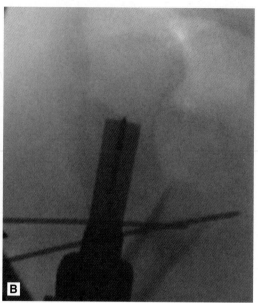

FIGURE 12-10

A. AP fluoroscopic view of the proximal femur confirms satisfactory placement of the blade plate. **B.** Lateral fluoroscopic view of the proximal femur confirms central placement of the blade plate.

the plate, with the initial screw inserted in a compressive mode. All screw holes should be filled with screws that have bicortical purchase (Fig. 12-12). If the bone quality is poor and screw fixation is tenuous, a nut used on the far side of the screw may allow for stronger fixation. Final fluoroscopic images are obtained to ensure that the femoral head is well reduced, the blade plate position is satisfactory, and the screws are the appropriate length (Figs. 12B and 12C).

The wound is then irrigated and closed. The vastus lateralis is sutured to the greater trochanter with nonabsorbable sutures while the hip is held in a mildly abducted position. The vastus lateralis fascia is closed with a running suture in its posterior margin. The fascia lata is closed with a running suture, with care being taken not to suture the vastus lateralis to the fascia lata. A suction drain is sometimes used deep to the fascia lata. Subcutaneous tissue closure and subcuticular absorbable sutures complete the closure, at which point adhesive skin closures (such as Steri-Strips) are placed.

The proximal femoral osteotomy used for toddlers with congenital hip dislocation differs from that described above to some degree. If the hip in DDH is irreducible after anesthesia and adductor tenotomy, then open reduction is needed. Once the hip capsule is opened and the femoral head is reduced, a decision is made as to whether the reduction is stable enough or whether femoral shortening is needed to help maintain the reduction. In general, in children over the age of 18 to 24 months, femoral shortening osteotomy has been useful in maintaining hip reduction. If the hip is irreducible even after capsulotomy, then femoral shortening is always advisable.

If femoral shortening is needed in DDH, the blade plate most commonly used to fix this osteotomy is basically the same as that described above. A major difference, however, is if the blade plate is

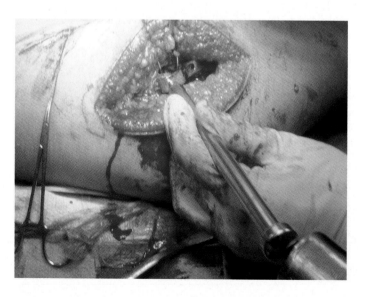

FIGURE 12-11

A tamp is used as the final insertion device to ensure that the side plate is against the bone in the proximal osteotomy fragment.

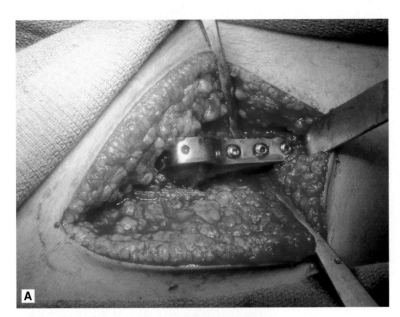

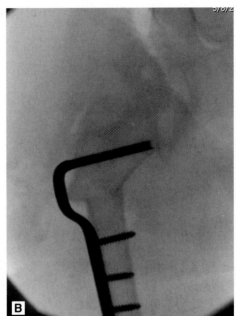

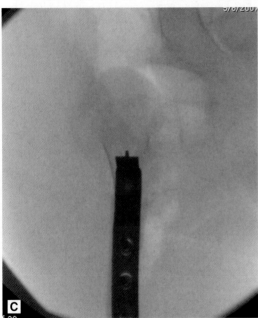

FIGURE 12-12   **A.** Clinical appearance of the blade plate and screw placement after insertion.
B. AP fluoroscopic view confirms satisfactory position of the blade plate and screws with reduced
femoral head. **C.** Lateral fluoroscopic view shows central position of the blade plate.

used for femoral shortening, the amount of varus correction is minimal and usually should be
limited to between 0 and 10 degrees. If marked femoral anteversion is present on the side of the dislocated hip, some external rotation correction is warranted.

Whereas the blade plate used in DDH is the same as that used in hip subluxation or neuromuscular dislocation, the position in which the proximal femur is held differs significantly. It is important
to emphasize that little or no varus correction is needed when the blade plate is used to hold a femoral
shortening osteotomy in DDH patients.

POSTOPERATIVE MANAGEMENT

Postoperative immobilization can range from none to a hip spica cast. In an older child or
teenager who can be trusted to walk with crutches using a toe-touch gait, no cast or brace is usually needed. In children with spastic CP, a hip spica cast is used to immobilize the VDO, to

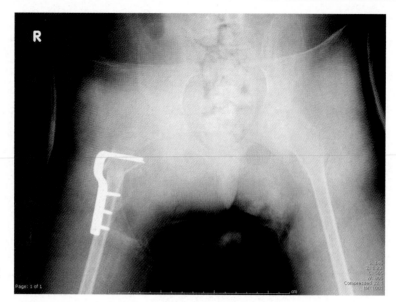

FIGURE 12-13

Postoperative immobilization in a hip spica cast. The anterior portion is cut down low enough to allow the child to sit up at least at a 45-degree angle.

protect the implant in bone that may be osteoporotic, and to stretch out muscles and tendons that have been lengthened in conjunction with the VDO. The femoral osteotomy should heal within 5 to 6 weeks (Fig. 12-13).

If a hip spica cast is used, it is usually removed at about 5 weeks after surgery. A hip abduction brace is then used to maintain hip symmetry, particularly in children with spastic CP. With VDO surgery for Legg-Perthes disease or for hip subluxation associated with DDH, hip abduction bracing is not usually necessary.

In ambulatory children, physical therapy is used following femoral osteotomy until hip motion and hip girdle muscle strength are regained. Hip abductor strength usually takes the longest to achieve. Full weight bearing can be started at about 5 to 6 weeks postoperatively. Full weaning off crutches is most dependent on the speed at which the patient regains muscle strength and control.

COMPLICATIONS TO AVOID

Complications associated with VDO can be either related to the underlying medical conditions that the child has or to the surgical procedure itself. VDO is used most commonly in children with spastic CP, who are prone to numerous medical problems with any operation. Seizure medications need to be given up to the time of general anesthesia and need to be restarted immediately postoperatively. Respiratory therapy treatments are instituted after general anesthesia to prevent atelectasis and pneumonia, particularly if a hip spica cast has been applied. The use of an epidural catheter for 2 to 3 days postoperatively has been shown to decrease the need for intravenous narcotics and to lessen pulmonary complications from oversedation. The hip spica cast may lead to an ileus, which delays feeding with or without a gastrostomy tube.

The main surgical complication of VDO is related to the insertion and stability of the blade plate implant used to fix the osteotomy. Because many of the spastic CP patients needing VDO are nonambulatory, the bone is often not strong. During insertion of the chisel for the blade plate, fracture of the femoral neck or fracture through the greater trochanter can occur either with suboptimal chisel insertion up the femoral neck or when moving the hip into a frog-leg lateral position to obtain fluoroscopic views. If these fractures occur intraoperatively, it is usually possible to obtain acceptable hip position and osteotomy fixation with a combination of wires, pins, blade plate, and screws to allow for satisfactory completion of the procedure. A hip spica cast should then be used postoperatively to maintain the position until bone healing is complete. If the femoral head cannot be held in a reduced position, the use of a large Steinmann pin through the greater trochanter into the supra-acetabular area (not across the hip joint) can be used with the hip spica cast until healing is complete, at which point the stout Steinmann pin is removed.

Once the patient is in the hip spica cast, the blade plate may move as it cuts through the poor-quality bone in the femoral neck. Thus, x-rays should be obtained every 2 weeks to monitor the bone healing for the first 6 weeks after surgery. Usually when plate migration occurs, it is minor and rarely requires reoperation.

Recurrence of hip subluxation and dislocation after VDO can occur if hip symmetry is not maintained. Any condition that will return the operated hip to an adducted position will lead to recurrence of hip instability. This can occur when the opposite hip has an abduction contracture, which will cause the windswept position to be assumed after surgery, or when there is severe pelvic obliquity associated with scoliosis. If these coexisting conditions are present, surgical treatment of the abducted hip and of the scoliosis is usually needed to prevent recurrences.

If the VDO is done when the child is relatively young, the blade plate will move distally relative to the hip joint as growth takes place in the proximal femur. In some instances, the blade plate can protrude through the medial cortex, leading to an increased risk of fracture at this level. In addition, in children with poor bone quality, there is a risk of fracture of the femoral shaft just distal to the side plate, which makes that portion of the femur more rigid than the child's own bone. These "stress risers" that may lead to later femoral shaft fracture can be eliminated by removing the blade plate and screws.

The question of whether routine implant removal is needed in children after VDO remains unanswered. Some surgeons routinely remove these implants any time after 6 months from the time of surgery, whereas others rarely remove the implant. Implant removal is more commonly done in children who were quite young when the blade plate was inserted, to minimize the risk of femoral fracture and to prevent the plate from being buried within the femoral shaft as growth takes place. If overgrowth of bone completely encases the plate, future surgery, such as total hip arthroplasty, becomes more difficult and complicated. If the blade plate and screws are removed, limited weight bearing on crutches is needed for 3 to 4 weeks to allow the screw holes and blade track to fill in with bone and to prevent fracture through these bone holes. If plate removal is done on ambulatory children without neuromuscular disease, physical therapy is needed for several weeks to regain hip abductor strength before full return to normal activity.

If a postoperative wound infection occurs, all attempts should be made to leave the blade plate in place until the osteotomy site is healed. Prompt diagnosis of an infection, followed by operative irrigation and debridement with wound closure over drains, plus a several-week course of appropriate antibiotics should allow healing of the infection without plate removal. If there continues to be some evidence of infection, suppressive antibiotics are used until bone union, at which point the blade plate and screws can be removed to allow full resolution of the infection.

ILLUSTRATIVE CASE

A 10-year-old boy with spastic diplegia had previously undergone selective dorsal rhizotomy for muscle tone reduction in the lower extremities. Approximately 4 years after rhizotomy, he was noted to have subluxation of the right femoral head (Fig. 12-14A). In addition, increased internal rotation of the left lower extremity was present due to excessive femoral anteversion. He underwent proximal femoral varus osteotomy on the right side with blade plate fixation (Fig. 12-14B). An arthrogram after the varus osteotomy demonstrated a superior dye pool (Fig. 12-14C); also, in 10 degrees of adduction, a medial dye pool was seen, leading to the intraoperative decision to add an acetabular procedure to increase hip stability. A Dega-type osteotomy was done to improve femoral head coverage and stability (Fig. 12-14D). The left hip was treated with an external rotation proximal femoral osteotomy with modest varus positioning, using blade plate fixation. Note that the level of osteotomy allows for the proximal osteotomy fragment to fit nicely into the plate offset, avoiding lateralization of the plate and distal femur (Figs. 14E and 14F). Six months following surgery, the osteotomies in the femurs and right acetabulum were well healed, and the hips were stable (Fig. 12-14G).

PEARLS AND PITFALLS

- Open reduction of the hip, accompanied by a VDO, is contraindicated in children with spastic cerebral palsy and long-standing hip dislocation due to femoral head erosions and deformation.
- Anteroposterior radiograph of the hip with the hip internally rotated will provide the best estimation of the true femoral neck-shaft angle, a value necessary when planning the required amount of varus correction.
- A dynamic hip arthrogram prior to the osteotomy will allow the surgeon to determine the optimal position of the femoral head within the acetabulum and will be the guide for the degrees of varus and rotational correction needed in the proximal femur to center the femoral head in the best position.
- Varus correction should result in a femoral neck-shaft angle of no less than 110 degrees in patients with spastic Cp.

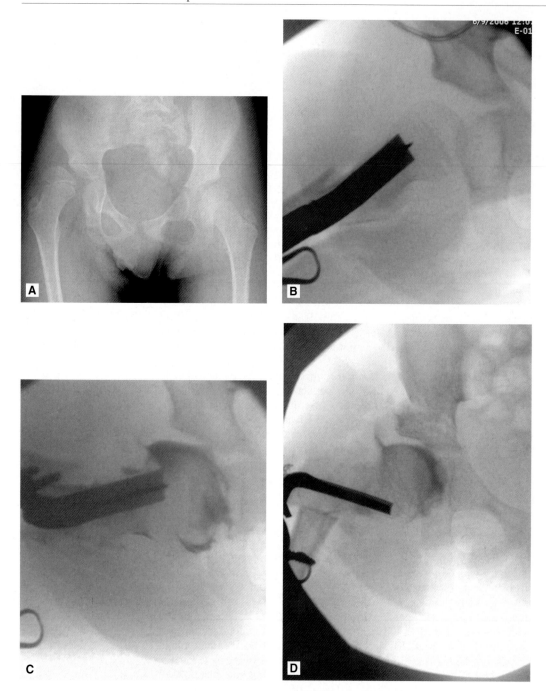

FIGURE 12-14   A. AP radiograph of the pelvis with lateral subluxation of the right femoral head in a 10-year-old boy with spastic diplegia who had a prior dorsal rhizotomy. Right VDO and left rotational osteotomy were recommended. **B.** Lateral fluoroscopic view of the right hip, demonstrating the central position of the blade plate in the femoral neck and reduction of the femoral head on hip abduction. **C.** Despite hip reduction with abduction, a superior dye pool is shown on this fluoroscopic view of an arthrogram after the VDO was completed. The decision was made to add an acetabular osteotomy to achieve more hip stability. **D.** AP fluoroscopic view of arthrogram after completion of Dega-type acetabular osteotomy demonstrates excellent femoral head coverage by the bony and cartilaginous acetabulum. AP **(E)** and lateral **(F)** fluoroscopic views of proximal left femur after rotational correction as treatment for excessive femoral anteversion. **G.** AP radiograph of the pelvis demonstrates healed femoral and acetabular osteotomies and improved position of the femoral heads in the acetabulum. *(continued)*

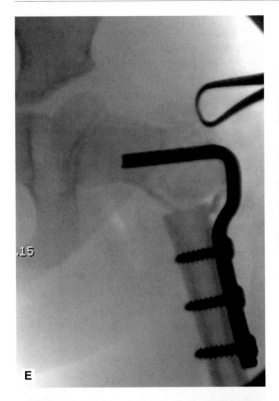

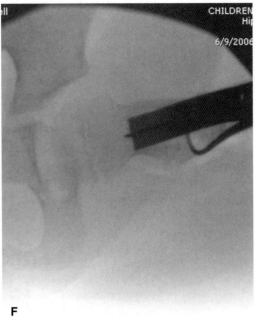

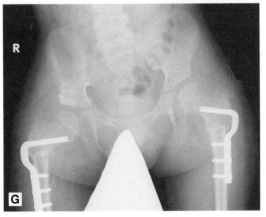

FIGURE 12-14   (*Continued*)

- The amount of varus correction should never exceed the amount of passive hip abduction with the hip in extension on preoperative examination.
- Rotational correction with the VDO should allow for nearly equal hip internal rotation and external rotation postoperatively.
- Because fixed angle plates are used for osteotomy fixation, insertion of the initial Steinmann pin to determine the position and direction of the cutting chisel is a very important step. The pin should be in perfect position, as judged fluoroscopically, prior to placement of the chisel and the osteotomy.
- Once the osteotomy is complete, a repeat dynamic arthrogram is helpful before wound closure to ensure that the femoral head, with the hip in a neutral position, is in the desired location within the acetabulum.
- Blade plate removal is more common the younger the patient is at the time of VDO. The blade plate moves distally with growth and becomes a stress riser for a possible femoral shaft fracture.

REFERENCES

1. Brunner R, Baumann JU. Long-term effects of intertrochanteric varus-derotation osteotomy on femur and acetabulum in spastic cerebral palsy: an 11- to 18-year follow-up study. *J Pediatr Orthop.* 1997;17:585–591.
2. Hess T, Esser O, Mittelmeier H. Combined acetabuloplasty and varus derotational osteotomy in congenital dislocation of the hip: long-term results. *Int Orthop.* 1996;21:350–356.
3. Inan M, Senaran H, Domsalski M, et al. Unilateral versus bilateral peri-ilial pelvic osteotomies combined with proximal femoral osteotomies in children with cerebral palsy: perioperative complications. *J Pediatr Orthop.* 2006;26:547–550.
4. Lahoti O, Turnbull TJ, Hinves BL. Separation of the proximal femoral epiphysis after derotation varus osteotomy of the femur. *J Pediatr Orthop.* 1998;18:662–664.
5. Leitch JM, Paterson DC, Foster BK. Growth disturbance in Legg-Calvé-Perthes disease and the consequences of surgical treatment. *Clin Orthop Relat Res.* 1991;262:178–184.
6. Nakamura M, Matsunaga S, Yoshino S, et al. Long-term result of combination of open reduction and femoral derotation varus osteotomy with shortening for developmental dislocation of the hip. *J Pediatr Orthop B.* 2004;13:248–253.
7. Noonan KJ, Walker TL, Kayes KJ, et al. Varus derotation osteotomy for the treatment of hip subluxation and dislocation in cerebral palsy: statistical analysis in 73 hips. *J Pediatr Orthop B.* 2001;10:279–286.
8. Song HR, Carroll NC. Femoral varus derotation osteotomy with or without acetabuloplasty for unstable hips in cerebral palsy. *J Pediatr Orthop.* 1998;18:62–68.
9. Suda H, Hattori T, Iwata H. Varus derotation osteotomy for persistent dysplasia in congenital dislocation of the hip: proximal femoral growth and alignment changes in the leg. *J Bone Joint Surg Br.* 1995;77(8);756–761.
10. Wilkinson AJ, Nattrass GR, Graham HK. Modified technique for varus derotation osteotomy of the proximal femur in children. *ANZ J Surg.* 2001;71:655–658.

13 Irrigation and Debridement of a Septic Hip

Frances A. Farley

A septic hip in a child requires emergent drainage. It should be distinguished from other pathologic hip conditions in a child by history, physical exam, a hip ultrasound, and laboratory data.[1] Recent publications support an algorithmic approach to the evaluation of a limping child to accurately distinguish a child with a septic hip from a child with toxic or transient synovitis. Kocher noted four risk factors—refusal to walk, fever, elevated white blood cell count (greater than 12,000 mm^3), and erythrocyte sedimentation rate (ESR) above 40 mm/hr—and validated these risk factors in a subsequent report.[3] However, other centers have found that these four factors may not have as high a predictive value in determining a septic hip as was originally thought.[4] The finding of a C-reactive protein (CRP) level above 1.0 is highly suggestive of infection as well.[5]

INDICATIONS/CONTRAINDICATIONS

A child with a history of fever who has an irritable hip is the classic presentation of a septic hip and requires a hip ultrasound. If there is greater than 2 cc of fluid in the hip, the hip is tapped under ultrasound guidance through an anterior or medial approach. The fluid is sent to the laboratory, where a cell count, gram stain, and culture are obtained. If the fluid appears as pus, the child is taken to the operating room at once for drainage. If the fluid appears purulent, has a white cell count of greater than 100,000 or a positive gram stain, or there is a positive culture requires drainage of the hip joint is required. Cell counts between 40,000 and 100,000 may require drainage, depending on the clinical picture and other laboratory findings, particularly the ESR and CRP values.

SURGICAL PROCEDURE

A septic hip in a child is preferably drained through an anterior approach. The superficial dissection is between the sartorius muscle, supplied by the femoral nerve, and the tensor fascia femoris muscle, supplied by the superficial gluteal nerve. The deep dissection is between the rectus femoris muscle, supplied by the femoral nerve, and the gluteus medius muscle, supplied by the superficial gluteal nerve.

A time-out, or surgical pause, is taken prior to anesthesia and again prior to the incision. Prior to anesthesia, the surgeon marks the affected leg with a felt-tip pen to reduce the risk of wrong site surgery. The child is placed supine on a radiolucent operating table. A bump is placed under the affected hip to facilitate exposure. The child's affected leg is prepped and draped free in the usual sterile fashion.

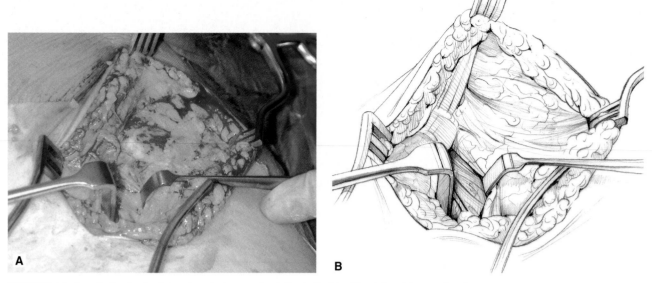

FIGURE 13-1   A, B. An incision for drainage of a left septic hip. The lateral femoral cutaneous nerve crosses the sartorius.

A bikini incision is made one finger's breadth below the anterior superior iliac spine, extending 2 cm lateral and medial from the anterior superior iliac spine (ASIS). The skin and soft tissues are sharply dissected with a knife. Scissors are used to bluntly dissect to identify the lateral femoral cutaneous nerve, which lies in the interval between the sartorius and the tensor fascia femoris muscles and crosses the sartorius muscle near the ASIS (Fig. 13-1). Once the lateral femoral cutaneous nerve is identified and retracted medially, the sartorius origin is detached from the ASIS with a sliver of cartilage and tagged with a Vicryl stitch. Distal and medial retraction of the sartorius protects the lateral femoral cutaneous nerve. The iliac apophysis is split sharply with a knife, and the soft tissue is subperiosteally elevated from the outer iliac wing with a Cobb elevator and retracted laterally. An alternative approach practiced by the editors is to leave the iliac apophysis and abductors intact, and proceed directly down to the retus femoris.

The rectus femoris origin is identified. Both the direct and the reflected heads are sharply dissected off the ASIS and are tagged with a Vicryl stitch to allow this muscle to be retracted distally. A Cobb elevator is used to clear any other soft tissue off the anterior hip capsule. A 1-cm × 1-cm square of anterior hip capsule tissue is removed and sent for culture and pathologic examination (Fig. 13-2). Fluid is sent for culture for aerobic and anaerobic bacteria, as well as for fungus and tuberculosis. An initial IV dose of antibiotic is given after cultures have been obtained. The cartilage of the femoral head is visually inspected. Several liters of pulsatile lavage are irrigated through the hip joint while rotating the femur and the femoral head. If there is suspicion of a coexisting femoral

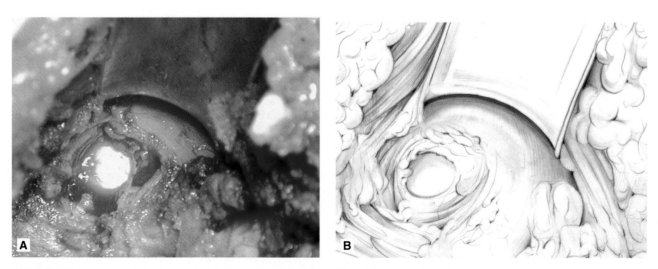

FIGURE 13-2   A, B. Anterior approach to the hip. The femoral head is exposed in the center of the picture.

neck osteomyelitis from preoperative imaging studies, the femoral neck can be drilled or a small cortical window can be removed to decompress the bone infection.

A drain is placed in the joint and exits through the incision. The rectus femoris tendons are repaired to the AIIS with a 0-Vicryl suture. The sartorius is repaired to the ASIS with a 0-Vicryl suture. The iliac apophysis is repaired with a 0-Vicryl suture. The wound is closed with interrupted 2-0-Vicryl sutures in the subcutaneous tissue. The skin is closed with a running subcuticular Monocryl suture, except for 1 cm for the drain to exit and drain.

Nonadherent and 4×4 sterile dressings are placed, and tape is applied to secure the dressing. The patient is awakened and taken to the recovery room.

POSTOPERATIVE MANAGEMENT

The drain is removed 2 days after surgery. An infectious disease consult is obtained for advice on antibiotic use. Antibiotics are usually given for 2 or 3 weeks, initially through an intravenous route. If the patient remains afebrile with decreasing pain, the patient is discharged when he or she has good oral intake and is comfortable on oral pain medicines.

If the patient remains febrile or has increasing hip pain, the hip is drained and irrigated again through the same approach. At the second drainage, the surgeon may elect to leave the wound open with wet to dry dressing changes. The hip should have repeated irrigation if the patient remains febrile or the hip remains increasingly irritable.

COMPLICATIONS TO AVOID

A delay in drainage of a septic hip may lead to severe damage to the femoral head articular cartilage. If there is coexisting femoral neck osteomyelitis, irreversible damage to the proximal femoral growth plate may also occur. The result of either or both of these complications is a hip with limited motion and eventually shortness of the involved lower extremity.

Avascular necrosis of the femoral head may also occur if there is delay in operative drainage. Avascular necrosis may also occur if inadequate drainage of a coexisting femoral neck osteomyelitis occurs when the surgeon is performing an incision and drainage of the hip for septic arthritis.

With the surge of community-acquired methicillin-resistant *Staphylococcus aureus,* the need for a second or third debridement of hip septic arthritis or osteomyelitis has become more commonly necessary. If the surgeon is not ready to do this reoperation on children who have this organism, later complications are more likely to occur.

ILLUSTRATIVE CASE

A 6-year-old boy presented with a 2-day history of right hip pain and a fever of 102°F. On the day of presentation, he was refusing to walk. His white blood cell count was 20,000 cm^3, and his ESR was elevated at 45 mm/hr. His hip exam demonstrated a positive log roll (limited hip rotation) and painful limited range of hip motion. Radiographs of the hip were normal. Hip ultrasound showed a moderate right hip effusion. Under ultrasound guidance, the right hip was tapped, revealing purulent fluid on aspiration.

The child was taken directly to the operating room, where the right hip was drained through an anterior approach. The hip had about 4 cc of purulent fluid, which was sent for culture. A small specimen of the joint capsule was sent for pathology examination. The cartilage appeared pristine and normal. Three liters of saline were irrigated through the wound. A Penrose drain was placed.

The boy continued to improve postoperatively. None of the cultures identified any bacterial growth. The histologic examination was normal joint capsular tissue. The child had the Penrose drain discontinued on postoperative day 2 and was discharged on postoperative day 3. He had a peripherally inserted central catheter line placed for 3 weeks of intravenous antibiotics to treat a presumed *S. aureus* infection. He continued to improve and had a normal range of hip motion, with return to all activities by 6 weeks after surgery.

PEARLS AND PITFALLS

- Septic arthritis of the hip is a surgical emergency. Do not delay in carrying out the surgery needed to drain the infected hip.
- The most important risk factors that help establish early diagnosis of septic arthritis include elevated C-reactive protein and erythrocyte sedimentation rate, refusal to walk, and decreased hip motion fever.

- If the diagnosis of septic hip arthritis is made, be sure to assess for possible coexisting involvement of the femoral neck with osteomyelitis.
- Children with septic hip arthritis treated late usually have long-term complications of hip stiffness and impaired proximal femoral growth.

REFERENCES

1. Jung ST, Rowe SM, Moon ES, et al. Significance of laboratory and radiologic findings for differentiating between septic arthritis and transient synovitis of the hip. *J Pediatr Orthop.* 2003;23(3):368–372.
2. Kocher MS, Mandiga R, Murphy JM, et al. A clinical practice guideline for treatment of septic arthritis in children: efficacy in improving process of care and effect on outcome of septic arthritis of the hip. *J Bone Joint Surg Am.* 2003;85A(6):994–999.
3. Kocher MS, Mandiga R, Zurakowski D, et al. Validation of a clinical prediction rule for the differentiation between septic arthritis and transient synovitis of the hip in children. *J Bone Joint Surg Am.* 2004;86A(8):1629–1635.
4. Luhmann SJ, Jones A, Shootman M, et al. Differentiation between septic arthritis and transient synovitis of the hip in children with clinical prediction algorithms. *J Bone Joint Surg.* 2004;86A:956–962.
5. Caird MS, Flynn JM, Millman JE, et al. Factors distinguishing septic arthritis from transient synovitis of the hip in children. A propective study. *J Bone Joint Surg Am.* 2006;88(6):1251–1257.

14 Shelf Arthroplasty of the Hip

Alvin H. Crawford and José A. Herrera-Soto

There are a wide variety of treatments for developmental hip conditions, such as congenital dislocations, growth alterations, and arthritic disorders, and complications of avascular necrosis, as well as conditions such as Legg-Calvé-Perthes disease and slipped capital femoral epiphysis. The index acetabular procedure for developmental dysplasia of the hips is the inominate osteotomy, as reported by Salter.[8] The treatment of Legg-Calvé-Perthes disease is still controversial but is focused on femoral head coverage and containment. There are instances in which femoral head coverage is not complete after femoral or pelvic osteotomies, requiring it to be augmented or substantiated by a shelf arthroplasty procedure.[6] Femoral head coverage is necessary in all pediatric hip conditions to avoid hip subluxation and instability.

The shelf arthroplasty procedure may contribute to acetabular coverage by primary or secondary implementation. The original description of a shelf was in 1891 by Konig.[4] Although several modifications have subsequently been developed, the basic concept of using bone graft to augment the acetabular roof and improve femoral head coverage has been maintained. Kuwajima et al.[6] combined a Salter osteotomy with a shelf operation to achieve greater acetabular coverage with a better hyaline-cartilage interface. Domzalski et al.[2] recently considered the shelf to be a labral support procedure, not designed to fully contain the head, though they did note an inducement of additional lateral acetabular growth after a shelf procedure, not seen after varus derotational femoral osteotomies.

INDICATIONS/CONTRAINDICATIONS

The primary indication for a shelf augmentation is in the patient with hip dysplasia with aspherical hip congruity not amenable to redirectional osteotomies. A shelf augmentation acetabuloplasty is secondarily warranted for anterolateral acetabular extension in dysplastic hips in which femoral head coverage cannot be achieved by the more commonly performed pelvic osteotomies. It is also indicated in patients aged 8 years or older with Legg-Calvé-Perthes disease[3,5,10] who typically present with coxa magna and early lateralization of the femoral head.

Shelf arthroplasty was once thought to be contraindicated in skeletally immature patients because of potential injury to the lateral acetabular growth center. However, this procedure now appears to augment the lateral acetabular rim. It is contraindicated in patients with spherical congruent joints where a redirectional osteotomy can adequately cover the femoral head. On occasion, the shelf arthroplasty is used to augment pelvic osteotomies and can be used with either a Salter innominate osteotomy (Fig. 14-1) or a Chiari osteotomy (Figs. 14-2 and 14-3).

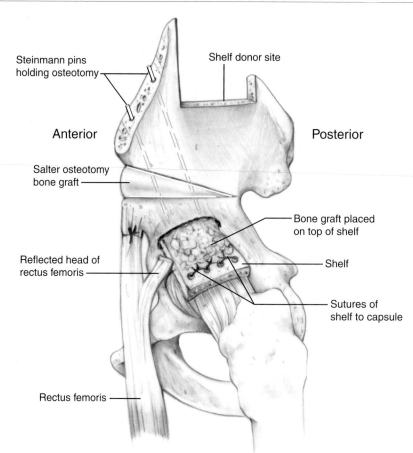

FIGURE 14-1

Shelf-augmented innominate osteotomy on left hip for Legg-Calvé-Perthes disease. This illustration shows the reflected head of the rectus femoris as well as capsular sutures holding the graft in place. Today, the rectus femoris is no longer sutured, but heavy sutures are still used to hold the graft to the capsule.

Steinmann pins holding osteotomy

Shelf donor site

Anterior

Posterior

Salter osteotomy bone graft

Bone graft placed on top of shelf

Reflected head of rectus femoris

Shelf

Sutures of shelf to capsule

Rectus femoris

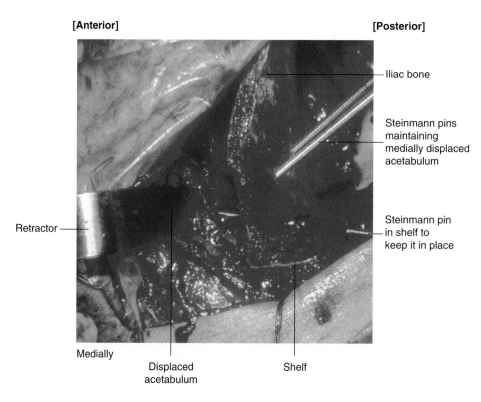

FIGURE 14-2

Operative photograph of fixation of shelf augmenting a Chiari osteotomy of the left hip. The inferior pelvic fragment (displaced acetabulum) has been secured to the ilium by two large, oblique Steinmann pins. A smaller Steinmann pin has been driven through the shelf into the inferior pelvic fragment to hold it in place. Abundant bone graft is then placed over the shelf after the pins have been cut.

[Anterior]

[Posterior]

Iliac bone

Steinmann pins maintaining medially displaced acetabulum

Steinmann pin in shelf to keep it in place

Retractor

Medially

Displaced acetabulum

Shelf

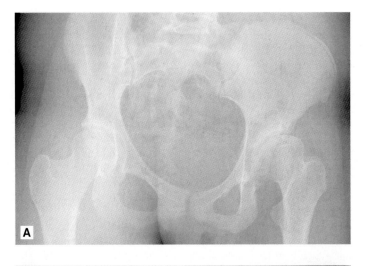

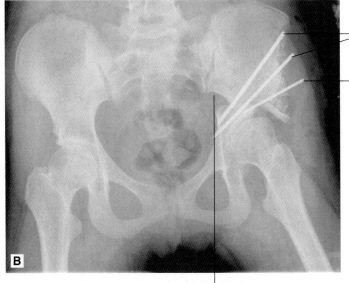

Steinmann pins
holding Chiari
medially displaced
acetabular fragment

Steinmann pin
holding shelf in place

Edge of Osteotomy

FIGURE 14-3

Acetabular dysplasia **(A)** treated by Chiari osteotomy with shelf augmentation. The smaller pin **(B)** is used to hold the shelf in place. The larger pins maintain the medially displaced acetabulum.

PREOPERATIVE PLANNING

Plain radiographs of the pelvis (anteroposterior in the standing position and frog lateral views) are needed to assess the amount of femoral head coverage needed. A supine abduction internal rotation (AIR) view is also warranted. The AIR view will help determine joint congruity and the need for either a redirectional osteotomy or a shelf procedure to add femoral head coverage. The segment of iliac bone harvested is enough to allow the femoral head to be completely covered; an extra centimeter of bone graft length is added to insert into a pelvic trough. However, excessive coverage is avoided to prevent loss of abduction and hip flexion. Achieving a center-edge angle of 35 degrees is optimal. The graft may be placed more anteriorly or posteriorly, according to an assessment of where femoral head coverage is most necessary, but usually anterolateral coverage is warranted.

In patients with Legg-Calvé-Perthes disease, physical therapy is encouraged prior to surgery. If there is a restricted range of hip motion and any evidence of femoral head extrusion or subluxation, the surgical treatment is staged. These patients initially undergo an adductor longus tenotomy, inferior capsulotomy with release of the transverse acetabular ligament, and Petrie casting 6 weeks before the shelf procedure.[6]

Recently, Rab presented an analysis of the direction of joint forces in Perthes computer models.[7] The area of femoral head collapse will tend to guide the direction of subluxation and extrusion. For example, purely lateral femoral head collapse will lead to lateral head subluxation. Thus placement of the shelf is determined with these principles in mind.

SURGICAL PROCEDURE

The patient is placed supine on a radiolucent table. A sandbag is placed in the ipsilateral lumbar region to elevate the affected hemipelvis. A bikini-type curvilinear incision is done about one-third the distance from the iliac brim to the greater trochanter, curving anteriorly to the midinguinal line. Below the incision, the intervals used for the Smith-Petersen approach between the sartorius and the tensor fascia femoris muscles are developed. Care must be taken not to injure the lateral femoral cutaneous nerve, which exits between the two muscles and becomes superficial to the sartorius muscle. The iliac crest apophysis is split with either a sharp knife or a cautery. A T-type cut is made in the apophysis at the anterior and posterior margins to decrease tension and allow better exposure and closure. The tensor fascia lata origin and gluteal musculature are elevated from the outer pelvic table subperiosteally down to the capsular margin. The iliacus muscle is elevated from the inner pelvis. Hemostasis of the perforating vessels is obtained with either bone wax or cautery. Packing several sponges under the periosteum decreases bleeding and improves exposure.

The reflected head of the rectus femoris is identified and detached from the attachment at the acetabulum. The groove where this tendon lies is the absolute lateral acetabular margin and is always directly above the capsular attachment to the acetabular wall above the labrum; this groove serves as an anatomical marker. Historically, the reflected head was detached anteriorly and, once the graft was placed, was sutured back to its origin to the direct head of the rectus femoris to maintain the shelf in place.[9] The technique described in this chapter obviates resuturing the reflected head into the main tendon. Complete lateral, anterolateral, and posterolateral exposure of the capsule is performed. For greater anterior capsular exposure, the tendon of the rectus femoris may need to be tagged and cut about 1 cm distal to the insertion in the anterior inferior iliac spine. Any redundant capsule attached to the ilium (pseudoacetabulum) needs to be elevated from the outer pelvic wall.

The periacetabular area is scored with several upwardly inclined drill holes that are made in line with the tendon of the reflected head attachment to the acetabular margin, avoiding joint penetration. It is most advantageous to start the holes from posterior to anterior to avoid blood overflow that would obstruct visualization posteriorly. These drill holes are then interconnected with a straight 1-cm osteotome and widened with a ronguer to create a one centimeter deep trough that is angulated cephalad about 15 degrees. Flouroscopy is encouraged to avoid joint penetration. The area to be covered by the graft is measured. An extra centimeter is added in length to accommodate insertion of the graft into a trough to be created. A trapezoidal graft is obtained by osteotomizing both cortices of the ilium. Bosworth[1] preferred to osteotomize the outer table only, whereas others have described using the inner table of the pelvis as graft. The shelf description by Staheli and Chew[9] used matchstick-like grafts obtained from the iliac outer table, inserted perpendicular first and then parallel to the iliac bone, just superior to the acetabular margin.

In the technique described in this chapter, the graft is provisionally inserted into the trough, and a fluoroscopic image is taken to assess femoral head coverage. The hip is ranged to allow at least 45 degrees of abduction with the graft in place. Hip flexion is also examined to avoid anterior impingement. The graft is then trimmed accordingly to ensure enough coverage but not excessive coverage, which would limit abduction and/or hip flexion. Four holes are then drilled in the peripheral aspect of the graft. Strong nonabsorbable sutures (Ethibond-0) are used to anchor the graft into the capsule. The anchors are about 5 to 10 mm more medial than the drill holes to ensure compression of the graft into the pelvis. The first suture goes from outside the graft to the capsule and back through the first hole. The second anchor goes from the first hole to the capsule and through the second hole. The third comes from the second hole to the capsule and through the third hole, and so forth, until the last hole is used. Each suture is tagged with different hemostats. The graft is then impacted into the supra-acetabular trough, and the sutures are tied from posterior to anterior. Rarely, but on occasion, a threaded Steinmann pin is used to add security to the graft. Freeze-dried bone graft and local cancellous bone from the pelvis are then used to augment and buttress the roof of the new acetabulum. A sterile compressed sponge (such as Gelfoam) may be used to constrain the loose fragments within the hematoma.

The gluteus minimus and medius will lie on top of the graft to maintain it in place. The straight rectus femoris tendon, if detached, is resutured to the AIIS. Any excess bone graft may be used to fill the harvested area. The apophysis is then closed anatomically. The wound is closed over drains in standard fashion. Because this type of graft is done in older children, rarely is there a need for spica casting.

POSTOPERATIVE MANAGEMENT

Drains are kept in place for 2 days. Intravenous antibiotics are maintained until the drains and the Foley catheter are removed.

The patient is not fully ambulatory until there is evidence of bone healing. Prior to discharge, physical therapy to include internal and external rotation of the hip is allowed and encouraged.

Hip flexion is allowed as well. Full abduction is discouraged to prevent fracture or upward displacement of the shelf at the pelvis-capsule juncture.

COMPLICATIONS TO AVOID

Carefully expose and avoid injuring the lateral femoral cutaneous nerve, which is usually found between the sartorius and the tensor fascia femoris muscles. Inadequate graft will be insufficient. Excessive coverage is a complication that may limit motion (impingement), especially in abduction and/or hip flexion. The acetabular trough must be near the joint line to allow adequate graft stress. Do not place the graft too high above the acetabulum. Superiorly placed grafts tend to resorb due to lack of bone stresses, which will lead to poor final femoral head coverage. Avoid joint penetration when preparing the trough and inserting the shelf to prevent cartilage injury and early osteoarthritis.

PEARLS & PITFALLS

- Adequate graft placement requires proper exposure.
- The capsule should be cleaned. If hypertrophic, it may be trimmed down to allow better contact with the femoral head.
- The graft should be sutured to the capsule as snugly (tightly) as possible.
- The groove of the reflected head of the rectus femoris is an excellent anatomic marker for the lateral acetabular margin.
- Fluoroscopic guidance should be used while preparing the trough to avoid joint penetration.
- Abundant autologous bone graft, as well as allograft, may be placed on the shelf. A sterile compressed sponge or absorbable hemostat (e.g., Gelfoam or Surgicel) will help maintain the shelf within the hematoma so the loose bone graft will not migrate proximally.

ILLUSTRATIVE CASES

Case 1

A 12-year-old child initially diagnosed as bilateral Legg-Calvé-Perthes disease. He was subsequently confirmed to have spondyloepiphyseal dysplasia. Bilateral varus derotational femoral osteotomies were augmented with shelf procedures (Fig. 14-4).

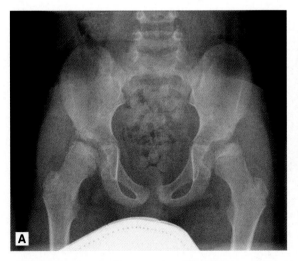 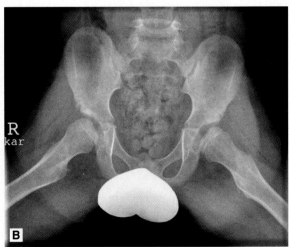

FIGURE 14-4 **A.** Preoperative AP pelvic x-ray, illustrating coxa valga and acetabular insufficiency. **B.** Frog-leg pelvic x-ray, illustrating ability of femoral heads to be centered into the acetabulum. **C.** Post-op x-ray at 3 years, illustrating containment of femoral heads. **D.** Frog-leg pelvic x-ray 3 years post-op, illustrating maintenance of shelves. *(Continued)*

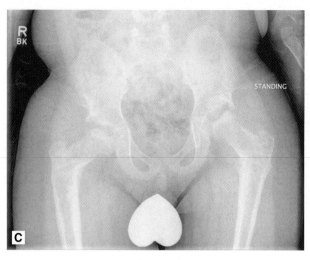

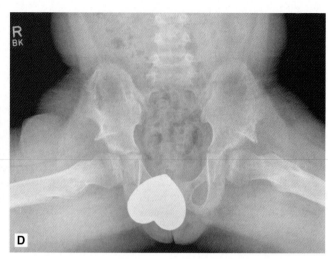

FIGURE 14-4   *(Continued)*

Case 2

A 14-year-old girl presented with bilateral hip dysplasia secondary to developmental dysplasia of the hip (DDH). Bilateral shelf procedures were augmented with abundant iliac crest bone graft (Fig. 14-5). After 2 years, the graft appeared to be consolidated, with excellent augmentation of the acetabulum.

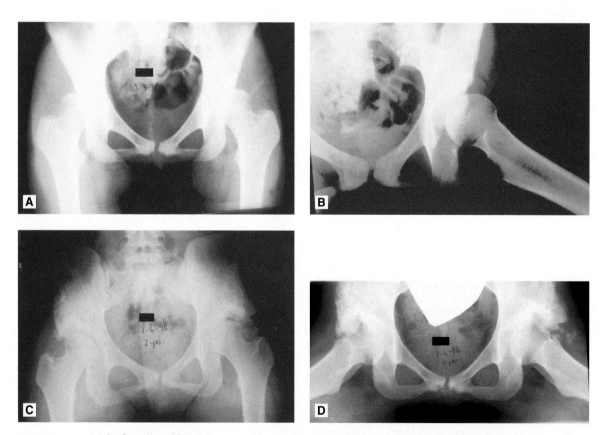

FIGURE 14-5   A. Standing AP pelvic x-ray, illustrating severe bilateral hip dysplasia with a less than 0-degree center edge angle. **B.** Frog-leg lateral of left hip, illustrating ability of head to center into the acetabulum. **C.** Standing AP pelvis 2 years post-op, illustrating result of acetabular augmentation and center edge angles of greater than 30 degrees. **D.** Frog-leg pelvis view 2 years post-op, illustrating symmetrical full abduction of both hips and abundant acetabular coverage.

Case 3

An 11-year-old girl had presented at 6 months of age with a right DDH. Attempts at correction with an abduction brace failed. At 18 months of age, she underwent a shelf-augmented Salter innominate osteotomy and was seen 9 years later. The shelf appeared to be enhanced rather than be resorbed over time (Fig. 14-6).

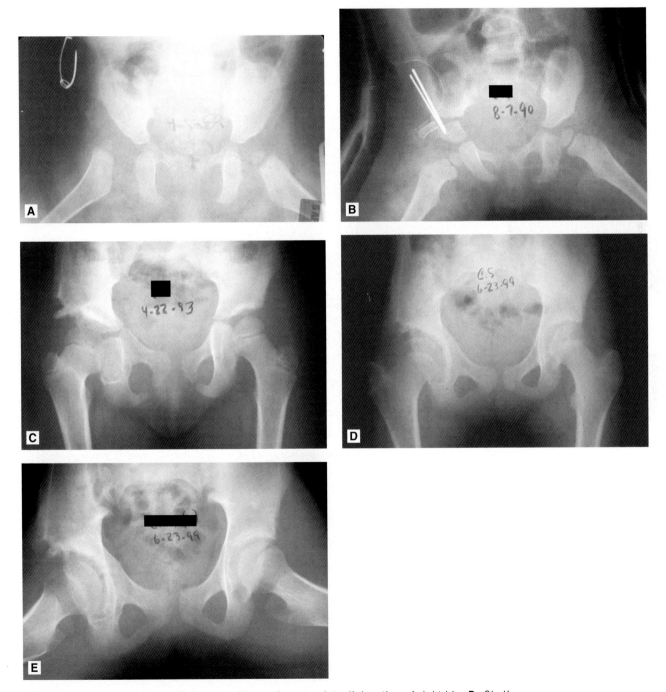

FIGURE 14-6   A. Frog-leg pelvic x-ray, illustrating complete dislocation of right hip. **B.** Shelf-augmented innominate osteotomy. **C.** AP pelvic x-ray 3 years after augmented innominate osteotomy. **D.** AP pelvis 9 years after augmented innominate osteotomy. **E.** Frog pelvis 9 years after augmented innominate osteotomy.

Case 4

This patient presented with severe avascular necrosis and was treated by augmentation acetabuloplasty and was followed for 1 year (Fig. 14-7). The augmentation appears to be consolidated, with excellent extension of the acetabular margins.

Case 5

A 15-year-old boy with unilateral right DDH had been treated by Pavlik harness as an infant (Fig. 14-8). The right hip reduced well, but he sustained bilateral avascular necrosis (AVN). At age 10, he was treated by bilateral augmentation acetabuloplasties. The left side also underwent an innominate osteotomy. The right side underwent a shelf only.

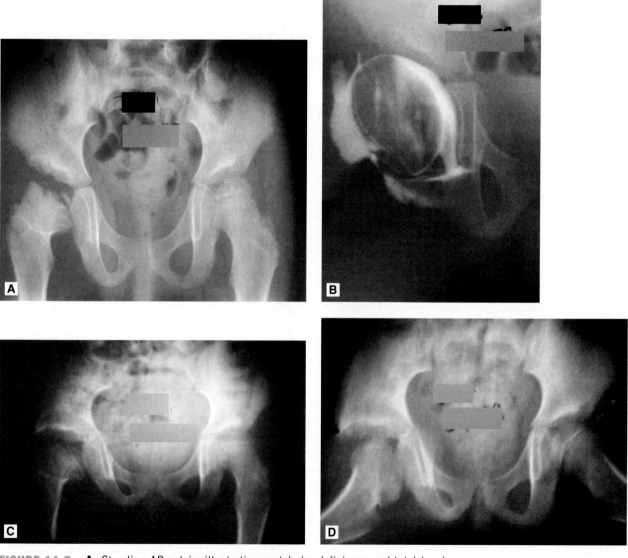

FIGURE 14-7   **A.** Standing AP pelvis, illustrating acetabular deficiency and total-head-involvement avascular necrosis. **B.** Intraoperative arthrogram, illustrating coxa plana and coxa brevia. **C.** Standing AP pelvis 1 year after surgery, illustrating abundant acetabular lateral extension. **D.** Frog pelvis 1 year after surgery, illustrating abundant acetabular lateral extension.

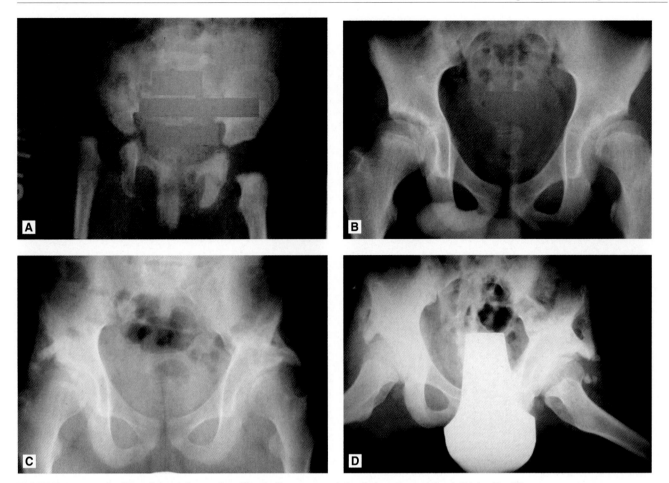

FIGURE 14-8 **A.** AP pelvis at 5 months, illustrating a complete dislocation of the left hip. **B.** AP pelvis at age 10, illustrating bilateral hip dysplasia with changes of AVN and left hip partial subluxation. **C.** Standing AP pelvis at age 15, illustrating results of left augmented innominate osteotomy and right shelf arthroplasty. **D.** Frog pelvis, illustrating full consolidation of shelves on both sides.

REFERENCES

1. Bosworth DM. Hip shelves in children. *J Bone Joint Surg Am.* 1960;42(7):1223–1238.
2. Domzalski ME, Glutting J, Bowen JR, et al. Lateral acetabular growth stimulation following a labral support procedure in Legg-Calvé-Perthes disease. *J Bone Joint Surg Am.* 2006;88(7):1458–1466.
3. Gill AB. Legg-Perthes disease of the hip: its early roentgen graphic manifestations and its clinical course. *J Bone Joint Surg.* 1940;22(4):1013–1047.
4. Konig F. Osteoplastische Behandlung der congenitalen Huftgelenksluxation (mit Demonstration eines Praparates). *Verh Dtsch Ges Chir.* 1891;20(1):75–80.
5. Kruse RW, Guille JT, Bowen JR. Shelf arthroplasty in patients who have Legg-Calvé-Perthes disease: a study of long-term results. *J Bone Joint Surg Am.* 1991;73(9):1338–1347.
6. Kuwajima SS, Crawford AH, Ishida A, et al. Comparison between Salter's innominate osteotomy and augmented acetabuloplasty in the treatment of patients with severe Legg-Calvé-Perthes disease: analysis of 90 hips with special reference to roentgenographic sphericity and coverage of the femoral head. *J Pediatr Orthop Br.* 2002;11(1):15–28.
7. Rab GT. Theoretical study of subluxation in early Legg-Calvé-Perthes disease. *J Pediatr Orthop.* 2005;25(6):728–733.
8. Salter RB. Role of innominate osteotomy in the treatment of congenital dislocation and subluxation of the hip in the older child. *J Bone Joint Surg Am.* 1966;48(7):1413–1439.
9. Staheli LT, Chew DE. Slotted acetabular augmentation in childhood and adolescence. *J Pediatr Orthop.* 1992;12(5):569–580.
10. Willett K, Hudson I, Catterall A. Lateral shelf acetabuloplasty: an operation for older children with Perthes' disease. *J Pediatr Orthop.* 1992;12(5):563–568.

15 Percutaneous Pinning of Slipped Capital Femoral Epiphysis

Laurel C. Blakemore

Slipped capital femoral epiphysis (SCFE), the most common hip disorder in adolescents, is defined as displacement of the proximal femoral epiphysis relative to the metaphysis. Displacement is nearly always posterior and inferior to the metaphysis. SCFE is associated with obesity as well as hypothyroidism, hyperparathyroidism, and end-stage renal disease. Two classification systems exist, with the more recent system categorizing SCFE as stable or unstable. Stability can be defined either clinically, as the ability to bear weight with or without crutches, or radiographically.

Symptoms of stable SCFE can be vague but usually include groin, thigh, or knee pain. An acute SCFE is characterized by sudden onset of pain and inability to bear weight. Plain radiographs are usually sufficient for diagnosis, though magnetic resonance imaging, computed tomography, or bone scan may occasionally be useful as well.

The goals of treatment include preventing further displacement and maintaining optimal hip function. Treatment options for unstable SCFEs are *in situ* screw epiphysiodesis, bone peg epiphysiodesis, and proximal femoral osteotomy. Recently, there has been enthusiasm for the use of hip dislocation, reduction, and internal fixation for an unstable SCFE. *In situ* screw epiphysiodesis, first described in 1990, is the recommended treatment of stable SCFE and, at present, the treatment of choice for unstable SCFE.

INDICATIONS/CONTRAINDICATIONS

The radiographic documentation of an SCFE is sufficient indication for percutaneous pinning in almost all cases. Anteroposterior (AP) and lateral views are obtained in stable slips; for unstable slips, frog lateral views are often too painful to obtain. Prophylactic pinning of a radiographically normal hip on the contralateral side is controversial; anatomic alignment is maintained, and the risk of iatrogenic complications is lower in prophylactic pinning than in risking a second SCFE.

Younger children (under age 10), those with endocrinopathies (including hypothyroidism, growth hormone deficiency, and secondary hyperparathyroidism), obese children, and African-American children have a higher risk of contralateral SCFE.

PREOPERATIVE PLANNING

The surgeon should verify the availability and good working order of the fracture table and C-arm fluoroscopy. A cannulated stainless steel screw system, measuring between 6.5 and 7.3 mm, must be available. Self-tapping screw systems are ideal. Although titanium systems are available, many surgeons no longer use them because of difficulty with later screw removal.

SURGICAL PROCEDURE

After induction of general anesthesia, the patient is transferred to the fracture table, and a perineal post is placed. The ipsilateral arm is usually positioned across the chest on a support or blanket rolls, and a safety belt is placed around the upper torso. For unilateral SCFE, the well leg is placed in a well-leg holder with the hip flexed and abducted; care is taken to avoid compression of the peroneal nerve. This may also be done for stable bilateral SCFE, with each side prepped and draped separately. Alternatively, both legs may be placed in extension, with the second side to be pinned abducted to allow the C-arm to enter between the legs. The operative side is placed in a traction boot holder, with the patella positioned anteriorly without excessive force. This positioning and traction may result in a partial or complete reduction of the slip, but no further efforts at reduction should be made, as forcible reduction is associated with a higher rate of avascular necrosis. The C-arm should be brought in before prepping, to verify that adequate AP and lateral views of the hip(s) can be obtained. In chronic slips, especially in these often-obese patients, the femoral head may be relatively osteopenic and difficult to visualize. It is essential that the outline of the epiphysis can be identified on both the AP and the lateral images. In particularly large patients, an arthrogram may be used to help visualize the femoral head.

The hip is prepped from iliac crest to knee. The operative side may be draped free, or a transparent curtain drape with Kocher clamps weighing down the free inferior margin can be used. After the C-arm is positioned, a guide pin (blunt tip leading) is used to mark the ideal trajectory, in both the AP and lateral projections. The meeting of the two virtual lines marks the skin incision site. However, the ideal starting point is sometimes just proximal to their crossing, so it is usually best to mark a 1- to 2-cm incision beginning at that point and extending proximally. A slender clamp can be used to bluntly dissect along the projected path to the anterior femoral cortex. Fluoroscopic guidance is used to aim the guide pin at the center of the epiphysis, passing perpendicular to the physis. This is usually performed first in the AP view, switching to the lateral view to confirm or fine-tune the starting point and angle. The starting point for severe slips may be surprisingly anterior on the femoral neck, making positioning of the guide pin challenging. The threaded guide pin is then passed across the physis and to the subchondral bone of the epiphysis, verifying by C-arm that the guide pin does not penetrate the joint on any view.

The screw length can be estimated using a calibrated drill, a pin depth gauge, or a second guide pin of equal length. In unstable slips, a second guide pin may be placed into the femoral head at this point to stabilize the epiphysis during drilling and screw passage; this second pin is placed inferomedially, if possible, to avoid the end arterial supply in the superior lateral margin. The guide pin is then overdrilled with a cannulated drill, and great care is taken to ensure that the pin does not pass into the joint during drilling or lose position as the drill is withdrawn. A second pin can be utilized to hold the joint in place as the drill is removed.

A self-tapping screw can then be passed over the guide pin under fluoroscopic guidance, which is used to verify that the screw does not penetrate the joint on any view. Most surgeons recommend placing three to five threads in the epiphysis, leaving some threads in the metaphysis. The operative surgeon may elect to remove the leg temporarily from the traction boot holder at this point and range the hip, feeling for crepitation that might indicate screw penetration. The guide pin is removed, or at least retracted, so that the end of the screw can be visualized. Live imaging may be performed while the hip is gently put through maximum range of motion to all extremes to make certain the screw is not outside the femoral head or closer than 5 mm to the articular surface in any position.

The wound is then irrigated and closed with absorbable sutures, and a small sterile dressing is applied.

POSTOPERATIVE MANAGEMENT

The child is typically placed on crutches and limited to partial weight bearing for 6 weeks. If both sides have been treated, a wheelchair is appropriate, with weight bearing for transfers on the more clinically stable side. Normal activity is gradually resumed, and the patient is monitored clinically and radiographically every 3 to 6 months until skeletal maturity to ensure physeal closure and to monitor for complications.

For patients with a unilateral slip, the need to seek urgent medical care is stressed to the family if similar symptoms arise on the other side.

COMPLICATIONS TO AVOID

Intraoperative complications mostly involve technical errors, including eccentric guide pin positioning, joint penetration, improper screw length, or loss of guide pin position. Unstable slips can be difficult to instrument and occasionally require a second screw.

Complications of SCFE include the following:

- Chondrolysis—possibly associated with joint penetration
- Loss of fixation—possibly due to screw ploughing in the metaphysis or epiphysis
- Slip progression—more common in younger patients, those with underlying endocrinopathies, and those with unstable slips; epiphysis "grows off" the screw and may require repeat pinning
- Pain from the screw head irritating soft tissues

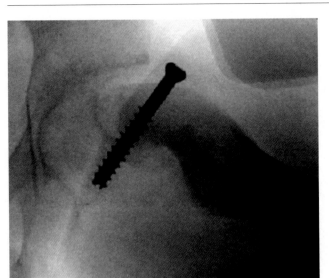

FIGURE 15-1   This screw was left a little proud; it abuts the acetabulum when the hip is flexed. This is particularly problematic when the SCFE is very posteriorly displaced and the screw head is on the anterior femoral neck. (From Flynn JM. Staying out of trouble with the hip: Legg-Calvé-Perthes, slipped capital femoral epiphysis, and transient synovitis versus septic arthritis. In: Skaggs DL, Flynn JM, eds. *Staying Out of Trouble in Pediatric Orthopaedics.* Philadelphia: Lippincott Williams & Wilkins, 2006, with permission.)

- If screw head is left too prominent, may result in catching of soft tissue or impingement of the screw on the acetabulum (Fig. 15-1)
- Avascular necrosis—much higher risk in unstable slips
- Residual deformity—causing external rotation, loss of flexion, and later degenerative changes; can be addressed with realignment osteotomy after healing

ILLUSTRATIVE CASE

This 12-year-old child presented to the orthopaedic clinic with a 2-month history of right thigh pain aggravated by ambulation. He denied any history of trauma or sudden worsening of his pain. Physical examination revealed an obese child whose weight was greater than 90% expected for height. The left hip was nonirritable to log roll in the extended position and mildly irritable in internal rotation. The right hip was mildly irritable to log roll in the extended position and painful at 40 degrees of gentle passive flexion. Radiographs revealed a bilateral SCFE, with the right more severe than the left (Fig. 15-2).

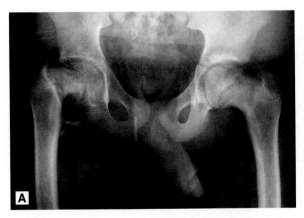
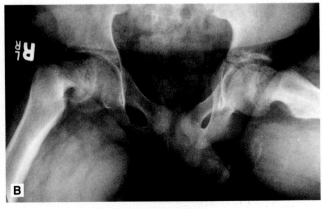

FIGURE 15-2   AP **(A)** and frog lateral **(B)** views of the hips, showing a moderately severe left SCFE and severe right SCFE. The deformity is more easily seen on the lateral views, as is usually the case.

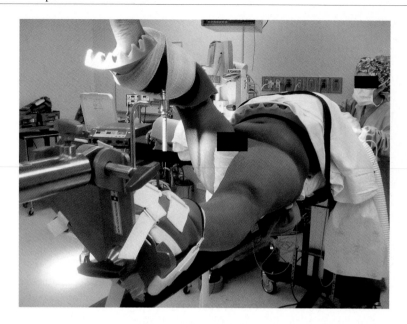

FIGURE 15-3

Positioning for fixation of the left hip.

The patient was made non–weight bearing and admitted to the clinic. He underwent bilateral percutaneous screw fixation the following day (Figs. 15-3 to 15-8). He was discharged on crutches and with a wheelchair and limited to partial weight bearing for 6 weeks. At 1 year postoperatively, he had no pain, had lost 10 pounds, and had increased in height. His internal rotation was limited to neutral on the left, and he lacked 15 degrees of internal rotation to neutral on the right. Both sides demonstrated obligate external rotation with hip flexion. The proximal femoral physes were not completely closed.

PEARLS AND PITFALLS

- Use fluoroscopic imaging frequently, as it is important to know right away if a guide wire or screw is about to enter the joint.
- If a cannulated drill stops advancing, suspect that the guide wire may be bent. Remove and inspect the drill bit for metal shavings and/or image the guide wire to look for a bend. If the guide wire is bent, remove it. Prolonged drilling over a bent guide wire could shear it off, usually at the cortex where it is difficult to remove.
- When backing out the cannulated drill bit, do not put the drill in reverse, as the drill bit may bind the guide wire and remove it.

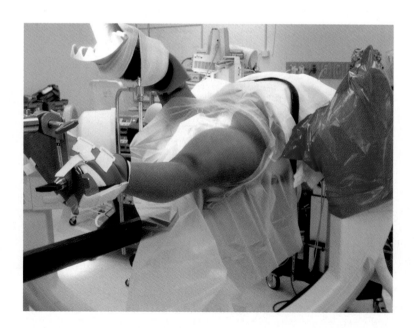

FIGURE 15-4

C-arm is brought in to confirm that good AP and lateral images can be obtained prior to prepping and draping.

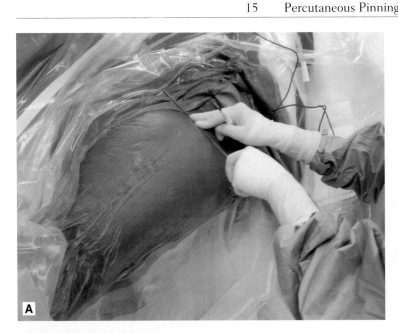

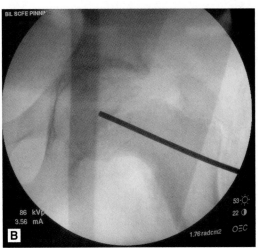

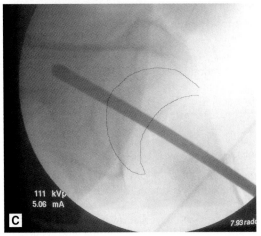

FIGURE 15-5   **A.** A guide pin is placed on the skin, and an AP image is obtained.
B. When the pin is properly positioned, aiming at the center of the epiphysis and crossing perpendicular to the physis, the skin is marked along the pin. **C.** The same procedure is performed on the lateral view.

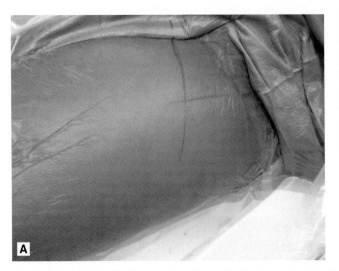

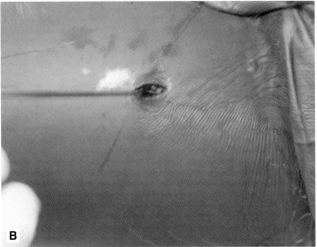

FIGURE 15-6   **A, B.** The incision is marked just proximal to the junction of the skin lines, and a threaded-tip guide pin is inserted to the femoral neck.

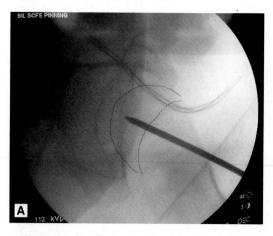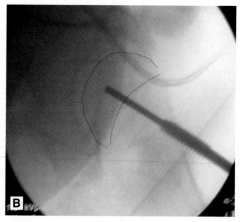

FIGURE 15-7 **A.** Under fluoroscopic guidance, the guide pin is inserted. **B.** After measuring the length and drilling with a cannulated drill, the screw is inserted under fluoroscopic guidance to ensure that the pin is not driven forward. (The head is outlined here for better visualization.)

- A hip arthrogram helps visualize the joint space in very large patients.
- The entrance point of the screw should be proximal to the lesser trochanter; otherwise, a fracture may occur through the hole (or multiple holes) of a missed attempt (Fig. 15-9).
- Before leaving the operating room, there should be no doubt that a screw is not in a joint. Live imaging while moving the leg in all positions is critical.
- Attempt to place a single screw in the center of the femoral head with the tip no less than 5 mm from the articular surface.

EDITORS' NOTE

Some surgeons, such as the editors DLS and VTT, prefer to pin an SCFE using a radiolucent table rather than a fracture table. In some institutions, it takes as long to set up a fracture table as it does to do the surgery. In addition, this technique allows bilateral SCFEs to be pinned without a second draping and positioning.

There are a few pitfalls to this approach. First, when getting a lateral image, the hip is moved into a frog lateral position. In very large patients, this may bend the guide wire (Pearls and Pitfalls). When using a 7.3-mm cannulated screw system, the guide wires are stout enough to avoid bending—most of the time. Second, it is absolutely essential that a guide

---

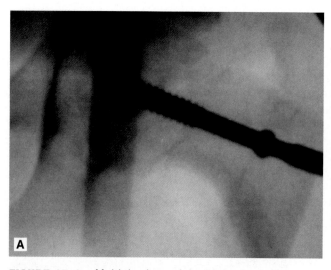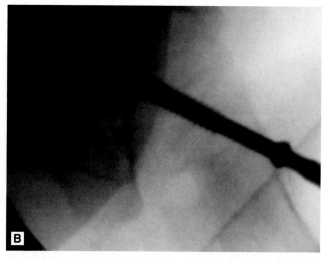

FIGURE 15-8 Multiple views of the final screw position are obtained to confirm that the screw is well positioned without joint penetration before removing the guide pin. AP **(A)** and lateral **(B)** views are obtained using a C-arm. Some surgeons also obtain plain films prior to discharge.

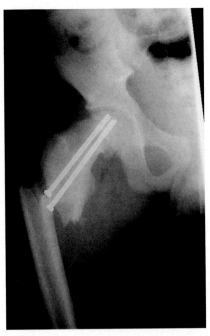

FIGURE 15-9   This SCFE was stabilized using an adult hip fracture technique, with a very low subtrochanteric starting point for two screws. The screws were not perpendicular to the physis, and they created a stress riser leading to a subtrochanteric fracture. (From Flynn JM. Staying out of trouble with the hip: Legg-Calvé-Perthes, slipped capital femoral epiphysis, and transient synovitis versus septic arthritis. In: Skaggs DL, Flynn JM, eds. *Staying Out of Trouble in Pediatric Orthopaedics.* Philadelphia: Lippincott Williams & Wilkins, 2006, with permission.)

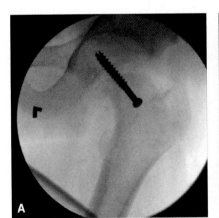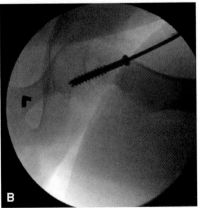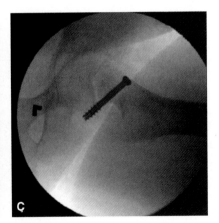

FIGURE 15-10   An essential part of staying out of trouble after SCFE fixation is careful intraoperative evaluation of the screw placement. This stresses the importance of a true lateral with the frog lateral position. A former fellow thought the screw was in good position on the AP **(A)** and frog lateral position **(B)** and was about to close. However, slight rotation of the hip in the frog lateral position demonstrated the screw tip was in poor position **(C).** The time to discover this is in the operating room, not months later in the office. (From Flynn JM. Staying out of trouble with the hip: Legg-Calvé-Perthes, slipped capital femoral epiphysis, and transient synovitis versus septic arthritis. In: Skaggs DL, Flynn JM, eds. *Staying Out of Trouble in Pediatric Orthopaedics.* Philadelphia: Lippincott Williams & Wilkins, 2006, with permission.)

wire or screw is not in the joint (or across the joint) when moving the hip into a frog lateral position. Be on the lookout for any crepitation when starting to move the hip. Finally, the frog lateral view looks different, depending on the amount of internal or external rotation of the hip. Make certain the screw looks good in the frog lateral position through a range of hip rotation (Fig. 15-10).

The editors have found that drawing lines on the skin gives a poor estimate of where to start the guide wire, particularly in large patients where the skin can be quite far from the bone. An alternative is to place a K-wire percutaneously into the femoral head, estimating where the guide wire should be. Under AP imaging, the K-wire is pierced through the skin in line with the femoral neck, starting the tip of the K-wire in the center of the lateral-most portion of the femoral neck. The amount of posterior aim (remember, the head slips posteriorly) is estimated from the preoperative radiographs. Once the K-wire is in the femoral head, AP and lateral images will help estimate where the final guide wire should be placed. A 1-cm incision should then be made in the skin at the appropriate location relative to the K-wire.

REFERENCES

1. Aronson DD, Carlson WE. Slipped capital femoral epiphysis: a prospective study of fixation with a single screw. *J Bone Joint Surg.* 1992;74:810–819.
2. Loder RT, Aronson DD, Dobbs MB, et al. Slipped capital femoral epiphysis. *J Bone Joint Surg.* 2000;82:1170–1188.
3. Morrissy RT. Slipped capital femoral epiphysis technique of percutaneous in-situ fixation. *J Pediatr Orthop.* 1990;10:347.
4. Sanders JO, Smith WJ, Stanley EA, et al. Progressive slippage after pinning for slipped capital femoral epiphysis. *J Pediatr Orthop.* 2002;22:239–243.

16 Chiari Osteotomy of the Pelvis

Charles T. Price and Bouchaib Yousri

A variety of pelvic osteotomies are available for management of hip dysplasia and other hip disorders. These osteotomies can be placed into three general categories: (a) redirectional (Salter innominate, double and triple pelvic osteotomies, and periacetabular osteotomies); (b) volume reducing (Pemberton, Dega, and San Diego osteotomies); and (c) greater load-bearing surface (shelf arthroplasty procedures and Chiari osteotomy). The first two categories attempt to place articular cartilage in a more favorable position for improving joint function. Concentric articular surfaces are required for redirectional osteotomies, whereas younger age groups are usually required for volume-reducing osteotomies. The Chiari osteotomy provides a greater load-bearing surface over the femoral head and also displaces the joint medially to decrease the body-weight moment arm force across the hip, thus reducing the joint load on the hip during weight bearing. The Chiari osteotomy and shelf arthroplasty procedures utilize an interposed hip capsule for weight bearing between the femoral head and the laterally augmented acetabulum. By providing this improved lateral acetabular coverage, the hip capsule can undergo fibrocartilaginous metaplasia to provide hyaline-like cartilage in contact with the femoral head.

INDICATIONS/CONTRAINDICATIONS

The Chiari osteotomy is unique because it is the only pelvic osteotomy that is indicated primarily when the hip is incongruous and when femoral head coverage cannot be achieved by other methods of reconstruction. This procedure is recommended when the femoral head is irregular or cannot be centered in the acetabulum by abduction and internal rotation of the hip. The Chiari osteotomy can also be performed in the presence of severe instability. However, patients should be advised that prevention or treatment of pain, rather than primary improvement in hip function, is the principal objective of this procedure. A Trendelenburg gait may persist following a Chiari osteotomy. Satisfactory outcomes have been reported for the Chiari osteotomy in the treatment of hip deformity and pain caused by developmental dysplasia, Legg-Calvé-Perthes disease, cerebral palsy, and skeletal dysplasias. Best results have been obtained in patients less than 45 years of age with mild or moderate hip dysplasia and early osteoarthritis. The procedure is more easily performed when the center-edge angle (CE angle) is less than −10 degrees. Poor results have been reported when Chiari osteotomy has been used for the management of hip displacement due to myelodysplasia. Poor results have also been reported when this procedure is performed for late-stage osteoarthritis of the hip. Chiari osteotomy is contraindicated for a hip with sufficient proximal migration of the femoral head, which would preclude an appropriate level of osteotomy, or for a hip in which there would be an inability to cover 80% of the femoral head following medial displacement of the distal osteotomy fragment.

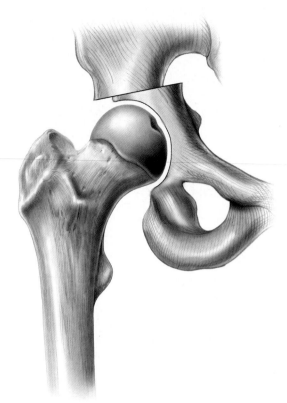

FIGURE 16-1

Oblique osteotomy is performed just proximal to the acetabular margin so that the acetabular roof supports the lateral hip capsule when the hip is displaced medially. The angle of the osteotomy should be approximately 10 degrees. (Redrawn after Colton, *J Bone Joint Surg Br.* 1972;54:578, with permission.)

PREOPERATIVE PLANNING

The objective is to perform an oblique osteotomy in a proximal and medial direction, beginning at the lateral margin of the dysplastic acetabulum. This allows lateral coverage of the femoral head when the joint is displaced medially (Fig. 16-1). One should avoid starting the osteotomy too proximal or too distal. An osteotomy that is too distal may enter the joint or place increased pressure on the femoral head when the hip is displaced medially. An osteotomy that is too proximal may fail to provide adequate load bearing for the femoral head. However, several authors have reported satisfactory results when the osteotomy is high, providing that medial displacement is adequate. The optimal location to begin the osteotomy is within 1 cm or less of the capsular insertion on the lateral margin of the dysplastic acetabulum.

One shortcoming of the Chiari osteotomy is that the insertions of the hip abductor muscles are displaced medially and proximally as the hip is displaced along the slope of the osteotomy (Fig. 16-2). This may reduce the strength of the hip abductor muscles and decrease their mechanical advantage. The degree of weakening of hip abductor function correlates to a greater slope of osteotomy and greater medial displacement. Some authors recommend distal and lateral transfer of the greater

FIGURE 16-2

Effect on hip abductor function. **A.** The position of the hip abductors prior to osteotomy. **B.** Effects of an osteotomy with high inclination and displacement. This reduces the strength of the abductors due to medial and proximal displacement of the greater trochanter.

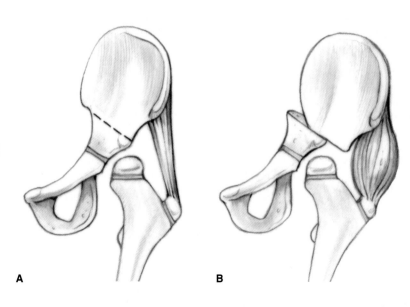

A   B

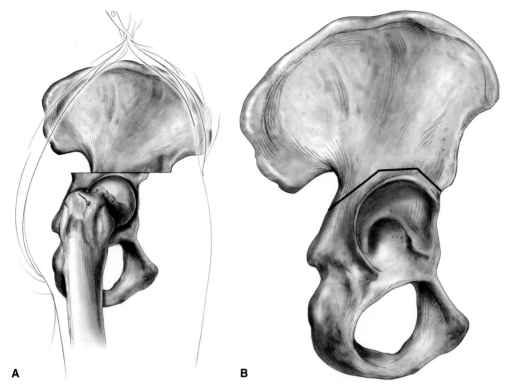

A   B

FIGURE 16-3
Illustration of transverse and dome-shaped osteotomies. **A.** Transverse osteotomy may displace posteriorly. (Redrawn after Colton, *J Bone Joint Surg Br.* 1972;54:578, with permission.) **B.** Dome-shaped osteotomy resists posterior displacement and provides more anterior and posterior support for the hip capsule. Three straight osteotomy cuts are sufficient, in the authors' experience.

trochanter or valgus osteotomy of the proximal femur to improve abductor function and to minimize the risk of persistent Trendelenburg gait.

A third technical consideration with this technique is avoidance of posterior displacement of the distal osteotomy fragment; there is a greater risk of this occurring when the osteotomy is more horizontal. An osteotomy that is curved from anterior to posterior will help resist posterior displacement of the acetabulum. A dome-shaped osteotomy also provides more anterior and posterior support to the hip capsule and femoral head (Fig. 16-3).

Another technical consideration is the amount of medial displacement that is needed. It is recommended that 80% of the femoral head should be covered following displacement. Colton suggested that because the pelvis is approximately triangular at the level of the osteotomy, greater medial displacement reduces the contact area of the osteotomy (Fig. 16-4A). However, anatomical models

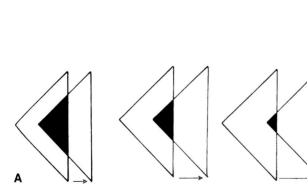

A

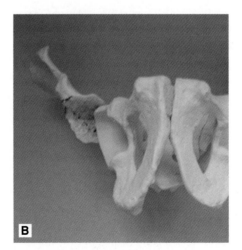

B

FIGURE 16-4   Surface area of osteotomy following displacement. **A.** Illustration from Colton suggests that the shape of the pelvis at the level of the osteotomy is triangular. This would result in decreased surface contact between the fragments as displacement is increased. (Redrawn after Colton, *J Bone Joint Surg Br.* 1972;54:578, with permission.) **B.** Anatomical model demonstrates that the osteotomy surfaces are broad and ovoid. This provides greater surface contact than estimated by Colton when more then 50% displacement is achieved. Up to 80% displacement can be safely performed.

demonstrate that the osteotomy surfaces are broad and ovoid (Fig. 16-4B). Several authors have noted that displacement of up to 80% heals satisfactorily and provides stability as the bone remodels around the capsule. When displacement is attempted, there is a tendency for the distal fragment to rotate on the pubic symphysis, whereas the proximal fragment tends to rotate at the sacroiliac joint. This should be avoided as much as possible by performing direct medial displacement of the distal fragment. Medial displacement is more difficult when the slope of the osteotomy is inadequate.

SURGICAL PROCEDURE

One of several surgical approaches may be used to expose the lateral acetabulum for Chiari osteotomy. It is helpful to have clear visualization of the lateral pelvis from the anterior inferior iliac spine (AIIS) to the sciatic notch. However, percutaneous osteotomy has been performed by one of the authors through a lateral, minimally invasive, muscle-splitting incision (Fig. 16-5). The senior author prefers the anterior-lateral approach described by Smith-Petersen, but the incision should be

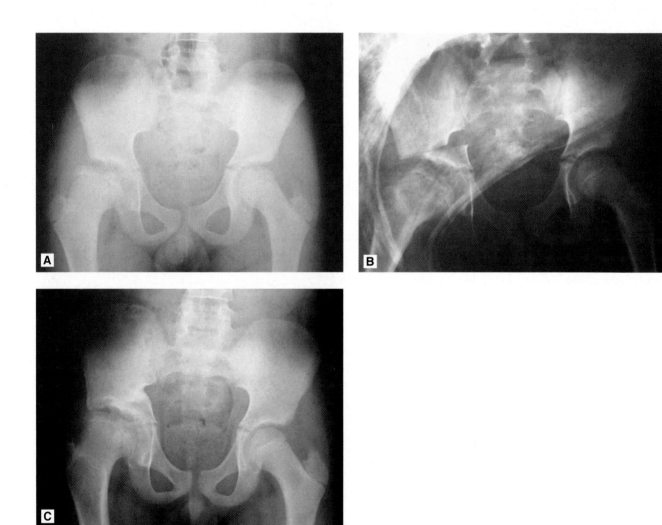

FIGURE 16-5   Radiographs of a child treated by percutaneous Chiari osteotomy. **A.** Radiograph of an 11-year-old boy with a painful hip following Legg-Calvé-Perthes disease. **B.** Chiari medial displacement osteotomy was performed through a small lateral incision under radiographic control. The hip was displaced medially by abducting the lower extremity with immobilization in a hip spica cast. **C.** Follow-up radiograph of the pelvis demonstrates remodeling with good coverage of the femoral head. Symptoms were relieved.

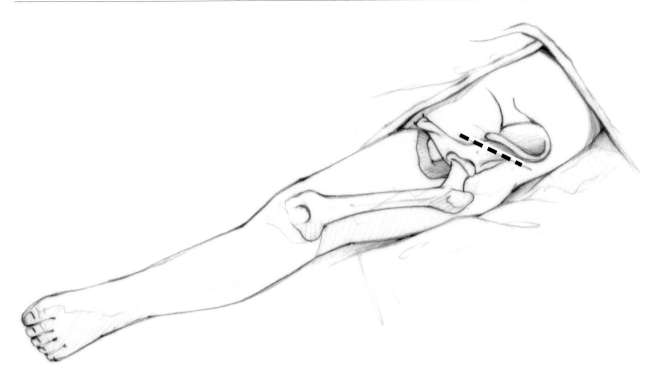

FIGURE 16-6   Exposure by the Smith-Peterson anterolateral approach. **A.** A more oblique incision than described by Smith-Peterson is recommended. The incision begins 2 cm medial and distal to the anterior superior iliac spine and is extended posterior and proximal along the distal boarder of the iliac crest to the junction of the middle and posterior thirds of the crest.

extended proximally along the iliac wing to allow posterior retraction of the tensor fascia femoris muscle and the gluteus medius and gluteus minimus muscles. The procedure is most easily performed on a fracture table the gluteal muscles are unsupported and so that imaging is facilitated. Alternatively, the patient may be positioned on an image-translucent operating table in the supine position, with a bolster under the sacrum to allow the soft tissues of the gluteal region to remain suspended for easier retraction.

The incision is oblique and begins 2 cm medial and distal to the anterior superior iliac spine (Fig. 16-6). It is extended posteriorly and proximally along the distal border of the iliac crest to the junction of the middle and posterior thirds of the crest. Subcutaneous tissue is divided until the fascia of the thigh is exposed. The interval between the sartorius and the tensor fascia lata is palpated in the distal portion of the wound. The fascia of the thigh is incised, and the lateral femoral cutaneous nerve is identified and protected as it exits deep to the inguinal ligament and passes over the sartorius on the medial side of the tensor fascia femoris. The iliac crest is exposed by releasing the lateral fibers of the external oblique muscle. The periosteum or apophysis of the iliac crest is then incised laterally, beginning at the posterior third of the ilium and proceeding anteriorly. At the anterior superior iliac spine (ASIS), the incision turns distally just lateral to the anterior superior and anterior inferior iliac spine and extends to the hip capsule, allowing subperiosteal exposure of the entire medial and lateral surfaces of the ilium. The origin of the sartorius and rectus femoris muscles are elevated and reflected medially, as is the periosteum of the ilium. In adults, these muscles are tagged and reflected individually for later reattachment. The medial and lateral surfaces of the ilium are exposed to the sciatic notch posteriorly. It is advisable to visualize the anterior margin of the notch for approximately 1 cm. In addition, the superior and lateral fibers of the hip capsule may have very proximal attachments on the ilium due to persistent subluxation. These attachments are released and elevated almost to the lateral margin of the dysplastic acetabulum. Fluoroscopic imaging is essential to determine the anatomic lateral margin of the dysplastic acetabulum.

Following exposure, a 2.5-mm Steinmann pin is inserted at the superior-lateral acetabular margin and is directed proximally at an angle of 10 degrees to the transverse plane of the pelvis. If the angle is too high, the sacroiliac joint may be violated. If the angle is directed inferiorly, then the osteotomy will not displace.

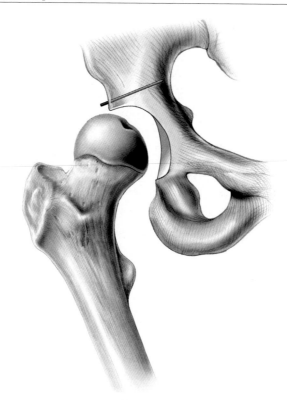

Following exposure, a 2.5-mm Steinmann pin is inserted at the superior-lateral acetabular margin and is directed proximally at an angle of 10 degrees to the transverse plane of the pelvis (Fig. 16-7). If the angle is too high, the pin may enter the sacroiliac joint. If the angle is directed distally, the osteotomy will not displace due to resisted elongation of the hemipelvis.

After the proper starting point and angle of the osteotomy have been identified, a 2-cm straight osteotome is driven into the ilium, just proximal to the Steinmann pin and along the same path (Fig. 16-8). Maintaining the appropriate slope can be difficult due to proximal migration of the femoral head; traction on the leg can assist in maintaining the proper angle of the osteotomy. The first osteotome is left in place while another similar osteotome is driven across the anterior ilium. This second osteotome has the same proximal slope but is tilted distally to approximately match the attachment of the anterior hip capsule (the capsule attaches more distally). A third osteotome is then driven across the posterior ilium to a point just anterior to the sciatic notch. This osteotome is also maintained at a proximal slope of 10 degrees but is tilted distally along the posterior hip capsule. (Although the transtrochanteric approach may permit better visualization and greater ease of osteotomy, the authors have no experience with this approach; the approach described above has worked well for the authors.)

After the three osteotomies have penetrated the medial cortex of the ilium, they are removed. The posterior cortex at the sciatic notch can be divided by a sharp osteotome while retractors protect the sciatic nerve, or a Gigli saw can be introduced to the sciatic notch to complete the division of the posterior cortex (Fig. 16-9). For the latter approach, the Gigli saw is held in place by an instrument until it begins to cut into the wall of the sciatic notch at the level of the posterior limb of the osteotomy. It is essential to have a clean and complete division of the margin of the sciatic notch. If this portion of the osteotomy is incomplete or has a spike of bone, medial displacement of the acetabulum will be difficult.

Following completion of the osteotomy, the acetabulum and hip joint are displaced medially by abducting the lower limb (Fig. 16-10). Approximately 50% displacement is usually adequate, though more displacement may be required to obtain coverage of 80% of the femoral head. At this point in the procedure, palpation of femoral head coverage is often more reliable than radiographs. Gaps between the cut surface of the ilium and the capsule can be filled with bone graft. Bone graft can also be placed medially to facilitate union when displacement is greater than 50%.

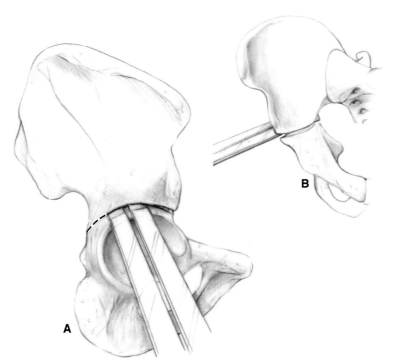

FIGURE 16-8   Osteotomy technique. **A.** After the proper starting point and angle have been identified, a 2-cm straight osteotome is driven into the ilium, just proximal to the Steinmann pin and along the same path. **B.** The first osteotome is left in place while another similar osteotome is driven across the anterior ilium. Although the same proximal slope is maintained, this second osteotome is tilted distally to approximately match the attachment of the anterior hip capsule as the capsule attaches more distal.

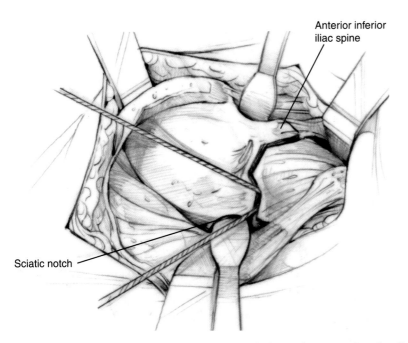

FIGURE 16-9   A Gigli saw is shown in the sciatic notch to complete the division of the posterior cortex. This is not always necessary. The Gigli saw is held in place by an instrument until it begins to cut into the wall of the sciatic notch at the level of the posterior limb of the osteotomy. (Redrawn after Betz RR, Kumar SJ, Palmer CT, et al. Chiari pelvic osteotomy in children and young adults. *J Bone Joint Surg Am.* 1988;70:182, with permission.)

FIGURE 16-10

Medial displacement of the acetabulum is accomplished manually or by abducting the lower limb. Approximately 50% displacement is usually adequate, though more displacement may be required to obtain coverage of 80% of the femoral head. Secure fixation may be used instead of cast immobilization.

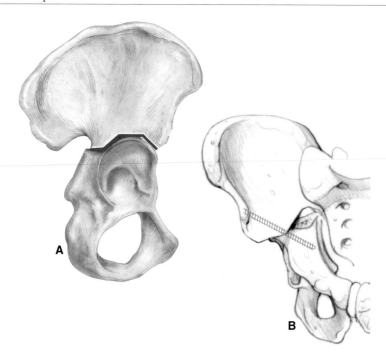

Stabilization of the osteotomy may be achieved by placing the patient in a hip spica cast without fixation, providing that the lower limb is abducted to maintain displacement. However, in the majority of cases, stabilization with large cannulated screws or large threaded Steinmann pins provides excellent fixation and obviates the need for postoperative cast immobilization.

Postoperatively, patients are advised to remain in bed or in a wheelchair for 2 weeks. Toe-touch weight bearing with a walker or crutches is then permitted until 6 weeks postoperative. Rehabilitation is recommended, beginning at about 6 weeks postoperatively, to increase abductor strength, weight bearing, and range of motion. Serial hip and pelvic radiographs are used to assess healing. Once the osteotomy is healed and rehabilitation is complete, full activity is resumed.

COMPLICATIONS TO AVOID

The major complication to avoid is injury to the sciatic nerve. It is advisable to minimize posterior displacement of the acetabulum during the procedure. Careful retraction in the sciatic notch for protection of the sciatic nerve is essential. Utilization of a Gigli saw to complete the posterior portion of the osteotomy may reduce the risk of injury to the sciatic nerve. Damage to the superior gluteal nerve or artery can also result from excessive retraction of the gluteal muscles or from an osteotome entering the sciatic notch too deeply. This may lead to permanent weakness of the abductors. Other complications include wound infections, delayed union, irritation from implants, and other complications that may occur with any major surgical procedure. Patients should be advised that postoperative groin swelling might be pronounced. Use of a Foley catheter may be necessary until the edema subsides.

ILLUSTRATIVE CASE

An 18-year-old ambulatory girl with spastic hemiplegia presented with pain, internal rotation, and limited abduction of her left hip. Anteroposterior radiographs of the hip demonstrated subluxation and proximal migration of the femoral head with a nonconcentric acetabulum (Fig. 16-11A). The abduction, internal rotation radiograph demonstrated an inability to reduce the hip into the acetabulum (Fig. 16-11B). This finding was subsequently confirmed by arthrography under general anesthesia prior to osteotomy. Chiari pelvic osteotomy was performed with screw fixation. Derotational osteotomy of the proximal femur was also performed with internal fixation. No postoperative immobilization was needed. Radiographs 6 months postoperative demonstrated excellent containment of the femoral head with remodeling of the osteotomy to conform to the shape of the capsule (Fig. 16-11C). The patient remained ambulatory and became pain free.

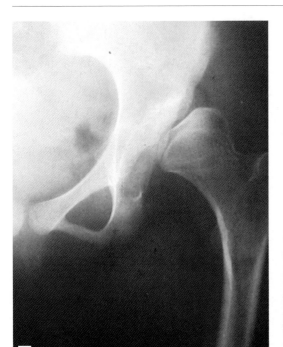

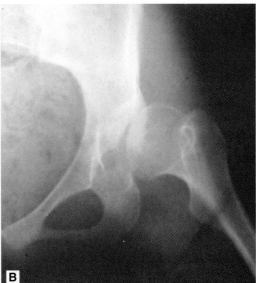

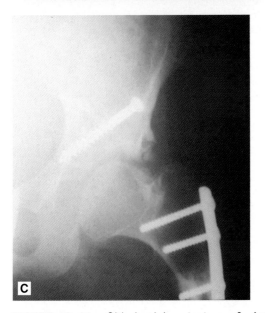

FIGURE 16-11   Chiari pelvic osteotomy. **A.** Anteroposterior radiograph of an 18-year-old ambulatory girl with spastic hemiplegia. Note the subluxation and proximal migration of the femoral head with a nonconcentric acetabulum. **B.** Abduction, internal rotation radiograph demonstrated inability to reduce the hip into the acetabulum. **C.** Radiograph 6 months following Chiari pelvic osteotomy. A derotational osteotomy of the proximal femur was also performed.

REFERENCES

1. Betz RR, Kumar SJ, Palmer CT, et al. Chiari pelvic osteotomy in children and young adults. *J Bone Joint Surg Am.* 1988;70:182–191.
2. Handelsman JE. The Chiari pelvic sliding osteotomy. *Orthop Clin North Am.* 1980;11:105–125.
3. Ito H, Matsuno T, Minami A. Chiari pelvic osteotomy for advanced osteoarthritis in patients with hip dysplasia. *J Bone Joint Surg Am.* 2005;87:212–225S.
4. Matsuno T, Ichioka Y, Kaneda K. Modified Chiari pelvic osteotomy: a long-term follow-up study. *J Bone Joint Surg Am.* 1992;74:470–478.
5. Scher MA, Jakim I. Combined intertrochanteric and Chiari pelvic osteotomies for hip dysplasia. *J Bone Joint Surg Br.* 1991;73:626–631.

17 Ponseti Technique in the Treatment of Clubfoot

Kenneth J. Noonan

The Ponseti method of clubfoot correction consists of a series of manipulations and cast applications designed to diminish the pathoanatomical abnormalities of the idiopathic clubfoot. In general, this method is well tolerated by almost all patients with idiopathic clubfoot. The results of this method almost completely obviate the need for extensive posterior medial and lateral release in greater than 97% of patients.[6,10]

This chapter outlines the pertinent pathoanatomy and method of clubfoot treatment as outlined by Professor Ignacio Ponseti.[13] The goal of treatment for idiopathic clubfoot is to produce a flexible, plantar-grade foot that is painless for the life of the individual and that does not require orthotics.

PREOPERATIVE PLANNING

To have success with the Ponseti method, the pathology and functional anatomy of the clubfoot must be well understood. The congenital clubfoot is a complicated, three-dimensional deformity with four components, as described by the acronym *CAVE:* (a) Cavus deformity refers to the increased height of the vault of the foot. (b) Adductus deformity refers to the medial deviation of the forefoot relative to the hind foot. (c) Varus deformity refers to the adducted and inverted positioning of the calcaneus under the talus. (d) Equinus deformity refers to the increased degree of plantar flexion of the foot (Fig. 17-1). The acronym CAVE also directs the order in which the four deformities are purposefully addressed via the Ponseti method. Cavus is corrected first, adductus and varus follow sequentially, and equinus is the last to be corrected. Fundamentally, all morphologic deformities can be described by the relationship of the forefoot on the midfoot and the relationship of the midfoot on the hind foot.

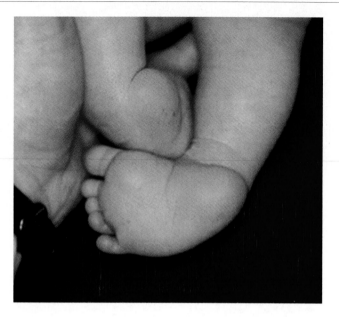

FIGURE 17-1

Bilateral clubfoot in a 4-week-old boy. This figure clearly demonstrates the cavus, adductus, and varus deformity. The hind-foot deformity is always stiffer than the forefoot deformity.

At birth, the whole clubfoot appears to be severely inverted and supinated; the forefoot is adducted and pronated relative to the midfoot and hind foot, the latter of which is in varus and equinus. Although the entire foot is supinated, the forefoot is pronated relative to the hind foot, thus resulting in the cavus. Anatomically, adductus is due to medial displacement and inversion of a wedge-shaped navicular that articulates with the medial aspect of the head of the talus (which has a medially directed neck) and that is in close proximity to the medial aspect of the tibia. The cuboid is also adducted in front of the calcaneus and along with the metatarsals, thus further adducting the midfoot. Hind-foot varus is due to the adducted and inverted position of the calcaneus under the talus (Fig. 17-2). As such, the distal end of the calcaneus lies directly beneath the talar head and not in the lateral position as normally seen.

Equinus deformity is due to the shortening of the extrinsic tendons, such as the gastrocsoleus, tibialis posterior, and long toe flexors. The talus is plantarflexed in the ankle plafond, and the posterior ankle and subtalar capsules are also tight. Midfoot breach resulting from hind-foot stiffness may lead to deceptive physical assessment of actual hind-foot deformity when the foot is dorsiflexed. In these cases, the foot may appear to dorsiflex up to 10 degrees; however, the true equinus deformity can be appreciated by palpating the heel fat pad, which feels empty due to proximal retraction of the calcaneal tuberosity. Radiographically, the tibial-calcaneal angle is increased, and a plantarflexed talus results in a rocker bottom deformity from the aforementioned midfoot breach.

FIGURE 17-2

Hind-foot varus is a result of adduction **(A)** and eversion **(B)** of the calcaneus underneath the body of the talus.

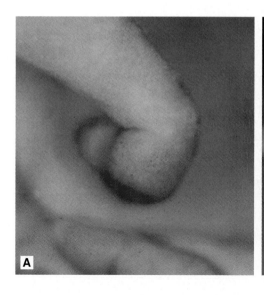

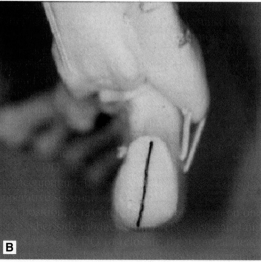

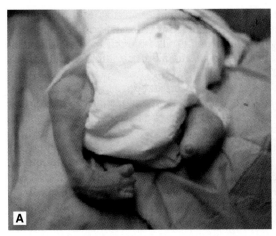 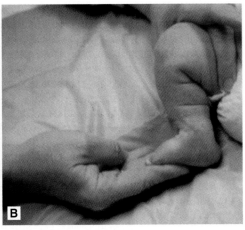

FIGURE 17-3

Constriction band syndrome results in a right clubfoot and a left foot amputation—pretreatment **(A)** and posttreatment **(B).** This child will require an ankle-foot orthotic to maintain correction.

INDICATIONS/CONTRAINDICATIONS

The Ponseti method is ideally suited for use in patients with idiopathic clubfoot. In the author's experience, this method may also have utility in patients with clubfeet secondary to chromosomal abnormalities or neuromuscular disorders or in patients with constriction band syndrome (Fig. 17-3). Although full correction of the teratologic clubfoot secondary to arthrogryposis and spina bifida is not likely, partial correction can be expected with improvement in the forefoot cavus and adductus. As such, the Ponseti method is beneficial for improving foot position and for decreasing the soft-tissue contracture and potential for wound tension following surgical correction of residual deformity. Great care is needed in performing the Ponseti method in children who have teratologic clubfoot, as the stiffness of these insensate feet may lead to skin sores or pressure ulcers when aggressive correction is attempted with the cast (Fig. 17-4).

Ten years ago, Dr. Ponseti taught that the results of his method were directly dependent upon the age at which the child began the treatment of manipulation and casting. Within the past 5 years, however, this philosophy has changed, as older children with neglected or incompletely treated clubfeet have been successfully treated with excellent results.[10] However, the Ponseti method should still ideally be started within a few weeks of delivery.

Special consideration is needed for those babies who are born premature. As a practical matter, it is difficult to perform the Ponseti method in an intensive care unit (ICU) due to the constraints of monitors and lines. In addition, the practitioner must anticipate what he or she plans to do with the corrected clubfoot in prenatal babies. The standard Ponseti method requires patients to be placed into an abduction orthosis with shoes attached to a bar. Unfortunately, there is no such device available for small premature babies who have full correction of their clubfoot deformity within 4 to 5 weeks of delivery. In general, it is often best to institute physiotherapy for preterm babies in the ICU. Therapists should be instructed on gentle manipulation and forefoot abduction as described by Dr. Ponseti. These exercises may be performed daily to maintain the suppleness of the foot prior to institution of casting once the child begins the treatment.

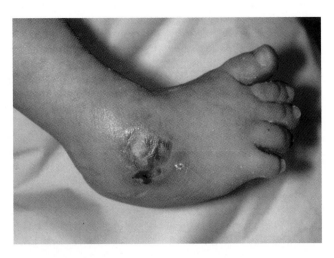

FIGURE 17-4

Pressure sore present on the head of the talus in an 8-week-old child with arthrogryposis. Patients with teratologic clubfeet are more prone to sores because of intrinsic foot stiffness. Greater care is needed during cast application in these children.

In patients with recurrent or undercorrected clubfoot, it is appropriate to begin the Ponseti method, no matter what age, and to continue treatment until no further correction can be obtained. Practitioners in third world countries report that the results from this method may yield partial correction in some toddlers and young children with idiopathic clubfeet who were untreated when infants.[15]

SURGICAL PROCEDURE

In the Ponseti method, the foot is manipulated in a defined manner that stretches ligaments and tendons of the malpositioned tarsal bones. A cast is then applied to hold the corrected position for at least 5 to 7 days. During the intervening days, the ligaments and tendons stretch. The tarsal bones have been noted to quickly readapt and remodel their articular surfaces.[11] Successful treatment of the clubfoot via this method depends on several important principles: The three tarsal joints—subtalar, calcaneocuboid, and talonavicular joints—move simultaneously, and the deformity is corrected during the manipulation. Despite this fact, it is helpful for the beginner to keep the CAVE concept in mind, as it will guide him or her to understand that the first deformity corrected is the cavus and then the adductus, which then leads to correction of the varus deformity. In the standard clubfoot, it is critical that the foot be maintained in equinus until full correction of cavus, adductus, and varus deformities but before heel-cord tenotomy. Premature dorsiflexion of the foot will block calcaneal abduction and eversion, thus decreasing varus correction and increasing the potential for a rocker bottom deformity.

Second, long-leg, bent-knee plaster casts are always used to prevent the child from kicking off the casts. These casts also maintain the forefoot abduction moment, which is required for correction of the adductus and varus deformities. Although some practitioners use synthetic cast material, the author continues to follow the principles as described by Ponseti, who described plaster of Paris applied over thin layers of cotton padding.

As classically taught, the Ponseti method involves a series of manipulations of the clubfoot (each for 1 to 2 minutes), followed by the application of a cast in the position of correction obtained via the manipulation. It is critical that the child remain somewhat relaxed to optimize cast application and to prevent inadvertent cast sores or skin irritations. It is beneficial for formula or breast milk to be withheld for a couple of hours prior to the treatment so that the infant may be fed during cast application. This strategy helps to relax the infant, greatly facilitating the casting. Other methods to relax the child include using warm blankets, soft lighting, or background music.

Casts are usually applied over thin layers of cotton webbing. In cases of bilateral deformities, it is advantageous to apply the cotton and to mold the plaster casts of the feet and lower legs first, as the agitated infant is more easily casted from below the knee than from above (Fig. 17-5). The popliteal fossa must be carefully inspected to ensure that no compression is present from the posterior proximal edge of the short-leg casts. Both casts are then finished by flexing the knee to 90 degrees and extending the upper thigh plaster over cotton roll. In general, manipulation and casting are performed on a weekly basis. An accelerated treatment protocol (5-day interval) may be considered in infants who live a great distance from the practitioner; however, more frequent sessions are likely to be poorly tolerated and may lead to significant foot edema.[9] The manipulations may be performed at 2-week intervals in children older then 6 months of age, but the ultimate time to correction may be longer.

Cavus Correction   The goal of the first casting session is to correct the cavus deformity. This will result in a more rigid forefoot lever arm, which is instrumental in reducing the metatarsus adductus through further forefoot abduction and casting. The pronated forefoot is supinated, and the first metatarsal is elevated. A well-molded plaster cast is then applied with a flat toe plate, thus maintaining all of the metatarsal heads in a row (Fig. 17-6). This maneuver corrects the cavus deformity, though it does result in a potentially alarming global increase in inversion of the foot that is of no consequence. Experienced practitioners may combine cavus correction with the *slight* forefoot abduction during the initial cast session to simultaneously correct some of the adductus deformity. In general, it is a good idea to avoid *aggressive* forefoot abduction during the first cast session so that infants can become used to the method. It is not uncommon for a child to be uncomfortable for the first 24 to 36 hours after casting and manipulation. If an infant is persistently inconsolable following application of a plaster cast, the cast should be removed and the skin inspected for irritation. Because cast sores are more likely to occur when the cast slips distal on the child's foot, parents need to be instructed to watch for proximal migration of the toes (Fig. 17-7). Hyperflexion of the knee to 120 degrees and immobilization with an anterior plaster splint may be needed in patients who have a history of atypical clubfoot or who have difficulty with frequent cast slippage.

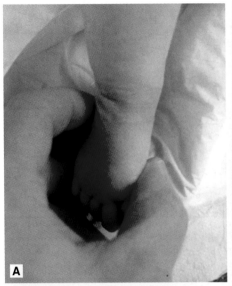
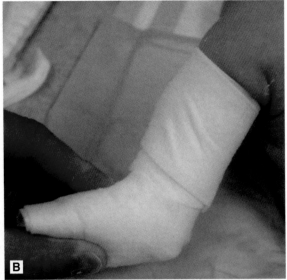
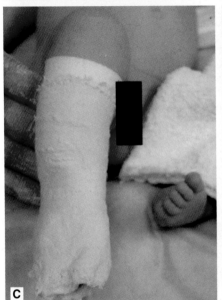
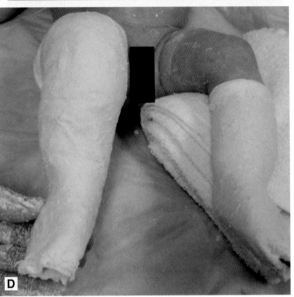
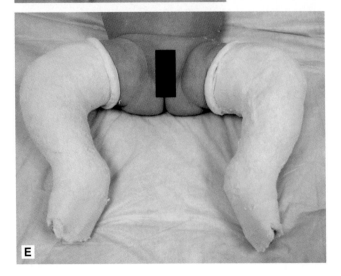

FIGURE 17-5

Casting sequence for 6-week-old girl with bilateral clubfeet. **A.** The right foot is manipulated prior to cast application. **B.** While the child is feeding on a bottle, the right short-leg portion is started with cotton padding. **C.** The plaster is hardening after being molded on the right short-leg portion. **D.** After the left short-leg cast has been applied, the upper portion of both legs can be applied. (In bilateral cases, casting the lower leg portions first is recommended to take advantage of the time when the child is distracted during feeding.) **E.** Completion of both casts. Note how the proximal thigh cotton is rolled down to decrease chafing. (Case donated by Dr. Blaise Nemeth.)

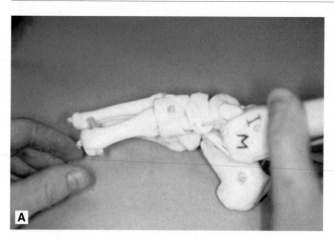
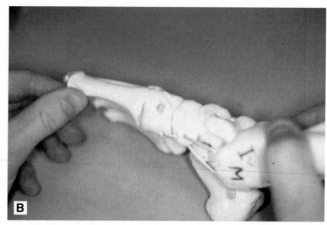

FIGURE 17-6   Correction of forefoot cavus. **A.** Cavus deformity is due to plantarflexion of the first metatarsal, resulting in a forefoot pronation relative to the remainder of the foot. **B.** In the first step, the first metatarsal is elevated, thus reducing the cavus and aligning the forefoot for more efficient future abduction of the foot.

Metatarsus Adductus and Varus Correction   Correction of adductus and varus deformities occur sequentially and are a result of the *predominant* manipulation in which the forefoot is abducted against counterpressure on the head of the talus (Fig. 17-8). The practitioner must be careful to place the counterpressure accurately—not on the fibula or the calcaneocuboid joint. Anatomically, this maneuver will correct the metatarsus adductus by reduction of the metatarsals and the navicular on the head of the talus and the cuboid on the calcaneus. With subsequent casting, the calcaneus will begin to evert and abduct under the talus. The hind foot will then convert from a varus to a neutral or valgus position. To promote efficient correction, it is critical that abduction be performed with the forefoot in supination, thus maintaining prior correction of forefoot cavus, and with the foot in equinus so that the calcaneus will not be prevented from everting and abducting underneath the talus. Dynamic forefoot abduction may be promoted by slightly externally rotating the previously molded and hardened short-leg portion of the cast while the upper thigh portion is applied and molded (Fig. 17-9).

At subsequent visits, the cast is removed with either a cast knife or a cast saw. If the latter is used, the technician must be aware that these casts are applied over thin layers of padding, thus exposing the infant to the risk of saw burns by the inattentive technician (Fig. 17-10). After cast removal, the

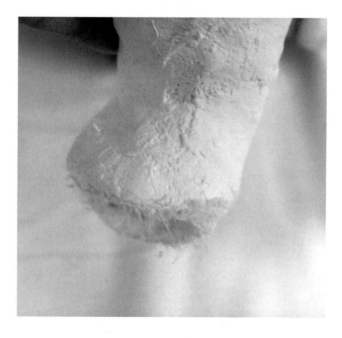

FIGURE 17-7

Families are instructed to look for retraction of the toes within the cast (shown here), which can predispose the foot to a pressure sore on the heel.

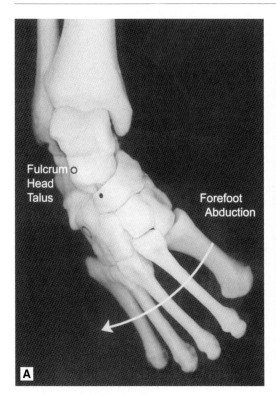 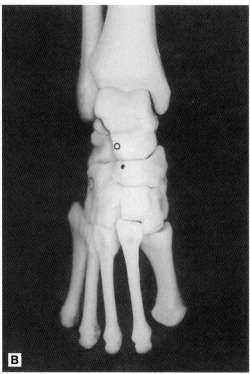

Fulcrum
Head
Talus

Forefoot
Abduction

A   **B**

FIGURE 17-8

Correction of metatarsus adductus via forefoot abduction. **A.** Medial deviation of the navicular and cuboid lead to metatarsus adductus. This is reduced with forefoot abduction against a fulcrum of pressure against the exposed talar head. **B.** When fully corrected, the head of the talus is covered by the reduced navicular. In addition, the cuboid has been reduced on the distal end of the calcaneus.

child undergoes manipulation of the forefoot against pressure over the talus. This time may be increased in children with stiffer feet. Weekly manipulations and castings are performed with the forefoot in slight supination and with the foot in equinus until full correction of forefoot adduction and hind-foot varus is obtained (Fig. 17-11). In general, the full correction of these two deformities can be expected when the thigh-foot axis is approximately 60 degrees externally rotated. Once this angle has been obtained, the final deformity that needs to be corrected is the equinus deformity.

Equinus Correction   The success of the Ponseti method depends on adequate correction of the Achilles contracture. Yet for the neophyte, it can be challenging to decide whether the foot being treated is deserving of a heel-cord release; this is because the apparent ability to dorsiflex the ankle may actually represent dorsiflexion through the midfoot (rocker bottom). In this case, failure to perform the heel-cord tenotomy will result in a recurrence of clubfoot deformity as the child ages. Some physicians are reticent to perform this procedure due to a perceived risk of overlengthening

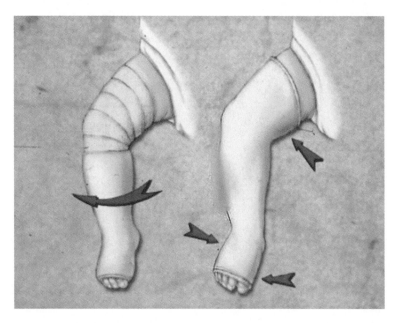

FIGURE 17-9

Slight external rotation (curved arrow) is performed when converting the short-leg portion to the long-leg cast. This leads to dynamic forefoot abduction (short arrows) while in the cast.

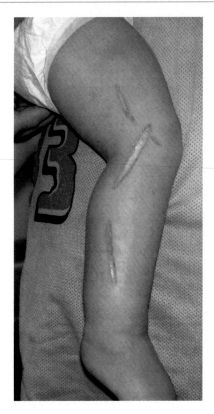

FIGURE 17-10

Cast saw burns may result from cast removal by neophyte cast technicians who are not aware of the thin cotton and the intimate mold that are utilized with the Ponseti method.

or infection. In the latter scenario, the risk of infection is exceedingly low. Likewise, in the former concern, the risk of overcorrection via heel-cord tenotomy with subsequent calcaneus positioning and heel-cord weakness has been shown to be exceedingly low in a long-term follow-up study from Iowa.[3] Ippolito et al.[7] have demonstrated greater weakness when posterior release was performed instead of the simpler heel-cord tenotomy.

Based on experience, the author performs percutaneous Achilles tenotomy in 99% of cases; in the rare and extremely mild foot, the final deformity may be corrected through sequential dorsiflexion casting. Although Ponseti recommended heel-cord sectioning in cases where the foot does not obtain 10 degrees of dorsiflexion at the end of casting, he also said that if there is any doubt about the appropriateness of performing a heel-cord tenotomy, then it should be performed.

FIGURE 17-11

Correction of hind-foot varus. **A.** Prior to varus correction, the calcaneus is abducted and inverted under the talus. One can easily see why premature dorsiflexion of the foot would prevent the distal end of the calcaneus from dorsiflexing, then leading to midfoot breech. **B.** Manipulation of the forefoot promotes adduction and eversion of the calcaneus and correction of the varus deformity.

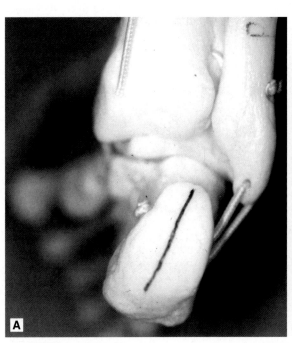

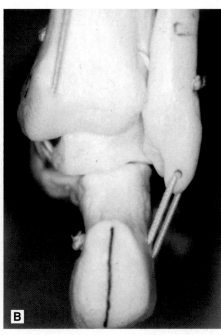

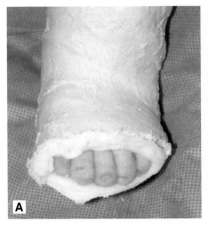 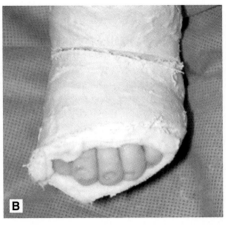 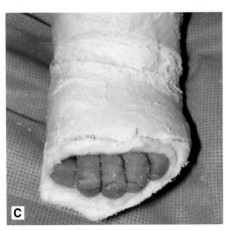

FIGURE 17-12   Intraoperative tenotomy and casting is often performed in children who have severe deformity or who have been difficult to cast. In these cases, a complete tenotomy can be ensured and maximal dorsiflexion obtained. **A.** After tenotomy, the foot is maximally dorsiflexed in the cast. Unfortunately the toes here are white due to poor blood supply. **B.** A cast saw splits the cast along the anterior ankle crease. **C.** The foot is gradually plantarflexed until brisk capillary refill is reestablished. The defect is then casted in this position.

Complete heel-cord tenotomy can be performed without concern of overlengthening or weakness in children up to 18 months of age. The author's institution performs heel-cord tenotomy in the clinic for those children with clubfeet who are up to 6 months of age. However, the operating suite is preferred in children who are older than 6 months of age or in children with a history of being very agitated during clubfoot casting. Furthermore, the operating suite may be the best location for any child who has a very stiff foot and who requires complete and certain tenotomy (Fig. 17-12).

When the Ponseti method is performed in the clinic, the parents are typically asked to leave the cast room suite so the tenotomy may be performed in their absence. In the clinic, topical anesthetic cream is applied to the posterior heel-cord region for 45 minutes prior to tenotomy. If desired, lidocaine without epinephrine may be injected, but care should be taken to prevent overinjection of the anesthetic, which could prevent accurate palpation of the tendon prior to the tenotomy. Pain is greatly decreased when the parents prophylactically administer an appropriate dose of acetaminophen 1 to 2 hours prior to tenotomy.

Heel-cord tenotomy is performed using a semisterile technique by prepping with sterile surgical soap. The knee is held by an assistant, and the foot is positioned to avoid excessive dorsiflexion, as this would obscure the tendon to palpation within the surrounding soft tissues. The practitioner should be aware of the location of the medial neurovascular bundle and remember the elevated calcaneal pitch. The author performs the tenotomy about 1.5 cm above the palpable tuberosity of the calcaneus (Fig. 17-13). A #6900 Beaver blade or a #11 blade is inserted medial to the tendon edge

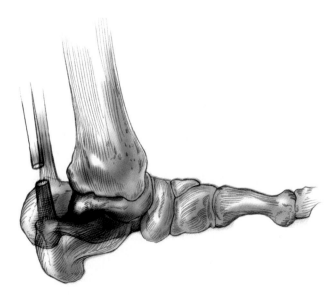

FIGURE 17-13

In more than 99% of clubfeet, equinus is corrected via a heel-cord tenotomy. It is important to recognize that the calcaneus is elevated in the fat pad; therefore, tenotomy needs to be more proximal than what seems intuitive.

and rotated laterally to lie partially anterior to the Achilles tendon. The contralateral index finger is then used to push the Achilles tendon against the knife blade, thus completing tenotomy. Complete tenotomy is heralded by a palpable pop and an increase in dorsiflexion of approximately 20 degrees. Whereas some have encountered significant bleeding from this procedure,[4] the author has found that all bleeding can be well controlled by applying pressure with sterile gauze. Once the tenotomy is performed, the sterile soap must be completely removed. A well-molded plaster cast is then applied over a sterile cotton roll placed over the tenotomy site. The cast is applied with maximum dorsiflexion and abduction of the foot. The foot must be carefully inspected to ensure that good blood flow is present. In children younger than 6 months of age, the cast is kept on for 3 weeks. Older children are maintained in a plaster dressing for up to 4 weeks to allow for full healing. Oral acetaminophen is given for 24 to 36 hours for post-tenotomy pain. Families are informed that a mild amount of blood (up to the size of a quarter) may be present on the posterior cast and are further instructed to call if the toes pull back in the cast, if the patient has inconsolable pain, or if the toes have inadequate blood flow.

POSTOPERATIVE MANAGEMENT

It is important that all concerned parties recognize that successful treatment of the idiopathic clubfoot via the Ponseti method is considered a two-stage process. In the first stage, the practitioner *obtains* correction through a series of manipulations, casting, and, in most cases, a heel-cord tenotomy. The infant's caregiver must then *maintain* the correction with the use of an appropriate orthosis and occasional physiotherapy. It is further important to emphasize that patient compliance with the bracing protocol is directly related to results.[4,8,14] Failure to follow recommendations for maintaining correction dramatically increases the recurrence rate by up to 17 times the recurrence rate seen in compliant patients.[10] In a recent follow-up study, Dobbs et al.[5] showed that noncompliance increases the recurrence rate by an odds ratio of 183 ($p < 0.00001$) and that noncompliance may be related to the parents' educational level. Results of treatment (recurrence) were not related to degree of deformity, age at treatment onset, or previous treatment.

In many respects, this is the most important section of this chapter. Once the procedure is complete, the physician no longer has complete control of the foot and is thus dependent on the caregiver to fully follow directions. Once the clubfoot is adequately corrected, the family is instructed in the importance of postcast bracing. In addition, a great deal of time is spent guiding the family on different strategies to obtain full compliance.

After correction of the deformity, the child is usually placed in a foot abduction orthosis, which consists of two shoes attached to a bar that maintains foot abduction (external rotation) and keeps the feet at shoulder width. The shoes are placed on the bar to the degree of external rotation obtained in the last cast—typically about 45 to 60 degrees of external rotation (Fig. 17-14). In unilateral cases, however, the unaffected foot is positioned at 35 degrees of external rotation. Parents are educated that after the treatment, the child's feet are usually hypersensitive; therefore, the parents should spend some time during the first few weeks washing and massaging the feet to desensitize them. In addition, the practitioner should use a pen to outline the position of the toes on the foot bed of the open-toed shoe. This will provide a quick reference so that parents can detect proximal migration of the foot in the shoe. This migration not only hinders control of the foot but also greatly increases the rate of heel sores. Parents are instructed that skin sores can result from improper shoe fit and that for the first week they should remove the shoes and check the feet for impending skin sores each time they change the diaper. Should problems arise, the patient can usually be managed by brace modification, by temporary use of moleskin, or by increasing the number of socks. Full-thickness sores are rare and must be managed by abstaining from brace use until fully healed, at which time the brace would be refitted.

The child returns to the clinic at intervals of 1 month, 3 months, 6 months, and 10 months from final cast removal. At each visit, the feet are inspected for recurrence and for proper brace fit. In general, one to two prescriptions will be required for new orthotic shoes within the first year of life due to growth. The family is taught that new shoes are needed when the toes overlap the edge of the open-toe shoe. The author's institution recommends full-time brace wear until the child starts to pull to a standing position, which may begin as early as 9 to 10 months. At this point, the patient is weaned from full-time brace wear to nighttime-only brace wear by 15 months of age. On average, brace wear is decreased to 4 hours per day for each month after the patient begins cruising. For example, by 13 months of age, an infant who began cruising at 1 year of age is placed in the brace at bedtime. The brace is removed by 4 p.m. the following day. At 14 months of age, the child has the brace removed at noon. At 15 months of age, the child is probably walking well, and thus the brace is removed when the child awakens. Nighttime brace wear is continued until 3 to 4 years of age.

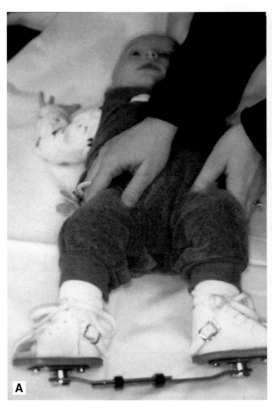
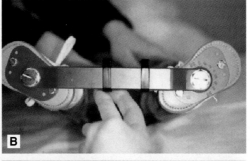
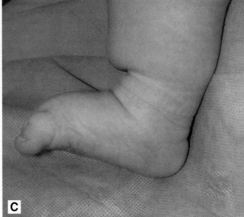

FIGURE 17-14
Abduction orthosis is worn to prevent recurrence and maintain correction in this boy with a left clubfoot. **A.** The orthosis is maintained at shoulder width. **B.** The left foot is externally rotated to 60 degrees, while the contralateral foot is rotated to 45 degrees. **C.** The left foot has slight narrowing above the ankle that is of no clinical significance and is a hallmark of a compliant family.

This brace-wearing protocol deviates slightly from Dr. Ponseti's recommendation, which is full-time brace wear for only 3 months. The author's institution has found that compliance is increased if the child wears the brace full time in the months that he or she is not likely to be walking. After the first few months of bracing, families are instructed to avoid removing the brace when the child is sporadically crying; however, if the child appears to be in pain and the crying is persistent, the brace needs to be removed and the foot inspected. Compliance appears to be greatly increased when full-time brace wear is maintained until cruising age and the infant learns that the brace is a non-negotiable aspect of his or her life.

One must determine whether recurrence of deformity is due to parents not fully following instructions or whether it results from a foot that is intrinsically stiffer and thus not fully corrected. In the latter instance, family compliance is likely to decrease due to the difficulty of maintaining such feet in off-the-shelf shoes. One strategy for improving brace wear in such cases is to decrease the foot's external rotation to a lesser degree for 1 month and then increase the external rotation as the child's foot acclimates to the brace. Other options for improving the fit, and thus the compliance, are also available to the physician and the orthotist. For instance, three different shoes are available—the Markell Corporation (Yonkers, New York) has modified its original shoe (which is still available) by offering one with the heel removed. This new shoe may be more effective in children with recurrent equinus who have a propensity for coming out of the shoe. More recently, a sandal style of shoe has been used in Iowa; despite good results, however, this shoe is not widely available. In addition, an orthotist may customize these shoes by applying plastizote heel counters or pads on the tongue portion for small feet, which tend to slide out.

Other methods may be used to maintain the correction in cases where a foot abduction orthosis cannot be used. For example, in children whose feet simply cannot be held in the foot abduction orthosis or in children with an amputation or a foot deformity on the contralateral foot (precluding adequate fitting), a custom-made polypropylene knee-ankle-foot orthotic (knee flexed to 90 degrees) may be used to maintain the foot in maximum dorsiflexion and foot abduction. Once the child is a good walker, the KAFO can be converted to an AFO.

Clearly there is a role for physical therapy in the management of clubfoot, as evidenced by the functional method used in France by Bensahel et al.[2] The author's clinic occasionally prescribes physiotherapy that is predominately home based and that teaches the caregiver to work on dorsiflexion stretching with forefoot abduction (Fig. 17-15). This referral is usually made to those patients who have incomplete correction of the deformity with residual equinus deformity. In rare cases, there has been improvement in foot position in children with completely unbraceable feet.

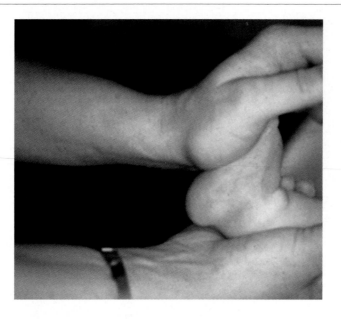

FIGURE 17-15

Physiotherapy. Parents may be shown how to stretch the heel cord when residual contracture is present. Care is used to place the force in the arch of the foot, thus diminishing the risk of a rocker bottom deformity.

COMPLICATIONS TO AVOID

The reported incidence of residual deformity following treatment with the Ponseti method is anywhere between 1% and 35% of feet.[3,10] This disparity is due in part to differing definitions of what comprises residual deformity that may or may not require treatment. *Persistent* foot deformity may result from an inability to obtain full correction following the removal of the last cast, or it may be a *recurrence* of deformity. Feet that are prone to persistent deformity include feet of children who are greater than 1 year of age at time of initial treatment onset or of children who are born with severe or atypical clubfoot. These children have short, fat feet with a persistent and deep plantar crease from the medial border to the lateral border of the foot; they also often have a shortened first ray in comparison with the other four rays. Recurrent deformity after full correction of the clubfoot is rare and is usually due to noncompliance from abduction bracing. Recurrent deformity may be more common in children with clubfeet and with only four toes on the affected foot. These individuals may have absence of the peroneal muscle group (similar to that seen in fibular hemimelia), thus leaving them more prone to recurrence.

Residual deformities are seen within the first year and include isolated equinus, metatarsus adductus, forefoot supination, or combinations of all three. Equinus is the most common persistent deformity and tends to precede other deformities if not addressed. For instance, when the foot is in equinus, abduction bracing is difficult due to the inability of the foot to be held appropriately. The progression and worsening of recurrence is expected with an unbraceable posterior contracture that then leads to recurrence of the midfoot adductus and supination. If left uncorrected, the residual hind-foot equinus leads to varus positioning when children begin to walk.

A subgroup of patients have recurrent metatarsus adductus and no equinus contracture. However, these children usually present after weaning of the abduction bracing and when patients are ambulatory. During the swing phase of gait, forefoot supination will develop due to persistent medial displacement of the navicular and subsequent medial pull of the anterior tibialis. In these instances, the tibialis anterior acts as a forefoot supinator as opposed to a foot dorsiflexor. This deformity may be detected in nonambulatory children who are braced—the practitioner scratches the plantar aspect of the foot and observes whether the foot completely dorsiflexes or supinates in response to the plantar stimulation.[12]

Treatment of residual deformity depends on location and severity and on the age of treatment. Recasting may be considered in children younger than 18 months of age who have residual deformity. In this instance, the feet are manipulated and casted in a fully corrected position (including dorsiflexion) for a 2-week period. After 2 weeks, the casts are removed and reapplied, usually for three casting sessions for a total of 6 weeks. After this, abduction bracing is reinstituted. As previously mentioned, the most common deformity that precludes adequate bracing is residual equinus deformity, which can be addressed by the stretching casts mentioned earlier. In older children, it can be difficult to effectively stretch the hind-foot contracture due to midfoot breech. In response, a repeat heel-cord tenotomy and casting may be beneficial in children who have midfoot breach or in children who have failed a repeat casting. Repeat heel-cord tenotomies consistently increase dorsiflexion 10 to 15 degrees, which may be just enough to maintain the feet in the abduction orthosis, thus preventing any further recurrence. Repeat heel-cord tenotomy, which can be done up to the age of 1.5 years, is more successful in children who have a clearly palpable and defined tendon. Those children with significant scarring and an indiscrete tendon, on the other hand, will likely have less improvement following a repeat percutaneous heel-cord tenotomy.

Children with significant recurrent deformity after 18 months of age uniformly require some open surgery to correct deformities that are persistent. The author strongly advocates the "a la carte" method of surgical treatment of idiopathic clubfoot as advocated by Bensahel et al.[1] To prevent overcorrection, it is important to carefully examine the foot clinically and radiographically before determining which deformity requires surgical treatment.

In infants with isolated and persistent hind-foot equinus; correction is attempted with an open Achilles tendon lengthening. If, after lengthening, there is residual posterior contracture, then a posterior release also needs to be performed. The author has found that release of the posterior ankle capsule; calcaneal fibular ligament and syndesmosis of the distal tibia and fibula are required to obtain adequate dorsiflexion. A K-wire is placed through the plantar aspect of the heel through the calcaneus and the talus and into the tibia to maintain correction in the cast for 6 weeks. Those patients with persistent equinus despite posterior release should be carefully inspected for forefoot cavus deformity, which will accentuate the apparent equinus deformity. These individuals are treated with a plantar fascia release and release of the abductor hallicus muscle through a medial incision.

Infants with persistent equinus, varus, and metatarsus adductus can be ameliorated with presurgical casting before correcting the hind-foot deformity. In some instances, however, this presurgical casting is ineffective at reducing the deformity, and a more extensive exposure is thus needed. A standard Turco incision is used in children with significant residual equinus, metatarsus adductus, and inversion. Posterior release is done through this incision to lengthen the tendons of the posterior tibialis, the flexor digitorum longus, and the flexor hallucis longus muscles. A midfoot release can also be performed through this incision by incising the navicular first cuneiform joint; occasionally, the talonavicular joint is also performed. Transfer of the anterior tibialis toward the midportion of the foot can also be performed in the capsulotomy defect when dynamic supination exists. The midfoot and hind foot are pinned, as described above, and placed in a cast for 6 weeks with the knee bent. Afterward, a short-leg cast is applied for weight bearing for 6 more weeks. Release of the subtalar joint is avoided in these children, as this would predispose the foot to growth arrest and overcorrection, with later implications for pain and disability.

In children older than 2 to 3 years of age, any residual deformity can be corrected using bony procedures and extrinsic tendon lengthenings as needed. Capsulotomy and significant soft-tissue releases in the older age group are more prone to recurrence and stiffness; thus the deformities should be corrected through appropriately planned osteotomies. Residual equinus deformity is corrected with a heel-cord tenotomy as needed; varus deformity can be corrected with an opening wedge or sliding calcaneus osteotomy. Persistent metatarsus adductus and dynamic supination are corrected through an opening wedge osteotomy of the first cuneiform and lateral transplantation of the anterior tibialis into the third cuneiform (Fig. 17-16). In these patients, it is important to ensure that the ossific nucleus of the third cuneiform is present in order to place the anterior tibialis tendon into an appropriate anchor site. A first cuneiform opening wedge osteotomy may be paired with a closing wedge cuboid osteotomy in patients with excessive metatarsus adductus (see Chapter 19). Once osteotomies have been done, the foot may be pronated to account for a supination deformity that may have been present from the unopposed anterior tibialis pull. Transfer of the anterior tibialis to the third cuneiform may then be performed to maintain correction. These individuals are placed in a long-leg cast for 6 weeks, with the knee bent at 90 degrees. Once the initial cast and pins are removed, a period of short-leg casting for 6 weeks is utilized.

Technique of Anterior Tibialis Transfer

A dorsal–medial incision is based over the first cuneiform and the palpable insertion of the anterior tibialis. The soft tissues and inferior extensor retinaculum are incised, and the tendon is detached from its insertion with as much tendon length as possible. The tendon is sutured with a modified Bunnell stitch, using 1 Vicryl suture (absorbable suture). The tendon is freed up to the inferior margin of the superior extensor retinaculum lying over the ankle joint. A lateral incision is made over the third cuneiform, and the toe extensors are retracted medially, while the extensor digitorum brevis is retracted laterally. The ossific nucleus of the third cuneiform is identified, and an appropriate drill hole is placed from dorsal to plantar through the ossific nucleus. The tendon is delivered into the lateral wound and pulled through the drill hole by the 1 Vicryl stitch delivered through the plantar aspect of the foot. The tendon is confirmed to easily *and reproducibly* slide into its new insertion under several trials. The suture is tied with a button *on the exterior* of the plantar aspect of the cast after the dressing has been applied (Fig. 17-17). Securing the tendon via a button under the plaster

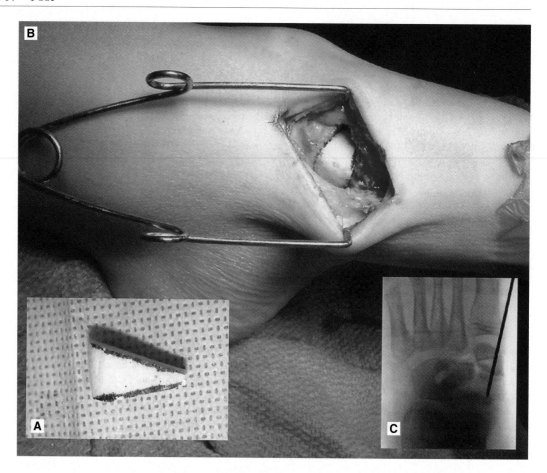

FIGURE 17-16

Correction of residual forefoot deformity in a 6-year-old boy. **A.** Tricortical allograft is fashioned to fit into an osteotomy of the first cuneiform. **B.** The allograft is placed medial, with the widest portion of the wedge placed plantarly (to correct cavus) and medially (to correct adductus). **C.** A single K-wire can be used to securely fix the osteotomy.

often results in pressure sores, even when a thick felt pad is used. The patient is kept non–weight bearing in the cast for 6 weeks. At the time of cast removal, the 1 Vicryl stitch breaks off at the skin margin as the cast is removed. Alternative methods of fixation of the anterior tibialis include suture to the peroneus tertius tendon and the use of suture anchors.

PEARLS AND PITFALLS

Pitfalls in Indications and Assessment of Deformity

One should be aware of the increased risk for pressure sores from manipulation and casting in patients with a particularly stiff clubfoot. In patients with spina bifida or arthrogryposis (as with all clubfoot patients), it is important to apply the cast only to the limits that may be obtained via manipulation.

Pitfalls in Manipulation

Errors in manipulation include hyperpronation of the first ray. The foot should remain supinated throughout the casting procedure; as increased correction is obtained, the supination is decreased to a more normal alignment. It is also important to maintain the foot in equinus during the sessions of manipulation and casting. As mentioned, the fulcrum of pressure should be positioned over the head of the talus. Errantly positioning pressure over the calcaneocuboid joint will block the reduction of the calcaneus under the talus and prevent subtalar correction.[12] The heel must not be touched, as doing so may prevent the normal eversion that is fundamental to correction of the hind-foot varus.

Pitfalls in Casting

Use of short-leg plaster casts is ineffective at obtaining and maintaining correction of the clubfoot; long-leg plaster casts are always used. Increased incidence of cast sores and difficulty with castings obviously occur in children who are agitated. Bottle feeding is recommended during casting. Two to three layers of cotton roll are sufficient before application of the cast—too much cotton will result in movement of the foot within the cast, increasing the risk for friction blisters and decreasing

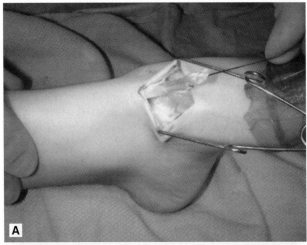

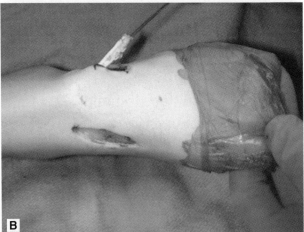

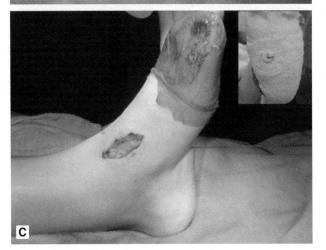

FIGURE 17-17

Anterior tibialis tendon transfer is useful in the older child with recurrent metatarsus adductus and dynamic supination of the forefoot. **A.** The whole anterior tibialis tendon is harvested from the midfoot, and a 1 Vicryl suture is attached with a Bunnell weave. **B.** The tendon is delivered into the lateral foot over the third cuneiform. **C.** The tendon is placed through a drill hole in the third cuneiform, and the suture is delivered through the plantar aspect of the foot. The suture is tied over a button on the *outside* of the cast (inset). The cast is maintained for 6 weeks until the tendon heals into its new insertion.

the ability to correct the foot. A plaster cast is used, as opposed to fiberglass cast material, as molding with fiberglass is more difficult. To prevent later problems, it is a good idea to send families home with a roll of cotton to pad the proximal margin of the cast should the skin on the thigh become irritated.

Molding is done so that large divots of the plaster, and thereby pressure sores, are not encountered. When converting a short cast to the long-leg cast, one must carefully examine the popliteal fossa to ensure there is no pressure on the neurovascular structures. When trimming the cast, it is important not to expose the dorsal aspect of the foot proximal to the metatarsal-phalangeal joints to a great degree, as this will often lead to a tourniquet effect and swelling of the toes.

The digits should always be inspected prior to patient discharge from the clinic. If the digits are discolored after trimming of the cast material to reveal and to allow movement of the toes, the cast should be inspected, reflecting upon the preceding application. Vascular compromise commonly occurs at one of two sites: The popliteal fossa and/or the midfoot. In addition, the foot in some patients is supplied only by the posterior tibial artery, which may become impinged on the medial malleolus from the increased dorsiflexion obtained following the Achilles tenotomy. If the pale digits are recognized during the casting and molding process, a slight relaxation of the forced dorsiflexion usually results in return of arterial flow. If not recognized until after the cast has set and been trimmed to reveal the toes, the anterior portion of the cast about the ankle may be split axially and the foot slightly plantarflexed to return arterial flow.

If vascular function is compromised and does not return following the previously described maneuvers, one should not hesitate to remove the cast and repeat the application.

Pitfalls During Heel-Cord Tenotomy

If the assistant holds the foot with maximum dorsiflexion, a tightening of the Achilles tendon will result in difficulty of palpation. Similarly, difficult palpation of the heel cord is encountered when large amounts of lidocaine are injected around the tendon. Tenotomy needs to be approximately 0.5 cm proximal to the distal heel crease, or about 1.5 cm proximal to the calcaneal tuberosity. Laceration of the posterior tibial nerve and artery is avoided by entry of the blade posterior to the bundle. After the blade is placed anteriorly to the Achilles tendon from the medial approach, pressure should be placed over the dorsal aspect of the tendon, pushing the tendon through the blade while keeping the blade stationary. Pulling the blade posteriorly, sweeping through the tendon, may result in lacerating the skin after the tendon is transected and resistance to the blade disappears.

Pitfalls in Abduction Bracing

Errors in fitting the abduction orthosis include deviation from the shoulder-width positioning of the shoes and from the standard external rotation of the feet of 50 to 60 degrees. Improper sizing of the shoes will result in pressure sores over the point of the heel. In those patients who have pressure sores or ill-fitting shoes due to poor sizing, an improved fit can be obtained with the placement of Plastazote heel counters, tongue liners, and foot beds on the interior aspect of the shoe. Typically, as children age and their feet grow, proper fit is more easily obtained. In those patients who have completely failed bracing due to compliance issues from poor fit, a combination of AFO use and aggressive physical therapy can help reduce rates of recurrence.

Atypical Clubfoot

Recently the Iowa group identified an "atypical clubfoot" within the idiopathic clubfoot designation. The atypical foot is usually shorter with a first ray that is proximally recessed from the later four toes. In addition, a deep plantar crease extends from the medial arch to the lateral border of the foot. These feet tend to be fatter with a higher cavus than normally seen and are much more difficult to treat as a result of the intrinsic stiffness. The atypical clubfoot has a deep heel crease with a very tight heel cord that is fibrotic up to the distal one-third of the calf. These feet are treated with standard manipulation and casting until they have 20 degrees of foot abduction (less than the usual 60 degrees obtained in the typical clubfoot). Then, instead of further foot abduction, these patients are started on correction of equinus through progressive dorsiflexion with both thumbs under the metatarsals. Heel-cord tenotomy is then performed when the foot reaches its limits of dorsiflexion. To prevent slippage in the cast, the knee must be in 120 degrees of flexion, which is obtained with a plaster splint in front of the knee. These atypical feet often require more extensive post-tenotomy casting to obtain maximal correction; a second tenotomy may eventually be needed.

CONCLUSIONS

The Ponseti method of clubfoot treatment has been recognized as the most effective way to treat idiopathic clubfoot. Physicians need to be familiar with the anatomy (and anatomical variants) of the clubfoot and the order of manipulation, reducing first the cavus, followed by the adductus and varus, while maintaining the hind foot in equinus. Physicians also must be facile in cast application and in performance of the percutaneous tenotomy. In addition, the family needs to be aware of the importance of compliance with, and appropriate fit of, the foot abduction orthosis to prevent recurrence.

Feet with residual deformity should be treated individually. No single treatment plan is appropriate for all feet. The practitioner must be astute in assessment of residual deformity and be prepared to initiate recasting, repeat tenotomy, or more extensive surgery. Despite the fact that the Ponseti method does not provide 100% success in every foot, the use of this method will result in improved correction of the bulk of deformity, thus decreasing the need for more extensive surgery.

REFERENCES

1. Bensahel H, Csukonyi Z, Desgrippes Y, et al. Surgery in residual clubfoot: one-stage medioposterior release "a la carte." *J Pediatr Orthop.* 1987;7:145–148.
2. Bensahel H, Guillaume A, Czukonyi Z, et al. Results of physical therapy for idiopathic clubfoot: a long-term follow-up study. *J Pediatr Orthop.* 1995;10:189–192.
3. Cooper DM, Dietz FR. Treatment of idiopathic clubfoot: a thirty-year follow-up. *J Bone Joint Surg Am.* 1995;77:1477–1489.
4. Dobbs MB, Gordon JE, Walton T, et al. Bleeding complications following percutaneous tendoachilles tenotomy in the treatment of clubfoot deformity. *J Pediatr Orthop.* 2004;24(4):353–357.
5. Dobbs MB, Rudzki JR, Purchell DB, et al. Factors predictive of outcome after use of the Ponseti method for the treatment of idiopathic clubfoot. *J Bone Joint Surg Am.* 2004;86(1):22–27.
6. Herzenberg JE, Radler C, Bor N. Ponseti versus traditional methods of casting for idiopathic clubfoot. *J Pediatr Orthop.* 2002;22:517–521.
7. Ippolito E, Farsetti P, Caterini R, et al. Long-term comparative results in patients with congenital clubfoot treated with two different protocols. *J Bone Joint Surg Am.* 2003;85(7):1286–1294.
8. Lehman WB, Mohaideen A, Madan S, et al. A method for the early evaluation of the Ponseti (Iowa) technique for the treatment of idiopathic clubfoot. *J Pediatr Orthop Br.* 2003;12:133–140.
9. Morcuende JA, Abbasi D, Dolan LA, et al. Results of an accelerated Ponseti protocol for clubfoot. *J Pediatr Orthop.* 2005;25(5):623–626.
10. Morcuende JA, Dolan LA, Dietz FR, et al. Radial reduction in the rate of extensive corrective surgery for clubfoot using the Ponseti method. *Pediatrics.* 2004;113(2):376–380.
11. Pirani S, Zeznik L, Hodges D. Magnetic resonance imaging study of the congenital clubfoot treated with the Ponseti method. *J Pediatr Orthop.* 2001;21:719–726.
12. Ponseti IV. Common errors in the treatment of congenital clubfoot. *Int Orthop.* 1997;21:137–141.
13. Ponseti IV. Congenital clubfoot: fundamentals of treatment. *Oxford Med Pub.* 1996.
14. Thacker MM, Scher DM, Sala DA, et al. Use of the foot abduction orthosis following Ponseti casts: is it essential? *J Pediatr Orthop.* 2005;25(2):225–228.
15. Tindall AJ, Steinlechner WB, Lavy C, et al. Results of manipulation of idiopathic clubfoot deformity in Malawi by orthopaedic clinical officers using the Ponseti method: a realistic alternative for the developing world? *J Pediatr Orthop.* 2005;25(5):627–629.

18 Operative Treatment of Resistant Clubfoot

Richard S. Davidson

A s early as 1890, Phelps described a one-stage medial plantar release, including lengthening of tendons, and an osteotomy of the talus neck with wedge resection of the talus. He recommended first treating with manipulation and force, then cutting "the contracted parts as they first offer resistance, cutting . . . the tendo-Achilles, plantar fascia, tibialis posticus, plantar skin, abductor hallucis, flexor brevis, long flexors, deltoid ligament, then linear osteotomy of the neck of the astragalus and lateral closing wedge osteotomy of the os calsis." This technique is reminiscent of the "posteromedial" and "complete subtalar release" advocated by Turco, McKay, Simons, Carroll, and others treating clubfoot in the latter half of the 20th century. The development and popularity of x-rays allowed measurement of the clubfoot, which resulted in competition among 20th-century surgeons to find the most extensive release with the best correction according to the radiographic measurements, particularly the talocalcaneal angles on anteroposterior (AP) and lateral radiographs.

It was not until 1992, when Ponseti described his technique and his long-term results, that the pediatric orthopaedic community began to accept his principles, which mainly consist of a specific method of closed manipulative clubfoot correction, combined in most cases with percutaneous tendo-Achilles lengthening. The technique has gained such popularity that most university centers today, and even third world physicians, are employing Ponseti's basic principles of manipulation, casting, and minimal operative treatment of the clubfoot. The Ponseti approach appears to provide adequate correction for most clubfeet, with the added advantage of better foot mobility than is often seen after extensive surgical release and correction.

A decade ago, most pediatric orthopaedic surgeons would surgically treat a child who had a clubfoot, claiming only about a 10% success rate when treating clubfoot with casting. Now most would claim that extensive surgical techniques are necessary in fewer than 5% of clubfoot cases. Clearly there will always be the recalcitrant clubfoot that resists methods such as the Ponseti technique; these clubfeet typically fall into the arthrogrypotic or teratologic categories. When this type of severe clubfoot deformity is encountered, it should prompt more thorough investigation and a search for other diagnoses, such as polio, spina bifida, cerebral palsy, arthrogryposis, spinal cord abnormalities, and muscular dystrophy, instead of treating these feet as idiopathic clubfeet.

INDICATIONS/CONTRAINDICATIONS

Most idiopathic clubfeet today are treated well in infancy with the Ponseti method of manipulation, casting, and percutaneous tendo-Achilles lengthening. With the Ponseti technique, extensive posteromedial or posterolateral soft-tissue release is avoided, although many of these patients later benefit from an anterior tibial tendon transfer as toddlers. The extensive soft-tissue releases employed a decade and more ago are contraindicated as an initial treatment of clubfeet in children under 1 year of age and even perhaps into toddler age.

The extensive soft-tissue surgical releases outlined in this chapter are currently primarily used for those clubfeet that are associated with syndromes, chromosomal abnormalities, and neurologic or muscle disorders. In a small number of patients with idiopathic clubfoot who are of an older age and/or resistant to the Ponseti treatment, part or all of the soft-tissue releases described here may be needed to obtain a plantigrade foot position.

PREOPERATIVE PLANNING

The list of anatomic structures that can be lengthened, released, transferred, or rotated is extensive. A review of the literature will reveal articles recommending alteration of any or all of the structures in the foot, ankle, and calf. Many excellent reviews of the anatomy around the subtalar joint are available; any surgeons treating clubfoot deformities must be thoroughly knowledgeable of this anatomy.

A thorough physical and radiographic examination of the foot must be performed to identify the deformities remaining after treatment with the Ponseti technique. Even if not fully successful in correcting the clubfoot deformity, a trial of manipulation and casting with the Ponseti technique is usually helpful prior to additional surgical treatment.

The author and editors agree that the goal of surgical treatment is first to release enough of the tight structures to bring the foot into an anatomically correct position without tension on the neurovascular structures or on the other soft tissue in the foot and ankle areas. Many will add that muscles should be balanced to help maintain the anatomic position obtained by this correction. This latter goal is often difficult to assess in the stiff and deformed clubfoot before surgery or even at the time of surgical release. Muscle balancing is probably better left for later, after rehabilitation from the extensive surgical soft-tissue release has been completed, at which time any abnormalities of muscle balance around the foot and ankle can be more accurately assessed. It is important to understand that neuromuscular abnormalities, growth disturbances, and simple muscular or mechanical imbalances can lead to recurrence or overcorrection throughout the growth period, at which time stretching, bracing, casting, and even additional surgery may be needed.

Henri Bensahel recommended the "a la carte" approach, in which intraoperative evaluation leads the surgeon to release any and all tight structures. The surgeon must be prepared to do as little or as much as needed to accomplish anatomic realignment. Overcorrection can lead to valgus deformity, which will need correction at a later time.

The child's age will play an important role in determining what must be done to restore anatomic alignment. In general, soft-tissue releases are adequate from age 2 months to 4 years, and in some cases to age 6 years. By the age of 4 years, many clubfeet are beginning to show bone deformity, which will block or prevent complete correction after soft-tissue releases alone. The presence of lateral column varus and equinus, heel varus, a triangular navicular, dorsolateral subluxation of the talonavicular joint, and forefoot varus may all require osteotomy or resection arthrodesis to obtain acceptable correction in older children.

Surgical release should begin posteriorly and then continue medially, as these are the areas with the tightest soft-tissue structures in an equinovarus foot. Failure to correct the clubfoot deformity after the posterior and medial release is likely due to contracted fibrous tissue on the lateral side of the hind foot, which blocks derotation and correction of the deformity at the subtalar joint. In this instance, release of the lateral soft-tissue structures should allow full correction of the clubfoot. In a clubfoot, the normally saddle-shaped subtalar joint is flattened, allowing derotation and correction after adequate soft-tissue release has been completed.

SURGICAL PROCEDURE

The three most popular incisions for surgical release of the resistant clubfoot are the Turco posteromedial incision, the Carroll medial and posterolateral incisions, and the Cincinnati incision (Fig. 18-1). The Turco approach allows medial and posterior access; the Carroll incision allows medial access and more posterolateral access; and the Cincinnati incision allows more extensive medial, posterior, and lateral access for the soft-tissue releases.

The Turco incision begins at the first metatarsomedial cuneiform joint medially, extends proximally just distal to the tip of the medial malleolus, then turns in a proximal direction up the calf to expose the Achilles tendon. To reach the lateral side, the surgeon must open the subtalar joint like a book or make a separate lateral incision.

The Carroll incision, which allows medial and more posterolateral access, consists of two incisions: (a) The medial incision is accurately placed by first determining a triangle demarcated by the center of the calcaneus, the front of the medial malleolus, and the base of the first metatarsal. This incision is started parallel at the base of the triangle, curves proximal-plantar, and finally curves distally over the dorsum of the foot. (b) The posterolateral incision runs obliquely from the midline of the distal

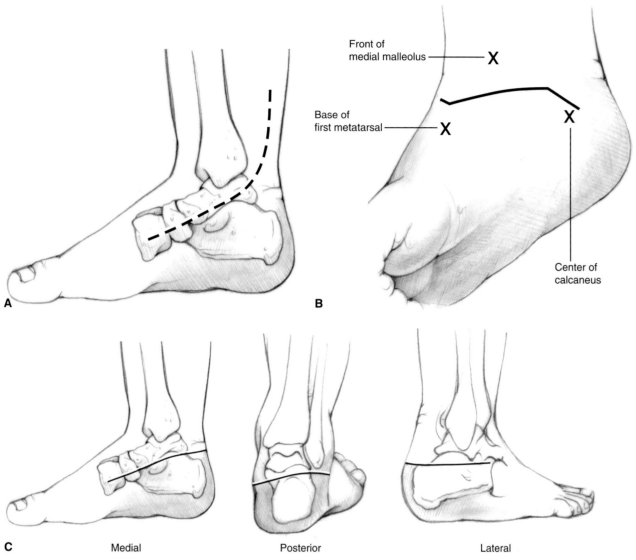

FIGURE 18-1 **A.** Turco incision. **B.** Carroll incision (medial incision is shown). See text for lateral incision location. **C.** Cincinnati incision.

posterior calf to a point between the tendo-Achilles and the lateral malleolus. An additional lateral incision may be required to reach the lateral talonavicular (TN) joint.

The Cincinnati incision allows the most extensive access to the foot and is the author's preference. This incision provides excellent medial, posterior, and lateral access. The incision begins medially over the TN joint, extends posteriorly at the level of the subtalar joint, and then continues distally to the lateral TN joint.

The incisions can be extended distally on both the medial and the lateral sides. The Cincinnati incision is most easily performed with the patient prone. Flexing the knee provides excellent access to the Achilles tendon for Z-lengthening. For severely deformed feet with marked equinus deformity, closure of the incision posteriorly may be difficult. In this situation, wound closure and positioning of the foot in the postoperative immobilization in some equinus for 2 weeks to allow wound healing can be followed by serial casting to stretch the soft tissues to dorsiflex the foot into a plantigrade position.

This chapter describes the total and extensive soft-tissue release. However, this complete release is not always needed. It is important to evaluate each foot after each step of the surgical release to determine whether the anatomy is corrected or whether additional release is necessary. The goal is to do as little or as much of the complete release as is necessary to place the foot in a corrected position without force. Lengthening tendons and then capsules and ligaments at each location will minimize scarring and stiffness. All tissues must be handled carefully. Damage to articular surfaces and physes must be avoided.

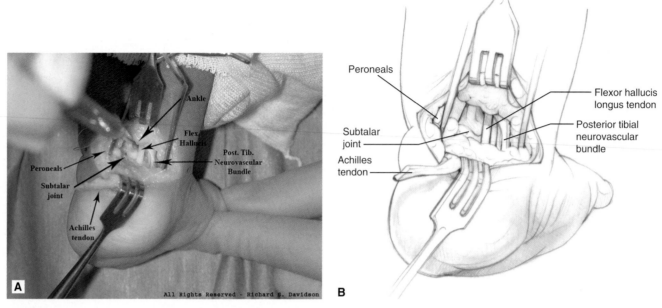

FIGURE 18-2 Posterior portion of the Cincinnati incision. The Achilles tendon has been cut for lengthening and retracted.

The author prefers performing this release with the patient in the prone position, as this provides optimal access to and visibility of the important structures in the foot (Fig. 18-2). A tourniquet is used during the soft-tissue releases.

First the posterior portion of the Cincinnati incision is made from the distal tip of the medial malleolus around the posterior ankle to the distal tip of the lateral malleolus. The Achilles tendon sheath is incised to expose the Achilles tendon. In the child under 18 months, the tendon can be lengthened by tenotomy; in the older child, however, this should be lengthened by Z-lengthening.

To facilitate visualization for a Z-lengthening of the Achilles through the Cincinnati incision, flex the prone patient's knee. With the Cincinnati incision, the surgeon is looking at the plantar aspect of the foot through the incision and up the calf. The Achilles tendon is lengthened in a notch fashion. The medial half of the Achilles insertion is lengthened distally to reduce the varus force. Fibrotic bands in this region and the tendon sheath should also be released.

If Achilles lengthening is not sufficient to correct the clubfoot deformity, the surgeon should sequentially release the capsules in the posterior aspect of the subtalar and ankle joints. First the sural nerve and vessels laterally and the posterior tibial neurovascular bundle medially are identified and protected. The flexor hallucis longus (FHL) tendon is identified posteromedially and retracted. The peroneal tendons are identified laterally and are protected.

The ankle capsule is identified and incised from the posteromedial to the posterolateral corners to allow dorsiflexion of the talus in the ankle mortise.

Next, the subtalar joint is identified and incised first posteriorly, then medially and laterally to the interosseus ligament. The fibulotalar and fibulocalcaneal ligaments are released as needed.

Following these releases, the foot at the ankle joint should be able to be dorsiflexed at least 20 degrees above the neutral position. If the great toe is tightly flexed when this ankle dorsiflexion is carried out, the FHL tendon can be lengthened through the incision by Z-lengthening.

If the posterior release described above does not fully correct the anatomy and the clubfoot deformity, the posterior portion of the Cincinnati incision is extended medially to the medial aspect of the navicular (Fig. 18-3).

The posterior tibial neurovascular bundle should be identified and protected before any thickened fascia is released. The FHL tendon, which may have been lengthened through the posterior part of the incision, is then identified and protected.

The posterior tibialis (PT) tendon is identified just distal to the flexor digitorum longus (FDL) tendon and is lengthened in a notch fashion as necessary. The FDL tendon is identified just anterior to the PT neurovascular bundle and is lengthened in notch fashion as necessary.

Next, the abductor hallucis muscle proximally or the abductor hallucis tendon distally is identified and lengthened to help improve correction of the forefoot varus.

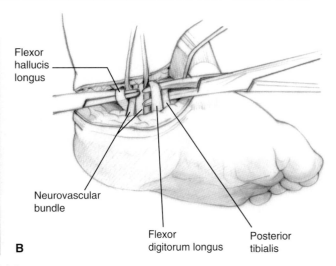

FIGURE 18-3   Medial portion of Cincinnati incision, superficial.

Failure to lengthen the tendons of the FHL, FDL, and PT may lead to failure to adequately rotate and correct the subtalar joint intraoperatively or to a rapid recurrence of deformity in the postoperative period. Preservation or repair of the sheaths of these tendons has been found to be of value. As long as all the tethers and blocks to motion are removed, a flexible foot and ankle can result.

Deciding whether to lengthen the anterior tibialis tendon can be difficult. Often the appearance of forefoot supination is related to overpull of the anterior tibialis. However, this imbalance may also be the result of positioning of the foot. Release and realignment (eversion and lateral rotation through the subtalar joint) of the foot may restore the balance without lengthening the anterior tibialis tendon. If the anterior tibialis tendon appears contracted after anatomic correction, this tendon should also be lengthened by Z-lengthening. Occasionally, the anterior tibialis tendon remains overactive and will need to be lengthened or transferred at a future time if the foot is still supinated.

When lengthening the tendons on the medial side of the foot, each end of the lengthened tendons should be tagged with a suture, which is then held in a paired color-coded "bulldog" clamp. Each group of proximal and distal sets of clamps can then be held in proper order by a safety pin. This will avoid confusion in identifying the proper tendon and will prevent tangling of the sutures when it is time to repair the tendons after anatomic realignment of the foot is accomplished.

Although release of the plantar fascia has been recommended by some, the author has rarely done so, as plantar fascia release at the time of clubfoot correction can contribute to later planovalgus foot position. If there is any evidence of rocker bottom foot deformity during the casting prior to surgery, the plantar fascia must not be released.

Care should be taken to avoid injury to the medial plantar vessels and nerve. If lengthening of these medial tendons does not permit anatomic alignment and full correction of the clubfoot deformity, further release of the following structures is needed.

The TN joint is identified and released. In a clubfoot, the navicular is medially displaced on the talar head so that the TN joint is oriented in an oblique plane, rather than in a transverse plane as in a normal foot. The surgeon should follow the distal stump of the Z-lengthened PT tendon to its insertion on the navicular. The TN capsule is released on the medial, plantar, and dorsal aspects, in addition to as far laterally as the surgeon can safely reach. The surgeon should be careful not to cut the talar neck in young children, as this may lead to avascular necrosis or growth disturbances.

Next, the medial subtalar capsule is released from the TN joint to the interosseus ligament medially, including a release of the spring ligament. The posterior subtalar capsule will have already been released in the posterior dissection. The surgeon should be careful not to damage the deep deltoid ligament. A Freer elevator placed into the ankle joint posteriorly can help identify the ankle and subtalar joints.

The medial aspect of the calcaneocuboid joint is reached by carefully dissecting the soft tissues from the plantar aspect of the talar neck. Release of the calcaneocuboid capsule will allow a wedge opening of the calcaneocuboid joint to straighten the lateral column. Another anatomic landmark in the area of the calcaneocuboid joint visualized from the medial side of the foot is the peroneus longus tendon, which crosses from a lateral to a plantar position. Although many authors have described release of the interosseus ligament through this incision, the author believes it is important to preserve the interosseous ligament as a pivot axis for subtalar correction and to preserve its associated blood supply to the talus.

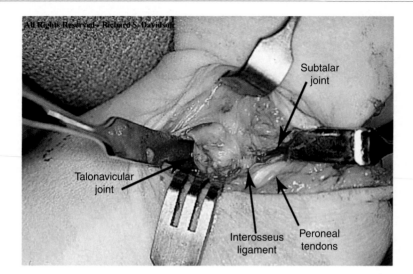

FIGURE 18-4

Lateral portion of Cincinnati incision, showing the lateral structures.

The calcaneus usually has rotated under the talus on the interosseus membrane and is often tethered by a stiff, fibrotic lateral capsule. If the posterior and medial releases do not permit anatomic alignment, a lateral soft-tissue release may be needed (Fig. 18-4).

The posterior portion of the Cincinnati incision, already made for the posterior release, is extended laterally at the level of the subtalar joint to the lateral TN joint. The extensor digitorum brevis muscle is identified over the sinus tarsi, and its plantar edge is detached from the lateral calcaneus, with the muscle elevated to expose the sinus tarsi and the neck and head of the talus.

The lateral capsule of the TN joint is exposed and released, completing the circumferential release of the TN joint. The beak of the calcaneus is then palpated. From the lateral aspect of the TN joint, the lateral subtalar capsule is cut between the beak of the calcaneus and the talar neck, proximally to the interosseous ligament, completing the circumferential release of the subtalar capsule.

Once the appropriate soft tissues have been released, the foot can be realigned. A finger is placed over the talar head dorsolaterally, and the foot is then laterally rotated as it is held in a position of slight supination. This is similar to the technique used for the Ponseti technique manipulation. A Freer elevator can be placed in the ankle joint in line with the dome of the talus (axis of the talus). The foot should be rotated until the first metatarsal is just lateral to the talar dome axis. This maneuver should correct the convex lateral border to a straight position. The heel is positioned in slight valgus, and the talar head is reduced under the navicular (the navicular should be slightly prominent to palpation, as in normal feet), without wedging open the subtalar joint (Fig. 18-5).

FIGURE 18-5

A. Subtalar rotation of the foot. The Freer elevator is in the ankle joint and demonstrates the alignment of the ankle joint. The foot is medially rotated through the subtalar joint. **B.** The reduced foot held in place with a pin through the talonavicular joint. Note the heel in slight valgus.

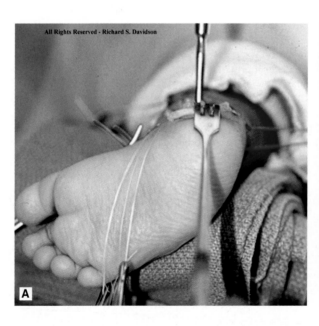
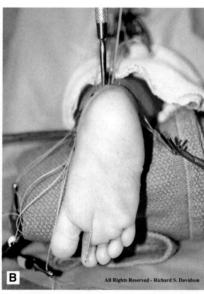

Holding the foot in the anatomically corrected position until the capsules and tendons heal is best done with a 0.62 Kirschner wire that is passed from the posteromedial talus, through the center of the talar head, into the navicular and medial cuneiform, and finally out the skin in the region of the first web space.

The TN joint must not be overreduced. Lateral overcorrection of this joint and release of the plantar fascia will cause postoperative valgus foot deformity. Dorsolateral subluxation of the TN joint will lead to a triangular shape of the navicular, which in turn will lead to supination, cavus, and metatarsus adductus foot deformities. Incomplete medial and plantar reduction will lead to undercorrection of the equinovarus deformity. Residual plantarflexion of the first metatarsal in relation to the axis of the talus can cause forefoot plantarflexion and hind-foot varus.

Intraoperative radiographic images should be obtained at this point to confirm that all components of the reduction have been obtained. The tarsal navicular does not usually ossify until 3 or 4 years of age and will not be seen directly on intraoperative radiographs obtained on children younger than this.

All the joints should be congruous. Wedged-open joints may indicate incomplete release of bone deformity, which may require osteotomy.

Proper reduction should result in near-normal motion of the ankle, though the fixation pin restricts foot motion when it is in place. Some authors do not use pin fixation of the corrected clubfeet following release and instead perform serial casting. The author prefers the use of K-wire fixation, however, as there is sometimes loss of alignment during postoperative casting once postoperative swelling is reduced and the cast becomes loose. Clubfeet that are resistant to the Ponseti method prior to surgery are often small and pudgy feet, which can also be difficult to control with casts alone following corrective surgery.

If division of the interosseous ligament (rarely needed in the author's experience) has been performed, a second pin should be placed from the calcaneus into the talus to maintain proper alignment of the subtalar joint.

Once the foot is anatomically aligned, the tendons are repaired with the foot at 90 degrees to the tibia—a position of neutral ankle dorsiflexion. Do not repair the tendons until the bones have been realigned anatomically. Repairing the tendons at too short a length will result in rapid recurrence.

Capsules and ligaments should not be repaired surgically, as these will heal on their own.

Intraoperative clinical and radiographic assessment prior to wound closure to ensure that full correction has been obtained (Fig. 18-6) should include all of the following:

- Lateral border of foot is straight.
- Heel is in slight valgus with the foot at 90 degrees to the tibia.
- Prior to repair of the tendons, the ankle range of motion should be 20+ degrees of dorsiflexion and 30+ degrees of plantarflexion.
- After repair of the tendons, the ankle dorsiflexion should be to neutral or 0 degrees.
- The talar head is reduced under the forefoot, with the navicular palpated to be slightly proud medially.
- The TN joint should be flush dorsally and plantarly.

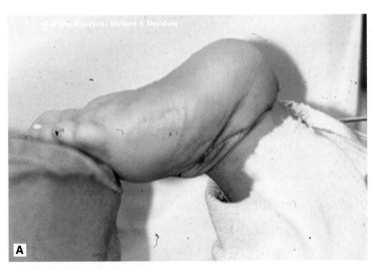
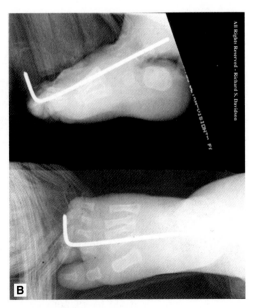

FIGURE 18-6   **A.** Foot of the prone patient positioned for AP and lateral intraoperative x-rays. **B.** AP and lateral intraoperative x-rays with internal fixation. Note that on the lateral view, the talus points into the first metatarsal, and on the AP, it points just medial to the first metatarsal.

- The first metatarsal should be in line with the talus on the lateral radiograph and should be in 0 to 30 degrees valgus relative to the talar axis on the anteroposterior (AP) radiograph.
- The talocalcaneal angle should be >25 degrees on the lateral and AP radiographs.

Severe, stiffly deformed clubfeet, particularly in the older child, may have bone deformity, which can prevent adequate anatomic correction with soft-tissue release alone. Posterior soft-tissue release will do little for ankle stiffness due to a "flat top" talus. AP and lateral radiographs (preferably standing if possible) should always be obtained preoperatively for these severely deformed stiff feet in order to carefully define the deformity present and the surgical techniques needed to provide optimum correction.

Metatarsal and talar neck osteotomies are rarely indicated in the young child.

POSTOPERATIVE MANAGEMENT

During the first postoperative week, the author prefers a Jones-type dressing to allow for postoperative swelling in children under the age of 6 months and bulky dressings and casts for children over 6 months of age.

Casts should be changed 1 week following surgery. Ponseti-type casting will help maintain alignment. Cast changes each month for 3 months postoperatively are advisable. Braces are helpful for prolonged periods following the 3 months of postoperative casting if recurrence occurs or if an underlying neuromuscular disease has been identified. Following clubfoot surgery, no weight bearing in the cast is continued for at least 1 month postoperatively or as long as any K-wires are in place crossing joints.

COMPLICATIONS TO AVOID

Most complications associated with extensive soft-tissue releases for clubfoot deformity have been noted in the Surgical Procedure section.

Because there is commonly absence of a portion of the peroneal or anterior tibial arterial supply to the foot, it is essential that the posterior tibial artery be carefully identified and protected during the entire clubfoot-release surgery. If the posterior tibial artery is cut during surgery, the tourniquet is deflated, and circulation to the foot is assessed. If adequate foot circulation is still present, the posterior tibial artery may be ligated. However, if there is inadequate foot circulation at this stage, microvascular repair of the posterior tibial artery should be attempted.

Overcorrection or undercorrection of the clubfoot needs to be avoided. Overcorrection leads to flat feet and weak gastrocnemius, resulting in poor pushoff for walking and running. Undercorrection leads to early recurrence, which may need further surgery; this in turn leads to a stiffer foot in the end.

Dorsal subluxation of the navicular will lead to a triangular shape of the navicular, a high midfoot, and difficulty with shoe fitting. The TN joint should be directly visualized during insertion of the K-wire; the foot should be held in a position of mild equinus during this pinning to prevent unrecognized dorsal subluxation of the navicular. As noted earlier, the navicular is not yet ossified at the usual age of this surgery and cannot be directly seen on the intraoperative radiographs.

SUMMARY

The goal of the soft-tissue releases described here is to produce anatomic alignment in one surgical procedure when less-invasive procedures have failed.

The Ponseti technique of manipulation and casting has dramatically and successfully redirected clubfoot treatment away from extensive surgical releases, which were preferred by many throughout the 20th century. Most pediatric orthopaedic surgeons who were once enamored by the technically challenging extensive releases for the clubfoot now realize that such extensive releases are very rarely needed. In most clubfeet, similar results to those obtained in the past by surgical intervention can be obtained with the Ponseti method and with fewer complications.

It is unfortunate that for those rare, stiff, deformed clubfeet that are not amenable to minimally invasive techniques, like the Ponseti method, there will be few surgeons with the experience needed to manage them. Stiffness, recurrence, and weakness are common, and no treatment known today can correct the underlying neuromuscular etiologies. It is advisable that these feet should be referred to centers with the most experience, as these clubfeet are not easy problems in anyone's hands.

REFERENCES

1. Adams W. *Clubfoot: Its Causes, Pathology, and Treatment.* London: J.& A. Churchill; 1866.
2. Atar D, Lehman WB, Grant AD. Complete soft-tissue clubfoot release with and without internal fixation. *Orthop Rev.* 1993;22:1015–1016.
3. Atar D, Lehman WB, Grant AD, et al. Fractional lengthening of the flexor tendons in clubfoot surgery. *Clin Orthop.* 1991:267–269.
4. Bensahel H, Csukonyi Z, Desgrippes Y, et al. Surgery in residual clubfoot: one-stage medioposterior release "a la carte." *J Pediatr Orthop.* 1987;7:145–148.
5. Bost FC, Schottstadt ER, Larsen LJ. Plantar dissection—an operation to release the soft tissues in recurrent talipes equinovarus. *J Bone Joint Surg Am.* 1960;42:15.
6. Brockman EP. *Congenital Clubfoot.* Bristol: J. Wright and Sons; 1930.
7. Brockman EP. Modern methods of treatment of club-foot. *BMJ.* 1937;2:572–574.
8. Carroll NC. Congenital clubfoot: pathoanatomy and treatment. *Instr Course Lect.* 1987;36:117–121.
9. Carroll NC. Pathoanatomy and surgical treatment of the resistant clubfoot. *Instr Course Lect.* 1988;37:93–106.
10. Carroll NC. Controversies in the surgical management of clubfoot. *Instr Course Lect.* 1996;45:331–337.
11. Carroll NC, Gross RH. Operative management of clubfoot. *Orthopedics* 1990;13:1285–1296.
12. Codivilla A. Sulla cura del piede equino varo congenitl: nuovo metodo di cura cruenta. *Archivo Orthopedica.* 1906;23:245.
13. Crawford AH, Gupta AK. Clubfoot controversies: Complications and causes for failure. *Instr Course Lect.* 1996;45:339–346.
14. Crawford A, Marxen J, Osterfeld D. The Cincinnati incision: a comprehensive approach for surgical procedures of the foot and ankle in childhood. *J Bone Joint Surg Am.* 1982;64:1355–1358.
15. Cummings RJ, Lovell WW. Operative treatment of congenital idiopathic club foot. *J Bone Joint Surg Am.* 1988;0:1108–1112.
16. Elmslie RC. Principles in treatment of congenital talipes equinovarus. *J Orthop Surg.* 1920;2:119.
17. Fripp AT, Shaw NE. *Club-Foot.* London: E. & S. Livingstone; 1967.
18. Hippocrates. The Loeb Classical Library. Cambridge: Harvard University Press; 1948. Jones WHS, translator.
19. Little WJ. *A Treatise on the Nature of Clubfoot and Analogous Distortions.* London: W Jeffs, S Higley; 1839.
20. McCauley JC Jr. Operative treatment of club feet. *New York State Journal of Medicine.* 1947;47P:255.
21. McKay D. New concept and approach to clubfoot treatment. Section I. Principles and morbid anatomy. *J Pediatr Orthop.* 1982;2:347–356.
22. McKay D. New concept and approach to clubfoot treatment. Section II. Correction of the clubfoot. *J Pediatr Orthop.* 1983;3:10–21.
23. McKay D. New concept and approach to clubfoot treatment. Section III. Evaluation and results. *J Pediatr Orthop.* 1983;3:141–148.
24. McKay DW. Surgical correction of clubfoot. *Instr Course Lect.* 1988;37:87–92.
25. Otremski I, Salama R, Khermosh O, et al. An analysis of the results of a modified one-stage posteromedial release (Turco operation) for the treatment of clubfoot. *J Pediatr Orthop.* 1987;7:149–151.
26. Peltier LF. *Orthopedics: A History and Iconography.* San Francisco: Norman Publishing; 1993.
27. Phelps. Present status of the open incision method. *Med Record.* 1890;38:593–598.
28. Porat S, Kaplan L. Critical analysis of results in club feet treated surgically along the Norris Carroll approach: seven years of experience. *J Pediatr Orthop.* 1989;9:137–143.
29. Scarpa A. *Memoir on Congenital Clubfeet.* Edinburgh: A. Constable; 1818.
30. Simons GW. Complete subtalar release in club feet. Part I A preliminary report. *J Bone Joint Surg Am.* 1985;67:1044–1055.
31. Simons GW. Complete subtalar release in club feet. Part II Comparison with less extensive procedures. *J Bone Joint Surg Am.* 1985;67:1056–1065.
32. Simons GW. The complete subtalar release in clubfeet. *Orthop Clin North Am.* 1987;18:667–688.
33. Simons GW. Calcaneocuboid joint deformity in talipes equinovarus: an overview and update. *J Pediatr Orthop Br.* 1995;4:25–35.
34. Turco V. Resistant congenital club foot. One-stage posteromedial release with internal fixation. A follow-up report of a fifteen year experience. *J Bone Joint Surg Am.* 1978;61:805–814.
35. Turco VJ. *Clubfoot.* New York: Churchill Livingston; 1981.
36. Turco V. Present management of idiopathic clubfoot. *J Pediatr Orthop Br.* 1994;3:149–154.
37. Yngve DA, Gross RH, Sullivan JA. Clubfoot release without wide subtalar release. *J Pediatr Orthop.* 1990;10:473–476.

19 Midfoot Osteotomies

Deirdre D. Ryan and Robert M. Kay

Midfoot deformities, a common source of morbidity during childhood, are often part of complex foot deformities involving the forefoot and hind foot. Examples include the association of midfoot supination with hind-foot valgus and midfoot pronation with hind-foot varus. Other foot deformities, including cavus and hind-foot deformities, are addressed in other chapters in this text.

Midfoot deformities, such as metatarsus adductus, may be present at birth. Recurrent or residual deformity following clubfoot treatment may also result in midfoot deformity. When deformities develop and progress during childhood (particularly when associated with pes cavus), they are often secondary to neuromuscular disorders, such as Charcot-Marie-Tooth disease or spinal cord tumor. As a result, any child who presents with a later-onset progressive deformity should be evaluated thoroughly to rule out such an underlying etiology.

Regardless of cause, midfoot deformities can cause pain, footwear problems, and decreased stability in stance phase. Conservative treatment with appropriate footwear and over-the-counter or custom orthotics may be sufficient to alleviate symptoms. If surgery is ultimately required, however, it is important to assess the flexibility of the deformity and to address the underlying soft-tissue imbalance. For flexible deformities, appropriate soft-tissue balancing will suffice. For rigid deformities, a combination of soft-tissue and bony surgery (typically one or more osteotomies) is needed.

METATARSUS ADDUCTUS/VARUS

Metatarsus adductus is a medial deviation of the forefoot. The foot may be described as being bean-shaped. Most children with metatarsus adductus are asymptomatic, though this deformity may be associated with pain, difficulty with footwear, and intoeing. The hind foot is neutral, while the forefoot is often slightly supinated. Radiographic findings include a trapezoidal-shaped medial cuneiform and medial deviation of the metatarsals.

Indications/Contraindications

Surgery is rarely indicated in congenital metatarsus adductus. Spontaneous resolution is common, and the majority resolve by six years of age. Surgical correction is warranted in the older child with pain, callus formation, and disability despite appropriate footwear. Foot orthotics may be helpful in those with supination associated with adductus.

Surgery is more commonly necessary in the case of relapsed clubfoot with persistent or recurrent metatarsus varus and supination recalcitrant to nonoperative measures. Surgery may also be indicated in a persistently painful skewfoot.

Such surgery is contraindicated in children less than 4 years old because of the high incidence of spontaneous resolution of congenital adductus. In addition, the small size of the tarsal bones (and their largely cartilaginous nature in young children) often precludes sufficient correction.

FIGURE 19-1

A dorsal lateral incision is made over the cuboid, extending from the base of the fifth metatarsal to the most distal end of the calcaneus.

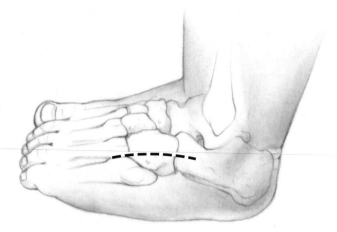

FIGURE 19-1

A dorsal lateral incision is made over the cuboid, extending from the base of the fifth metatarsal to the most distal end of the calcaneus.

Preoperative Planning

- Weight-bearing AP and lateral radiographs of the feet should be taken.
- Gait analysis is an excellent adjunct, especially in children with neuromuscular disease.
- The following should be requested:
  - Fluoroscopy
  - Tourniquet
  - Oscillating saw
  - 1/4-in. and 1/2-in. osteotomes
  - 1.6-mm and/or 2.0-mm smooth Steinmann pins
  - Bone staples (manual or power driven)
  - Chandler retractors
  - Hohman retractors

Surgical Procedure

Mild/Moderate Adductus: Closing-Wedge Osteotomy of the Cuboid   The patient is placed supine on a radiolucent table, and a bump is placed under the ipsilateral hip to internally rotate the leg and facilitate access to the lateral foot. A thigh tourniquet is used. Fluoroscopic imaging confirms the location of the cuboid, and a longitudinal incision is made over the dorsal lateral border. (Fig. 19-1). Full-thickness flaps are developed. Retractors are placed plantarly and dorsally to protect the soft tissues—namely, the toe extensors dorsally and the peroneals plantarly (Fig. 19-2). The cuboid's periosteum is incised in an H shape, with a longitudinal cut and two transverse cuts (proximally and distally), staying away from the calcaneocuboid (CC) joint proximally and the cuboid-fifth metatarsal joint distally. The periosteum is elevated proximally and distally.

FIGURE 19-2

Hohman retractors are placed dorsally and plantarly over the cuboid, protecting the toe extensors dorsally and the peroneal tendons plantarly. Care is taken not to disrupt the capsules of the calcaneocuboid joint and the cuboid fifth metatarsal joint.

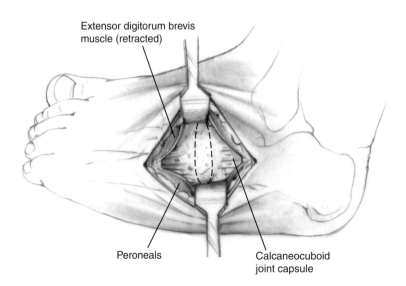

Extensor digitorum brevis muscle (retracted)

Peroneals

Calcaneocuboid joint capsule

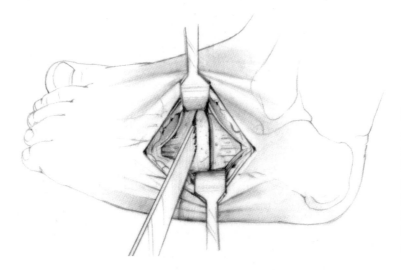

FIGURE 19-3

An oscillating saw is used to make a laterally based closing-wedge osteotomy of the cuboid bone. To mobilize the osteotomy site, the medial cortex of the cuboid should be cut.

A small oscillating saw or a 1/2-in. osteotome is used to remove a laterally based triangle of bone. An oscillating saw generally makes a more precise cut and facilitates harvesting the excised bone in one piece, which is particularly important when harvesting bone graft for an opening-wedge osteotomy of the medical cuneiform (Fig. 19-3). The osteotomy usually removes majority of the cuboid's ossific nucleus. The medial cortex of the cuboid should be cut to facilitate mobilization as well as closure of the osteotomy. If closure of the osteotomy results in appropriate correction, no other bony procedure is needed. If there is insufficient correction of the adductus, then an opening-wedge osteotomy of the medial cuneiform may be needed. The cuboid osteotomy site can be fixed using 1.6- or 2.0-mm smooth Steinmann pins or bone staples (Fig. 19-4). Placement of the pins eccentrically in the cuboid (close to the lateral cortex) helps hold the osteotomy closed during the healing phase. The Steinmann pins are left percutaneous, allowing for pin removal in the office 4 weeks postoperatively. The wound is closed, and the child is placed in a well-padded short-leg nonwalking cast.

Severe Adductus: Closing-Wedge Osteotomy of the Cuboid and Opening-Wedge Osteotomy of Medial Cuneiform

In cases in which a medial cuneiform osteotomy is needed for persistent adductus following cuboid osteotomy, a straight longitudinal medial incision is made overlying the medial medial cuneiform (Fig. 19-5A). Dissection is carried down with tenotomy scissors. The anterior tibialis tendon is identified over the first medial cuneiform. The tendon is gently dissected free, without disrupting its attachments, and is retracted dorsally (Fig. 19-5B). (If a split anterior tibial tendon transfer [SPLATT] is being performed in conjunction with the osteotomies, it is preferable to split the tendon and remove its plantar limb at this point, allowing

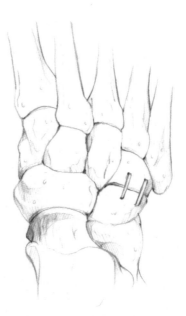

FIGURE 19-4

Bone staples are used to secure the osteotomy site after closure. Alternatively, Steinmann pins can be used.

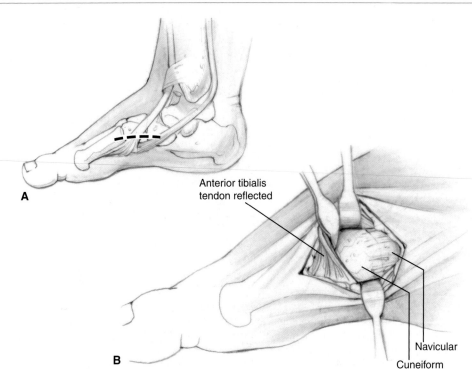

FIGURE 19-5

A. A medial incision is made over the medial cuneiform, extending from the base of the first metatarsal over the cuneiform to the navicular. **B.** The anterior tibialis tendon is retracted dorsally, keeping it out of harm's way.

Anterior tibialis tendon reflected

Navicular

Cuneiform

easier access to the medial cuneiform.) The center of the cuneiform is identified, and the periosteum is incised using either electrocautery or a #15 blade from dorsal to plantar. The periosteum is elevated proximally and distally approximately 5 mm in each direction. Care is taken not to disrupt the capsules of the proximal and distal joints. The joints can be identified with a small-gauge needle or needle electrocautery tip. Small Chandler retractors are placed dorsally and plantarly at the cuneiform. An osteotomy is performed at the center of the cuneiform and should be parallel with the distal articular surface. Because this surface is often sloped, the direction of the osteotomy should be confirmed under fluoroscopy. Again the osteotomy can be performed using an oscillating saw or a 1/2-in. osteotome. The authors prefer the osteotome, as the excursion of the oscillating saw could place the anterior tibialis tendon and other structures at risk (Fig. 19-6). The lateral cortex can be left closed. The osteotomy site is opened using a laminar spreader within the osteotomy site or by spreading against Steinmann pins placed on either side of the osteotomy. The wedge of bone from the cuboid is then inserted (Fig. 19-7A). The medial cuneiform osteotomy site is often inherently stable following placement of the autograft bone; if not, the osteotomy and graft can be fixed using 1.6- or 2.0-mm smooth Steinmann pins, or it can be held using staples (Fig. 19-7B). Of note, if the fascia of the abductor hallucis muscle is too tight, it may need to be released with lengthening of the medial column of the foot.

FIGURE 19-6

A 1/4-in. straight osteotome is used to make the osteotomy cut in the medial cuneiform. Care is taken to protect the anterior tibialis tendon. The osteotomy extends across the majority of the bone, but the lateral cortex is left intact.

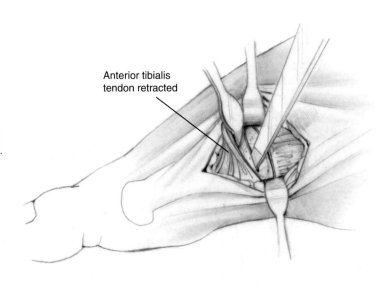

Anterior tibialis tendon retracted

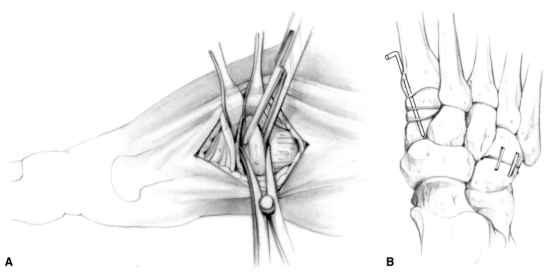

A   **B**

FIGURE 19-7   A. A lamina spreader is used to open the osteotomy site. The wedge of bone taken from the cuboid is inserted. **B.** The medial cuneiform osteotomy site can be held using a smooth Steinmann pin if the site is felt to be unstable.

Metatarus Varus: Complete Midfoot Osteotomy   In cases in which there is a supination deformity of the midfoot, causing metatarsus varus, the supination needs to be addressed as well. For flexible supination deformities (i.e., cases in which passive pronation of the midfoot is possible), transfer of the anterior tibial tendon is needed to correct the soft-tissue imbalance. A SPLATT may be preferred for children with neuromuscular causes of the supination/adductus deformities, though a whole-tendon transfer may be considered in young children with recurrent or residual supination and adductus following clubfoot treatment. (The split anterior tibial tendon transfer [SPLATT] technique is discussed in Chapter 9.)

If the supination deformity is rigid, the osteotomy should extend across the entire midfoot, including the cuboid and all three cuneiforms, and exit the middle of the medial cuneiform (Fig. 19-8). During this osteotomy, it is crucial that soft-tissue retractors are placed plantar and dorsal across the midfoot immediately adjacent to the tarsal bones to protect neurovascular structures (e.g., the dorsal pedis artery and superficial and deep peroneal nerves) and tendons. Once the osteotomy is completed across the midfoot, the foot distal to the osteotomy can easily be pronated until it is perpendicular to the long axis of the tibia. At this point, the forefoot can be placed in almost any position desired. Several 1.6- to 2.0-mm smooth wires are used to fix the foot in the corrected position. These pins are removed in the office 4 weeks postoperatively (Fig. 19-9). The duration of casting is 6 to 8 weeks, with the first 4 weeks in a non-weight-bearing short-leg cast and the remaining time in a short-leg walking cast. A SPLATT is typically performed in conjunction with these osteotomies to minimize the risk of recurrent supination deformity.

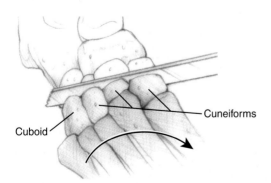

FIGURE 19-8   For forefoot varus, the osteotomy is extended across the midfoot. A 1/2-in. osteotome is used to cut across the midfoot, starting at the cuboid and exiting the middle of the medial cuneiform. Note: It is crucial to protect the dorsal and plantar soft tissues with retractors when making this cut.

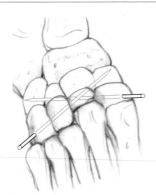

FIGURE 19-9

The midfoot osteotomy site is held using two to four smooth Steinmann pins. Note: The forefoot is now perpendicular to the long axis of the tibia.

Pearls and Pitfalls

- As with other deformities, metatarsus adductus only requires surgical treatment if the child is significantly symptomatic and has failed conservative management.
- The cuboid osteotomy should remove the majority of the ossified cuboid to achieve sufficient correction.
- Medial cuneiform osteotomy—or even osteotomies of all cuneiforms and the cuboid—may be necessary in moderate to severe deformities.
- If there is no ossific nucleus of the medial cuneiform, there is a higher rate of graft extrusion.
- If supination deformity is also present, the anterior tibial tendon should be transferred (in part or whole) to minimize the risk of recurrent deformity.

Postoperative Management

A well-padded short-leg nonwalking cast is placed at the time of surgery. The pins are pulled 4 weeks postoperatively, at which time the child is allowed to weight bear as tolerated in a short-leg walking cast. Casting is continued for a total of 6 to 8 weeks postoperatively.

Complications to Avoid

Undercorrection most typically occurs if a sufficient amount of cuboid is not removed at the time of surgery or if the cuboid osteotomy "opens up" due to loss of fixation postoperatively. Extrusion of the medial cuneiform graft can occur and can contribute to undercorrection. Recurrent deformity most commonly occurs in the presence of ongoing soft-tissue imbalance that was not addressed at surgery with anterior tibial tendon transfer. Wound complications may occur, particularly in children who have had previous ipsilateral foot surgeries. Vascular injury is minimized by maintaining the retractors immediately adjacent to bone.

SKEWFOOT

Skewfoot is a rare, complex foot deformity combining medial deviation of the forefoot (adductus) with lateral translation of the midfoot and hind-foot valgus. The cause is generally unknown, but some cases are felt to be iatrogenic from improper casting of metatarsus adductus and clubfoot. X-rays demonstrate two deformities between the first metatarsal and the talus in both the frontal and the sagittal plane. Mosca provided the best description of the deformity: "The navicular is abducted and dorsiflexed on the head of the talus. The first metatarsal is adducted and plantarflexed on the medial cuneiform."

Indications/Contraindications

Because the true natural history of skewfoot is not well described, conservative management is used in asymptomatic cases.

Surgery is indicated in children who have skewfeet and persistent pain, callosities, and difficulty wearing shoes if they have failed conservative measures such as heel-cord stretching, appropriate shoes (wide, soft shoes with sufficient padding), and orthotics.

Surgery is contraindicated in children less than 4 years of age, as obtaining and maintaining correction is difficult in children this young.

Preoperative Planning

- Weight-bearing AP and lateral films of the feet should be taken.
- The following should be requested:
  - Fluoroscopy
  - Tourniquet
  - Allograft (unless the family chooses autograft)
  - 1/4-in. and 1/2-in. osteotomes
  - 1.6-mm or 2.0-mm smooth Steinmann pins
  - Bone staples (manual or power driven)
  - Chandler retractors
  - Hohman retractors

Surgical Procedure

The child is positioned supine on the operating table with a bump under the ipsilateral hip to internally rotate the foot. After the leg is exsanguinated and the thigh tourniquet is inflated, the hind-foot valgus deformity is addressed through a modified Evans approach. A longitudinal incision is made just plantar to the peroneal tendons, starting at the junction of the proximal and middle thirds of the calcaneus and ending at the CC joint (Fig. 19-10A). The sural nerve is sought and protected. The peroneal tendon sheath is opened, and the tendons are retracted plantarly (Fig. 19-10B). The osteotomy site is selected between the anterior and middle facet. Slipping a Freer elevator over the dorsum of the calcaneus and into the space between the two facets localizes this space (Fig. 19-10C). The periosteum of the calcaneus is elevated in a dorsal-to-plantar direction using cautery; this is generally 2 to 2.5 cm proximal to the CC joint. Care is taken not to violate the capsule of the CC joint. The lateral third of the plantar fascia must be released off the plantar aspect of the calcaneus to facilitate later opening of the osteotomy site. A portion of the abductor digiti minimi may need to be released as well.

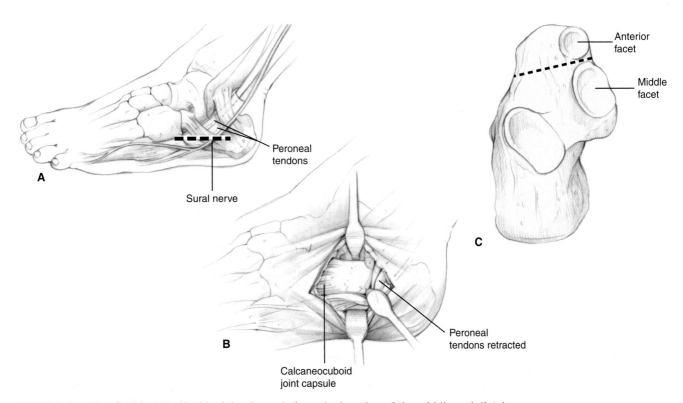

FIGURE 19-10   A. A longitudinal incision is made from the junction of the middle and distal third of the calcaneus to the calcaneocuboid joint. **B.** The peroneal tendons are retracted plantarly, and the extensor digitorum brevis is retracted dorsally. Care is taken not to violate the calcaneocuboid joint. **C.** The plane of the osteotomy should follow the plane between the anterior and middle facets of the calcaneus.

The osteotomy is made with a straight osteotome. It is necessary to cut a small portion of the abductor digiti minimi and the plantar fascia to allow the osteotomy site to open up.

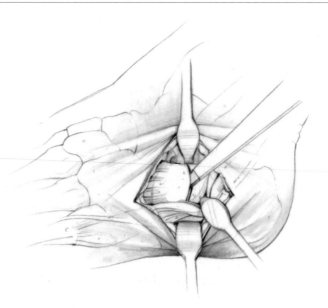

The calcaneal osteotomy is usually inherently stable once bone graft has been placed; pin fixation is rarely needed. However, fixation may be considered in order to stabilize the CC joint during distraction of the osteotomy to prevent CC joint subluxation. It may also be considered if there is concern about potential loss of fixation. If the decision is made to use fixation, a Steinmann pin suffices for fixation: A 2.0-mm smooth Steinmann pin is placed from distal to proximal across the CC joint to stabilize it prior to the osteotomy. A Hohman or Chandler retractor replaces the Freer elevator and is placed on the plantar aspect of the calcaneus at the osteotomy site. Care must be taken to stay extraperiosteal and not to enter the plantar surface of the calcaneus, as the bone is easily penetrated here. The plane of the osteotomy runs parallel to the space between the anterior and middle facets. This can be checked under fluoroscopy. The osteotomy is performed using a 1/2-in. osteotome, taking care not to penetrate the talar neck (Fig. 19-11).

To open up the osteotomy site, a 1.6- or 2.0-mm smooth Steinmann pin may be placed in the calcaneus (perpendicular to its long axis) proximal and distal to the site. Alternatively, a broad, flat laminar spreader can be used without the pins (Fig. 19-12A).

A trapezoidal-shaped bone graft, either autologous or allograft, is inserted. The authors have had good results using a cancellous allograft block. The size of the graft is selected after opening the osteotomy site and measuring the amount of lengthening that is required to shift the navicular over the talar head, usually as much opening as can be obtained (Fig. 19-12B). This length is the base of the trapezoid. Grafts are typically twice as long laterally as medially, with measurements 14 to 16 mm laterally and 7 to 8 mm medially. The bone graft is inserted, and the pin that was stabilizing the CC joint is driven across the bone graft site to stabilize it, while continuing to stabilize the CC joint if a pin was placed (Fig. 19-12C).

At this point, attention turns to the forefoot. After lengthening the lateral column, the metatarsus adductus will appear even more pronounced. A straight longitudinal incision is made overlying the medial cuneiform. Dissection is carried down with tenotomy scissors. The anterior tibialis tendon is identified over the first cuneiform bone. The tendon is gently dissected free, without disrupting its attachments, and is retracted dorsally using a Hohman retractor. The center of the cuneiform is identified, and the periosteum is incised using either cautery or a #15 blade from dorsal to plantar. The periosteum is elevated proximally and distally approximately 5 mm in each direction. Care is taken not to disrupt the capsules of the proximal and distal joints. Small Chandler retractors are placed dorsal and plantar at the cuneiform. An osteotomy (1/2-in. osteotome) is performed at the center of the cuneiform and should be parallel with the distal articular surface. Because this surface is often sloped, the direction of the osteotomy should be confirmed under fluoroscopy. The osteotomy site is opened using laminar spreaders. A wedge of bone graft is then inserted and held using a 2.0-mm smooth Steinmann pin from distal to proximal (if a pin is needed for stability). The pin is left percutaneous distally. Of note, if the abductor hallucis muscle is too tight, it may need to be released with lengthening of the medial column of the foot (Figs. 19-4 to 19-6). If the correction is still not adequate after a generous wedge of bone has been placed, the osteotomy may be continued across the middle and even lateral cuneiform, and/or a closing-wedge osteotomy can be

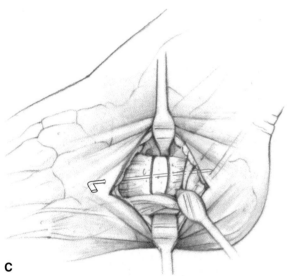

FIGURE 19-12   **A.** A lamina spreader is used to open the osteotomy site. **B.** As the lateral column is lengthened, coverage of the talar head improves. The size of the bone graft selected depends on the amount of opening required to cover the talar head. **C.** A trapezoidal-shaped piece of bone graft is placed in the osteotomy site and can be secured with the Steinmann pin that was placed to secure the calcaneocuboid joint, if necessary.

performed at the cuboid as previously described (Fig. 19-13). Dorsiflexion should be checked upon completion of the procedure; if dorsiflexion is less than 10 degrees with the knee extended, a tendo-Achilles lengthening or gastrocnemius recession should be performed. Frequently, the peroneus brevis tendon needs to be Z-lengthened if it is found to be taut after lateral column lengthening. The peroneus longus rarely requires lengthening.

Pearls and Pitfalls

- Equinus is commonly present in conjunction with skewfoot. Gastrocnemius recession or Achilles tendon lengthening is often requisite for complete correction of the skewfoot.
- When surgery is undertaken for a skewfoot, preservation of range of motion is important. Joint-preserving procedures, such as the osteotomies noted above, are preferable to fusions.
- Release of the plantar fascia should be performed in conjunction with calcaneal lengthening osteotomy to allow for sufficient lengthening to correct hind-foot valgus. Complete plantar fascia release may be needed to permit concomitant lengthening of the medial column, which occurs with medial cuneiform opening wedge.

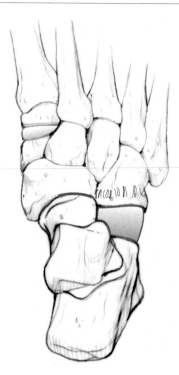

FIGURE 19-13

Skewfoot corrected with lateral column lengthening of the calcaneus, opening-wedge osteotomy of the medial cuneiform.

- There is excellent correction and graft incorporation with allograft cancellous bone blocks if used for the hind-foot and midfoot osteotomies described. Autograft may be used if the family desires, though this increases surgical time and introduces the risk of chronic pain at the bone graft harvest site. Tricortical iliac crest graft can also crush the adjacent osteopenic bone in patients with neuromuscular disease.

Postoperative Management

A well-padded, short-leg nonwalking cast is placed at surgery. Four weeks postoperatively, pins (if used) are removed in the office. The child is then placed into a short-leg walking cast for an additional 2 to 4 weeks. If a foot orthotic (such as a University of California at Berkeley Laboratory [UCBL]) is to be used, it is measured at the time of the cast change and delivered when the second cast is removed. Such an orthotic may be used for 4 to 6 months following cast removal.

Complications to Avoid

Continued pain and/or callus following surgery most commonly result from undercorrection of the deformity. Pain or numbness from injury to the sural nerve may occur. Wound problems can be minimized by using nonabsorbable simple skin sutures for the lateral calcaneal wound.

Nonunion of the bone graft site is extremely rare. Donor site morbidity (if autograft is used) is more common.

ILLUSTRATIVE CASES

A 16-year-old boy with cerebral palsy presented with a painful equinovarus foot despite treatment with orthotics and footwear modifications (Fig. 19-14). He underwent a closing-wedge osteotomy of the cuboid for forefoot adductus and cuneiform osteotomies for fixed-forefoot supination. Soft-tissue balancing was performed as well and included a SPLATT, posterior tibialis lengthening, and tendo-Achilles lengthening.

A 6-year-old boy with a skewfoot (Figs. 19-15 and 19-16) had persistent pain despite orthotic wear. He underwent a calcaneal lengthening osteotomy and medial cuneiform lengthening osteotomies (Figs. 19-18 and 19-19).

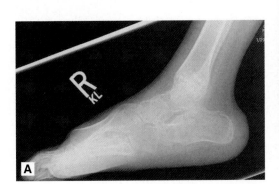
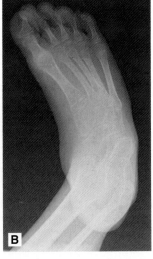

FIGURE 19-14

Preoperative lateral **(A)** and AP **(B)** radiographs of the patient. The supination is evident on the lateral radiograph, demonstrating stacking of the metatarsals.

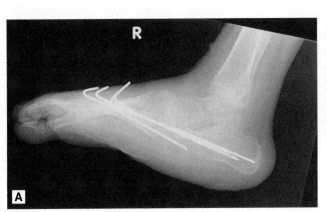
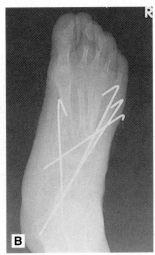

FIGURE 19-15

Lateral **(A)** and AP **(B)** radiographs were taken 4 weeks after surgery. The pins were removed in the office on this day, and the patient was placed in a short-leg walking cast.

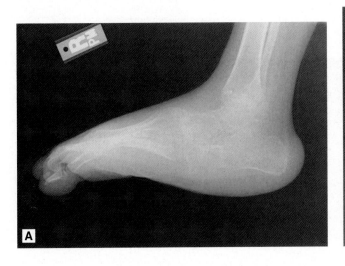
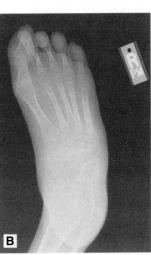

FIGURE 19-16

A, B. Two months postoperatively, the varus and equinus are nicely corrected, and the osteotomies are healed.

FIGURE 19-17

Preoperative lateral **(A)** and AP **(B)** radiographs of the patient. Note the lateral displacement of the navicular on the talus and the associated metatarsus adductus.

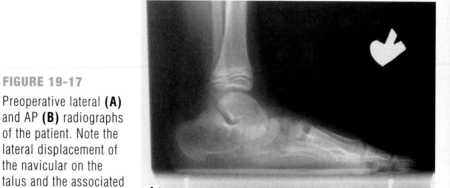

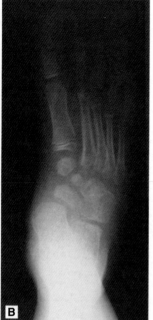

FIGURE 19-18

A, B. Intraoperative radiographs. On the radiograph, the graft for the medial cuneiform looks larger than the cuneiform; this is misleading, as radiographs only show the ossified portion of the bone. The graft lengthens the cuneiform well, correcting the adductus.

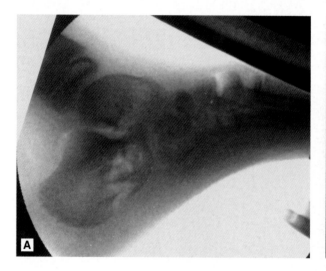

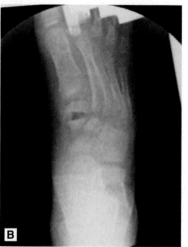

FIGURE 19-19

A, B. Radiographs taken 8 years after surgery. There is a mild talar sag, but overall good maintenance of correction. The patient is active in sports, is pain free, and no longer requires orthotics.

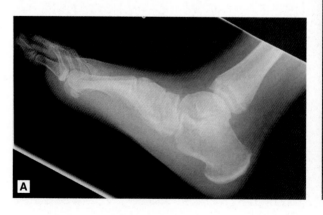

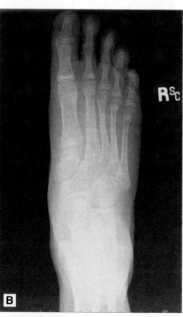

SUMMARY

Midfoot deformities are a common cause of pain and footwear problems. For children who have failed conservative management, surgery may be necessary to allow a return to age-appropriate activities.

REFERENCES

1. Evans D. Relapsed clubfoot. *J Bone Joint Surg Br.* 1961;43:722.
2. Evans D. Calcaneovalgus deformity. *J Bone Joint Surg Br.* 1975;57:270.
3. Gordon JE, Luhmann SJ, Dobbs MB, et al. Combined midfoot osteotomy for severe forefoot adductus. *J Pediatr Orthop.* 2003;23:74–78.
4. McHale KA, Lenhart MK. Treatment of residual clubfoot deformity—the bean shaped foot—by opening wedge medial cuneiform osteotomy and closing wedge cuboid osteotomy: clinical review and cadaver correlations. *J Pediatr Orthop.* 2003;23:70–73.
5. Mosca VS. Calcaneal lengthening for valgus deformity of the hindfoot: results in children who had severe, symptomatic flatfoot and skewfoot. *J Bone Joint Surg Am.* 1995;77:500.
6. Pohl M, Nicol RO. Transcuneiform and opening wedge cuneiform osteotomy with closing wedge cuboid osteotomy in relapsed clubfoot. *J Pediatr Orthop.* 2003;23:70–73.

20 Cavus Foot

David P. Roye and Jaime A. Gómez

INTRODUCTION

The subject of claw-foot (pes cavus, hollow foot, etc.) has been so well covered in the literature, especially during the last twenty years, that it is unnecessary and, of course, impossible to review the condition in detail.

—Wallace H. Cole, M.D., 1940

Cavus foot, or pes cavus, is a complicated and difficult problem. The best definition of the condition is the simplest: "a foot deformity characterized by an unusually high arch" (Merriam-Webster Medline Plus online dictionary). Due to the complex and varying nature of the etiology and pathologies that cause pes cavus, a more specific definition requires discussion and qualifications. Because of the wide range of pes cavus pathogeneses, it is impossible to condense a comprehensive examination of this deformity into one chapter. If Dr. Cole was overwhelmed by the literature on pes cavus close to 70 years ago, one can imagine the plethora of information on the topic that is available now. Because most pes cavus is of neurogenic origin,[1] this discussion will focus on neurogenic cavus foot.

Though they will not be directly addressed in this chapter, nonneurogenic etiologies include arthrogryposis, residual of talipes equino varus, posttraumatic deformity (residual of compartment syndrome, crush syndrome, fracture malunion, and burn contracture), and idiopathic cavovarus.

Multiple neurogenic conditions can cause pes cavus, including poliomyelitis, cerebral palsy, spinal dysraphism, degenerative diseases of the central and peripheral nervous system such as Friedreich ataxia, and hereditary motor sensory neuropathies. Of the neurogenic causes for pes cavus, hereditary motor sensory neuropathy (HMSN, types I and II), otherwise known as Charcot-Marie-Tooth (CMT) disease, stands out as the most frequent underlying diagnosis.

Most contemporary authors agree that neurogenic pes cavus is caused by some sort of muscle imbalance. Different studies have cited different muscle pairs. One common interpretation involves a combination of intrinsic and extrinsic weaknesses. In this scenario, the intrinsic foot muscles and the tibialis anterior are weak. The tibialis posterior and the peroneus longus, however, have normal strength. The triceps surae is also weak and may be contracted. Tynan et al. postulated that overaction of the peroneus longus in comparison to its antagonist, the tibialis anterior, is an ultimate factor in the pathogenesis of the majority of symptomatic cases of forefoot pes cavus. Progression from insidious atrophy of the intrinsic musculature of the foot to fixed soft tissue and bone deformity occurs. In HMSN, insidious atrophy of the lumbricals and the interossei would cause dorsiflexion at the metatarsophalangeal joint.

Whatever the pathogenesis, cavus foot in the neurogenic population tends to have a few other accompanying deformities affecting foot stability. First, the ray of the first metatarsal becomes

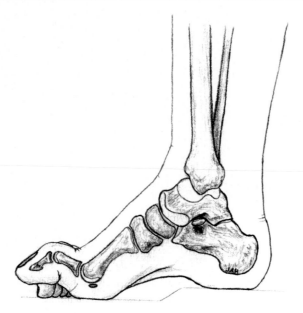

FIGURE 20-1

Cavus foot with claw toe. (Courtesy of Javier Avendano, M.D.)

plantarflexed, bringing the forefoot into supination. That process is worsened as the long toe extensors try to help the weak tibialis anterior and hyperextend the toes. To compensate, the calcaneus turns inward, causing an overall cavovarus deformity. Finally, the tightened plantar fascia pulls the toes inward via a windlass effect, leading to clawing of the toes (Fig. 20-1).

INDICATIONS/CONTRAINDICATIONS

The pes cavus patient often presents with fatigue and discomfort of the foot. Thick callosities over the overburdened first and fifth metatarsal heads are also common. Because there is frequently toe clawing, fat pads can be pulled distally, increasing the metatarsalgia.

Another sign of pes cavus is multiple lateral ankle sprains. The inverted hind foot puts extra pressure on the foot's lateral border, which may predispose to lateral ankle sprains. Roentgenograms will confirm the cavus foot diagnosis by showing the earlier-described bone deformities and the high arch. The high arch, is pathognomonic for the condition (Fig. 20-2). To determine the rigidity of the deformity, the block test can be performed. Developed by Dr. Coleman in 1977, the block test is quite simple: A wooden block is placed under the heel and the lateral border of the foot, with the first metatarsal hanging free to neutralize the forefoot pronation. If the hind foot returns to neutral or to valgus, the deformity can be classified as flexible; otherwise, it is rigid (Fig. 20-3). The results of the block test will affect treatment plans, as described in the following section.

PREOPERATIVE PLANNING

Nonoperative procedures for treating pes cavus have been developed, including casting, bracing, special shoes, and exercise. However, none of these treatments are usually definitive. Most are used only in the minimally deformed foot or in the cavus foot early in the deformity's evolution.

The supple early cavus foot is more easily treated than is the late rigid foot. The rigidity of the deformity can easily be tested with the block test described above. When a flexible hind foot is present and the patient is under 12 years of age, soft-tissue releases can be used alone to flatten the foot. However, more rigid deformities in older patients often need bony procedures. For the purposes of this chapter, the surgical procedures are classified into three categories: soft tissue, osteotomies, and arthrodesis. Most often, the surgeon decides on a combination of procedures from the three categories. Depending on the patient's condition, the procedures can be staged.

SURGICAL PROCEDURES

Soft-Tissue Procedures

Plantar Fasciotomy   The plantar release is always used when surgical treatment is indicated. Its main objective is to decrease the arch height, thus correcting the cavus foot. In young patients with flexible cavus foot, the fasciotomy may be enough to correct the deformity, flattening the arch.

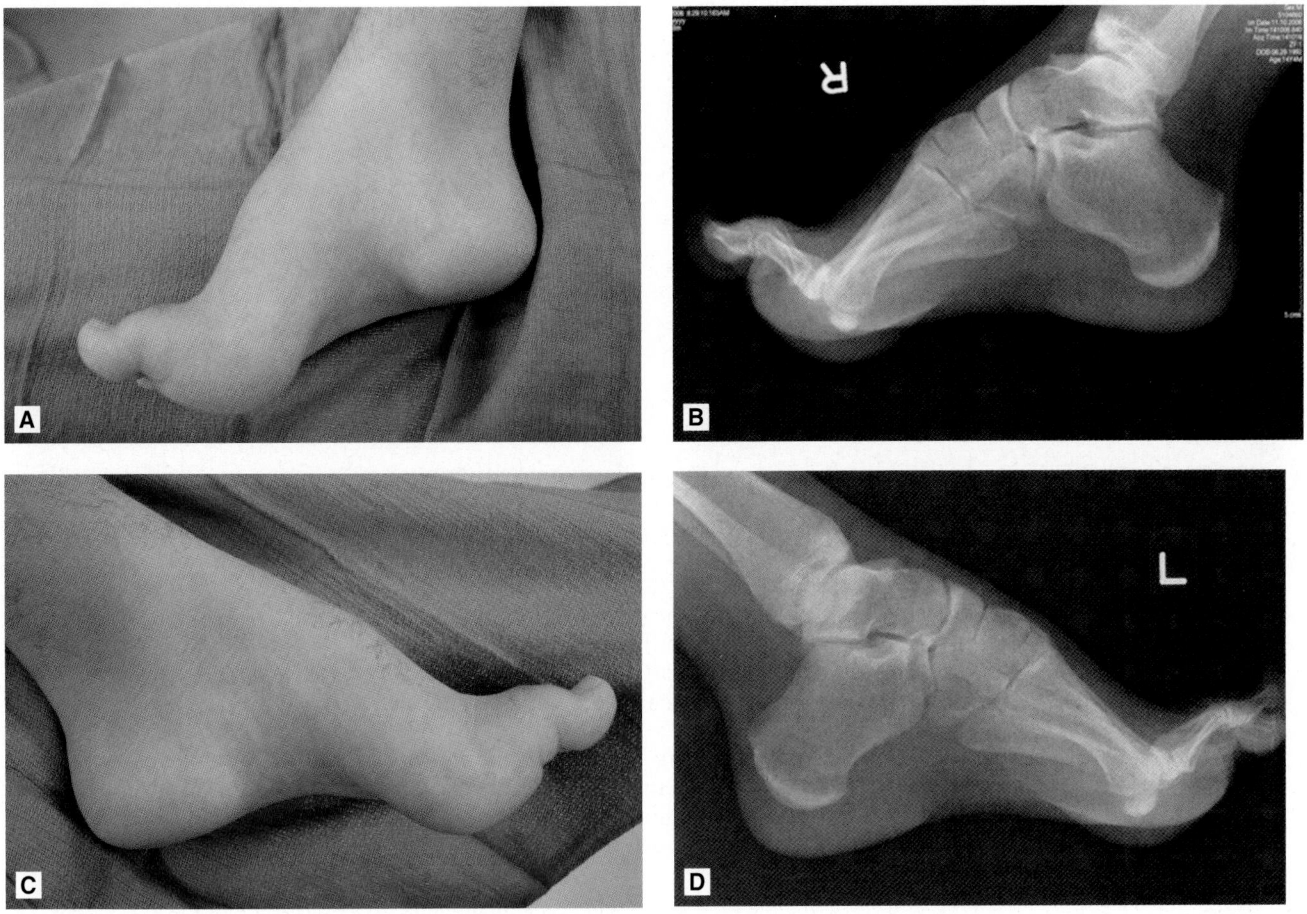

FIGURE 20-2   A. Lateral clinical picture of cavus right foot. **B.** Lateral x-ray of cavus right foot.
C. Lateral clinical picture of cavus left foot. **D.** Lateral x-ray of cavus left foot.

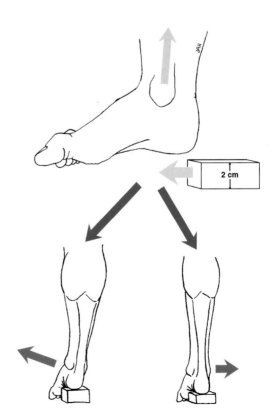

FIGURE 20-3

Coleman's block test for assessing rigidity. (Courtesy of Javier Avendano, M.D.)

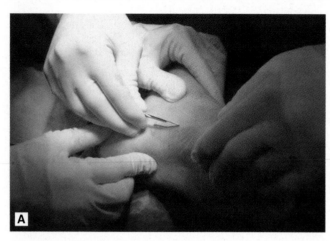
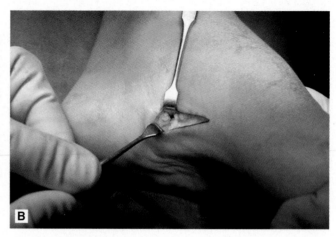

FIGURE 20-4   **A.** Initial incision for plantar fasciotomy. **B.** Approach to the plantar fascia for release.

A 2-cm incision is made over the internal border of the plantar surface of the midfoot (Fig. 20-4). The plantar fascia is identified, and two transverse incisions separated by 3 cm are made with a scalpel. This elongates the fascia, bringing the forefoot to dorsiflexion (Fig. 20-5). A cast is applied and changed every 2 weeks. Plantar fascial release is frequently employed in mild or moderate pes cavus, but it cannot correct severe deformity without other added procedures.

Achilles Tendon Lengthening   If a varus deformity is present the Z-lengthening can be performed leaving the lateral aspect of the insertion of the Achilles tendon intact. In the absence of significant varus a coronal plane lengthening can be performed. The authors recommend an oblique incision as opposed to a straight vertical incision. This approach provides excellent exposure and better cosmesis. (Fig. 20-6).

The Achilles lengthening is performed as a complementary procedure in those cavus feet that present with equinus deformity of the hind foot. When an Achilles lengthening is needed, it should be saved for last so that the midfoot and forefoot can be forcefully dorsiflexed during the necessary releases in those areas. Although others report using a Steinmann pin through the ankle joint to accomplish the same thing, the authors do not like to violate the joint.

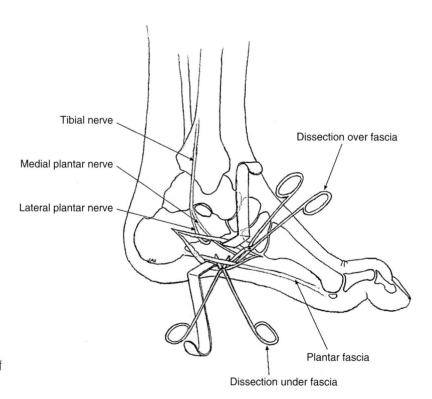

FIGURE 20-5

Plantar fascia dissection. (Courtesy of Javier Avendano, M.D.)

Tibial nerve

Medial plantar nerve

Lateral plantar nerve

Dissection over fascia

Plantar fascia

Dissection under fascia

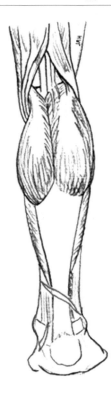

FIGURE 20-6

Posterior incisions for Achilles lengthening. (Courtesy of Javier Avendano, M.D.)

Steindler Stripping   A medial incision is usually recommended, though some authors prefer the approach through a median or a lateral plantar incision from the calcaneus tuberosity distally to the base of the metatarsus. The plantar fascia is then identified and detached from the calcaneus. Then, from medial to lateral, the abductor hallucis, flexor digitorum brevis, and abductor digiti quinti are detached. The surgeon must keep the dissection close to the bone to avoid neurovascular injuries. Releasing the section of the long plantar ligaments that go from the calcaneus to the cuboid, scaphoid, and calcaneonavicular spring ligament is optional. It has been the authors' experience that in moderate or severe feet, all those structures will need to be released to achieve adequate correction.

Closure is achieved after homeostasis, and a short-leg cast is used to maintain the obtained correction. This cast may be changed every 2 weeks during 8 weeks of immobilization.

In addition to the plantar stripping, when a varus component is present, a medial stripping must also be performed. The posterior tibial tendon is detached from its insertions, because it is responsible for the fixed equinus of the first metatarsal bone. Also released is the master knot of Henry (the fascia investing the crossing of the flexor digitorum longus and flexor hallucis longus tendons on the medial side of the foot) and the Y ligament. The plantar aspect of the cuneometatarsal capsules should be opened through the medial approach.

Some authors do not recommend the Steindler release procedure because of the retractile scarring that may appear with the medial incision and because of the possibility of a neurovascular injury. Again, it has been the authors' experience that this procedure is necessary in most moderate and all severe feet.

Anterior Tibial Transfer   This surgery aims to improve the foot's eversion strength. The whole tendon can be transferred, or to avoid the risk of overcorrection, the lateral half only can be transferred. When performing the whole-tendon transfer, great care must be taken not to transfer the new insertion too lateral, as doing so can potentiate the plantarflexion strength of the peroneus longus, resulting in a pronated, overcorrected midfoot and forefoot.

A 2-cm incision is performed over the base of the first metatarsal bone. Then the anterior tibial tendon is identified. Either half or all of this tendon is detached and retracted with a whip suture.

A second incision is made over the distal third of the anterior face of the leg. The anterior compartment fascia is divided, and the muscle-tendon junction of the anterior tibialis is identified and retracted, obtaining the distal part of the tendon that is going to be transferred. It may be useful to use an Ober tendon passer for this maneuver.

Finally a third incision is made over the cuboid or over the base of the fourth metatarsal. A tendon passer or a clamp is used to bring the tendon from the second incision site. The transfer is made posterior to the extensor retinaculum of the ankle. At this point, the tendon is fixed to the bone through two convergent perforations that create a tunnel for the tendon, which is sutured over itself. If this is not possible, the tendon can pass through a perforation to the plantar aspect of the foot, where gauze or a button can be used for fixation.

The forefoot must be left in dorsiflexion and immobilized in a short-leg cast after hemostasis and incision closure.

Posterior Tibial Tendon Transfer This procedure can be performed to diminish the plantarflexion strength of the tendon over the first metatarsal and to improve dorsiflexion. However, the surgeon must keep in mind that this transfer is not ideal because the tendon is transferred to produce an antagonistic (out-of-phase) function.

A first incision is made over the scaphoid bone; the tendon is identified, detached, and dissected free. Care must be taken to achieve as much length as possible. A scalpel is used to incise the sheath as far proximally as possible, and a whip suture is inserted in the tip of the tendon.

The second posterior, medial, and oblique incision is performed on the medial face of the distal third of the leg, just posterior to the tibia. With the help of a Langenbeck retractor and a headlight, the fascia is divided, and the tibialis posterior tendon is identified, extracted, and tagged (Fig. 20-7).

The third incision is made over the anterior aspect of the leg on the distal third. The tibial ridge must be palpated. The longitudinal incision is performed 1.5 cm lateral to the tibia's subcutaneous border. If the incision is made over the tibia, the scar may be painful and adherent. The fascia of this compartment is sectioned, and a space between the anterior tibialis and the extensor digitorum longus is dissected distally to the interosseous membrane. The surgeon must be aware of the neurovascular bundle that lies immediately posterior to the interosseous membrane. A window is made in the interosseous membrane through which the tendon is passed from the site of the second incision. At this point, authors recommend making the longitudinal sides of the window first and then the transverse sides (Fig. 20-8A).

Finally an incision is made over the dorsal aspect of the foot at the level of the third cuneiform or the third metatarsal. The tendon is identified where the third incision was made. With a tendon passer, the tendon is guided, passing posterior to the extensor retinaculum, and is fixed to the

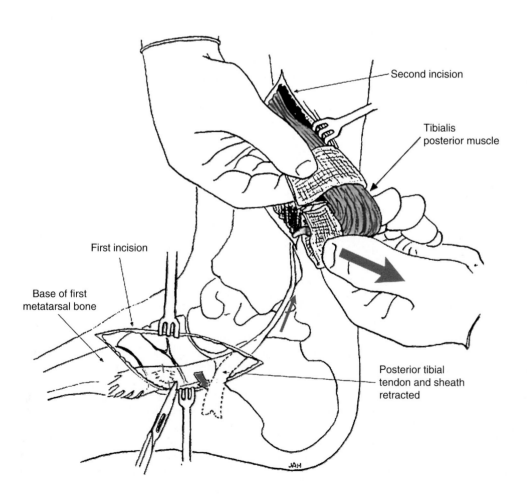

FIGURE 20-7

Anterior transfer of posterior tibial tendon through interosseous membrane. (Courtesy of Javier Avendano, M.D.)

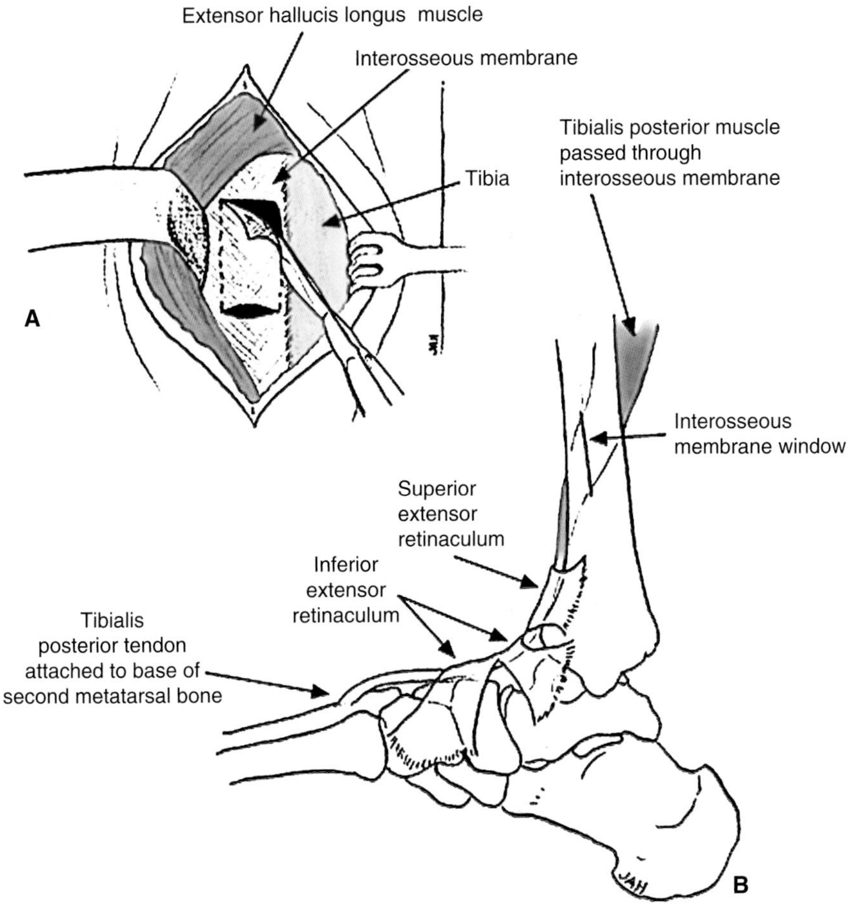

Extensor hallucis longus muscle

Interosseous membrane

Tibialis posterior muscle
passed through
interosseous membrane

Tibia

A

Interosseous
membrane window

Superior
extensor
retinaculum

Inferior
extensor
retinaculum

Tibialis
posterior tendon
attached to base of
second metatarsal bone

B

FIGURE 20-8
A. Rectangular window on interosseous membrane. **B.** Anterior transfer of posterior tibial tendon and attachment to second metatarsal. (Courtesy of Javier Avendano, M.D.)

cuneiform or the metatarsal with a double convergent perforation (Fig. 20-8B). The tunnel may also be made to the plantar aspect of the foot, and a button or gauze can be used to fix the tendon as Cole[4] described.

Hemostasis is achieved. Wounds are irrigated and closed, and the foot is immobilized with a short-leg cast. Management of this condition requires a well-fitted cast. However, after such an extensive dissection, the surgeon may be reluctant to apply such a cast. In this case, a splint or thickly padded bivalved cast should be applied, with plans to bring the patient back for casting after swelling has subsided, even if another anesthesia is required.

Transfer of Long Toe Extensors to Heads of Metatarsals

The goal of this procedure is to enhance the foot's dorsiflexion strength and to elevate the metatarsal heads when claw toes are present with pes cavus.

A dorsal incision is made over the metatarsophalangeal joint. The extensor hallucis longus and the extensor hallucis brevis are identified and sectioned distally (Fig. 20-9A–9B). The extensor hallucis longus is then passed from medial to lateral through a perforation on the head of the first metatarsal, and the tendon is sutured on itself (Fig. 20-9C–9D). The distal stump of the extensor hallucis longus is then sutured to the detached brevis to preserve the extension function of the interphalangeal (IP) joint, thus avoiding a flexion deformity.

In the other toes, the extensor digitorum longus is used the same way, passing it through a proximal metatarsal perforation and avoiding the physis in children younger than 12 years of age. The extremity must be immobilized with a cast for 6 weeks when the IP arthrodesis is performed.

Peroneus Longus Tendon Transfer

A centered incision over the insertion of the peroneus brevis tendon is made. Blunt dissection is performed until the peroneus tendons are identified. The peroneus longus tendon is sectioned, and its proximal fragment is sutured to the peroneus brevis tendon. After homeostasis and wound closure, the tenorrhaphy is protected with a short-leg cast for 6 weeks.

The goal of this procedure is to decrease the plantarflexion strength of the peroneus longus over the first metatarsal and increase the eversion strength of the peroneus brevis.

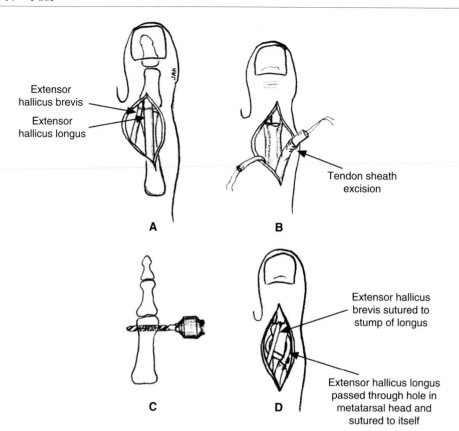

FIGURE 20-9

Transfer of long toe extensors to heads of metatarsals (Jones transfer).
A. Identification of hallux extensor tendons. **B.** Hallucis longus and brevis are sectioned.
C. Perforation on first metatarsal bone.
D. Extensor hallucis longus passed from medial to lateral and sutured to itself. (Courtesy of Javier Avendano, M.D.)

Within figure: Extensor hallicus brevis / Extensor hallicus longus / Tendon sheath excision / Extensor hallicus brevis sutured to stump of longus / Extensor hallicus longus passed through hole in metatarsal head and sutured to itself

Osteotomies

First Metatarsal Osteotomy   Commonly the first metatarsal requires an osteotomy to correct the equinus intrinsic to the first ray. This type of osteotomy may be performed at the base of the first metatarsal, creating a dorsally based closing wedge (Figs. 20-10 to 20-16). The dorsalis pedis vessels and the extensor tendons are carefully retracted, and the first tarsometatarsal joint is palpated and/or located with imaging. The authors prefer not to open the capsule or expose the joint so as to preserve motion.

An alternative procedure which avoids injury of the first metatarsal proximal physis in children is a dorsally based closing wedge osteotomy of the medial cuniaform.

Osteotomies of Metatarsals Two Through Five   Osteotomies of metatarsals two through five are occasionally necessary. However, the authors are reluctant to recommend these osteotomies routinely, as they may result in substantial stiffness of the midfoot. When this procedure is performed, the osteotomy is located in the proximal metaphysis and is described being performed through two parallel incisions. The metatarsal heads are forced into dorsiflexion (Fig. 20-15) and fixed in the corrected position with two Steinmann pins or a screw (Fig. 20-16).

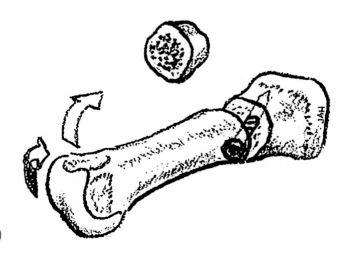

FIGURE 20-10

First metatarsal osteotomy and screw fixation. (Courtesy of Javier Avendano, M.D.)

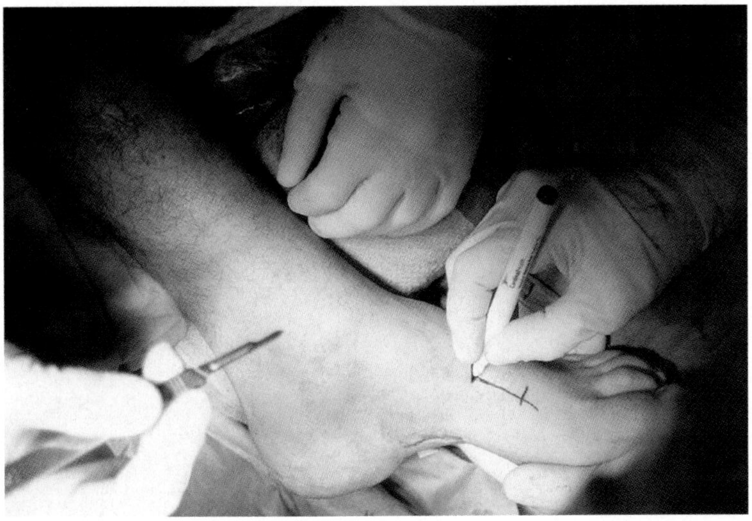

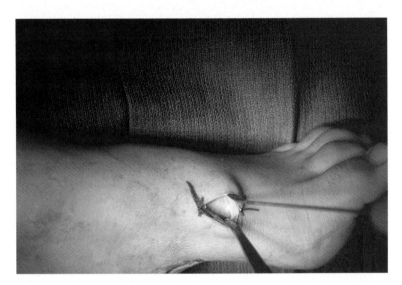

FIGURE 20-11
Dorsal incision over first metatarsal.

FIGURE 20-12
Dissection to first metatarsal diaphysis.

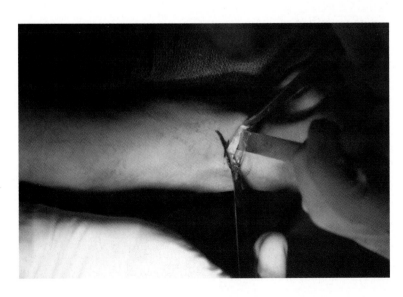

FIGURE 20-13
First metatarsal osteotomy.

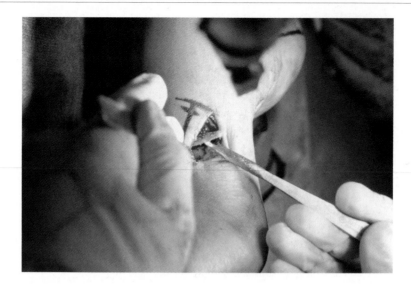

FIGURE 20-14
Removing dorsally
based metatarsal
wedge.

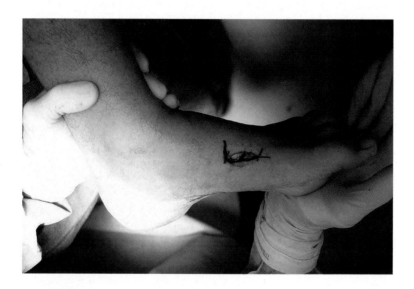

FIGURE 20-15
Closing wedge with
dorsiflexion maneuver.

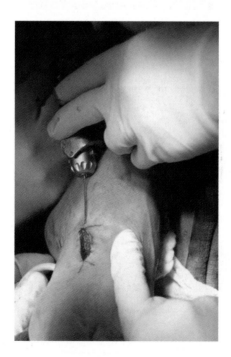

FIGURE 20-16
Osteotomy fixation
using Steinmann pins.

The extremity is then immobilized with a short-leg cast. Although others have recommended that if the patient is skeletally mature, all metatarsals should be osteotomized, the authors do not agree. Instead they recommend using combinations of midfoot soft-tissue releases and osteotomies to achieve correction.

Midfoot Wedge Osteotomy   This procedure is the authors' preferred osteotomy for treating rigid cavus feet that definitively need an osteotomy. Two dorsal incisions are made to expose the cuboid and the naviculocuneiform joint. Through the medial incision, the extensor hallucis longus, the dorsalis pedis vessels, and the anterior tibial tendon are identified and retracted medially to expose the naviculocuneiform joint. Through the lateral incision, the extensor brevis and the peroneus brevis tendons are retracted laterally, exposing the cuboid.

Subsequently a wedge with a dorsal base is performed with an osteotome (Fig. 20-17). This must include the naviculocuneiform joint and the cuboid; the size of the wedge depends on the magnitude of the deformity and the amount of correction needed (Fig. 20-18). The corrected foot position is then fixed with two Steinmann pins, staples, or cannulated screws. This fixation may be difficult to perform because the distal fragment is often osteoporotic. The osteotomy is subsequently protected with a short-leg cast.

Japas V-Osteotomy of the Tarsus   This osteotomy is performed through a 6- to 8-cm longitudinal incision made on the midline of the foot over the tarsal bones. The dorsalis neurovascular bundle, the extensor hallucis longus, and the anterior tibial tendon are identified and retracted medially and laterally. The extensor digitorum brevis and the peroneal tendons are identified and retracted. The talonavicular joint must be clearly identified to avoid injury to the midtarsal joints.

The osteotomy is started with an oscillating saw. Most cases should be continued with osteotomes. The surgeon starts the osteotomy medially, just proximal to the cuneometatarsal joint. The osteotomy is then continued through the body of the navicular. At this point, the lateral part of the V is continued, redirecting the osteotomes and leaving an apex or preferably a dome-shaped figure proximally to end the osteotomy close to the fifth metatarsal-cuboid joint (Fig. 20-19).

With longitudinal traction and using a periosteal elevator as a lever, the distal segment is depressed toward the plantar aspect of the foot. This maneuver corrects the cavus deformity and elongates the concave surface of the foot's sole. From the authors' experience, even a complete cut is usually not enough to allow for complete correction. In most cases, bone resection from the dorsum of the osteotomy is needed. The obtained correction is maintained with a Steinmann pin that is best passed from medial and distal to lateral and proximal. Wounds are closed after homeostasis, and a short-leg cast is used to immobilize the limb for 6 weeks.

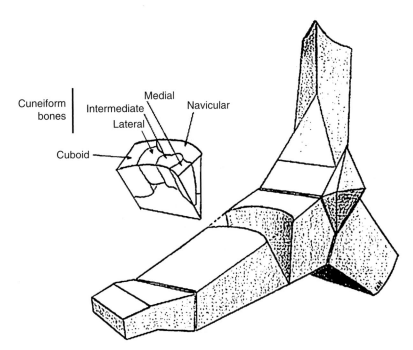

FIGURE 20-17

Osteotomy of the tarsus and midfoot dorsally based wedge. (Courtesy of Javier Avendano, M.D.)

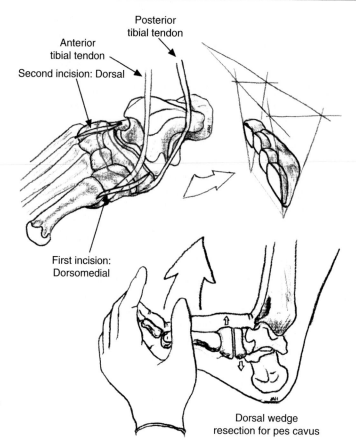

Posterior
tibial tendon

Anterior
tibial tendon

Second incision: Dorsal

First incision:
Dorsomedial

Dorsal wedge
resection for pes cavus

Calcaneal Osteotomy A lateral oblique incision is made just posterior to the peroneal tendons, exposing the calcaneus (Figs. 20-20 and 20-21). The fibulocalcaneal ligament is identified and sectioned along with the periosteum. A lateral-based wedge is performed on the calcaneus, immediately posterior to the peroneus longus tendon (Fig. 20-22).

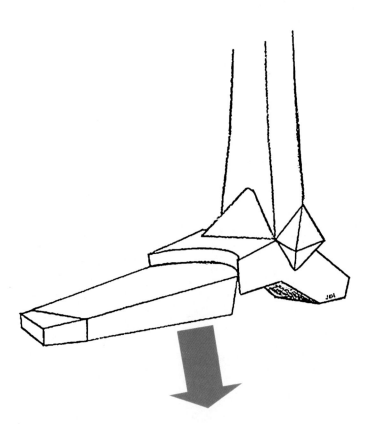

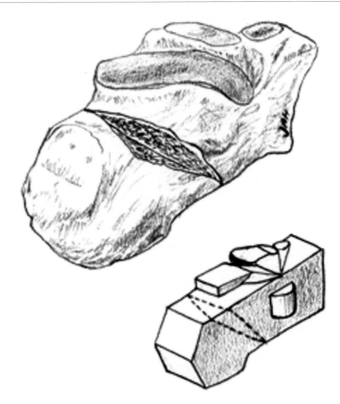

FIGURE 20-20
Wedge osteotomy of the calcaneus. (Courtesy of Javier Avendano, M.D.)

The wedge is closed and fixed with a Steinmann pin or a cannulated 7.3-mm screw (Figs. 20-23, 20-24, and 20-26). The screw can be introduced percutaneously in a trajectory that is close to perpendicular to the osteotomy and buried. The distal fragment may be moved into a more valgus position by the closing wedge; it can also be translated dorsally to help correct the cavus. Using the guide pin for the 7.3-mm cannulated screw is an effective way to achieve correction.

This osteotomy is rarely performed in isolation. The patient should be non–weight bearing for 4 weeks in a short-leg cast. Subsequently the cast can be changed to a weight-bearing cast until healing is observed.

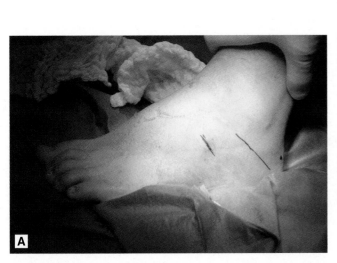
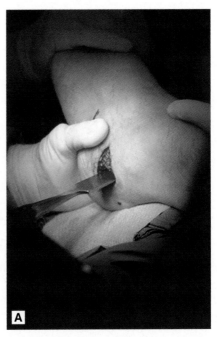

FIGURE 20-21   **A.** Lateral incision for calcaneus osteotomy. **B.** Osteotomy of the calcaneus.

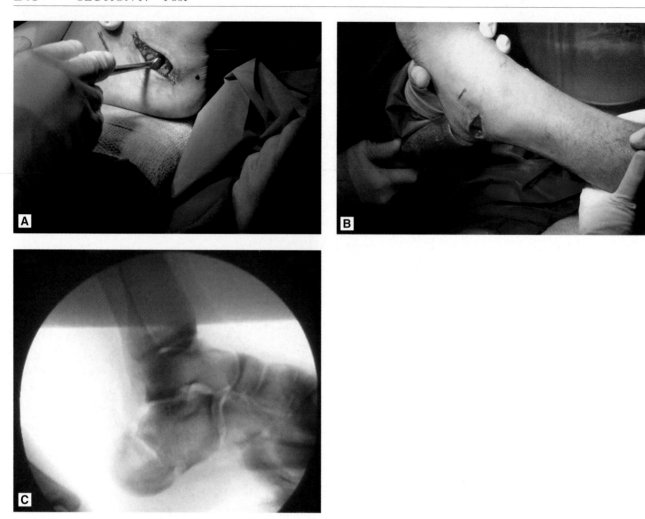

FIGURE 20-22 **A.** Lateral-based wedge on the calcaneus posterior to the peroneus longus tendon. **B.** Proximal segment of the calcaneus displaced cephalad. **C.** Postosteotomy lateral x-ray.

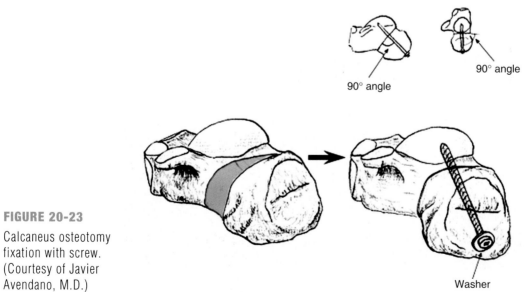

FIGURE 20-23

Calcaneus osteotomy fixation with screw. (Courtesy of Javier Avendano, M.D.)

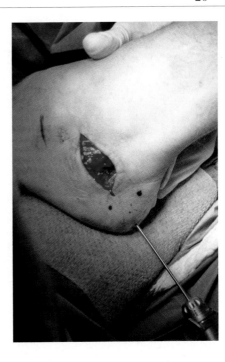

FIGURE 20-24
Calcaneus osteotomy fixation with Steinmann pin.

Variations of this technique have been described, including sliding the posterior fragment laterally without resection or, as Mitchell suggested, sliding the fragment superiorly and posteriorly. The Mitchell variation is useful in calcaneus cavus feet.

Triple Arthrodesis   When considering arthrodesis, the surgeon should attempt to limit the fusion to those areas that he or she has been unable to control with soft-tissue surgeries and/or osteotomies (i.e., performing only a subtalar fusion or limiting it to a subtalar and calcaneocuboid fusion). The triple arthrodesis should be regarded as a salvage procedure; however, it is a powerful procedure when combined with appropriate soft-tissue correction and with resection of appropriate wedges in the articulations among the calcaneus, talus, cuboid, and tarsal navicular. This procedure puts extra stress on the nonfused joints and may be a cause of later degenerative arthritis in the tibial talar joint and the midfoot joints. Fusions should be avoided in patients with impairment of sensory function. That said, many of the most difficult cavus feet (e.g., HMSN, myelomeningocele) have such deficiencies. Fusions in feet with impaired sensation and proprioception can lead to skin breakdown and Charcot joints. In any event, this procedure is often the only one available for an older patient with a stiff cavus foot.

A Kocher-type incision centered over the sinus tarsi is made, and the short toe extensors are taken down proximally from their origin and reflected distally. The midtarsal and the subtalar joints are exposed through blunt dissection. The peroneal tendons and the sural nerve are retracted laterally with a small Homan retractor placed on the plantar aspect of the foot. The toe extensors and the dorsalis pedis bundle are identified and retracted medially. Dorsal wedges are performed on the midtarsal joints (talonavicular and calcaneocuboid), and a lateral-based wedge is taken from the subtalar joint when the cavus is accompanied by a varus deformity. Most deformity can be accommodated by customizing the wedges.

POSTOPERATIVE MANAGEMENT

Casting after surgery is a vital element of the treatment. The authors' usual technique is splinting for approximately 1 week to allow for swelling, followed by casting and manipulation under anesthesia. This technique avoids skin complications and enhances correction. Frequently the authors will change the cast at about 3 weeks, without anesthesia, aiming for more correction after ensuring that the skin is intact and wound healing is progressing (Fig. 20-25).

Bracing and splinting are at best temporizing measures in these patients. If there is a foot drop, a brace is needed for function. After surgery, an insert may help hold the surgically achieved correction. According to the authors' experience, bracing as the primary treatment or as an attempt at prophylaxis has not been successful.

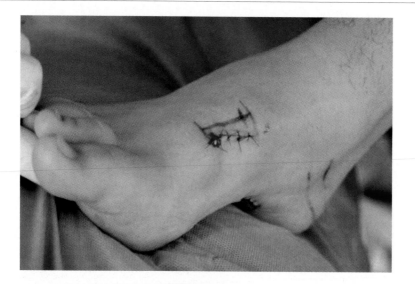

FIGURE 20-25
Immediately postoperatively after cavus foot correction.

COMPLICATIONS TO AVOID

The most common problems are related to wound complications. Avoiding excessive retraction, particularly with Homan retractors, is a must. Meticulous hemostasis, including achieving hemostasis by lowering the tourniquet prior to closure, will also help. Tourniquet time should be kept to a minimum.

Swelling after long, complex foot surgery with subsequent cast complications is a well-known problem. A splint that is easily removed should be considered for initial management. A circular cast can be applied at 7 to 10 days after swelling has been reduced. If further manipulation is indicated, general anesthesia should be used at this stage.

Misplaced or maloriented osteotomies of the midfoot or calcaneus can be avoided with the use of fluoroscopy. The combination of a preoperative computed tomography scan and intraoperative fluoroscopy are very effective at giving precise guidance to the corrective osteotomy.

Nonunion of an osteotomy or an attempted arthrodesis is best avoided by meticulous preparation of the surface and attention to the contact surfaces. It is often difficult to obtain adequate surface contact when correcting a complex three-dimensional deformity. The use of rigid internal fixation when possible is helpful.

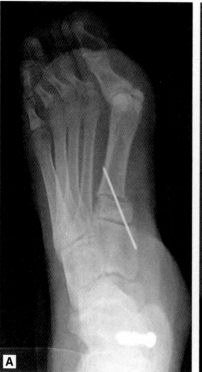
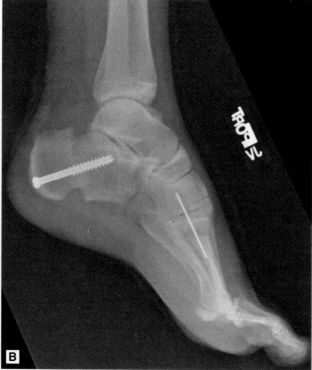

FIGURE 20-26

A) Post-op AP x-ray of left foot. **B)** Post-op lateral x-ray of left foot.

PEARLS AND PITFALLS

Treatment of pes cavus is not straightforward. Careful examination of the individual patient and knowledge of the details of a patient's deformity are key. Depending on the shape and severity of the deformity, the age of the patient, and the prognosis, any of the various soft-tissue, bony, or tendon release procedures may be used. As mentioned, bony procedures are usually not recommended in children under 12 years of age. The complications associated with cavus foot treatment are varied and usually increase with time.[5,6] This risk, however, is difficult to measure, as improvements in procedure and imaging, long-term complications, and recurrence may not be the same now as they were in past long-term studies. Because cavus feet are symptomatic and impair function, they deserve correction, despite the risk of complications associated with the procedures.

The treatment of the early-onset HMSN cavus foot is controversial. The authors' preferred technique is to perform early soft-tissue surgery in an attempt to avoid the extreme cavus deformities seen in teenagers and young adults. If the deformities are allowed to persist and progress, there is growth accommodation of the tarsal bones and more soft-tissue contracture, making correction progressively more difficult to achieve. Early tibialis posterior transfer with plantar fascial releases and any necessary toe releases give a plantar-grade foot that is more easily braced, more comfortable, and more functional.

In treatment of the cavus foot, it is rare that application of one of the single procedures described in this chapter will be adequate to correct all of the deformity. In almost every case, a careful clinical and radiographic analysis of the foot will lead to the conclusion that more than one procedure will be necessary.

REFERENCES

1. Aktas S, Sussman MD. The radiological analysis of pes cavus deformity in Charcot Marie Tooth disease. *J Pediatr Orthop Br.* 2000;9(2):137–140.
2. Amiot R, Coulter T, Nute M, et al. Surgical treatment of adult idiopathic cavus foot. *J Bone Joint Surg Am.*2003;85(7):1400–1401.
3. Azmaipairashvili, Z.; Riddle, E. C.; Scavina, M.; and Kumar, S. J.: Correction of cavovarus foot deformity in Charcot-Marie-Tooth disease. *Journal of Pediatric Orthopaedics,* 25(3): 360–365, 2005.
4. Burns J, Crosbie J, Hunt A, et al. The effect of pes cavus on foot pain and plantar pressure. *Clin Biomech (Bristol, Avon).* 2005; 20(9):877–882.
5. Carranza-Bencano A, Gonzalez-Rodriguez E. Unilateral tibial hemimelia with leg length inequality and varus foot: external fixator treatment. *Foot Ankle Int.* 1999;20(6):392–396.
6. Cole, W. H.: The classic. The treatment of claw-foot. By Wallace H. Cole. 1940. *Clinical Orthopaedics and Related Research,* (181): 3–6, 1983.
7. Coleman, S. S., and Chesnut, W. J.: A simple test for hindfoot flexibility in the cavovarus foot. *Clinical Orthopaedics and Related Research,* (123): 60–62, 1977.
8. Correction of multiplanar hindfoot deformity with osteotomy, arthrodesis, and internal fixation [review]. *Instr Course Lect.* 2005;54:269–276(review).
9. Giannini S, Ceccarelli F, Benedetti MG, et al. Surgical treatment of adult idiopathic cavus foot with plantar fasciotomy, naviculocuneiform arthrodesis, and cuboid osteotomy: a review of thirty-nine cases. *J Bone Joint Surg Am.* 2002;84 [Suppl 2]:62–69.
10. Herring J. *Tachdjian's Pediatric Orthopaedics.* 3rd ed. Philadelphia: WB Saunders; 2001.
11. Ibrahim K. Pes cavus. In: Evarts CM. *Surgery of the Musculoskeletal System.* 2nd ed. New York: Churchill Livingstone; 1990:4015–4034.
12. Joseph, T. N., and Myerson, M. S.: Correction of multiplanar hindfoot deformity with osteotomy, arthrodesis, and internal fixation. *Instructional course lectures,* 54: 269–276, 2005.
13. Mann RA. *Surgery of the Foot.* 5th ed. St. Louis: Mosby; 1986.
14. Mosca VS. The cavus foot [review]. *J Pediatr Orthop.* 2001;21(4):423–424.
15. Oh CW, Satish BR, Lee ST, et al. Complications of distraction osteogenesis in short first metatarsals. *J Pediatr Orthop.* 2004;24(6):711–715.
16. Olney B. Treatment of the cavus foot. Deformity in the pediatric patient with Charcot-Marie-Tooth [review]. *Foot Ankle Clin.* 2000;5(2):305–315.
17. Paley D, Lamm BM. Correction of the cavus foot using external fixation [review]. *Foot Ankle Clin.* 2004;9(3):611–624.
18. Paulos, L.; Coleman, S. S.; and Samuelson, K. M.: Pes cavovarus. Review of a surgical approach using selective soft-tissue procedures. *Journal of Bone and Joint Surgery—Series A,* 62(6): 942–953, 1980.
19. Price AE, Maisel R, Drennan JC. Computed tomographic analysis of pes cavus. *J Pediatr Orthop.* 1993;13(5):646–653.
20. Ramcharitar SI, Koslow P, Simpson DM. Lower extremity manifestations of neuromuscular diseases [review]. *Clin Podiatr Med Surg.* 1998;15(4):705–737, vi–vii.
21. Sammarco GJ, Taylor R. Cavovarus foot treated with combined calcaneus and metatarsal osteotomies. *Foot Ankle Int.* 2001;22(1):19–30.
22. Schwend RM, Drennan JC. Cavus foot deformity in children [review]. *J Am Acad Orthop Surg.* 2003; 11(3):201–211.
23. Solis, G.; Hennessy, M. S.; and Saxby, T. S.: Pes cavus: A review. *Foot and Ankle Surgery,* 6(3): 145–153, 2000.
24. Statler TK, Tullis BL. Pes cavus [review]. *J Am Podiatr Med Assoc.* 2005;95(1):42–52.
25. Sullivan RJ, Aronow MS. Different faces of the triple arthrodesis [review]. *Foot Ankle Clin.* 2002;7(1):95–106.
26. Teunissen LL, Notermans NC, Franssen H, et al. Disease course of Charcot-Marie-Tooth disease type 2: a 5-year follow-up study. *Arch Neurol.* 2003;60(6):823–828.

27. Tullis BL, Mendicino RW, Catanzariti AR, et al. The Cole midfoot osteotomy: a retrospective review of 11 procedures in 8 patients. *J Foot Ankle Surg.* 2004;43(3):160–165.
28. Turek SL, Buckwalter JA. *Orthopaedics: Principles and Their Applications.* 4th ed. Philadelphia: JB Lippincott Co; 1984:1450–1464.
29. Tynan, M. C.; Klenerman, L.; Helliwell, T. R.; Edwards, R. H. T.; and Hayward, M.: Investigation of muscle imbalance in the leg in symptomatic forefoot pes cavus: A multidisciplinary study. *Foot and Ankle,* 13(9): 489–501, 1992.
30. Watanabe RS. Metatarsal osteotomy for the cavus foot. *Clin Orthop Relat Res.* 1990;(252):217–230.
31. Wu KK. *Surgery of the Foot.* Philadelphia: Lea & Febiger; 1986:98–111.

21 Anterior Tibial Tendon Transfer

Ken N. Kuo

Anterior tibial tendon transfer has been utilized as treatment for supination foot deformity from a variety of causes. It has also been used as an adjunctive procedure in clubfoot management for both the prevention of recurrent deformity and the correction of dynamic supination and adduction deformities.

In 1940, Garceau[1] first described anterior tibial tendon transposition for the treatment of recurrent congenital clubfoot, reporting 77% good and excellent results in forefoot adduction correction and 93% good and excellent results for inversion deformity correction. Since then, the anterior tibial tendon transfer has been used widely in management of residual clubfoot deformity.[2,4–6,8]

In 1974, Hoffer et al.[3] first described a split anterior tibial tendon transfer in cerebral palsy children with spastic varus hind-foot deformity. The procedure has also been used in the treatment of residual dynamic clubfoot deformity.[4]

In 2001, Kuo et al.[4] published comparative results of a full anterior tibial tendon transfer and a split anterior tendon transfer (SPLATT) for residual functional clubfoot deformity. Both the full tendon transfer and the split tendon transfer obtained similar results in this series. Although the full anterior tibial tendon transfer obtains better correction for severe foot deformity, it also has a higher possibility of overcorrection. The split anterior tibial tendon transfer also can preserve some inversion function of the foot. However, in small children with a small anterior tibial tendon, splitting of the tendon is impractical; a full anterior tibial tendon transfer is recommended. In addition to correction of the dynamic supination foot deformity, ankle and foot range of motion, as well as leg and foot muscle function, definitely improved with either procedure.[4]

INDICATIONS AND CONTRAINDICATIONS

In general, anterior tibial tendon transfer is indicated for dynamic forefoot supination or varus foot deformity. The following are prerequisite conditions before this procedure is done:

- The foot must have supple subtalar motion or supination and pronation and must be able to be passively placed in a neutral position.
- The foot has rigid subtalar motion, but the heel is in a neutral position.
- The foot can be dorsiflexed to at least a neutral position.
- The foot has adequate dorsiflexion muscle strength from the anterior tibialis tendon, preferably a grade 4 or 5 by the Jones classification.

The best age for the procedure is between 4 and 8 years old due to the size of anterior tibialis tendon and better remodeling of tarsal bone growth. However, this procedure can be done in younger or older children if indicated.

The surgical indications for anterior tibial tendon transfer are as follows:

- Varus foot position and forefoot supination, either static or dynamic, in children with cerebral palsy
- Residual forefoot supination, adduction, or varus deformity, either static or dynamic, with overpowering of anterior tibial tendon function after initial clubfoot treatment
- Overpowering of anterior tibial tendon that causes dynamic foot deformity in children with other neurologic problems
- Loss of eversion power of the foot due to previous trauma

The surgical contraindications for anterior tibial tendon transfer are as follows:

- Rigid foot deformity so that the foot cannot be passively placed in a neutral position
- A weak anterior tibialis muscle of grade 3 or less
- Progressive neurologic disease in which weakness of the anterior tibialis muscle is expected (e.g., Charcot-Marie-Tooth disease)

SURGICAL PROCEDURES

Full Anterior Tibial Tendon Transfer

There are two types of full anterior tibial tendon transfer. The author prefers the technique of pulling the anterior tibial tendon proximally to the distal tibial area and rerouting the tendon to the lateral aspect of the foot. The other technique transfers the tendon subcutaneously at the dorsum of the foot.

The child is placed in a supine position under anesthesia. An appropriate-sized tourniquet is applied and inflated. A 1.5-cm oblique incision is made at the insertion of the anterior tibial tendon at the medial cuneiform. The anterior tibial tendon is exposed after incising the tendon sheath. The tendon is dissected to the insertion at the medial cuneiform and first metatarsal and is detached by sharp dissection (Fig. 21-1). A Bunnell suture is placed in the cut end of the tendon using 1.0 Vicryl sutures.

The second 1-cm incision is made at the anterior distal tibia, directly over the anterior tibial tendon and just lateral to the tibial crest. The tendon location can be easily palpated by pulling the distal end. After the tendon sheath is incised, the anterior tibial tendon is exposed. The tendon is pulled with a hemostat until its distal end is pulled all the way into the proximal incision (Fig. 21-2). The tendon is then protected with a wet sponge wrap.

The third incision of about 1 cm is made at the dorsum of the foot, directly over the lateral cuneiform. The extensor tendons of the toes are retracted to expose the lateral cuneiform. A large, curved hemostat is used to make a tunnel subcutaneously from the distal wound to the proximal wound. The hemostat is then used to widen the tunnel and to grasp the tendon suture strings. The tendon is pulled distally and laterally into the third incision (Fig. 21-3).

A drill bit slightly larger than the transferred tendon is used to make a drill hole through the lateral cuneiform in a dorsal-to-plantar direction (Fig. 21-4). It is important to keep a finger on the plantar area to prevent penetration of the drill bit through the skin. The two ends of the suture in the anterior tibial tendon are then separately attached to two long, straight Keith needles. The Keith needles are pushed through the drilled holes from the dorsal to the plantar surface. It is desirable to ensure that the exits of the two Keith needles at the plantar surface of the foot are 3 to 5 mm apart. With needles attached to the two sutures, the surgeon pierces through a small square of felt pad and a sterile button. With gentle pulling distally, the tendon is pulled into the drilled hole in the lateral

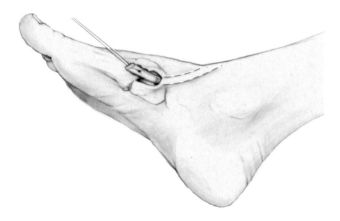

FIGURE 21-1

The first incision is on the medial side of the foot over the insertion of the anterior tibial tendon at the medial cuneiform and first metatarsal, where the tendon is divided at its insertion.

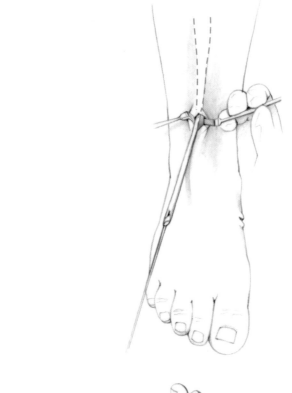

FIGURE 21-2

The second incision is at the anterior distal tibia, where the distal end of the tendon is pulled through into this anterior incision.

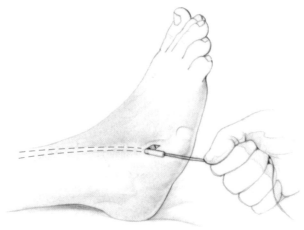

FIGURE 21-3

The third incision is over the lateral cuneiform. The tendon is passed subcutaneously into this distal incision.

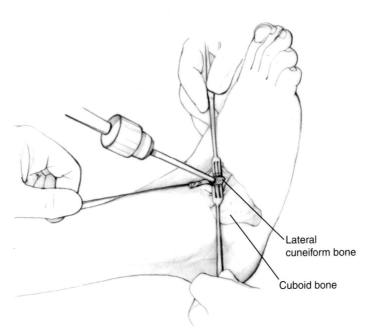

Lateral
cuneiform bone

Cuboid bone

FIGURE 21-4

A drill hole is made in the lateral cuneiform in a dorsal-to-plantar direction.

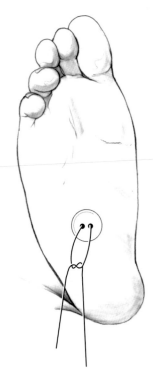

FIGURE 21-5

Using two Keith needles, the sutures are passed through the drill hole in the lateral cuneiform, and the sutures are tied at the plantar surface over the top of a button and a felt square.

cuneiform. The foot is held in neutral or mild dorsiflexion and eversion as the sutures are tied on top of the button (Fig. 21-5).

Simple closure of the wounds is adequate. It is important to watch the foot position during closure to prevent inadvertent loss of tendon tension. The tension of the transferred tendon should be palpable at the dorsum of the foot at the end of the procedure.

With the alternative technique, the distal end of the tendon is released, pulled back to the proximal foot, and then transferred laterally through a subcutaneous tunnel in the dorsal foot through the incision over the lateral cuneiform bone. The tendon-anchoring procedure is the same as described above (Fig. 21-6).

Spilt Anterior Tibial Tendon Transfer

The patient is placed in a supine position under anesthesia. An appropriate-sized tourniquet is applied and inflated. A 1.5-cm oblique incision is made at the insertion of the anterior tibial tendon at the medial cuneiform. The anterior tibial tendon is exposed after incising the tendon sheath. The tendon is traced to the insertion at the medial cuneiform and first metatarsal. The majority of feet have an equal insertion of this tendon onto each bone, and the distal part of the tendon already shows

FIGURE 21-6

The distal end of the tendon is passed subcutaneously from the medial wound directly to the lateral wound without pulling the tendon proximally. The tendon is then anchored the same way as described in Figure 21-5.

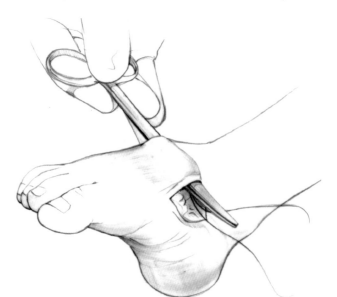

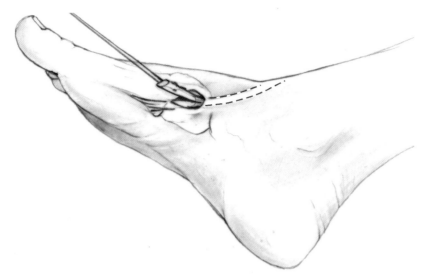

FIGURE 21-7
The first incision is at the medial side of the foot over the insertion of the anterior tibial tendon onto the medial cuneiform. The tendon is split equally, and the lateral half is divided and released from its insertion.

an equal division line anatomically.[7] The tendon can either be divided along this anatomical line or be split into two equal parts. The lateral half of the tendon is detached from the medial cuneiform (Fig. 21-7). A Bunnell suture is placed in the cut end of the split tendon using 1.0 Vicryl suture.

The second 1-cm incision is made at the anterior distal tibia, directly over the anterior tibial tendon and just lateral to the tibial crest. The tendon location can be easily palpated by pulling the distal end. After the tendon sheath is incised, the anterior tibial tendon is exposed. A tendon passer is inserted from the proximal wound toward the distal wound inside the tendon sheath. It is most important to watch the tip of the tendon passer exit at the distal wound inside the tendon sheath. The strings of the tendon suture are attached to the tendon passer, which is then pulled out from the proximal wound. By gently pulling the suture into the proximal wound, the tendon is spilt equally throughout the distance between the two incisions until it appears in the proximal wound (Fig. 21-8). The tendon is then protected with a wet sponge wrap.

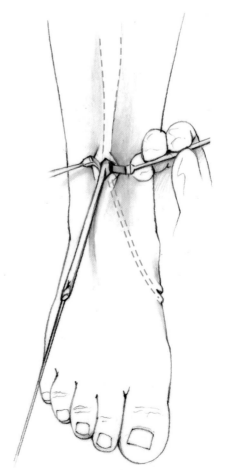

FIGURE 21-8
The second incision is at the anterior distal tibia. After passing the sutures proximally with gentle pulling, the distal end of the split tendon continues to split proximally in an even fashion.

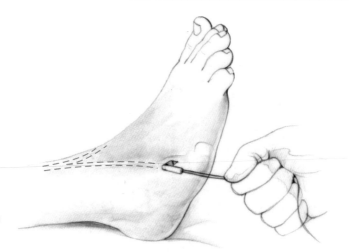

The third incision of about 1 cm is made at the dorsum of the foot, directly over the cuboid. The extensor digitorum brevis muscle fibers are split to expose the cuboid. A large, curved hemostat is used to make a subcutaneous tunnel from the distal wound into the proximal wound. The hemostat is then used to widen this tunnel and to pull the suture as the split tendon is passed distally and laterally into the third incision (Fig. 21-9).

A drill bit slightly larger than the transferred tendon is used to make a drill hole through the cuboid in a dorsal-to-plantar direction (Fig. 21-10). It is important to keep a finger on the plantar area to prevent penetration of the drill bit through the skin. The two ends of the suture in the split anterior tibial tendon are then separately attached to two long, straight Keith needles. The Keith needles are pushed through the drilled hole from the dorsal to the plantar surface. It is desirable to ensure that the exits of the two Keith needles at the plantar surface of the foot are 3 to 5 mm apart. With needles attached, two strings pierce through a small square of felt pad and a sterile button. With gentle pulling distally, the tendon is pulled into the drilled hole in the cuboid. The foot is held in neutral or mild dorsiflexion and eversion as the sutures are tied on top of the button (Fig. 21-11).

Simple closure of the wounds is adequate. It is important to watch the foot position during closure to prevent inadvertent loss of tendon tension. The tension of the transferred lateral half of the tendon should be palpable at the dorsum of the foot at the end of the procedure, while the medial half of the original tendon is usually not under tension.

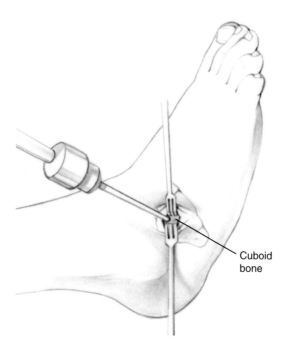

Cuboid
bone

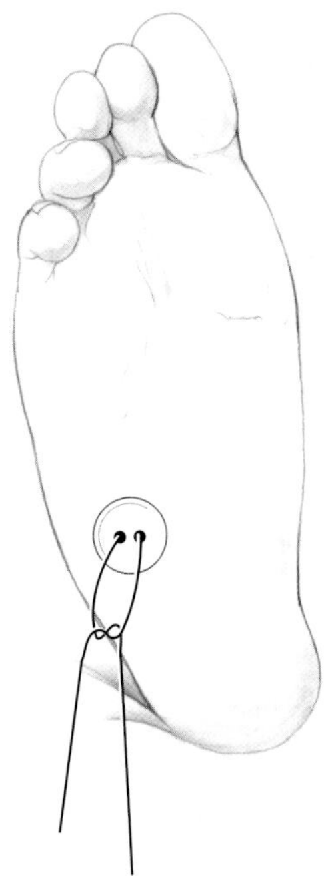

FIGURE 21-11

Using two Keith needles, the sutures are passed through the drill hole in the cuboid and are tied under tension at the plantar surface over a button and a felt square.

POSTOPERATIVE MANAGEMENT

At the end of surgery while the patient is still under anesthesia, the foot is placed in a short-leg walking cast. It is desirable to place the foot in a neutral position with a tendency toward dorsiflexion and eversion. The patient is allowed to bear weight on the second day postoperatively. The cast and the plantar anchoring button are removed 6 weeks following surgery. A hinged ankle-foot orthotic (AFO) with a plantarflexion stop at neutral and free dorsiflexion is used for 6 months.

RESULTS

- This procedure improves effective dorsiflexion and eversion motion of the foot, thereby improving total functional ankle motion.
- This procedure does not decrease the muscle strength of the anterior tibial tendon, because the transferred muscle function remains in the same axial direction and has the same phasic activity during walking. With better action direction of the transferred tendon, the strength of the muscle will actually become more effective, while the eversion strength of the leg and foot musculature also improves.
- This procedure corrects functional dynamic supination and adduction deformity.
- This procedure improves the plantigrade position of the foot during walking.

COMPLICATIONS TO AVOID

- The surgeon should watch for an inadvertent rupture of the transferred and inserted tendon by poor positioning of the foot and retraction intraoperatively during wound closure.
- A felt pad cushions the skin pressure from the button for the pull-out sutures, minimizing the risk of a pressure sore at the foot's plantar surface.
- It is important to have appropriate casting during the healing stage to prevent transferred tendon pull-off during the healing stage.
- Insufficient tension of the tendon transfer at the time of tying the sutures over the button must be avoided. It is desirable to have overtightening rather than not enough, as the tendon transfer always loses some tension as the tendon heals.

ILLUSTRATIVE CASE

Three cases are presented in Figures 21-12, 21-13, and 21-14.

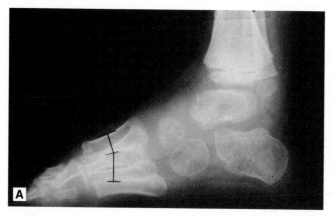
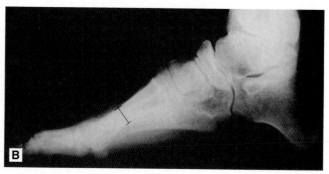

FIGURE 21-12 **A.** A preoperative standing lateral foot radiograph demonstrates a separation of the metatarsals, indicative of supination of the forefoot. **B.** A lateral foot radiograph 6 years after surgery demonstrates overlapping of the metatarsals, indicative of correction of the former supination deformity.

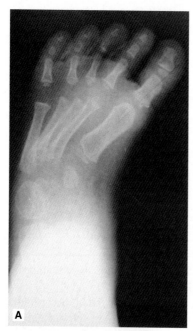

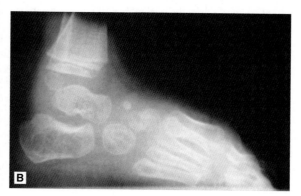

FIGURE 21-13

AP **(A)** and lateral **(B)** standing radiographs of a 5-year-old boy with a history of clubfoot surgical releases during his first year of life, with residual supination adduction deformity of the foot. AP **(C)** and lateral **(D)** standing radiographs 7 years after full anterior tibial tendon transfer show excellent correction of the forefoot adduction and the supination deformity.

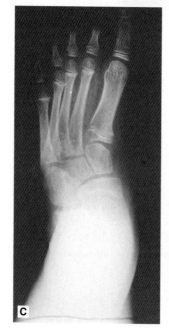

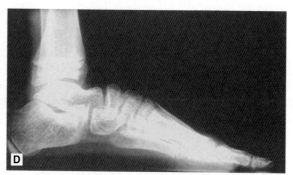

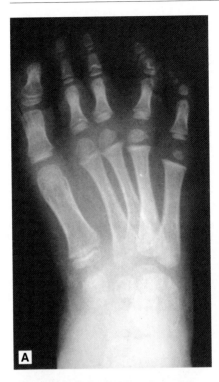

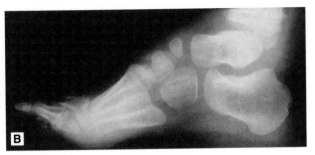

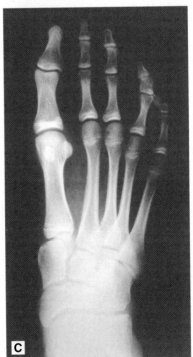

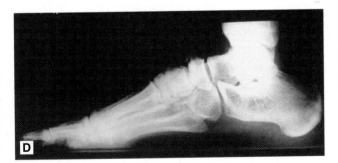

FIGURE 21-14

Standing AP **(A)** and lateral **(B)** radiographs of a 6$^1/_2$ year-old boy with a history of clubfoot surgical releases during his first year of life, but with residual supination and adduction of the foot. Standing AP **(C)** and lateral **(D)** radiographs 6 years after SPLATT show excellent correction of the forefoot adduction and the supination deformity.

PEARLS AND PITFALLS

- Anterior tibial tendon transfer is an excellent procedure for dynamic supination and varus deformity of the foot.
- A grade 4 or 5 anterior tibialis muscle strength by the Jones classification is a must to achieve a good result.
- The foot should be passively correctable to neutral position.
- During wound closure, always watch for intact tendon anchoring to avoid pull-off of the transferred tendon.

REFERENCES

1. Garceau GJ. Anterior tibial tendon transposition in recurrent congenital club-foot. *J Bone Joint Surg Am.* 1940;22:932.
2. Garceau GJ, Palmer RM. Transfer of the anterior tibial tendon for recurrent club foot. *J Bone Joint Surg Am.* 1967;49:207.
3. Hoffer MM, Reiswig JA, Garrett AM, et al. The split anterior tibial tendon transfer in the treatment of spastic varus hind-foot of childhood. *Orthop Clin North Am.* 1974;5:31.
4. Kuo KN, Hennigan SP, Hastings ME. Anterior tibial tendon transfer in residual dynamic clubfoot deformity. *J Pediatr Orthop.* 2001;21:35.
5. Laaveg SJ, Ponseti IV. Long-term results of treatment of congenital club foot. *J Bone Joint Surg Am.* 1990;62:23.
6. Ponseti IV. *Congenital Clubfoot: Fundamentals of Treatment.* New York: Oxford Medical Publications; 1996:84.
7. Sarrafian SH. *Anatomy of the Foot and Ankle.* Philadelphia: JB Lippincott Co; 1983:201.
8. Thompson GH, Hoyen HA. Tibialis anterior transfer after clubfoot surgery. 2nd International Congress on Clubfoot, Amsterdam. *J Pediatr Orthop.* 1997;6:298.

22 Calcaneal Lengthening Osteotomy

Vincent S. Mosca

INDICATION/CONTRAINDICATIONS

The calcaneal lengthening osteotomy is indicated for the flexible flatfoot with a short Achilles tendon when prolonged attempts at conservative management fail to relieve the pain under the head of the plantarflexed talus or in the sinus tarsi area.

This procedure is not indicated to change the shape of a pain-free flexible flatfoot. Surgery should not be performed in young children with flexible flatfeet who have nonlocalized, activity-related aching foot pain or nighttime pain in the lower extremities. Surgery should also not be carried out for incongruous signs or symptoms. In such situations, the flatfoot may be an incidental finding and not the cause of the symptoms. Finally, the calcaneal lengthening osteotomy is contraindicated in the iatrogenic flatfoot created by overcorrection of a clubfoot in which the talonavicular joint is well aligned and the thigh-foot angle is neutral p. despite the valgus alignment of the hind foot.

PREOPERATIVE PLANNING

Physical examination includes evaluation of the foot in weight bearing and non–weight bearing. In weight bearing, the surgeon should note the hind foot's valgus alignment, the depression of the longitudinal arch, and the outward rotation of the foot in relation to the flexion/extension plane of the knee as referenced from the alignment with the patella (Fig. 22-1). Flexibility of the flatfoot is confirmed by observing the creation of the longitudinal arch and conversion of hind-foot valgus to varus with toe standing.

On the examining table, the Silfverskiöld test is performed to determine whether the equinus contracture is in the gastrocnemius alone or involves the entire triceps surae. The thigh-foot angle and the transmalleolar axis are assessed with the patient prone (Fig. 22-2). Most commonly, the thigh-foot angle is abnormally positive (excessively turned out in relation to the thigh), whereas the transmalleolar axis (assessing tibial torsion) is normal. Further, the surgeon should determine whether the subtalar joint can be inverted to neutral; the calcaneal lengthening osteotomy can correct hind-foot valgus even in a rigid deformity.

Radiographs must be taken with full weight bearing to correlate with the physical examination findings. Anteroposterior and lateral views are required (Fig. 22-3). Oblique and Harris axial views of the foot can be added to confirm absence of a tarsal coalition. Anteroposterior, mortise, and lateral ankle radiographs are useful to determine whether any of the valgus deformity is in the tibiotalar joint.

The family should be informed of the risks and complications of allograft versus autograft for the required tricortical (bicortical) iliac crest bone graft. They should also be told of the possible need for a medial cuneiform, plantar-based closing-wedge osteotomy. The need for this additional procedure can only be accurately determined intraoperatively following correction of the hind foot and lengthening of the heel cord.

Discussion about staged versus concurrent correction of bilateral deformities should include issues relating to the need for strict non–weight bearing on the operated foot/feet for 8 weeks. Most

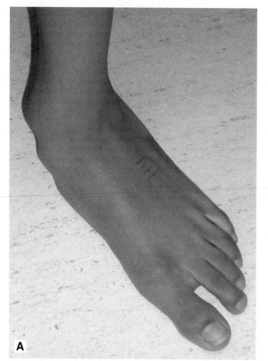

A

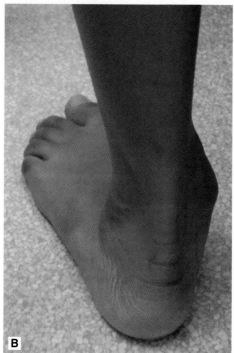

B

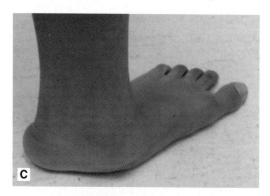

C

FIGURE 22-1

Flatfoot. **A.** Top view shows outward rotation of the foot in relation to the lower extremity. The patella is facing forward in this photograph. **B.** Back view shows valgus alignment of the hind foot and "too many toes" seen laterally. **C.** Medial view shows depression of the longitudinal arch and a convex medial border of the foot.

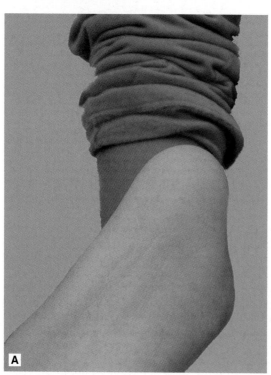

A

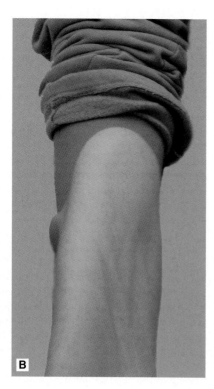

B

FIGURE 22-2

Prone thigh-foot angle assessment. **A.** Markedly positive (externally rotated) thigh-foot angle. **B.** Neutral thigh-foot angle created by inverting the subtalar joint. All of the outward rotation is, therefore, due to the everted subtalar joint. Following the calcaneal lengthening osteotomy, the thigh-foot angle will be straight.

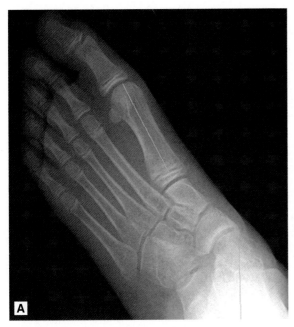

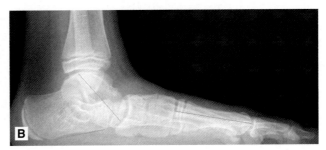

FIGURE 22-3   Standing radiographs of the foot. **A.** AP image demonstrates the external rotation component of eversion or valgus of the subtalar joint. **B.** The lateral image reveals plantar flexion of the talus, sag at the talonavicular joint, and a low calcaneal pitch.

adolescents choose the correction of one foot first, with correction of the other foot 6 months later. This interval allows adequate rehabilitation for the operated foot to function comfortably while non–weight bearing on the second foot.

SURGICAL PROCEDURE

Special equipment includes a narrow sagittal saw, smooth Steinmann pins, straight osteotomes, a lamina spreader with smooth teeth, Joker elevators and narrow Crego retractors (Fig. 22-4), and a mini-fluoroscope.

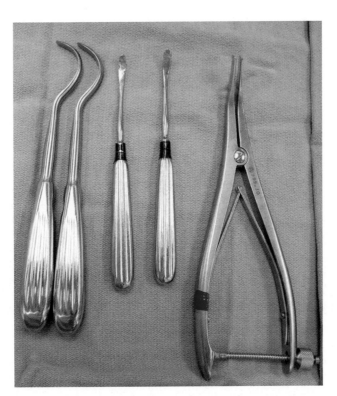

FIGURE 22-4

Narrow Crego retractors (left), Joker elevators (center), and lamina spreader with smooth teeth (right).

FIGURE 22-5

Modified Ollier incision marked in a Langer line, halfway between the tip of the lateral malleolus and the beak of the calcaneus (two dots) and extending from the superficial peroneal nerve (dotted line) to the sural nerve.

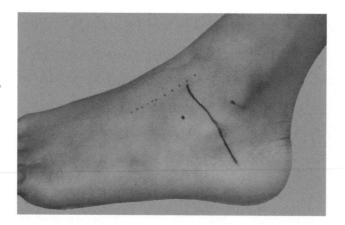

The patient is placed supine, with a folded towel under the ipsilateral buttock. If autograft is used, the patient is prepped and draped from the iliac crest to the toes, and a sterile tourniquet is used. If using allograft, only the lower extremity is prepped, and a nonsterile tourniquet is used.

A modified Ollier incision is made in a Langer skin line from the superficial peroneal nerve to the sural nerve (Fig. 22-5). The soft tissues are elevated from the sinus tarsi, avoiding exposure of or injury to the capsule of the calcaneocuboid joint.

The peroneus longus and the peroneus brevis are released from their tendon sheaths on the lateral surface of the calcaneus (Fig. 22-6A). The intervening tendon sheaths are resected, as is the peroneal tubercle if it is large. The peroneus brevis tendon is Z-lengthened. The surgeon must *not* lengthen the peroneus longus. The aponeurosis of the abductor digiti minimi is divided at a point approximately 2 cm proximal to the calcaneocuboid joint (Fig. 22-6B).

The interval between the anterior and middle facets of the subtalar joint is identified with a Freer elevator (Fig. 22-7). It is inserted into the sinus tarsi, perpendicular to the lateral cortex of the calcaneus at the level of the isthmus (i.e., the lowest point of the dorsal cortex in the sinus tarsi proximal to the beak and distal to the posterior facet). The middle facet will be encountered. The Freer is slowly angled distally until it falls into the interval between the anterior and middle facets. The Freer is replaced with a curved Joker elevator. A second Joker elevator is placed around the

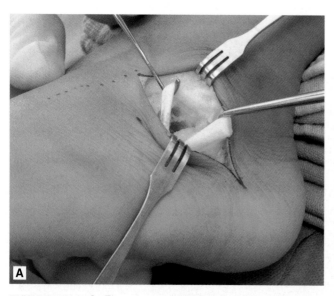

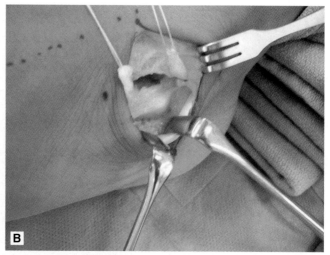

FIGURE 22-6 A. The peroneus brevis (above) and the peroneus longus (below) have been released from their tendon sheaths. **B.** The soft-tissue contents have been elevated from the isthmus of the calcaneus. The peroneus brevis is lengthened, and the peroneus longus is retracted. The aponeurosis of the abductor digiti minimi is exposed for release.

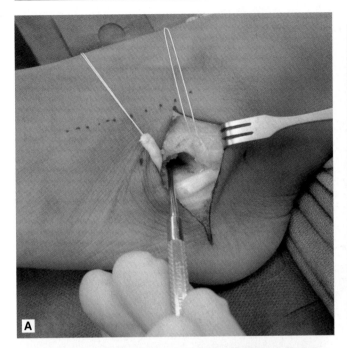

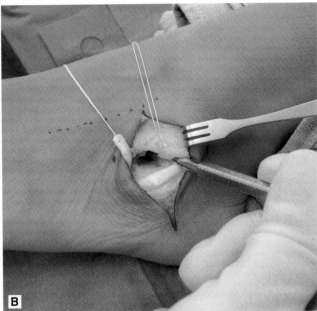

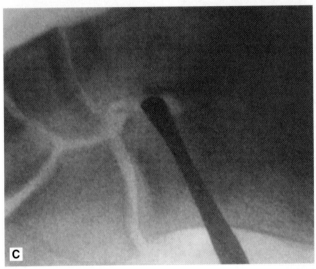

FIGURE 22-7   Finding the interval between the anterior and middle facets of the subtalar joint.
A. A Freer elevator is inserted perpendicular to the lateral border of the calcaneus just proximal to the beak of the calcaneus, making contact with the middle facet. **B.** The Freer is rotated distally until the tip falls into the interval between the anterior and middle facets. **C.** This is confirmed with the mini-fluoroscope.

plantar aspect of the calcaneus in an extraperiosteal plane in line with the dorsal Joker. The Jokers are then removed, and the exposures are prepared for the other procedures before the calcaneal osteotomy is performed.

A longitudinal incision is made along the medial border of the foot, starting at a point just distal to the medial malleolus and continuing to the base of the first metatarsal. The tibialis posterior is released from its tendon sheath. The tendon is cut in a Z-fashion, releasing its *dorsal* half from the navicular (Fig. 22-8). The stump of tendon remaining attached to the navicular contains the *plantar* half of the fibers.

The talonavicular joint capsule, including the spring ligament, is incised from dorsal-lateral to plantar-lateral. A 5- to 7-mm wide strip of capsule is resected from the medial and plantar aspects of this redundant tissue (Fig. 22-9).

The equinus contracture is assessed by the Silfverskiöld test, with the subtalar joint inverted to neutral and the knee both flexed and extended. A gastrocnemius recession is performed if

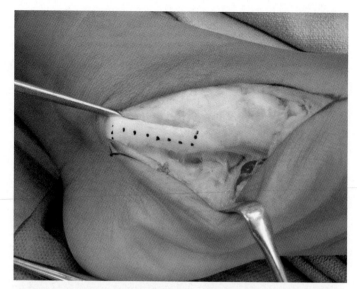

FIGURE 22-8

The tibialis posterior is cut in a Z-fashion, releasing the dorsal slip from the navicular.

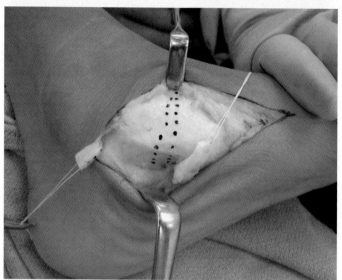

FIGURE 22-9

The talonavicular joint capsule is released from dorsolateral to plantar-lateral, including release of the spring ligament. A 5- to 7-mm-wide strip of redundant capsule is resected from its plantar-medial aspect.

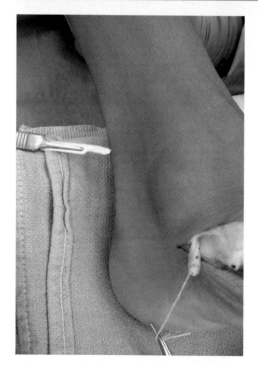

FIGURE 22-10

The Achilles tendon or the gastrocnemius tendon is lengthened based on the results of the Silfverskiöld test.

268

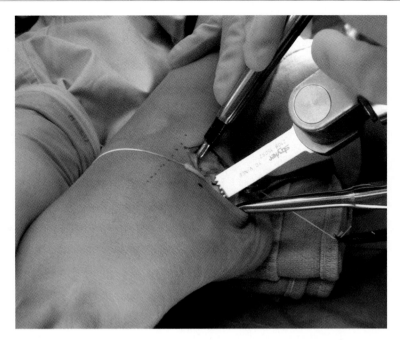

FIGURE 22-11

With Joker and Crego retractors surrounding the isthmus of the calcaneus and meeting in the interval between the anterior and middle facets, the osteotomy is performed with a sagittal saw in line with the retractors.

10 degrees of dorsiflexion cannot be achieved with the knee extended, even if this can be achieved with the knee flexed. An open or percutaneous Achilles tendon lengthening is performed if 10 degrees of dorsiflexion cannot be obtained even with the knee flexed (Fig. 22-10).

The Joker elevators, or Crego retractors, are replaced both dorsal and plantar to the isthmus of the calcaneus, meeting in the interval between the anterior and middle facets of the subtalar joint. An osteotomy of the calcaneus is performed using a sagittal saw or osteotome (Fig. 22-11). This is an oblique osteotomy from proximal-lateral to distal-medial that starts approximately 2 cm proximal to the calcaneocuboid joint (at the lowest point of the calcaneus proximal to the beak) and exits between the anterior and middle facets (Fig. 22-12). It is a complete osteotomy through the medial cortex. The plantar periosteum and long plantar ligament (*not* the plantar fascia) are cut under direct vision if necessary (i.e., if these soft tissues resist distraction of the bone fragments).

A 2-mm smooth Steinmann pin is inserted retrograde from the dorsum of the foot passing through the cuboid, across the center of the calcaneocuboid joint, and stopping at the osteotomy (Fig. 22-13). This insertion is performed with the foot in the original deformed position *before* the osteotomy is distracted. By doing so, the pes acetabulum (navicular, spring ligament, and anterior facet of calcaneus) will be maintained intact, and the distal fragment of the calcaneus will not subluxate dorsally on the cuboid during distraction of the osteotomy.

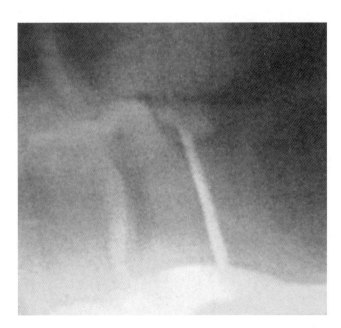

FIGURE 22-12

Fluoroscopic appearance of the osteotomy in the proper location.

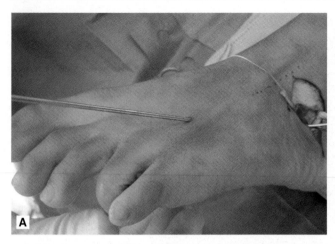
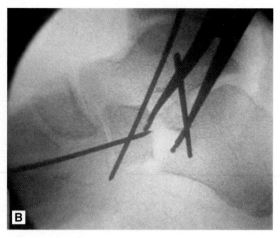

FIGURE 22-13   **A.** With the foot in the original flat and everted position, a 2-mm smooth wire is inserted retrograde from the dorsum of the foot through the middle of the calcaneocuboid joint, stopping at the osteotomy. **B.** The position of the wire is confirmed at the calcaneocuboid joint with fluoroscopy.

A 0.062-in. smooth Steinmann pin is inserted from lateral to medial in both of the calcaneal fragments immediately adjacent to the osteotomy. These will be used as joysticks to distract the osteotomy at the time of graft insertion. A smooth-toothed lamina spreader is placed in the osteotomy and distracted maximally, avoiding crushing the bone (Fig. 22-14). Deformity correction of the hind foot is assessed both clinically and with a mini-fluoroscope. The deformity is corrected when the axes of the talus and first metatarsal are collinear in both the AP and the lateral planes (Fig. 22-15). The distance between the lateral cortical margins of the calcaneal fragments is measured; this is the lateral length dimension of the trapezoid-shaped iliac crest graft that will be obtained either from the child's iliac crest or from the bone bank. The trapezoid should taper to a medial length dimension of 20% to 30% of the lateral length (Fig. 22-16). The calcaneal lengthening osteotomy is a distraction-wedge rather than a simple opening wedge, as the center of rotation is the center of the talar head and not the medial cortex of the calcaneus.

The lamina spreader is then removed, and the Steinmann pin joysticks are used to distract the calcaneal fragments. The graft is inserted and impacted, with the cortical surfaces aligned from proximal to distal in the long axis of the foot (Fig. 22-17). This places the cancellous bone of the graft in direct contact with the cancellous bone of the calcaneal fragments. The previously inserted 2-mm

FIGURE 22-14

Steinmann pins in the proximal and distal calcaneal fragments can be used as joysticks to distract the osteotomy during graft insertion. The lamina spreader is used to determine the necessary graft size.

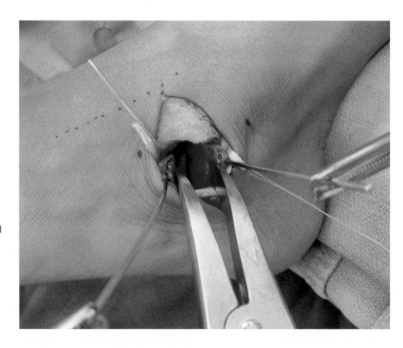

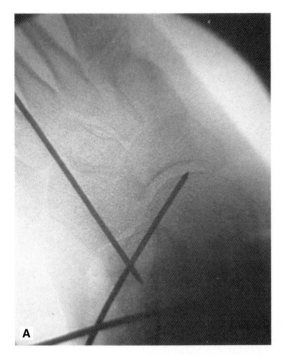
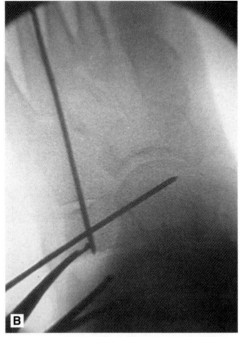

FIGURE 22-15

Fluoroscopy can help confirm the required graft size by showing, with the lamina spreader opened, when the talonavicular joint is aligned and the talus and first metatarsal axes are collinear **(A)** before, and **(B)** after opening the lamina spreader.

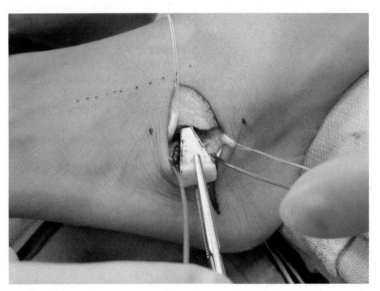

FIGURE 22-16

The tricortical iliac crest bone graft is frequently 11 to 15 mm in lateral length and 3 to 5 mm in medial length. The cortical surfaces are aligned with the dorsal, lateral, and plantar cortical surfaces of the calcaneus.

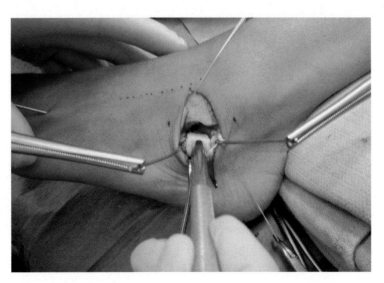

FIGURE 22-17

The graft is impacted and is usually inherently stable. Nevertheless, the 2-mm Steinmann pin can be advanced retrograde through the graft and into the posterior calcaneal fragment for additional stability.

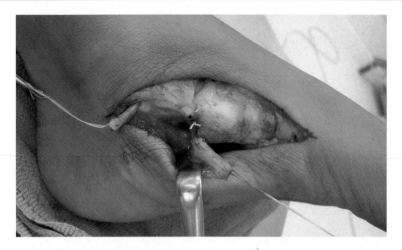

FIGURE 22-18

The plantar and medial aspects of the talonavicular joint capsule are repaired side to side with large-gauge dissolving suture material, having already resected the redundant capsule.

Steinmann pin is advanced retrograde through the graft and into the proximal calcaneal fragment. The pin is bent at its insertion site on the dorsum of the foot for later ease of retrieval in the clinic. No additional fixation is required. In fact, were the pin not needed to prevent subluxation at the calcaneocuboid joint, no graft fixation would be needed. The peroneus brevis tendon is repaired with an absorbable suture after a 5- to 7-mm lengthening.

The talonavicular joint capsule is plicated plantarmedially but not dorsally (Fig. 22-18). The proximal slip of the tibialis posterior is advanced approximately 5 to 7 mm through a slit in the distal stump of the tendon using a Pulvertaft weave with an absorbable suture material (Fig. 22-19).

The forefoot is assessed for structural supination deformity by holding the heel with the ankle in neutral dorsiflexion and viewing in line with the axis of the foot from toes to heel. The plane of the metatarsal heads is visualized in relation to the long axis of the tibia (Fig. 22-20). The dorsal-plantar mobility of the first metatarsal-medial cuneiform joint is also assessed. A plantarflexion osteotomy of the medial forefoot/midfoot is required if the metatarsals are supinated. A plantar-based closing-wedge osteotomy in the midportion of the medial cuneiform is an effective procedure to correct this deformity (Fig. 22-21). The plantar base of the resected wedge generally measures 4 to 7 mm in length. The osteotomy is closed and internally fixed with a 0.062-in. smooth wire staple that is inserted from plantar to dorsal. Correction of the forefoot deformity should be checked (Fig. 22-22).

The incisions are closed with absorbable sutures. A well-padded, short-leg, non-weight-bearing cast is applied and bivalved to allow for swelling overnight. Radiographs in the cast are obtained (Fig. 22-23). The patient is discharged from the hospital the following day after the bivalved cast is overwrapped with cast material.

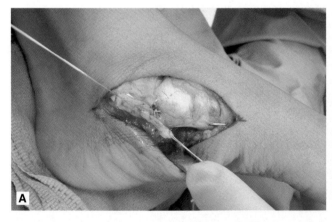
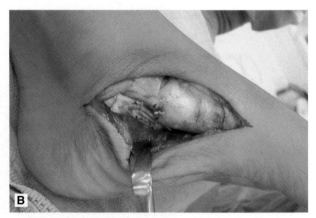

FIGURE 22-19   **(A)** The proximal slip of the tibialis posterior is advanced distally through a slit in the distal stump of the tendon and **(B)** repaired with large-gauge dissolving sutures.

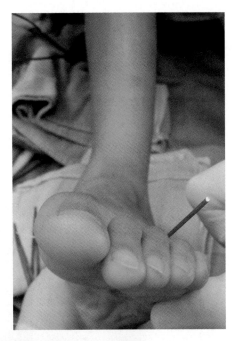

FIGURE 22-20

The rotational alignment of the forefoot is assessed following correction of the hindfoot deformity and heelcord contracture. If, as in this case, the forefoot is supinated, an osteotomy of the forefoot is required.

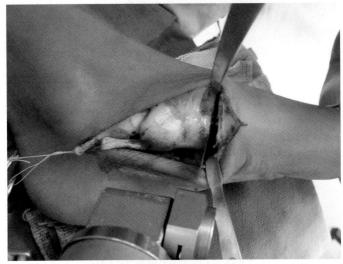

FIGURE 22-21

A medial cuneiform, plantar-based closing-wedge osteotomy will correct the supination deformity of the forefoot.

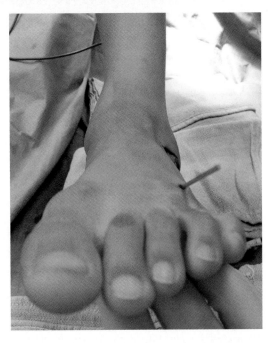

FIGURE 22-22

Forefoot deformity has been corrected.

FIGURE 22-23
Final radiographs in the bivalved cast. **A.** On the AP view, note the correction of the external rotation deformity at the talonavicular joint as also assessed by the talo–first metatarsal angle. **B.** The lateral view demonstrates dorsiflexion of the talus, alignment at the talonavicular joint, correction of the talo–first metatarsal angle, and normalization of the calcaneal pitch.

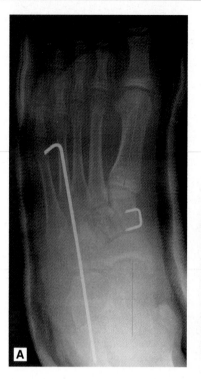

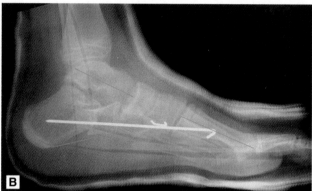

POSTOPERATIVE MANAGEMENT

The patient is immobilized in a below-the-knee cast and is not permitted to bear weight on the operated extremity for 8 weeks. At 6 weeks, the cast is removed to obtain simulated standing AP and lateral radiographs and to remove the Steinmann pin. Another below-the-knee, non-weight-bearing cast is applied. Upon removal of this cast 2 weeks later, final simulated standing AP and lateral radiographs are obtained. Over-the-counter arch supports are used indefinitely. Physical therapy is rarely needed.

COMPLICATIONS TO AVOID

- Subluxation of the calcaneocuboid joint when the calcaneal osteotomy is distracted
  - This is avoided by lengthening the peroneus brevis, releasing the aponeurosis of the abductor digiti minimi, releasing the plantar calcaneal periosteum and long plantar ligament (*not* the plantar fascia), and pinning the calcaneocuboid joint in a retrograde fashion *before* the osteotomy is distracted.
- Incomplete deformity correction
  - This is avoided by performing the procedures listed above and by releasing the entire dorsal talonavicular joint capsule. A graft that is large enough to make the axes of the talus and the first metatarsal collinear in both planes should be used. Correction is confirmed with intraoperative imaging, such as mini-fluoroscopy.
- Persistent equinus
  - This is avoided by lengthening the contracted Achilles tendon or gastrocnemius tendon.
- Persistent supination deformity of the forefoot on the hind foot
  - This is avoided by identifying the deformity following the calcaneal lengthening and heel-cord lengthening. It is treated with a medial cuneiform, plantar-based closing-wedge osteotomy.

ILLUSTRATIVE CASE

A 12-year-old boy with flexible flatfeet had a 4-year history of increasing activity-related pain under the head of the talus bilaterally. He was an avid and competitive soccer player and cross-country runner. Over-the-counter and custom-molded arch supports actually increased his pain. Twice daily heel-cord stretching exercises with his knees extended and his subtalar joints inverted to neutral did not relieve his symptoms. He tried to ignore the pain and complete his games and practice sessions, but he suffered for increasingly long periods of time after the workouts. This was unacceptable to the boy and his family.

The boy was tall and thin, with an athletic build. The torsional profile of his lower extremities was normal, in that he had greater lateral than medial rotation of his hips and his transmalleolar axes were normal. His thigh-foot angles and foot-progression angles were excessively out-turned.

His feet appeared to have longitudinal arches when he was sitting with his feet hanging dependently over the edge of the examination table, but they manifested flattening of the arches when he stood. One observed the "too many toes" sign when he was viewed from behind. His arches elevated and his hind-foot alignment changed from valgus to varus with toe standing and with the Jack toe-raise test. He had difficulty standing on his heels with his metatarsal heads off the ground unless he flexed his hips and leaned back.

There was thick callus formation with mild surrounding erythema and tenderness under the medial aspect of the midfoot, particularly under the plantar-medial aspect of the talar head. The subtalar joints were supple, with at least 35 degrees of both active and passive motion. His ankles dorsiflexed 10 degrees above neutral with his subtalar joints inverted to neutral and his knees flexed, but he lacked 10 degrees of dorsiflexion from neutral with his subtalar joints inverted to neutral and his knees extended. All of his muscles, including the tibialis posterior, had normal strength.

Standing AP, lateral, oblique, and axial radiographs demonstrated characteristic findings of flatfeet. There was no evidence of a tarsal coalition or an accessory navicular.

Because the boy was unable to relieve the pain under the plantarflexed head of the talus by prolonged attempts at conservative management, he was a candidate for surgical management. He was given the choice of having either both feet corrected concurrently or one at a time, with the knowledge that he would need to remain non–weight bearing on the operated foot/feet for 8 weeks. He chose the latter to enable independent mobility on crutches during the postoperative periods. He underwent reconstruction of his somewhat more symptomatic right foot by means of a calcaneal lengthening osteotomy with allograft, lengthening of the peroneus brevis tendon, plication of the talonavicular joint, advancement of the tibialis posterior tendon, plantar-based closing-wedge osteotomy of the medial cuneiform, and gastrocnemius recession. Six months later, he was pain free and completely rehabilitated on the right foot. He had returned to soccer, noting pain only in the left foot and was anxious to have it corrected. The same technique was used to correct the left foot at that time, and he bore weight only on the right foot during the 8 postoperative weeks.

Six years later, he remains pain free and functional in all activities, including competitive and endurance sports.

PEARLS AND PITFALLS

In the symptomatic flexible flatfoot for which surgery is indicated, there are at least two, and possibly three, deformities to treat. The most obvious is the valgus deformity (excessive eversion) of the hind foot. The second deformity, which is actually the source of the pain, is the contracted Achilles tendon, or at least its gastrocnemius component. A third deformity that is most accurately assessed intraoperatively, after the hind foot is corrected, is the supination of the forefoot in relation to the hind foot. The forefoot deformity should not be ignored, as significant uncorrected residual forefoot supination deformity will transform the compensated tripod of a flatfoot to an uncompensated bipod with lack of support under the first metatarsal head. This will lead to recurrence of the hind-foot valgus deformity.

One should concurrently balance the muscle forces when correcting the deformities, though this is perhaps less important for the flatfoot than for the cavus foot. The muscles of the midfoot and hind foot become unbalanced during calcaneal lengthening. Initially, the peroneus brevis is relatively contracted and becomes effectively further contracted after the lateral column is lengthened. It should be lengthened. The tibialis posterior is initially relatively elongated and becomes effectively further elongated as the navicular is rotated plantarmedially around the head of the talus. The tibialis posterior should be shortened, or plicated.

A published study of cadaver bones has raised concern that the calcaneal lengthening osteotomy could lead to early degenerative arthritis in the subtalar joint, because it violates the subtalar joint and is intra-articular in the roughly 60% of feet that were found to have conjoined anterior and middle facets. Only about 40% of the specimens had separate anterior and middle calcaneal facets. This is a theoretic conclusion based on a study of cadaver bones for which neither the anatomy nor the postsurgical arthritis has been suggested or confirmed by clinical studies. Arguments in favor of the calcaneal lengthening osteotomy for valgus deformity of the hind foot, despite the apparent anatomy of the subtalar joint, are many:

- There is no evidence that the same ratio of separate to conjoined anterior and middle calcaneal facets exists for flatfeet as for all feet.
- The subtalar joint complex is unlike any other joint in the body, except the hip joint, and it is more open and unconstrained than the hip. The anterior and middle facets act as a small and partial platform that supports the head of the talus. In the flatfoot, the platform is rotated dorsolaterally around the talar head, and the support is lost. The calcaneal lengthening osteotomy rotates the so-called acetabulum pedis (including the anterior facet) plantarmedially around the head of the talus in the axis of the subtalar joint. This replaces the anterior facet to its anatomic alignment, where it can again provide the needed support for the talar head.
- The actual separation of the calcaneal fragments along the medial column of the calcaneus is small—perhaps 1 to 3 mm. As long as the fragments do not translate vertically, the linear separation should be well tolerated as a simple, small enlargement of the platform that follows the shape and contour of the talar head and subtalar joint.
- In clinical studies, the alternatives of arthroereisis, arthrodesis, and soft-tissue plications have higher reported complication rates than does calcaneal lengthening. The posterior calcaneal displacement osteotomy creates a compensating deformity rather than correcting the primary deformity. It does not have the power to correct severe deformities and to realign the talonavicular joint.

By adhering strictly to the appropriate indications for surgery and by following the details of the procedure(s) as presented here, short- and long-term success should be consistently achieved.

REFERENCES

1. Anderson A, Fowler S. Anterior calcaneal osteotomy for symptomatic juvenile pes planus. *Foot Ankle.* 1984;4:274–283.
2. Evans D. Calcaneo-valgus deformity. *J Bone Joint Surg Br.* 1975;57:270–278.
3. Morrissy RT. Calcaneal lengthening osteotomy for the treatment of hindfoot valgus deformity. In: Morrissy RT, Weinstein SL, eds. *Atlas of Pediatric Orthopaedic Surgery.* 3rd ed. Philadelphia: Lippincott Williams & Wilkins; 2001:775–783.
4. Mosca VS. Calcaneal lengthening for valgus deformity of the hindfoot. Results in children who had severe, symptomatic flatfoot and skewfoot. *J Bone Joint Surg Am.* 1995;77:500–512.
5. Mosca VS. The foot. In: Morrissy RT, Weinstein SL, eds. Lovell and Winter's Pediatric Orthopedics. 5th ed. Philadelphia: Lippincott Williams & Wilkins; 2001:1151–1215.
6. Murphy GA. Pes planus. In: Canale ST, ed. *Campbell's Operative Orthopaedics.* 10th ed. St. Louis: Mosby; 2003:4025–4027.
7. Ragab AA, Stewart SL, Cooperman DR. Implications of subtalar joint anatomic variation in calcaneal lengthening osteotomy. *J Pediatr Orthop.* 2003;23:79–83.

SECTION V
KNEE

23 ACL Reconstruction in the Skeletally Immature Patient

Mininder S. Kocher and Jennifer M. Weiss

Intrasubstance anterior cruciate ligament (ACL) injuries in children and adolescents are being seen with increased frequency and have received increased attention. ACL injury has been reported in 10% to 65% of pediatric knees with acute traumatic hemarthroses in series ranging from 35 to 138 patients.[11,19,20,24,38,40] Management of these injuries is controversial. Nonoperative management of *complete tears* in skeletally immature patients generally has a poor prognosis, with recurrent instability leading to further meniscal and chondral injury, which has implications in terms of development of degenerative joint disease.[1,13,17,27,30,31,33] A variety of reconstructive techniques have been utilized, including physeal-sparing, partial transphyseal, and transphyseal methods using various grafts. Conventional adult ACL reconstruction techniques used in children risk potential iatrogenic growth disturbance due to physeal violation. Growth disturbances after ACL reconstruction in skeletally immature patients have been reported.

This chapter discusses an approach to ACL reconstruction in the skeletally immature patient based on physiological age (Fig. 23-1). In prepubescent patients, a physeal-sparing, combined intra-articular and extra-articular reconstruction with autogenous iliotibial band is performed. In adolescent patients with significant growth remaining, transphyseal ACL reconstruction is performed with autogenous hamstring tendons and fixation away from the physes. In older adolescent patients approaching skeletal maturity, conventional adult ACL reconstruction is performed with interference screw fixation using either autogenous central third patellar tendon or autogenous hamstrings.

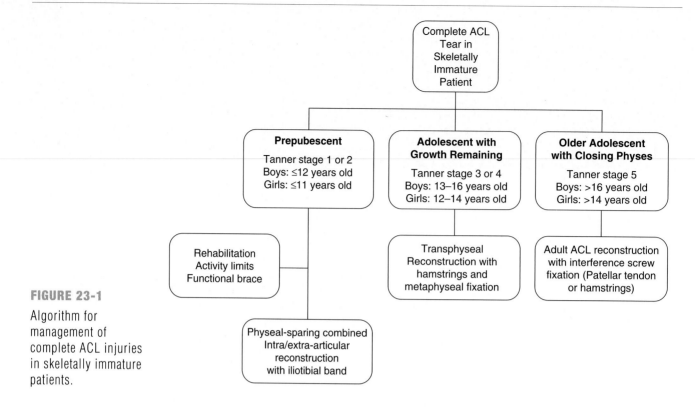

FIGURE 23-1

Algorithm for management of complete ACL injuries in skeletally immature patients.

INDICATIONS/CONTRAINDICATIONS

All skeletally immature patients are not the same. Some have a tremendous amount of growth remaining, while others are essentially done growing. The consequences of growth disturbance in the former group would be severe, requiring osteotomy and/or limb lengthening. However, the consequences of growth disturbance in the latter group would be minimal.

The vast majority of ACL injuries in skeletally immature patients occurs in adolescents. Management of these injuries in *preadolescent* children is particularly vexing, given the poor prognosis with nonoperative management, the substantial growth remaining, and the consequences of potential growth disturbance.

In the prepubescent patient with a complete ACL tear without concurrent chondral or repairable meniscal injury, nonreconstructive treatment with a program of rehabilitation, functional bracing, and return to non-high-risk activities is attempted first. Although the results of nonreconstructive treatment are generally poor, with subsequent functional instability and risk of injury to meniscal and articular cartilage, surgical reconstruction poses the additional risk of growth disturbance. Furthermore, some patients are able to cope with their ACL insufficiency or modify their activities, allowing for further growth and aging such that an adolescent-type reconstruction can later be performed with transphyseal hamstring tendons in a more anatomic manner.

For prepubescent patients with concurrent chondral or repairable meniscal injury, or those with functional instability after nonreconstructive treatment, a physeal-sparing, combined intra-articular and extra-articular reconstruction with autogenous iliotibial band is performed. This procedure is a modification of the combined intra-articular and extra-articular reconstruction described by MacIntosh and Darby.[25,29] This technique provides knee stability and improves function in prepubescent skeletally immature patients with complete intrasubstance ACL injuries, while avoiding the risk of iatrogenic growth disturbance through violation of the distal femoral and/or proximal tibial physes. In the authors' opinion, the consequences of potential iatrogenic growth disturbance caused by transphyseal reconstruction in these young patients are prohibitive. Because this reconstruction is nonanatomic, patients and families are counseled that patients may require revision reconstruction if they develop recurrent instability. However, they are also told that this procedure may temporize for further growth such that patients may then undergo a more conventional reconstruction with drill holes at a later date.

For adolescent patients with growth remaining who have a complete ACL tear, initial nonreconstructive treatment is not advised, because (a) the risk of functional instability with injury to the meniscal and articular cartilage is high, (b) the risk and consequences of growth disturbance from ACL reconstruction are less, and (c) the transphyseal technique is an anatomic reconstruction. In these patients, transphyseal ACL reconstruction with autogenous hamstring tendons with fixation away from the physes is performed.

For older adolescent patients who are approaching skeletal maturity and who have a complete ACL tear, conventional adult ACL reconstruction is performed with interference screw fixation, using either autogenous central third patellar tendon or autogenous hamstrings.

PREOPERATIVE PLANNING

When treating a skeletally immature athlete with an ACL injury, it is important to know his or her chronologic, skeletal, and physiologic age. Skeletal age can be determined from an anteroposterior radiograph of the left hand and wrist per the atlas of Greulich and Pyle.[14] Alternatively, it can be estimated from knee radiographs per the atlas of Pyle and Hoerr.[34] Physiologic age is established using the Tanner and Whitehouse[39] staging system (Table 23-1). In the office, the patient can be informally staged by questioning. In the operating room, after the induction of anesthesia, Tanner staging can be confirmed.

In skeletally immature patients, as in adult patients, acute ACL reconstruction is not performed within the first 3 weeks after injury, to minimize the risk of arthrofibrosis. Prereconstructive rehabilitation is performed to regain range of motion, decrease swelling, and resolve the reflex inhibition of the quadriceps. If there is a displaced, bucket-handle tear of the meniscus that requires extensive repair to protect it from the early mobilization prescribed by ACL reconstruction, then ACL reconstruction may be staged. Skeletally immature patients must be emotionally mature enough to actively participate in the extensive rehabilitation required after ACL reconstruction.

TABLE 23-1 Tanner Staging Classification of Secondary Sexual Characteristics

Tanner Stage		Boy	Girl
Stage 1 (prepubertal)	Growth	5–6 cm/yr	5–6 cm/yr
	Development	Testes <4 ml or <2.5 cm No pubic hair	No breast development No pubic hair
Stage 2	Growth	5–6 cm/yr	7–8 cm/yr

	Development	Testes 4 ml or 2.5–3.2 cm
		Minimal pubic hair at
		  base of penis
			Breast buds
			Minimal pubic hair on
			  labia

Stage 3	Growth	7–8 cm/yr	8 cm/yr

	Development	Testes 12 ml or 3.6 cm
		Pubic hair over pubis
		Voice changes
		Muscle mass increases
			Elevation of breast;
			  areolae enlarge
			Pubic hair on mons
			  pubis
			Axillary hair
			Acne

Stage 4	Growth	10 cm/yr	7 cm/yr
	Development	Testes 4.1–4.5 cm Pubic hair as adult Axillary hair Acne	Areolae enlarge Pubic hair as adult
Stage 5	Growth	No growth	No growth
	Development	Testes as adult Pubic hair as adult Facial hair as adult Mature physique	Adult breast contour Pubic hair as adult

Other		Peak height velocity:
		  13.5 years
			Adrenarche: 6–8 years
			Menarche: 12.7 years
			Peak height velocity:
			  11.5 years

SURGICAL PROCEDURE

In older adolescent patients who are approaching skeletal maturity who have a complete ACL tear, conventional adult ACL reconstruction with interference screw fixation is performed, using either autogenous central third patellar tendon or autogenous hamstrings. This is a standard, one-incision, arthroscopically assisted technique that will not be further detailed in this chapter.

Physeal-Sparing, Combined Intra-/Extra-articular Reconstruction with Autogenous Iliotibial Band

In prepubescent patients, physeal-sparing, combined intra-articular and extra-articular reconstruction with autogenous iliotibial band is performed under general anesthesia as an overnight observation procedure. Local anesthesia with sedation may not be reliable in prepubescent children who have the potential for a paradoxical effect of sedation. The child is positioned supine on the operating table, with a pneumatic tourniquet about the upper thigh; this tourniquet is used routinely. Examination under anesthesia is performed to confirm ACL insufficiency.

First, the iliotibial band graft is obtained. An incision of approximately 6 cm is made obliquely from the lateral joint line to the superior border of the iliotibial band (Fig. 23-2A and Fig. 23-3A). Proximally, the iliotibial band is separated from subcutaneous tissue using a periosteal elevator under the skin of the lateral thigh. The anterior and posterior borders of the iliotibial band are incised and the incisions carried proximally under the skin using curved meniscotomes (Fig. 23-2A). The iliotibial band is detached proximally under the skin using a curved meniscotome or an open tendon stripper. Alternatively, a counterincision can be made at the upper thigh to release the tendon. The iliotibial band is left attached distally at the Gerdy tubercle. Dissection is performed distally to separate the iliotibial band from the joint capsule and from the lateral patellar retinaculum (Fig. 23-2B). The free proximal end of the iliotibial band is then tubularized with a Ethibond-5 whipstitch.

Arthroscopy of the knee is then performed through standard anterolateral viewing and anteromedial working portals. Management of meniscal injury or chondral injury is performed if present. The ACL remnant is excised. The over-the-top position on the femur and the over-the-front position under the intermeniscal ligament are identified. Minimal notchplasty is performed to avoid iatrogenic injury to the perichondral ring of the distal femoral physis, which is in very close proximity to the over-the-top position.[6] The free end of the iliotibial band graft is brought through the over-the-top position using a full-length clamp (Fig. 23-2C) or a two-incision rear-entry guide (Fig. 23-3B) and out the anteromedial portal (Figs. 23-2D and 23-3C).

A second incision of approximately 4.5 cm is made over the proximal medial tibia in the region of the pes anserinus insertion. Dissection is carried through the subcutaneous tissue to the periosteum. A curved clamp is placed from this incision into the joint under the intermeniscal ligament (Fig. 23-2E). A small groove is made in the anteromedial proximal tibial epiphysis under the intermeniscal ligament using a curved rat-tail rasp to bring the tibial graft placement more posterior. The free end of the graft is then brought through the joint (Fig. 23-2F), under the intermeniscal ligament in the anteromedial epiphyseal groove, and out the medial tibial incision (Fig. 23-2G). The graft is fixed on the femoral side through the lateral incision with the knee at 90 degrees flexion and 15 degrees external rotation. Mattress sutures to the lateral femoral condyle at the insertion of the lateral intermuscular septum are used to effect an extra-articular reconstruction (Fig. 23-2H). The tibial side is then fixed through the medial incision with the knee flexed 20 degrees and tension applied to the graft. A periosteal incision is made distal to the proximal tibial physis as checked with fluoroscopic imaging. A trough is made in the proximal tibial medial metaphyseal cortex, and the graft is sutured to the periosteum at the rough margins with mattress sutures (Fig. 23-3D).

Postoperatively, the patient is maintained with touch-down weight bearing for 6 weeks. Range of motion is limited from 0 to 90 degrees for the first 2 weeks, followed by progressive full range of motion. A continuous passive motion (CPM) from 0 to 90 degrees and cryotherapy are used for 2 weeks postoperatively. A protective postoperative brace is used for 6 weeks postoperatively.

Pearls and Pitfalls
- Consider making a second proximal incision when harvesting the iliotibial band.
- Perform a *limited* notchplasty, just enough to visualize the over-the-top position.
- Avoid harvesting a short graft that is insufficient to reach the medial tibial incision.
- Passing the graft through the posterior joint capsule can be challenging.
- Passing the graft under the intermeniscal ligament can be challenging.

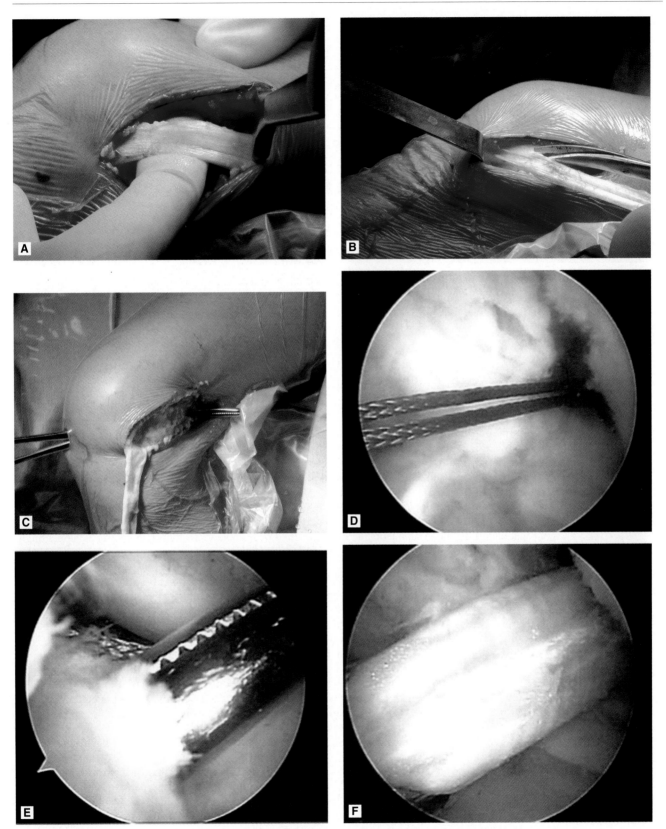

FIGURE 23-2   Physeal-sparing, combined intra-articular and extra-articular reconstruction utilizing autogenous iliotibial band for prepubescents. **A.** The graft is harvested through the lateral incision. **B.** The graft is left attached to the Gerdy tubercle distally. **C, D.** The graft is brought through the knee in the over-the-top position, using a full-length clamp. **E.** The graft is brought under the intermeniscal ligament. A groove can be made in the epiphysis in this region with a rasp. **F.** Intra-articular reconstruction component. *(Continued)*

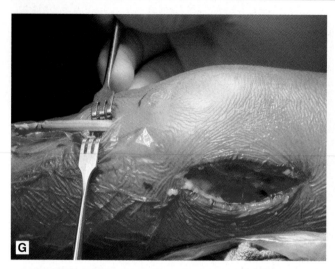
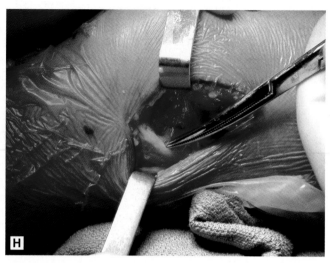

FIGURE 23-2 *(Continued)* **G.** The graft is brought out the medial tibial incision and fixed to a trough in the periosteum. **H.** Extra-articular reconstruction component.

Transphyseal Reconstruction with Autogenous Hamstrings with Metaphyseal Fixation

In adolescents with growth remaining, transphyseal ACL reconstruction with autogenous hamstring tendons with metaphyseal fixation away from the physes is performed. This is a fairly standard, one-incision, arthroscopically assisted technique that uses a four-stranded gracilis/semitendinosus graft with endobutton fixation on the femur. On the tibial side, the graft may be fixed with a soft-tissue interference screw if there is adequate tunnel distance (at least 30 mm) below the physis to ensure metaphyseal placement of the screw. Or it may be fixed with a post and a spiked washer.

The procedure is performed under general anesthesia as an overnight observation procedure. Local anesthesia with sedation may be performed in the emotionally mature adolescent child. The patient is positioned supine on the operating table with a pneumatic tourniquet about the upper thigh; this tourniquet is not used routinely. Examination under anesthesia is performed to confirm ACL insufficiency.

First, the hamstring tendons are harvested. If the diagnosis is in doubt, arthroscopy can be performed to confirm an ACL tear. A 4-cm incision is made over the palpable pes anserinus tendons on the medial side of the upper tibia (Fig. 23-4A). Dissection is carried through the skin to the sartorius fascia. Care is taken to protect superficial sensory nerves. The sartorius tendon is incised longitudinally, and the gracilis and semitendinosus tendons are identified. The tendons are dissected free distally, and their free ends are whipstitched with Ethibond-2 or Ethibond-5 sutures. The tendons are dissected proximally using sharp and blunt dissection. Fibrous bands to the medial head of the gastrocnemius should be sought and released. A closed tendon stripper is used to dissect the tendons free proximally. Alternatively, the tendons can be left attached distally, with an open tendon stripper used to release the tendons proximally. The tendons are taken to the back table, where excess muscle is removed, and the remaining ends are whipstitched with Ethibond-2 or -5 sutures. The tendons are folded over a closed-loop endobutton. The graft diameter is sized, and the graft is placed under tension.

Arthroscopy of the knee is then performed through standard anterolateral viewing and anteromedial working portals. Management of meniscal injury or chondral injury is performed if present. The ACL remnant is excised. The over-the-top position on the femur is identified. Minimal notchplasty is performed to avoid iatrogenic injury to the perichondral ring of the distal femoral physis, which is in very close proximity to the over-the-top position.[6]

A tibial tunnel guide (set at 55 degrees) is used through the anteromedial portal (Fig. 23-4B). A guide wire is drilled through the hamstring harvest incision into the posterior aspect of the ACL tibial footprint. The guide-wire entry point on the tibia should be kept medial to avoid injury to the tibial tubercle apophysis. The guide wire is reamed with the appropriate diameter reamer. Excess soft tissue at the tibial tunnel is excised to avoid arthrofibrosis. The transtibial, over-the-top guide (with the appropriate offset to ensure a 1- or 2-mm back wall) is used to pass the femoral guide pin

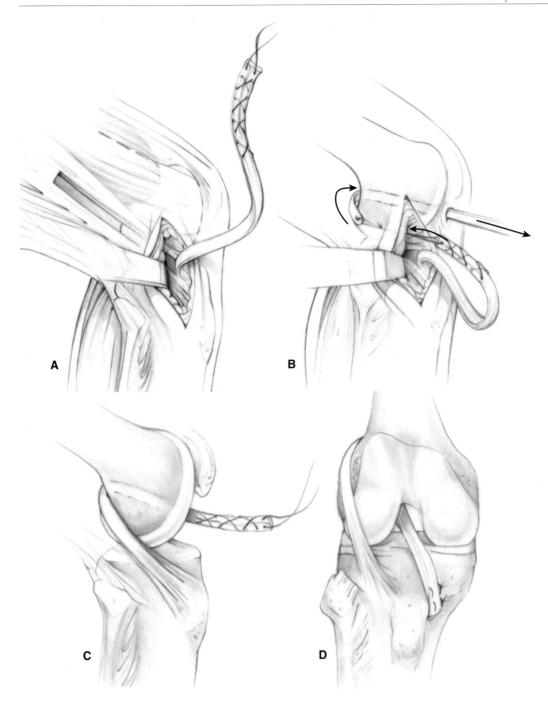

FIGURE 23-3   Physeal-sparing, combined intra-articular and extra-articular reconstruction utilizing autogenous iliotibial band for prepubescents. **A.** The iliotibial band graft is harvested free proximally and left attached to the Gerdy tubercle distally. **B.** The graft is brought through the knee in the over-the-top position posteriorly. **C.** The graft is brought through the knee and under the intermeniscal ligament anteriorly. **D.** Resulting intra-articular and extra-articular reconstruction.

(Fig. 23-4C). The femoral guide pin is overdrilled with the endobutton reamer, both of which are removed in order to measure the femoral tunnel length with a depth gauge. The guide pin is then replaced and brought through the distal lateral thigh. The femur is reamed to the appropriate depth (femoral tunnel length—endobutton length + 6–7 mm to flip the endobutton).

The Ethibond-5 sutures on the endobutton are placed in a slot of the guide wire and pulled through the tibial tunnel, then the femoral tunnel, and out the lateral thigh. These sutures are then pulled to bring the endobutton and graft through the tibial tunnel and into the femoral tunnel; one set of sutures

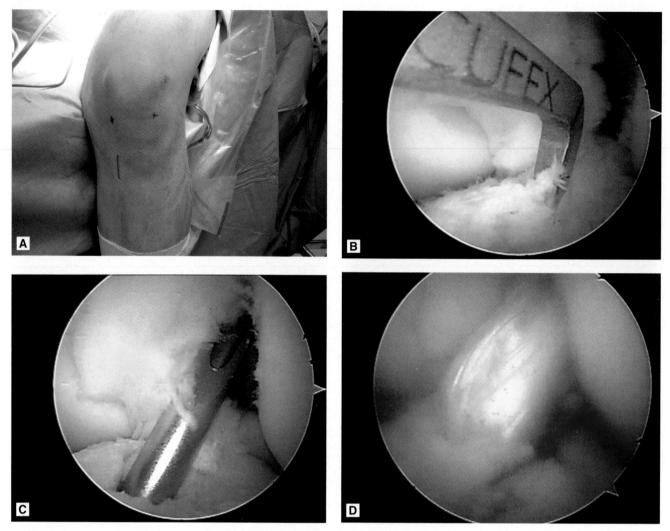

FIGURE 23-4 Transphyseal reconstruction with autogenous hamstrings for adolescents with growth remaining. **A.** The gracilis and semitendinosus tendons are harvested through an incision over the proximal medial tibia. **B.** The tibial guide is used to drill the tibial tunnel. **C.** The transtibial over-the-top offset guide is used to drill the femoral tunnel. **D.** Hamstrings graft after fixation.

is used to "lead" the endobutton, while the other set is used to "follow." Once the graft is fully seated in the femoral tunnel, the "follow" sutures are pulled to flip the endobutton. The flip can be palpated in the thigh. Tension is applied to the graft to ensure no graft slippage. The knee is then extended to ensure no graft impingement. The knee is cycled approximately 10 times with tension applied to the graft. The graft is fixed on the tibial side with the knee in 20 to 30 degrees of flexion, tension applied to the graft, and a posterior force placed on the tibia. On the tibial side, the graft may be fixed with a soft-tissue interference screw if there is adequate tunnel distance (at least 30 mm) below the physis to ensure metaphyseal placement of the screw. Or it may be fixed with a post and a spiked washer. Fluoroscopy can be used to ensure that the fixation is away from the physes. Postoperative radiographs are shown in Figure 23-5.

Postoperatively, the patient is maintained with touch-down weight bearing for 2 weeks. Range of motion is limited from 0 to 90 degrees for the first 2 weeks, followed by progressive full range of motion. CPM from 0 to 90 degrees and cryotherapy are used for 2 weeks postoperatively. A protective postoperative brace is used for 6 weeks postoperatively.

Pearls and Pitfalls
- Check for graft impingement.
- Keep tunnels small.
- Be careful not to amputate the hamstring grafts.
- Beware of poor tunnel placement.
- Do not place hardware in the physis.

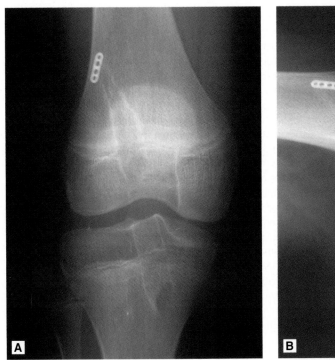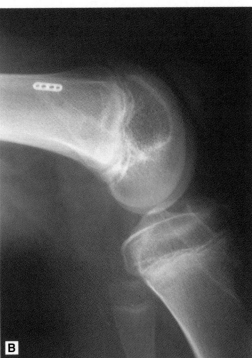

FIGURE 23-5   Transphyseal reconstruction with autogenous hamstrings for adolescents with growth remaining. Postoperative anteroposterior **(A)** and lateral **(B)** radiographs.

Technical Alternatives

Transphyseal reconstruction, partial transphyseal reconstruction, and physeal-sparing reconstruction techniques have been described to address ACL insufficiency in skeletally immature patients.

In prepubescent patients, physeal-sparing techniques have been described that utilize hamstring tendons under the intermeniscal ligament and over the top on the femur, through all-epiphyseal femoral and tibial tunnels, and with a femoral epiphyseal staple.[2,8,9,15,18,29,32,40]

In adolescent patients with growth remaining, transphyseal reconstructions have been performed with hamstrings autograft, patellar tendon autograft, and allograft tissue.[1,4,5,10,12,26–28,35–37,41] In addition, partial transphyseal reconstructions have been described with a tunnel through the proximal tibial physis and over-the-top positioning on the femur or a tunnel through the distal femoral physis with an epiphyseal tunnel in the tibia.[3,7,16,23]

POSTOPERATIVE MANAGEMENT

Rehabilitation after ACL reconstruction in skeletally immature patients is essential to ensure a good outcome, allow return to sports, and avoid reinjury. Rehabilitation in prepubescent children can be challenging. A therapist who is used to working with children and who can make therapy interesting and fun is very helpful. Compliance with therapy and restrictions should be carefully monitored.

After physeal-sparing iliotibial band reconstruction in prepubescent patients, full weight bearing is restricted for 6 weeks to allow for graft healing. After transphyseal hamstring reconstruction in adolescents with growth remaining, full weight bearing is restricted for 2 weeks. A CPM machine is used for 2 weeks postoperatively. A postoperative brace is then used for 6 weeks postoperatively.

Progressive rehabilitation consists of range-of-motion exercises, patellar mobilization, electrical stimulation, pool therapy (if available), proprioception exercises, and closed-chain strengthening for the first 3 months post-op, followed by straight-line jogging, plyometric exercises, sport cord exercises, and sport-specific exercises.

Return to full activity, including cutting sports, is usually allowed at 6 months postoperatively. A functional knee brace is used routinely during cutting and pivoting activities for the first 2 years after return to sports.

COMPLICATIONS TO AVOID

Complications of physeal injury can be avoided by performing only a limited notchplasty. Aggressive notchplasty could violate the distal femoral physis. Fixation of transphyseal graft should not violate either physis. Physeal injury to the proximal tibia is avoided by securing the graft distal to the physis. Pitfalls to avoid with the physeal-sparing iliotibial band reconstruction in prepubescents include harvesting a short graft insufficient to reach the medial tibial incision, difficulty passing the graft through the posterior joint capsule, and difficulty passing the graft under the intermeniscal ligament.

Pitfalls to avoid with the transphyseal hamstrings reconstruction in adolescents with growth remaining include amputation of the hamstring grafts, poor tunnel placement, and graft impingement. Based on the 15 cases of growth disturbance after ACL reconstruction in skeletally immature patients that the authors reported, as well as on anatomical studies in cadaveric pediatric knees, the authors recommend careful attention to technical details during ACL reconstruction in skeletally immature patients, particularly the avoidance of fixation hardware across the lateral distal femoral epiphyseal plate.[21,22] Care should also be taken to avoid injury to the vulnerable tibial tubercle apophysis. Given the cases of growth disturbances associated with transphyseal placement of patellar tendon graft bone blocks, the authors recommend the use of soft-tissue grafts. Large tunnels should be avoided as the likelihood of arrest is associated with greater violation of epiphyseal plate cross-sectional area. The two cases of genu valgum without arrest associated with lateral extra-articular tenodesis raise additional concerns about the effect of tension on physeal growth. Finally, care should be taken to avoid dissection or notching around the posterolateral aspect of the physis during over-the-top nonphyseal femoral placement to avoid potential injury to the perichondral ring and subsequent deformity.

OUTCOMES AND FUTURE DIRECTIONS

The authors have reviewed the results of physeal-sparing iliotibial band reconstruction in prepubescent patients in a preliminary series of eight patients.[29] More recently, they have reviewed the minimum 2-year results in 44 prepubescent patients. Between 1980 and 2002, 44 skeletally immature preadolescent children who were Tanner stage 1 or 2 (mean chronologic age: 10.3 years old; range: 3.6–14.0 years old) underwent physeal-sparing combined intra-articular and extra-articular ACL reconstruction using autogenous iliotibial band. Of those patients, 24 had additional meniscal surgery. Functional outcome, graft survival, radiographic outcome, and growth disturbance were evaluated at a mean of 5.3 years (range: 2.0–15.1 years old) after surgery. Two patients underwent revision ACL reconstruction for graft failure at 4.7 and 8.3 years after initial surgery (revision rate: 4.5%). In the remaining 42 patients, the mean International Knee Documentation Committee (IKDC) subjective knee score was 96.7 6.0 (range: 88.5–100) and the mean Lysholm knee score was 95.7 6.7 (range: 74–100). Per IKDC criteria, Lachman examination was normal in 23 patients, nearly normal in 18 patients, and abnormal in 1 patient. Pivot-shift examination was normal in 31 patients and nearly normal in 11 patients. Four patients who underwent concurrent meniscus repair had repeat arthroscopic meniscal repair or partial meniscectomy. Mean growth in total height from the time of surgery to final follow-up was 21.5 cm (range: 9.5–118.5 cm). There were no cases of significant angular deformity measured radiographically or of leg-length discrepancy measured clinically. Thus, physeal-sparing combined intra-articular and extra-articular ACL reconstruction using iliotibial band in preadolescent skeletally immature patients appears to provide for excellent functional outcome with a low revision rate and a minimal risk of growth disturbance.

RECOMMENDED READINGS

1. Kocher MS, Micheli LJ. The pediatric knee: evaluation and treatment. In: Insall JN, Scott WN, eds. *Surgery of the Knee.* 3rd ed. New York: Churchill Livingstone; 2001:1356–1397.
2. Stanitski CL. Anterior cruciate ligament injury in the skeletally immature patient: diagnosis and treatment. *J Am Acad Orthop Surg.* 1995;3:146–158.

REFERENCES

1. Aichroth PM, Patel DV, Zorrilla P. The natural history and treatment of rupture of the anterior cruciate ligament in children and adolescents: a prospective review. *J Bone Joint Surg Br.* 2002;84(1):618–619.
2. Anderson AF. Transepiphyseal replacement of the anterior cruciate ligament in skeletally immature patients: a preliminary report. *J Bone Joint Surg Am.* 2003;85(7):1255–1263.
3. Andrews M, Noyes FR, Barber-Westin SD. Anterior cruciate ligament allograft reconstruction in the skeletally immature athlete. *Am J Sports Med.* 1994;22(1):48–54.

4. Angel KR, Hall DJ. Anterior cruciate ligament injury in children and adolescents. *Arthroscopy.* 1989;5(3):197–200.
5. Aronowitz ER, Ganley TJ, Goode JR, et al. Anterior cruciate ligament reconstruction in adolescents with open physes. *Am J Sports Med.* 2000;28(2):168–175.
6. Behr CT, Potter HG, Paletta GA Jr. The relationship of the femoral origin of the anterior cruciate ligament and the distal femoral physeal plate in the skeletally immature knee: an anatomic study. *Am J Sports Med.* 2001;29:781–787.
7. Bisson LJ, Wickiewicz T, Levinson M, et al. ACL reconstruction in children with open physes. *Orthopedics.* 1998;21(6):659–663.
8. Brief LB. Anterior cruciate ligament reconstruction without drill holes. *Arthroscopy.* 1991;7:350–357.
9. DeLee J, Curtis R. Anterior cruciate ligament insufficiency in children. *Clin Orthop Relat Res.* 1983; 172:112–118.
10. Edwards PH, Grana WA. Anterior cruciate ligament reconstruction in the immature athlete: long-term results of intra-articular reconstruction. *Am J Knee Surg.* 2001;14:232–237.
11. Eiskjaer S, Larsen ST, Schmidt MB. The significance of hemarthrosis of the knee in children. *Arch Orthop Trauma Surg.* 1988;107(2):96–98.
12. Fuchs R, Wheatley W, Uribe JW, et al. Intra-articular anterior cruciate ligament reconstruction using patellar tendon allograft in the skeletally immature patient. *Arthroscopy.* 2002;18(8):824–828.
13. Graf BK, Lange RH, Fujisaki CK, et al. Anterior cruciate ligament tears in skeletally immature patients: meniscal pathology at presentation and after attempted conservative treatment. *Arthroscopy.* 1992;8(2):229–233.
14. Greulich WW, Pyle SI. *Radiographic Atlas of Skeletal Development of the Hand and Wrist.* 2nd ed. Palo Alto: Stanford University Press; 1959.
15. Guzzanti V, Falciglia F, Stanitski CL. Physeal-sparing intraarticular anterior cruciate ligament reconstruction in preadolescents. *Am J Sports Med.* 2003;31(6):949–953.
16. Guzzanti V, Falciglia F, Stanitski CL. Preoperative evaluation and anterior cruciate ligament reconstruction technique for skeletally immature patients in Tanner stages 2 and 3. *Am J Sports Med.* 2003;31(6):941–948.
17. Janarv PM, Nystrom A, Werner S, et al. Anterior cruciate ligament injuries in skeletally immature patients. *J Pediatr Orthop.* 1996;16(5):673–677.
18. Kim SH, Ha KI, Ahn JH, et al. Anterior cruciate ligament reconstruction in the young patient without violation of the epiphyseal plate. *Arthroscopy.* 1999;15(7):792–795.
19. Kloeppel-Wirth S, Koltai JL, Dittmer H. Significance of arthroscopy in children with knee joint injuries. *Eur J Pediatr Surg.* 1992;2(3):169–172.
20. Kocher MS, DiCanzio J, Zurakowski D, et al. Diagnostic performance of clinical examination and selective magnetic resonance imaging in the evaluation of intraarticular knee disorders in children and adolescents. *Am J Sports Med.* 2001;29(3):292–296.
21. Kocher MS, Hovis WD, Curtin MJ, et al. Anterior cruciate ligament reconstruction in skeletally immature knees: an anatomical study. *Am J Orthop.* 2005;34(6):285–290.
22. Kocher MS, Saxon HS, Hovis WD, et al. Management and complications of anterior cruciate ligament injuries in skeletally immature patients: survey of the Herodicus Society and the ACL Study Group. *J Pediatr Orthop.* 2002;22(4):452–457.
23. Lo IK, Kirkley A, Fowler PJ, et al. The outcome of operatively treated anterior cruciate ligament disruptions in the skeletally immature child. *Arthroscopy.* 1997;13(5):627–634.
24. Luhmann SJ. Acute traumatic knee effusions in children and adolescents. *J Pediatr Orthop.* 2003;23(2):199–202.
25. MacIntosh DL, Darby DT. Lateral substitution reconstruction in proceedings and reports of universities, colleges, councils, and associations. *J Bone Joint Surg Br.* 1976;58:142.
26. Matava MJ, Siegel MG. Arthroscopic reconstruction of the ACL with semitendinosus-gracilis autograft in skeletally immature adolescent patients. *Am J Knee Surg.* 1997;10(2):60–69.
27. McCarroll JR, Rettig AC, Shelbourne KD. Anterior cruciate ligament injuries in the young athlete with open physes. *Am J Sports Med.* 1988;16(1):44–47.
28. McCarroll JR, Shelbourne KD, Porter DA, et al. Patellar tendon graft reconstruction for midsubstance anterior cruciate ligament rupture in junior high school athletes: an algorithm for management. *Am J Sports Med.* 1994;22:478–484.
29. Micheli LJ, Rask B, Gerberg L. Anterior cruciate ligament reconstruction in patients who are prepubescent. *Clin Orthop Relat Res.* 1999;(364):40–47.
30. Millett PJ, Willis AA, Warren RF. Associated injuries in pediatric and adolescent anterior cruciate ligament tears: does a delay in treatment increase the risk of meniscal tear? *Arthroscopy.* 2002;18(9):955–999.
31. Mizuta H, Kubota K, Shiraishi M, et al. The conservative treatment of complete tears of the anterior cruciate ligament in skeletally immature patients. *J Bone Joint Surg Br.* 1995;77(6):890–894.
32. Parker AW, Drez D, Cooper JL. Anterior cruciate ligament injuries in patients with open physes. *Am J Sports Med.* 1994;22(1):44–47.
33. Pressman AE, Letts RM, Jarvis JG. Anterior cruciate ligament tears in children: an analysis of operative versus nonoperative treatment. *J Pediatr Orthop.* 1997;17(4):505–511.
34. Pyle SI, Hoerr NL. A Radiographic Standard of Reference the Growing Knee. Springfield, IL: Charles Thomas; 1969.
35. Shelbourne KD, Gray T, Wiley BV. Results of transphyseal anterior cruciate ligament reconstruction using patellar tendon autograft in Tanner stage 3 or 4 adolescents with clearly open growth plates. *Am J Sports Med.* 2004;32(5):1218–1222.
36. Simonian PT, Metcalf MH, Larson RV. Anterior cruciate ligament injuries in the skeletally immature patient. *Am J Orthop.* 1999;28(11):624–628.
37. Stanitski CL. Anterior cruciate ligament injury in the skeletally immature patient: diagnosis and treatment. *J Am Acad Orthop Surg.* 1995;3(3):146–158.
38. Stanitski CL, Harvell JC, Fu F. Observations on acute knee hemarthrosis in children and adolescents. *J Pediatr Orthop.* 1993;13(4):506–510.
39. Tanner JM, Whitehouse RH. Clinical longitudinal standards for height, weight, height velocity, and stages of puberty. *Arch Dis Child.* 1976;51:170–179.
40. Vahasarja V, Kinnunen P, Serlo W. Arthroscopy of the acute traumatic knee in children: prospective study of 138 cases. *Acta Orthop Scand.* 1993;64(5):580–582.
41. Volpi P, Galli M, Bait C, et al. Surgical treatment of anterior cruciate ligament injuries in adolescents using double-looped semitendinosus and gracilis tendons: supraepiphysary femoral and tibial fixation. *Arthroscopy.* 2004;20(4):447–449.

24 Discoid Lateral Meniscus Saucerization and Stabilization

Jennifer M. Weiss

INDICATIONS/CONTRAINDICATIONS

A discoid lateral meniscus is reported to be present in 7% of the population.[5] Much of the time, the discoid meniscus is asymptomatic. If the discoid meniscus is noted as an incidental finding and is asymptomatic, no intervention is recommended.

Surgery is indicated for a discoid meniscus if it is symptomatic. Knees signs and symptoms include pain, extension lag, clunking, and locking about the knee. Both a torn discoid meniscus and an unstable discoid meniscus can cause all of these signs and symptoms.

Surgery for a discoid lateral meniscus includes saucerization, or removal of the abnormal meniscus, with possible meniscal stabilization. Every discoid meniscus, whether complete or incomplete, needs to be probed at the anterior horn, in the middle, and at the posterior horn. If probing determines that the lateral meniscal is unstable, surgical stabilization to the capsule is necessary.

A study of peripheral rim stability of the discoid lateral meniscus by Klingele et al.[4] evaluated 128 knees and found that a complete discoid meniscus was present 62% of the time, with an incomplete discoid meniscus present 38% of the time. A complete discoid meniscus is more likely to be unstable than is an incomplete discoid meniscus. Peripheral rim instability was present 28% of the time. Anterior horn instability was most common (47%), with middle instability being present in 11% and posterior horn instability in 39%.

PREOPERATIVE PLANNING

The most important part of preoperative planning is a full discussion of the condition and the planned surgical procedure with the family. It is often difficult to determine from the magnetic resonance imaging (MRI) scan whether the discoid is complete, stable, or torn. The family should be comfortable with the fact that the surgeon will need to make treatment decisions based on intraoperative findings.

Radiographs are not always helpful in diagnosing a discoid lateral meniscus, though flattening of the lateral femoral condyle can be seen.[8] MRI diagnosis of a discoid lateral meniscus is made when three consecutive 5-mm sagittal cuts show meniscal tissue between the center of the femoral condyle and the tibial surface. This should correspond to a midportion measurement of the meniscus of greater than 14 mm.[1,6] Coronal views may also show a meniscal height difference of 2 mm or more.[6] Although MRI is more sensitive than arthroscopy in diagnosing intrasubstance tears and degeneration, it is not always reliable in diagnosing a clinically relevant tear of a discoid meniscus. Therefore, the family needs to be prepared for treatment of a meniscal tear seen intraoperatively, even if it is not evident on the preoperative MRI.[6]

The family should be informed that meniscal tears may or may not be reparable and that any meniscus that is removed will not grow back. The family should also be prepared for the different postoperative protocols that will follow either stabilization surgery or saucerization surgery—or both.

The surgeon should be prepared to operatively stabilize the posterior, middle, and/or anterior portions of the meniscus. Meniscal repair instruments for all of these possibilities should be made available prior to anesthesia.

SURGICAL PROCEDURE

Examination under Anesthesia

A complete examination of the patient's knee should be performed once the patient is under anesthesia. Specifically the surgeon should feel for clunking of the knee and protrusion of the discoid meniscus into the lateral joint line. If these findings are present, reassessment for these same findings should be done after surgery to be certain that they are absent.

Probing for Stability and Tears

In the arthroscopic surgery, the initial assessment of the discoid meniscus involves probing the entire lateral meniscus for tears. Stability should be assessed on the posterior, middle, and anterior portions. Normal excursion of the lateral meniscus is 11.2 ± 3.27 mm; excursion greater than this should raise concern for meniscal instability.[7] Peripheral meniscal detachment is also present if the lateral meniscus can be everted or if the anterior horn of the meniscus can be translated to the posterior half of the tibial plateau.[3] If a meniscal tear is present, its location and configuration should be noted. Like a tear of a nondiscoid meniscus, the tear should be assessed for repair depending on its anatomical location and the tear pattern. If the tear is complex and involves the meniscal rim, the meniscus may not be salvageable, in which case meniscectomy may be needed. Every effort should be made, however, to save the meniscus if it is considered to be salvageable.

Saucerization

Before removal of the abnormal central portion of the discoid lateral meniscus is begun, a probe is used to measure the peripheral rim that will be left intact. Saucerization is most reliably performed using basket biters. The surgeon starts with a straight biter, with the knee in neutral, to find the medial edge of the discoid meniscus. The knee is placed into a figure-of-four position to gain access to the midportion of the lateral meniscus. Right- and left-angled biters are used to remove the abnormal central tissue posteriorly and anteriorly. The remaining rim is measured frequently with a probe. If an intrasubstance tear is encountered, there may be multiple layers of tissue. At least a 6- to 8-mm rim of lateral meniscus should be left intact.[8] Carefully use a nonaggressive shaver to smooth the remaining tissue. Do not thin the remaining rim. Reassess for stability after saucerization.

Stabilization of the Anterior and Middle Horns of the Meniscus

If meniscal rim instability is present, the anterior and middle horns can be stabilized using an outside-in technique. The knee capsule and meniscal edge are rasped to stimulate bleeding. The lateral meniscus is reduced and held in place with a grasper. An 18-gauge spinal needle is inserted through the capsule and meniscus. A 2-0 Prolene (Johnson and Johnson) suture is introduced into the spinal needle. A microsuture lasso (e.g., Arthrex) is inserted 5 mm adjacent to the first needle through another spinal needle. The 2-0 Prolene is then hooked by the suture lasso and pulled out. The suture is then passed under the skin with a small hemostat and tied over the capsule. This is repeated until stability is achieved—usually four to five sutures (Fig. 24-1).

Stabilization of the Posterior Horn—Inside-Out Technique

To avoid injury to the common peroneal nerve, dissection must be carried down to the knee capsule. An incision is made just behind the lateral collateral ligament at the joint line. To determine the exact location of the joint line, the light of the camera can be observed through the skin when it is inserted into the lateral compartment. The interval between the iliotibial band and the biceps femoris tendon is identified. Placing the retractor anterior to the biceps protects the peroneal nerve. A periosteal elevator can then be used to elevate the lateral head of the gastrocnemius tendon from the posterior knee joint capsule. The assistant surgeon continues to hold the retractors and prepares to "catch" the needles as they are passed for the repair. The Zone Specific Meniscal Repair System (Linvatec) is preferred. During operation on the right knee, the left posterior cannula is used; for the left knee, the right posterior cannula is used. The lateral meniscal and capsular edges are rasped to promote bleeding tissue. The cannula is pushed up against the posterior horn of the lateral meniscus and is used to reduce the meniscus to the capsule. The inferior suture of the vertical mattress suture is passed first using a double-arm meniscal repair needle (e.g., Linvatec). The first needle is inserted through the cannula

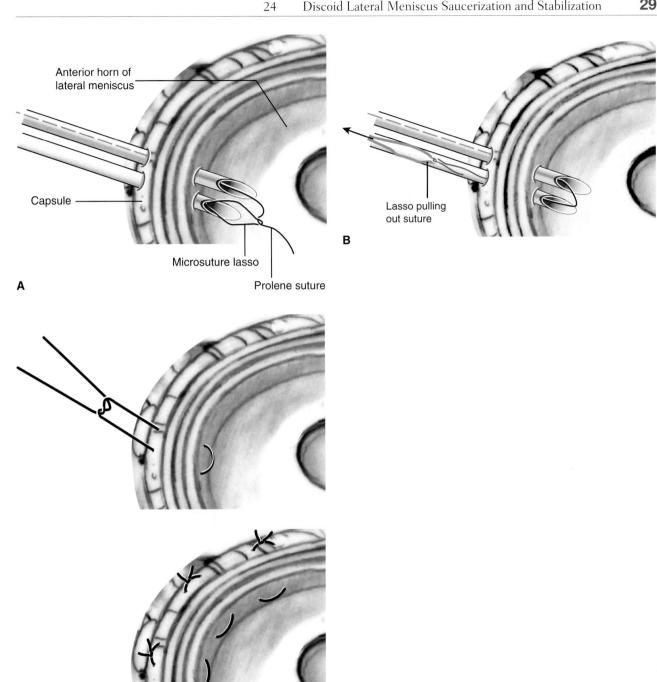

FIGURE 24-1 **A.** Spinal needle is inserted through capsule and meniscus. Prolene suture (2-0) is inserted through the spinal needle into the joint. Microsuture lasso is inserted, and the prolene suture is retrieved. **B.** Prolene suture is brought out through the microsuture lasso, and both needles are removed. **C.** Prolene suture is passed under the skin but over the capsule and tied.

and is retrieved by the assistant with a needle driver. The cannula is then moved superiorly on the lateral meniscus, and the second suture of the vertical mattress suture is passed. The needles are removed, and the suture strands are managed with hemostats until all sutures are passed with approximately a 5-mm space between them. The sutures are then tied over the knee capsule. The surgeon must not suture through the popliteal hiatus. Consideration may instead be given to using "all inside" stabilization of the posterior horn of the unstable discoid meniscus, as the biomechanics of the FasT-Fix implant (Smith and Nephew) has compared favorably with the gold standard—vertical mattress—suture.[2] Further study needs to be done in this arena (Fig. 24-2).

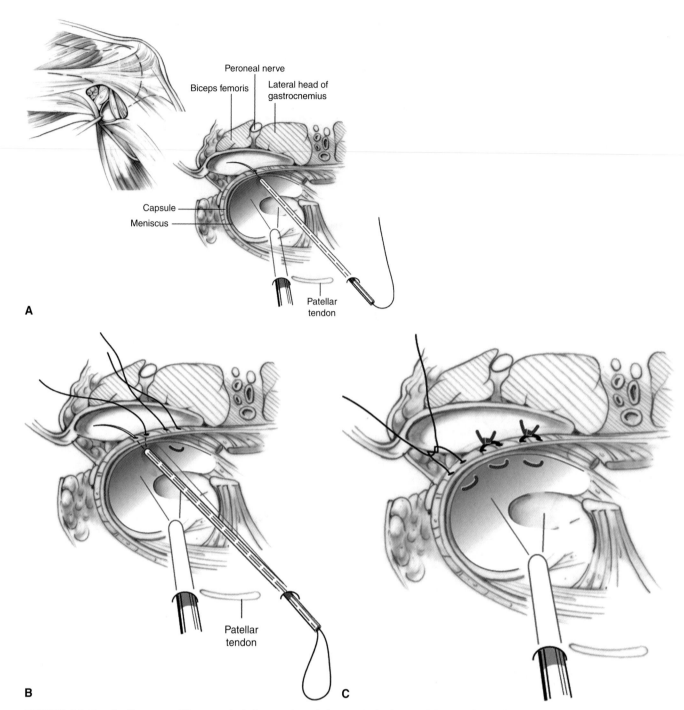

FIGURE 24-2   **A.** Zone-specific cannula is inserted, and the posterior horn of the meniscus is reduced to the capsule. The first arm of the suture is passed and caught by the assistant. **B.** The cannula is moved 0.5 cm, and the second arm of the suture is passed and caught. **C.** The sutures are tied over the capsule under direct visualization.

POSTOPERATIVE MANAGEMENT

If saucerization is performed without the need for meniscal stabilization, the patient can weight bear as tolerated and should begin knee range-of-motion exercises without precautions as soon as possible. The patient can return to sports as soon as his or her knee range of motion and lower extremity strength are comparable to the contralateral leg. If meniscal stabilization is performed, weight bearing should be protected for 6 weeks. A hinged knee brace is used to limit knee range of motion from 0 to 90 degrees for 4 weeks, after which full knee motion is encouraged.

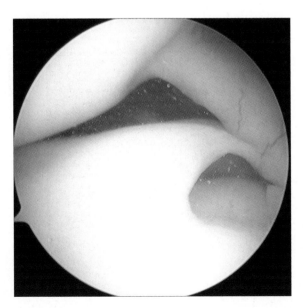

FIGURE 24-3
A complete discoid
meniscus as viewed
from the lateral
compartment.

COMPLICATIONS TO AVOID

The surgeon must be very careful not to remove too much of the discoid lateral meniscus. Measuring the peripheral rim repeatedly as the central tissue is removed is necessary to avoid this complication. If the remaining meniscal tissue is jagged or unstable, the patient will likely remain symptomatic, and repeat arthroscopic surgery will be necessary. When performing an inside-out repair technique, the surgeon should avoid injury to the common peroneal nerve by using careful retraction and visualization of all needles.

ILLUSTRATIVE CASE

A 13-year-old boy complained of locking and clunking in his right knee. MRI scan was suspicious for a torn discoid meniscus. Arthroscopic evaluation revealed a complete discoid meniscus with stable meniscocapsular attachments (Figs. 24-3 and 24-4). Saucerization was performed (Figs. 24-5 to 24-9).

FIGURE 24-4
A complete discoid
meniscus as viewed
from the notch.

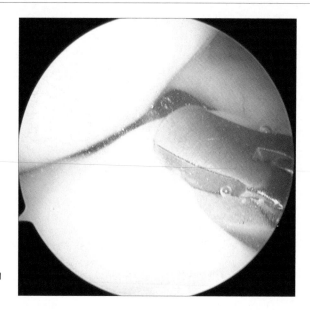

FIGURE 24-5
The saucerization begins with a biter, with the knee in neutral.

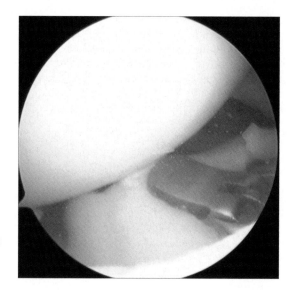

FIGURE 24-6
Saucerization continues with the knee in a figure-of-four position.

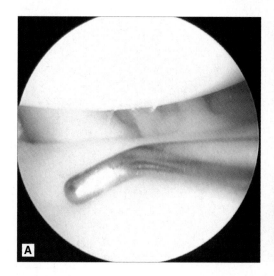
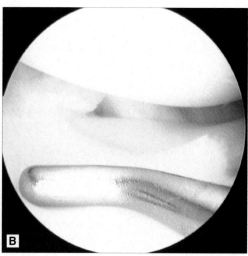

FIGURE 24-7
A–C. The probe is frequently inserted to measure the remaining rim. *(Continued)*

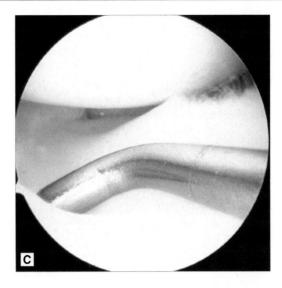

FIGURE 24-7
(Continued)

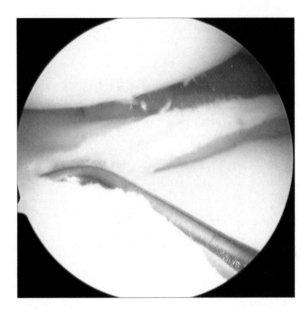

FIGURE 24-8
An 8-mm rim remains.

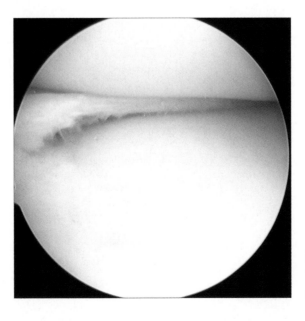

FIGURE 24-9
The edges are smooth after a shaver was used.

PEARLS AND PITFALLS

- If the patient has a clunk on physical exam, repeat the exam after surgery is complete but before breaking the sterile field. If the clunk remains, more work may need to be done.
- Start the saucerization of a complete discoid lateral meniscus with the knee in neutral to give easier access to the midportion.
- For children under the age of 8, consider using a small joint camera and tools.
- Do not use a shaver that is too big or too aggressive, as this can remove too much tissue and can damage the articular cartilage.
- Do not thin out the remaining rim.
- Do not propagate tears by moving too quickly or aggressively.
- Do not retract too hard on the peroneal nerve during an inside-out repair, as this can lead to peroneal nerve palsy.

REFERENCES

1. Araki Y, Yamamoto H, Nakamura H, et al. MR diagnosis of discoid lateral menisci of the knee. *Eur J Radiol.* 1994;18(2):92–95.
2. Borden P, Nyland J, Caborn DN, et al. Biomechanical comparison of the FasT-Fix meniscal repair suture system with vertical mattress sutures and meniscus arrows. *Am J Sports Med.* 2003;31(3):374–378.
3. Good CR, Green DW, Griffith MH, et al. Arthroscopic treatment of symptomatic discoid meniscus in children: classification, technique, and results. *Arthroscopy.* 2007;23(2):157–163.
4. Klingele KE, Kocher MS, Hresko MT, et al. Discoid lateral meniscus: prevalence of peripheral rim instability. *J Pediatr Orthop.* 2004;24(1):79–82.
5. Noble J. Lesions of the menisci: autopsy incidence in adults less than fifty-five years old. *J Bone Joint Surg.* 1977;59(4):480–483.
6. Silverman JM, Mink JH, Deutsch AL. Discoid menisci of the knee: MR imaging appearance. *Radiology.* 1989;173(2):351–354.
7. Thompson WO, Thaete FL, Fu FH, et al. Tibial meniscal dynamics using three-dimensional reconstruction of magnetic resonance images. *Am J Sports Med.* 1991;19(3):210–215, 5–6(disc).
8. Woods GW, Whelan JM. Discoid meniscus. *Clin Sports Med.* 1990;9(3):695–706.

25 Hemiepiphysiodesis

Peter M. Stevens

INTRODUCTION

As orthopaedists deal with growing children, they are frequently consulted about angular deformities, particularly of the weight-bearing extremities. Mindful of the natural history of physiologic genu varum (up to age 2) and genu valgum (ages 2–6), the orthopaedist's role for those patients is most often to educate parents and to withhold treatment because spontaneous resolution is the rule. However, myriad conditions, ranging from idiopathic to dysplastic, traumatic, metabolic, or genetic, may produce angular deformities that progress and become symptomatic or even disabling if left unchecked. These conditions vary with respect to the age of onset and speed of progression, compromising gait and joint stability. Although the knee is most often affected, remote problems at the hip or ankle may also ensue.

The traditional orthopaedic approach has been to consider a corrective osteotomy (or multiple osteotomies) to realign the limb and restore function. Despite the perception that this is a definitive approach, the underlying condition may lead to recurrent deformity. Furthermore, an osteotomy is a major undertaking that is associated with significant pain, risks, and immobility while the bone heals. Supplemental casts or external frames may prove to be bulky and not well tolerated.

Hemiepiphysiodesis, by comparison, represents a minimally invasive approach that avoids many of the aforementioned drawbacks. The available methods include the following:

- **Stapling:** Introduced by Walter Blount around 1950, this technique has waxed and waned in popularity, mainly due to concerns regarding surgical trauma to the physis and to hardware migration or fatigue failure.
- **Percutaneous drilling:** Popularized in the 1980s; proponents cite the main advantages of a small scar and no retained hardware. However, because this drilling causes permanent physeal closure, it demands precise timing and meticulous follow-up. Over- or undercorrection are inherent risks, necessitating an osteotomy if calculations are incorrect or patients are noncompliant.
- **PETS:** Percutaneous epiphysiodesis using transphyseal screws was introduced in the 1980s and became more popular in the late 1990s. Most of these patients are adolescents who require relatively precise timing to achieve optimal results. Although the instrumentation is simple, there is a calculated risk of screw breakage or of producing a physeal bone bridge, thus making this method inappropriate for younger patients. No series has documented consistent physeal growth following screw removal.
- **Guided growth:** Plate hemiepiphysiodesis, which uses the 8-plate and a flexible construct of a nonlocking plate and two screws, allows one to achieve angular correction around a focal hinge that is typically at or near the level of deformity Center of Rotational Axis of Deformity (CORA).[9] The extraperiosteal plate serves as a tension band without risk of direct damage to the physis. Consequently, this technique can be applied even for very young children, including those with "sick" physes. Because of the relative ease and safety of this method, the remainder of this chapter will focus on this technique.

INDICATIONS/CONTRAINDICATIONS

Any surgically accessible physis (knee, ankle, elbow, wrist) and any direction of deformity (frontal, sagittal, oblique) may be considered for guided growth. Bilateral and multilevel deformities may be addressed simultaneously without requiring immobilization or hospitalization. Any size or age patient is a candidate, provided that there is at least 1 year of growth remaining.

The only contraindication to guided growth would be an unresectable physeal bar or physeal closure due to damage or maturity.

PREOPERATIVE PLANNING

Because guided growth is reversible, the timing of surgery is elective and does not require precise calculation—a major advantage of this technique over other techniques. Once the surgeon obtains a detailed history, including the duration and age of onset, functional limitations, prior treatment, and family history, he or she should carefully observe the gait pattern. The magnitude and direction of deformity should be noted, along with symmetry (or lack thereof), limb lengths, and spinal deformity. A neuromuscular examination should be undertaken, and concomitant rotational deformities, ligamentous laxity, patellar instability, or joint contracture should be sought and documented.

Radiographic assessment should include a weight-bearing, full-length, anteroposterior (AP) view of the legs with the patellae neutral. If there is a perceived length discrepancy, it is helpful to level the pelvis with blocks. Lateral radiographs of the extremities are warranted, as is consideration of a Merchant or similar patellar view if there are anterior knee pain symptoms.

On the AP view of the legs, the mechanical axis deviation and the various joint/shaft or metaphyseal/diaphyseal angles should be determined. Orienting the radiograph so that the femoral condyles rest on a horizontal axis should make it readily apparent whether to address the femur, the tibia, or both (Fig. 25-1A–1B). If deformity is at both levels, then a single plate per physis will afford the most rapid and appropriate correction.

The goal of treatment is to achieve equal limb lengths, neutral mechanical axes, and horizontal knee joints. This may require guided growth of the femur, the tibia, or both (Fig. 25-1C–1D). If this goal can be achieved solely with hemiepiphysiodesis and without osteotomies, then guided growth may be the method of choice for deformity correction. In general, approximately 1 cm of hemiphyseal growth around the knee will correct 10 degrees of deformity; this effect is amplified for taller individuals.

SURGICAL PROCEDURE

The following description pertains to frontal-plane knee deformities. With the patient supine under a general anesthetic, a thigh tourniquet is applied and inflated. The image intensifier is centered over the knee. A 3-cm incision is marked over the distal femoral and/or proximal tibial physis at the apex of the deformity. The skin is infiltrated with 0.25% bupivacaine with epinephrine. The incision is deepened by sharp dissection, dividing the fascia (e.g., iliotibial band, vastus medialis fascia) parallel to its fibers, leaving the underlying periosteum *undisturbed*. A Keith or hypodermic needle is inserted into the physis (Fig. 25-2), and its position is checked with the C-arm. Ideally this is placed in or slightly posterior to the midsagittal plane (unless the surgeon is treating an oblique plane deformity) so as not to produce or exacerbate recurvatum.

FIGURE 25-1 **A.** With the knee in the horizontal position, the mechanical axis should bisect the knee at an angle of 87 degrees. **B.** Although the obvious clinical deformity is at the knee, disturbed gait mechanics and the shear force imparted by gravity are producing collateral damage at the hip and ankle. If the surgeon chooses to only correct one level (femur vs. tibia), a sloping knee and physes will result. **C.** Six osteotomies (femur/tibia/fibula—bilateral) would be required to realign the limbs. This patient's father underwent such treatment and was anxious to avoid the same scenario if possible. **D.** Guided growth, using four individual plates and screws, is an alternative to osteotomies. The comparative safety and reduced cost make this biologic solution appealing (See Fig. 25-3).

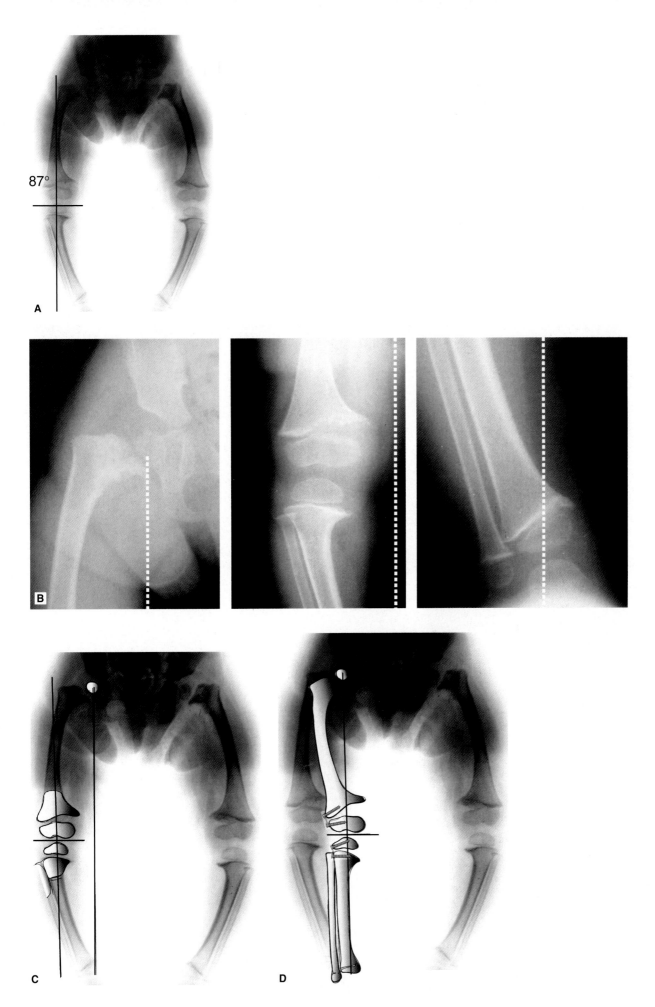

A

B

C

D

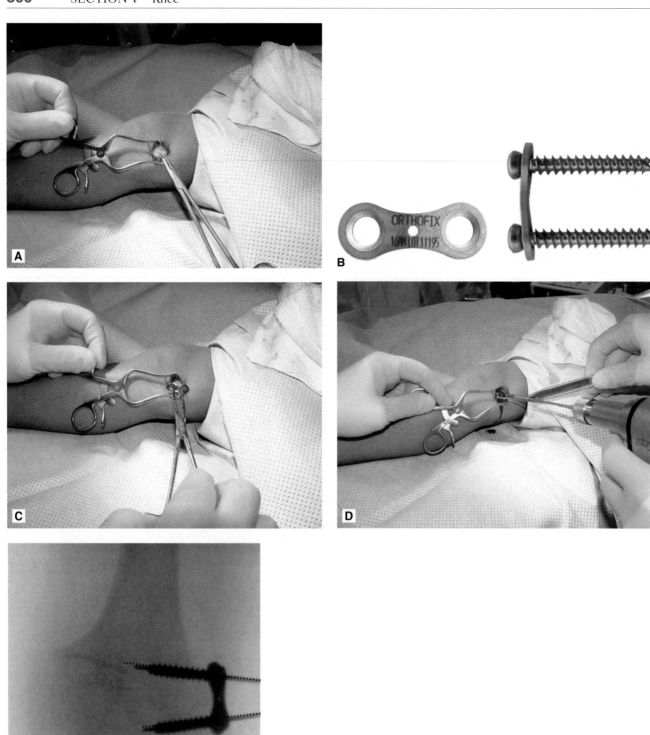

FIGURE 25-2   The 8-plate technique. **A.** A Keith needle is introduced into the physis and the plate is inserted **(B)** over the needle **(C). D.** Guide pins and screws are inserted. **E.** Screws are set above and below the physis. The screws do not need to be parallel.

The plate is centered on the needle and corresponding physis. The epiphyseal guide pin is inserted first, followed by the metaphyseal guide pin. It is not necessary for these to be parallel; however, it is critical that neither violates the adjacent joint or the physis. A 3.2-mm cannulated drill creates a "starter hole" (depth, 5 mm); drilling too deep may cause the guide pin to back out and/or may reduce the purchase afforded by the self-tapping screw-over. A 4.5-mm cannulated screw is inserted over each guide pin and is sequentially tightened. Usually only one plate is needed per physis. The exception to this would be inserting two anterior plates in the distal femur to correct fixed-knee flexion deformity. For this particular application, one plate is placed on each side of the patellofemoral sulcus, allowing the knee to gradually straighten.

POSTOPERATIVE MANAGEMENT

This is an outpatient procedure. A soft dressing is applied, and immediate weight bearing is encouraged, using crutches only for comfort as needed. The child may return to full activities and sports as motion and comfort permit. Follow-up is recommended at 3- to 4-month intervals to monitor the rate of correction. When the legs are straight, radiographs are repeated to document the normalization of the mechanical axis. When this axis is neutral, the plate is removed. Follow-up is continued periodically until maturity, repeating guided growth as needed.

COMPLICATIONS TO AVOID

Compared with osteotomy, the complications related to guided growth are negligible. Because the correction is gradual, there is no neurovascular risk. Because the bone is not cut, there is no need to await bone healing before resuming activities. There is no risk of malunion, loss of fixation, cast sores, compartment syndrome, or other conditions that may accompany an osteotomy. Furthermore, the aggregate cost of treatment is reduced accordingly.

Problems that sometimes accompany stapling, such as hardware fatigue or migration, are also averted. In addition, the speed of correction is faster with the plate technique because the flexible construct accommodates, rather than confronts, the physis. Typically most deformities correct within 12 months (±6), which is well within the stated guidelines of removing physeal restraints within 2 years of instrumentation, as is often stated in the stapling literature. Permanent physeal closure will not occur provided the periosteum is not surgically traumatized.

The only complication observed in more than 100 children treated since 2000 has been migration of 3.5-mm screws. When 4.5-mm screws were used instead, no loss of fixation occurred.

ILLUSTRATIVE CASE

A 21-month-old boy with hereditary metaphyseal dysplasia had varus of both the femora and the tibia, causing lateral knee thrust and pain with ambulation (Fig. 25-1). The patient was treated with guided growth, using four individual plates and screws. One year following pan genu–guided growth, he has experienced significant correction of genu valgum (Fig. 25-3). He is pain-free and fully active. His mechanical axis is improving, and his plates will be removed when the mechanical axis bisects the knee.

PEARLS/PITFALLS

- Pathologic angular deformities, regardless of the direction, etiology, or severity, may respond to guided growth using a two-hole plate and screws.
- It is imperative to *preserve the integrity of the periosteum* to avoid permanent and premature physeal closure.
- Guided growth offers a modular approach that may be applied for multilevel and even recurrent deformities in children of all ages.
- The relative ease, safety, and cost-benefit ratio all favor guided growth over the traditional osteotomy, which may be reserved for later correction of residual rotational deformities or length discrepancies.

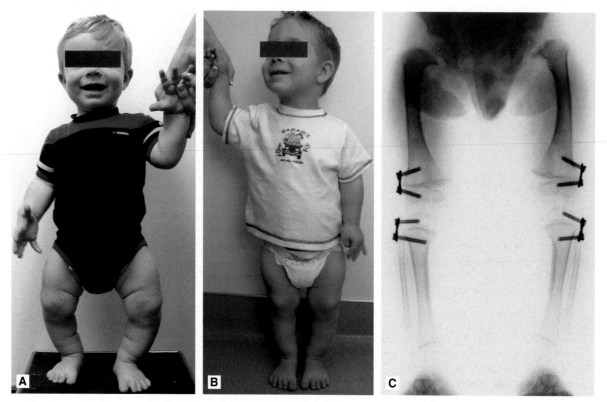

FIGURE 25-3   A. The patient is seen preoperatively at 21 months. **B, C.** Twelve months postoperatively. When the mechanical axes are netural, the plates are removed.

REFERENCES

1. Blount W, Clarke G. Control of bone growth by epiphyseal stapling. *J Bone Joint Surg Am.* 1949;464–478.
2. Bowen R, Johnson W. Percutaneous epiphysiodesis. *Clin Orthop Relat Res.* 1984;190:170–173.
3. Kramer S, Stevens P. Anterior femoral stapling. *J Pediatr Orthop.* 2001;21:804–807.
4. Metazeau J, Wong-Chung J, Bertrand H. Percutaneous epiphysiodesis using transphyseal screws (PETS). *J Pediatr Orthop.* 1998;18:363–369.
5. Mielke C, Stevens P. Hemiepiphyseal stapling for knee deformities in children younger than ten. *J Pediatr Orthop.* 1996;16:423–429.
6. Phemister D. Operative arrestment of longitudinal growth of bone in the treatment of deformities. *J Bone Joint Surg.* 1933;5:1–15.
7. Stevens P, MacWilliams B, Mohr A. Gait analysis of stapling for genu valgum. *J Pediatr Orthop.* 2004;24(1):70–74.
8. Stevens P, Maguire M, Dales M, et al. Physeal stapling for idiopathic genu valgum. *J Pediatr Orthop.* 1999;19:645–649.
9. Paley D. Principles of Deformity Correction, Springer-Verlag 2002.
10. Stevens P. Guided Growth for Angular Correction. *Journal of Pediatric Orthopaedics.* 2007; 27:253–259.
11. Stevens P. Guided Growth: 1933 to the Present. *Strat Traum Limb Recon.* 2006; 1:29–35.

26 Epiphysiodesis

William Warner

INDICATIONS/CONTRAINDICATIONS

Epiphysiodesis is a technique used to stop the growth of an open-growth plate or physis. The indications for epiphysiodesis, either complete or partial, are treatment of a leg-length inequality, correction of angular deformities, or prevention of a progressive limb-length inequality in a growing child. Several methods have been described to treat limb-length inequalities (Fig. 26-1). These methods range from a simple shoe lift to limb lengthening or limb shortening.[11,23,30] Although limb shortening can consist of an acute shortening of the femur or tibia, the most common method is slowing or stopping the growth of the longer extremity by epiphysiodesis.

Several methods have been described. Phemister[26] is credited with the first description of the epiphysiodesis technique. With the Phemister technique, a 1-cm rectangular bone block is removed from the lateral and medial aspects of the bone, with the bone block centered on the physis. The physis is curetted, and the bone block is reinserted after being rotated 180 degrees. White and Stubbins[35] described a technique using an osteotome or mortising chisel to remove intact a 1-in.-deep cube of bone containing the physis. A large portion of the remaining physis is removed with curettes. After the physis is curetted, the cube of bone is rotated 90 degrees and replaced in its original bed. Blount and Clarke[5] described the use of staples to obtain an epiphysiodesis, noting that three staples on each side (medial and/or lateral) were needed to stop growth of the physis. When one staple was used, the staple would break; when two staples were used, the staples would bend, leading to separation of the staple prongs. Indications for this technique have narrowed due to complications related to loosening or breakage of the staples and an often-unpredictable arrest of growth. Stevens reported the use of a single plate and screw construct that is based on the same principles of growth arrest as stapling but that has not reported the same complication from hardware failure as seen with stapling. Both Stevens technique and stapling have the theoretical advantage of normal growth resumption once correction has been achieved and hardware removed. However, this growth may not be fully predictable. Metaizeau et al.[19] described a technique for performing epiphysiodesis using screws placed percutaneously with fluoroscopic imaging across the physis in a diagonal or longitudinal fashion. The role of plate, screws, and staples in an epiphysiodesis is still evolving; as such, these techniques are used mainly for a hemiepiphysiodesis to treat an angular deformity.

The open Phemister technique of epiphysiodesis was the standard technique for obtaining growth arrest of the physis. However, it has currently been largely replaced by a percutaneous technique reported separately by Canale and Christian[6], Ogilvie and King[24], and Timperlake et al.[33] This new technique offers an attractive alternative to the traditional open procedures. Using image intensification, the growth plate is ablated with drills and curettes through small medial and lateral incisions. This technique, which has the advantage of giving reliable results with little morbidity, can be performed through small incisions, thus giving a better cosmetic result. The percutaneous technique for complete epiphysiodesis is the surgical technique described below.

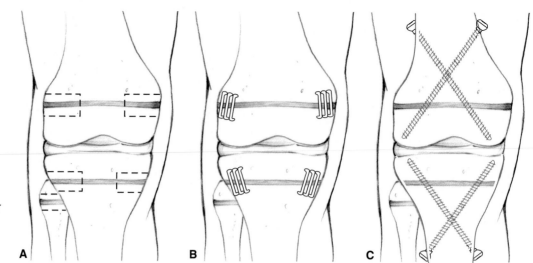

FIGURE 26-1

Epiphysiodesis can be done by several techniques. **A.** Phemister technique. **B.** Blount staples. **C.** Metaizeau technique.

PREOPERATIVE PLANNING

Several authors have reported that an error in timing the epiphysiodesis remains the main problem with using this technique for limb equalization.[4,7,8,14,16] The treating surgeon *must* be able to accurately predict the expected leg-length discrepancy at skeletal maturity. Remaining growth in the long leg and the short leg must be predicted accurately, and any growth inhibition in the involved extremity must be accounted for to ensure a successful result. Moseley[23] described three steps that must be done before recommending treatment for a leg-length discrepancy: (a) assessment of past growth, (b) prediction of future growth, and (c) prediction of the effect of surgery.

Several methods can be used to predict the growth remaining in the lower extremities. The four most-accepted methods of predicting the final leg-length discrepancy at maturity (Fig. 26-2) are (a) the growth-remaining charts of Anderson, Green, and Messner[2,3]; (b) the arithmetic method reported by Menelaus[18,34]; (c) Moseley's[21,22] straight-line graph; and (d) the multiplier method described by Paley et al.[1,25]

Potential inaccuracies certainly exist in the calculation of extremity growth remaining that is made to determine the timing of an epiphysiodesis. These inaccuracies can affect the final outcome obtained from surgery. The two most common sources of error are predictions of the exact date of skeletal maturity and the presence of any significant growth inhibition in the involved shorter extremity. Skeletal maturity or determination of the time that growth in the lower extremities will cease has been based on the patient's chronologic age or on the skeletal bone age as assessed radiographically. The inaccuracies of using only the chronologic age become obvious when one considers treatment of two 12-year-old girls. One 12-year-old girl can have a bone age of 14 years and be postmenarchal, with little growth remaining in the lower extremities. Another 12-year-old girl can have a bone age of 10 years and be premenarchal, with significant growth left in the lower extremities. Using the skeletal age as determined by a left hand and wrist anteroposterior (AP) radiograph for bone age, based on Gruelich and Pyle's[10] atlas of standards, may improve the accuracy of determining skeletal maturity, though this is still somewhat of an approximation. Menelaus[18] noted that if the bone age was within 1 year of the chronologic age, then the chronologic age would give an accurate assessment of skeletal maturity.

Growth inhibition of the involved extremities is another source of error. Shapiro[29] reported on five different patterns of growth inhibition. Yet even with these different patterns of growth inhibition, most evidence supports the assumption that the percentage of growth inhibition will remain constant throughout the growing years (i.e., if there is a 5% difference in limb lengths at birth, there will be a 5% difference in limb lengths once growth is complete).

The growth-remaining method of Anderson, Green, and Messner[2,3] is derived from data on the longitudinal growth of the femur and tibia, with a resultant estimation of the growth remaining in the femur and tibia. These data can be used to appropriately time an epiphysiodesis, as the study related leg-length growth to both chronologic and skeletal age. Describing leg length as a function of age allows one to determine the growth percentile of the child (e.g., 75th percentile on pediatric growth chart) and the amount of expected future growth of the femur and tibia. Although this method has been demonstrated to be accurate, the steps in calculating the final leg-length discrepancy and the percentage of growth inhibition must be followed as described by the authors. Proper use of this

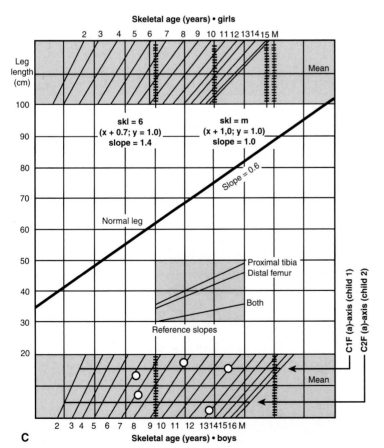

FIGURE 26-2 **A.** Growth-remaining charts of Anderson, Green, and Messner. **B.** Prerequisite growth information for the arithmetic method. **C.** Graph of Moseley straight-line method. **D.** Table of multiplier method for predicting limb length.

method requires the physician to estimate the percentage of growth inhibition based on at least two separate radiographic limb-length measurements taken at least 3 months apart.

The arithmetic method is based on the chronologic age and an estimation of the growth remaining in the distal femoral and proximal tibial physes. With this method, it is assumed that girls stop growing at 14 years of age and boys at 16 years of age. The distal femoral physis grows about 3/8 in. (10 mm) per year, and the proximal tibial physis grows about 1/4 in. (6 mm) per year. Menelaus[18] suggested that this method be used only in children whose skeletal age and chronologic age are less than 1 year apart.

Moseley[21,22] described a straight-line graph method for calculating leg-length discrepancy in the skeletally immature child and for determining the timing of long-leg epiphysiodesis to correct a leg-length inequality. This straight-line method is easy to use and gives a visual assessment of a leg-length discrepancy and of the predictive effect of a femoral and/or tibial epiphysiodesis. The graph is based on the data of the Anderson, Green, and Messner chart. By mathematically manipulating the original data, Moseley determined that a straight-line graph could be used. The difference in the slope of the two lines representing the long leg and the involved extremities represents the percentage of growth inhibition. The Moseley graph also uses a nomogram to help determine the growth percentile of the patient based on the skeletal age and the leg lengths. This method has been demonstrated to be accurate and relatively easy to use.[11,22]

Paley et al.[25] developed a multiplier method for predicting limb-length discrepancy at skeletal maturity. Using the Anderson, Green, and Messner data, these authors divided the expected femoral and tibial lengths at skeletal maturity by the femoral and tibial lengths at each age for each growth percentile group, resulting in a number called the *multiplier*. This multiplier is used in formulae to predict the expected final untreated limb-length discrepancy and the amount of growth remaining, thus allowing calculation of the timing of an epiphysiodesis. This method correlates closely with the Moseley straight-line graph and allows for a quick calculation of the predicted limb-length discrepancy at maturity.

Even with these four methods of determining leg-length discrepancy at maturity, however, the calculations remain an approximation and not an absolute value. Epiphysiodesis is recommended if the final leg-length discrepancy expected at skeletal maturity is between 2 and 6 cm. If the discrepancy at maturity is projected to be greater than 6 cm, a combination of epiphysiodesis and leg lengthening or limb lengthening only may need to be considered.[13,23]

SURGICAL PROCEDURE

The operation is performed under general anesthesia. Because this technique depends on intraoperative fluoroscopic imaging, a radiolucent operating table is usually used. Alternatively, a fracture table may be used with the limbs secured and draped free.

The longer limb is prepped and draped in a sterile fashion. A tourniquet can be used if desired. The limb is elevated off the operating table with a stack of towels or a sterile pillow beneath the calf (Fig. 26-3). A smooth K-wire is held over the skin, and the physis is localized fluoroscopically

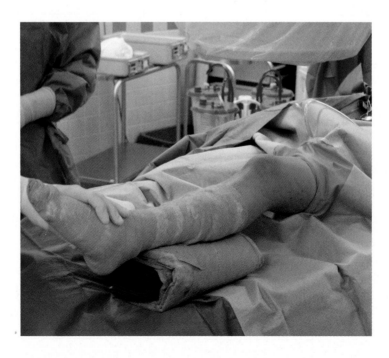

FIGURE 26-3

Patient set up on operating table.

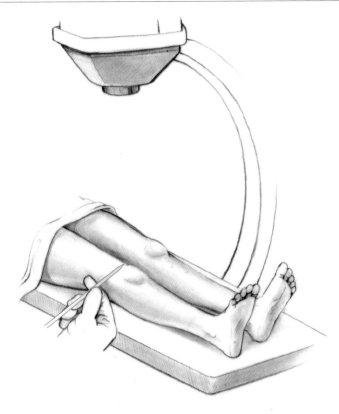

FIGURE 26-4

A smooth K-wire is used to localize the physis under image intensification.

(Fig. 26-4). A line is drawn along the skin with a skin marker to indicate the level of the physis on the AP projection (Fig. 26-5). The middle of the physis is identified on a lateral fluoroscopic projection, and another line is marked on the skin (Figs. 26-6 and 26-7). The intersection of these two lines will indicate where the skin incision should be made. A small incision, approximately 1.5 cm in length, is made.

A smooth guide wire is placed into the physis and drilled into the side of the distal lateral femoral physis. Correct positioning of the pin is confirmed on both AP and lateral fluoroscopic images (Fig. 26-8). Once the correct position of the guide wire is confirmed, a cannulated reamer and soft-tissue protector are placed over the guide wire. The physis is drilled to the midline, but *not across* the midline, with the guidance of fluoroscopy (Figs. 26-10). After removal of the reamer, a high-speed drill with a dental burr is introduced into the physeal area. The burr should be swept anteriorly and posteriorly and then superiorly and inferiorly to destroy a rectangular area of the lateral physis (Fig. 26-11). The skin should be protected with a skin guard to prevent damage from heat necrosis. Care should be taken not to cross the midline or enter the intercondylar notch of the femur.

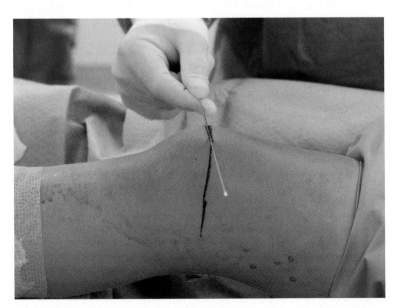

FIGURE 26-5

Physis is identified with a K-wire in the AP plane.

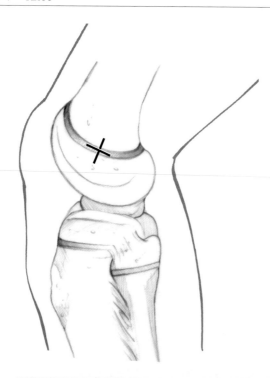

FIGURE 26-6

Lines are drawn on the skin on the AP and lateral to localize the incision.

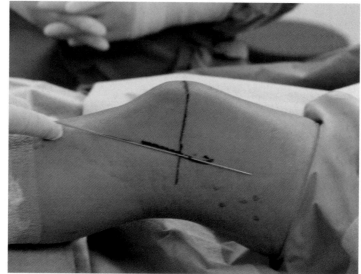

FIGURE 26-7

Physis is identified with a K-wire in the lateral plane.

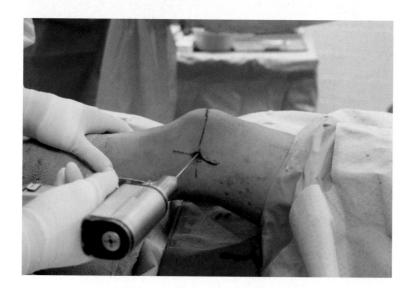

FIGURE 26-8

K-wire is drilled into the physis.

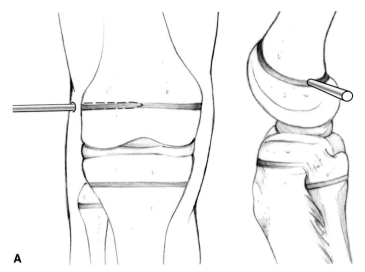

FIGURE 26-9

A. Smooth guide wire is placed in the physis in the AP plane. **B.** The position of the K-wire in the center of the physis is confirmed on the lateral radiographic image.

A

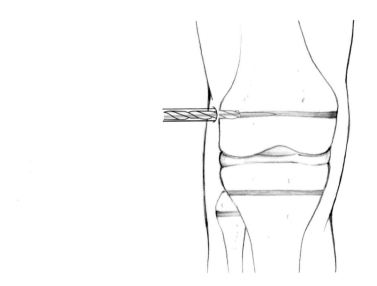

FIGURE 26-10

A cannulated reamer is used to destroy the physis over the smooth K-wire.

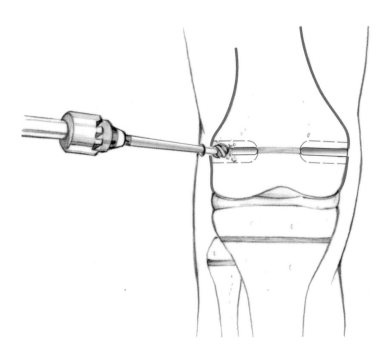

FIGURE 26-11

A burr is swept anterior and posterior and then inferior and superior to remove at least 50% of the involved physis.

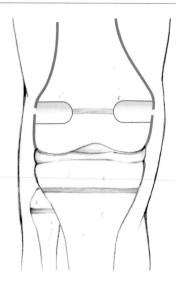

FIGURE 26-12

A rectangular area of the involved physis is removed.

At least 50% of the lateral physis should be removed either with the burr or with straight and angled curettes. A lucent area or blackout effect will be noted on fluoroscopic examination where the physis and surrounding bone have been removed (Fig. 26-12). The wound is thoroughly irrigated to remove all loose pieces of cartilage and cancellous bone. Thrombin and gel foam may be used to help decrease bleeding from the exposed bone. The wound is then closed with subcutaneous sutures.

The same technique is performed to remove the medial distal femoral physis. A similar technique may also be used to perform a proximal tibial epiphysiodesis. When the proximal fibula physis needs to be included in the epiphysiodesis, this can be done through the same incision for the lateral tibial physis or through a separate incision to avoid damage to the peroneal nerve. The fibula should be approached in an anterior-to-posterior direction to decrease the risk of damage to the peroneal nerve. Stephens et al.[31] recommended that the proximal fibular physis does not need epiphysiodesis if the patient has fewer than 3 to 4 years of skeletal growth remaining.

McCarthy[17] noted that fibular overgrowth of at least 1 cm was needed before the fibula became prominent and was usually not symptomatic unless overgrowth was greater than 2 cm, leading to the recommendation that proximal fibular epiphysiodesis be done if the expected overgrowth would exceed 1 to 2 cm.

POSTOPERATIVE MANAGEMENT

A compression dressing with an elastic wrap is applied. The family should be given instructions for loosening the elastic bandage in case distal leg and foot swelling occur in the limb. A knee immobilizer is fitted to the leg, and the patient is mobilized to bear weight as tolerated with crutches. Instructions for straight leg raise exercises to strengthen the quadriceps muscle in the immobilizer are given to the patient. One week postoperatively, range-of-motion exercises for the knee are begun and muscle strengthening is continued. Once knee range of motion is full and the quadriceps are strong, the knee immobilizer may be discontinued. Partial weight bearing with crutches is continued for 2 to 3 weeks after surgery. Sports are restricted for 8 weeks after surgery and are resumed only once there is a normal range of motion of the knee and normal quadriceps muscle function.

RESULTS

The Phemister technique has been the standard epiphysiodesis technique. Studies comparing the percutaneous technique with the Phemister technique have reported a shorter hospital stay, better cosmetic incisions, and a less frequent need for postoperative physical therapy.[6,9,15,24,27,28,33] One author noted that with the percutaneous technique, there may be increased bleeding from the bone into the soft tissue that may delay rehabilitation of the knee.[20] However, this problem can be avoided by use of a small drill and curette, as well as of thrombin and gel foam to help decrease the amount of bleeding.

Most studies have reported nearly a 100% closure rate of the physis after percutaneous epiphysiodesis, with few or no complications. Horton and Olney[12] did note continued growth after percutaneous epiphysiodesis in 13% of cases, compared with 15% of cases using the Phemister technique.

Correct timing continues to be the single most common cause for not obtaining the desired final correction with an epiphysiodesis.

COMPLICATIONS TO AVOID

Percutaneous epiphysiodesis has been shown to be a reliable method for obtaining a surgical growth arrest. Relatively few complications have been reported with this technique.

As with any surgery, however, postoperative infection is always a possibility. If there is an incomplete or asymmetric growth arrest, an angular deformity may develop.[32]

Excessive bleeding into the soft tissue from the exposed cancellous bone may occur but can be avoided by using a small drill and curette along with thrombin and gel foam. Fracture through the drill holes and the area of the physis removed is another possibility; this can be avoided with adherence to postoperative care recommendations.

Overcorrection or failure to obtain the desired correction can occur, but this is not a complication of the epiphysiodesis technique itself. Rather, it is a problem with the analysis of the available limb length and growth-remaining data and the timing of surgery prior to the percutaneous epiphysiodesis.

REFERENCES

1. Aguilar JA, Paley D, Paley J, et al. Clinical validation of the multiplier method for predicting limb length discrepancy and outcome of epiphysiodesis, part II. *J Pediatr Orthop.* 2005;25(2):192–196.
2. Anderson M, Green WT, Messner MB. Growth and predictions of growth in the lower extremities. *J Bone Joint Surg Am.* 1963;45:1–14.
3. Anderson M, Messner MB, Green WT. Distribution of lengths of the normal femur and tibia in children from one to eighteen years of age. *J Bone Joint Surg Am.* 1964;46:1197–1202.
4. Blair VP III, Walker SJ, Sheridan JJ, et al. Epiphysiodesis: a problem of timing. *J Pediatr Orthop.* 1982;2(3):281–284.
5. Blount WP, Clarke R. Control of bone growth by epiphyseal stapling: a preliminary report. *J Bone Joint Surg Am.* 1949;31:464–478.
6. Canale ST, Christian CA. Techniques for epiphysiodesis about the knee. *Clin Orthop Relat Res.* 1990(255):81–85.
7. Cundy P, Paterson D, Morris L. Skeletal age estimation in leg length discrepancy. *J Pediatr Orthop.* 1988;8(5):513–515.
8. Dewaele J, Fabry G. The timing of epiphysiodesis. A comparative study between the use of the method of Anderson and Green and the Moseley chart. *Acta Orthop Belg.* 1992;58(1):43–47.
9. Gabriel KR, Crawford AH, Roy DR, et al. Percutaneous epiphysiodesis. *J Pediatr Orthop.* 1994;14(3):358–362.
10. Greulich WW, Pyle SI. *Radiographic Atlas of Skeletal Development of the Hand and Wrist.* Palo Alto: Stanford University Press; 1959.
11. Herring JA. Limb length discrepancy. In: Herring JA, ed. *Tachdjian's Pediatric Orthopaedics.* 3rd ed. Philadelphia: WB Saunders; 2002:1039–1118.
12. Horton GA, Olney BW. Epiphysiodesis of the lower extremity: results of the percutaneous technique. *J Pediatr Orthop.* 1996;16(2):180–182.
13. Johnston CE II, Bueche MJ, Williamson B, et al. Epiphysiodesis for management of lower limb deformities. *Instr Course Lect.* 1992;41:437–444.
14. Kemnitz S, Moens P, Fabry G. Percutaneous epiphysiodesis for leg length discrepancy. *J Pediatr Orthop Br.* 2003;12(1):69–71.
15. Liotta FJ, Ambrose TA II, Eilert RE. Fluoroscopic technique versus Phemister technique for epiphysiodesis. *J Pediatr Orthop.* 1992;12(2):248–251.
16. Little DG, Nigo L, Aiona MD. Deficiencies of current methods for the timing of epiphysiodesis. *J Pediatr Orthop.* 1996;16(2):173–179.
17. McCarthy JJ, Burke T, McCarthy MC. Need for concomitant proximal fibular epiphysiodesis when performing a proximal tibial epiphysiodesis. *J Pediatr Orthop.* 2003;23(1):52–54.
18. Menelaus MB. Correction of leg length discrepancy by epiphyseal arrest. *J Bone Joint Surg Br.* 1966;48(2):336–339.
19. Metaizeau JP, Wong-Chung J, Bertrand H, et al. Percutaneous epiphysiodesis using transphyseal screws (PETS). *J Pediatr Orthop.* 1998;18(3):363–369.
20. Morrissy RT, Weinstein SL. *Percutaneous Distal Femoral Epiphysiodesis Atlas of Pediatric Orthopaedic Surgery.* 4th ed. Philadelphia: Lippincott Williams & Wilkins; 2006:550–554.
21. Moseley CF. A straight-line graph for leg-length discrepancies. *J Bone Joint Surg Am.* 1977;59(2):174–179.
22. Moseley CF. A straight-line graph for leg-length discrepancies. *Clin Orthop Relat Res.* 1978(136):33–40.
23. Moseley CF. Leg-length discrepancy. In: Morrissy RT, Weinstein SL, eds. *Lovell and Winter's Pediatric Orthopaedics.* 6th ed. Philadelphia: Lippincott Williams & Wilkins; 2006:1213–1256.
24. Ogilvie JW, King K. Epiphysiodesis: two-year clinical results using a new technique. *J Pediatr Orthop.* 1990;10(6):809–811.
25. Paley D, Bhave A, Herzenberg JE, et al. Multiplier method for predicting limb-length discrepancy. *J Bone Joint Surg Am.* 2000;82(10):1432–1446.
26. Phemister DB. Operative arrestment of longitudinal bone growth in the treatment of deformities. *J Bone Joint Surg Am.* 1933;15:1.
27. Porat S, Peyser A, Robin GC. Equalization of lower limbs by epiphysiodesis: results of treatment. *J Pediatr Orthop.* 1991;11(4):442–448.
28. Scott AC, Urquhart BA, Cain TE. Percutaneous vs. modified Phemister epiphysiodesis of the lower extremity. *Orthopedics.* 1996;19(10):857–861.
29. Shapiro F. Longitudinal growth of the femur and tibia after diaphyseal lengthening. *J Bone Joint Surg Am.* 1987;69(5):684–690.

30. Stanitski DF. Limb-length inequality: assessment and treatment options. *J Am Acad Orthop Surg*. 1999;7(3):143–153.
31. Stephens DC, Herrick W, MacEwen GD. Epiphysiodesis for limb length inequality: results and indications. *Clin Orthop Relat Res*. 1978(136):41–48.
32. Surdam JW, Morris CD, DeWeese JD, et al. Leg length inequality and epiphysiodesis: review of 96 cases. *J Pediatr Orthop*. 2003;23(3):381–384.
33. Timperlake RW, Bowen JR, Guille JT, et al. Prospective evaluation of fifty-three consecutive percutaneous epiphysiodeses of the distal femur and proximal tibia and fibula. *J Pediatr Orthop*. 1991;11(3):350–357.
34. Westh RN, Menelaus MB. A simple calculation for the timing of epiphysial arrest: a further report. *J Bone Joint Surg Br*. 1981;63(1):117–119.
35. White JW, Stubbins SG. Growth arrest for equalizing leg lengths. *J Am Med Assoc*. 1944;126:1146.

27 Operative Treatment of Tibia Vara

Perry L. Schoenecker and J. Eric Gordon

EARLY-ONSET/INFANTILE TIBIA VARA

Indications/Contraindications

The indication for a proximal tibial varus-correcting osteotomy in the treatment of infantile tibia vara (Blount disease) is the presence of pathologic Langenskiöld radiographic changes involving the proximal medial tibial epiphysis, physis, and metaphysis. These patients typically have had a bow-legged deformity noted since they began walking. Following a proximal varus-correcting osteotomy, sustained restoration of normal proximal medial physeal growth is more predictable if surgery is performed earlier in childhood (≤4 years of age) and the Langenskiöld stage is less than IV.[8]

Contraindications for proximal tibial osteotomy include lack of radiographic evidence of true tibia vara (i.e., the diagnosis of physiologic bowing).

Preoperative Planning

In the preoperative planning for treating infantile tibia vara in children 3 to 6 years of age, it is assumed that the deformity will be definitively corrected with a proximal osteotomy of the tibia and fibula. The osteotomy is performed in a transverse plane, allowing correction of frontal, sagittal, and rotational deformities. Fixation in this younger age group is provided with K-wires. Intraoperative correction of the varus deformity is assessed both visually and radiographically.[9]

Older children (≥7–8 years of age) with long-standing infantile Blount disease often have a varus deformity that may also include early medial proximal tibial physeal closure, medial tibial plateau depression, internal tibial torsion, shortening in the proximal tibia, and, occasionally, distal femoral valgus deformity.[4,9] For these deformities, additional surgical procedures, as well as a proximal tibial varus osteotomy, will usually be necessary to comprehensively treat the increasingly complex deformity.

Surgical Procedure

Children undergoing a proximal tibial fibular osteotomy are positioned supine on a radiolucent operating room table. *Both* lower extremities are prepped and draped, exposing each from the level of the proximal thigh to the toes. In unilateral procedures, exposure of both extremities allows for comparison of the intraoperative correction of the involved leg to the alignment of the uninvolved extremity. A sterile tourniquet is applied on the upper thigh, and prophylactic antibiotics are administered prior to inflation of the tourniquet.

The proximal tibia is approached through a longitudinal incision centered over the anteromedial tibia overlying the anticipated site of the tibial osteotomy. Subcutaneous flaps are raised medially, exposing the tibia's anteromedial surface. The overlying periosteum is incised, and the tibia is subperiosteally exposed circumferentially distal to the tibial tubercle. An image intensifier is helpful in selecting the appropriate site of the tibial osteotomy (Fig. 27-1).

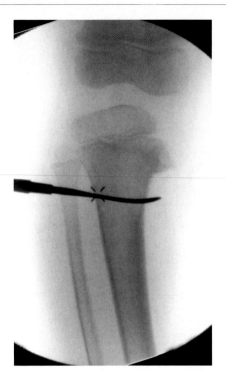

FIGURE 27-1

Intraoperative image intensifier anteroposterior (AP) views of the proximal tibia, showing the intended site of osteotomy.

Once the site of the tibial osteotomy has been selected, the wound is packed with a moist sponge while the fibular osteotomy is done. The fibula is approached through a 3- to 4-cm longitudinal incision centered over the lateral intramuscular septum. The anatomic interval between the posterior edge of the lateral compartment and the posterior compartment is developed, providing the most direct approach to the proximal fibula. The deepest portion of the peroneal muscle that surrounds the fibula and the underlying periosteum is incised and elevated, exposing the fibular diaphysis. Small subperiosteal retractors are carefully placed around the entire fibula. The fibula osteotomy is then done in a transverse plane with an oscillating saw, 2 cm distal to the intended site of the tibial osteotomy. Caution must be taken to avoid directly or indirectly injuring neurovascular structures (peroneal nerve motor branches to the anterior compartment and adjacent veins) lying just medial to the fibula. The fibular wound is then packed with a moist sponge.

An oscillating saw is used to perform a transverse tibial osteotomy distal to the tibial tubercle (Fig. 27-2A). The bone ends at the osteotomy site are aligned. The goal is to both correct the varus deformity and realign the tibia so the mechanical axis of the lower extremity is translated from its pathologic medial location to a point lateral to the center of the knee joint. Any sagittal-plane deformity (recurvatum or procurvatum) is corrected. The correct rotational alignment is achieved by aligning the second toe of the foot with the proximal tibial tubercle. Two or three 5/64-in. smooth K-wires are used for fixation of the tibial osteotomy (Fig. 27-2B).

FIGURE 27-2

A. Transverse osteotomy performed distal to the tibial apophysis. **B.** Smooth K-wires are used for fixation.

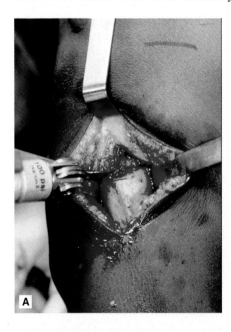
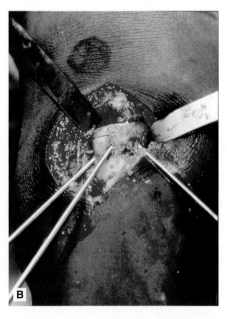

The correction is assessed visually and radiographically. If the varus deformity has been adequatel corrected, the tibia should assume a position of slight valgus alignment without any assistance. If the leg has to be manually held in a position of slight valgus at the knee but, when released, resumes a varus position at the knee, then the lower-extremity alignment is undercorrected. Sufficient correction is essential, so that after healing, as the patient begins weight bearing, the lower extremity will assume a slight valgus position. If the leg is undercorrected at the time of surgery, tibia vara will persist when the patient resumes weight bearing. In unilateral deformities, the correction obtained on the involved extremity can be compared with the prepped, but uninvolved, extremity. However, the surgeon should keep in mind that there is often some physiologic bowing present in the uninvolved extremity.

The most definitive intraoperative assessment of correction is done radiographically and can be obtained with the electrocautery cord and fluoroscopic evaluation (Fig. 27-3). The electrocautery cord is stretched from the center of the hip joint to the center of the ankle joint, simulating the lower extremity's mechanical axis. While the electrocautery cord is held in this position, it should be seen in the center of the knee joint on the AP fluoroscopic view. With the leg at rest, satisfactory correction of varus deformity into a slight valgus position has been obtained if the electrocautery cord courses lateral to the center of the knee joint on this AP image. This technique for assessing the mechanical axis allows for repositioning of the osteotomy and the K-wires as necessary.

The fibular osteotomy is palpated to ensure that the fragments are displaced, overriding, and not interfering with correction of the tibial deformity. No fixation is used on the fibular osteotomy. A suction drain is placed at the tibial osteotomy site and brought out through a stab incision. Tibial periosteal tissues are reapproximated as possible. The fascial opening into the anterior compartment that occurs during both exposure and/or osteotomy of the tibia is not closed. In some cases, a prophylactic anterior compartment fasciotomy distal to the tibial osteotomy site is used. Similarly, the interfascial dissection used to expose the fibula is not closed with sutures.

The subcutaneous tissues and skin are closed; the K-wires are left outside the skin and are bent over. A sterile dressing is placed, the drain is attached to a suction apparatus, and the tourniquet is deflated.

A long-leg cast is applied, with the foot in neutral dorsiflexion and the knee slightly bent. The undercast padding is split before applying the cast. The cast is bivalved and spread before bringing the patient to the postoperative recovery area.

Postoperative Management

The drain is typically removed on postoperative day 1 or 2, and the patient is then discharged. Patients are evaluated postoperatively at 2 weeks with a clinical assessment, including radiographs, to verify that the intraoperative correction has been maintained. The cast is removed at approximately 6 weeks in the operating room, and radiographs are taken at this time to assess healing. The K-wires are removed, and a new long-leg cast is applied, with planned removal in 3 weeks as an outpatient procedure. The patient is allowed to bear weight on the operated leg after cast removal. For very severe deformities (typically with associated ligamentous laxity), consideration may be given to measuring for a knee-ankle-foot orthosis (KAFO) at the time of cast change and pin removal in the operating room. For these patients, the KAFO is applied at the time of final cast removal.

The same osteotomy fixation technique is used for obese patients age 7 and younger. However, because of the disproportionately large thigh girth of these children, the best-applied long-leg cast is often not enough to satisfactorily protect the osteotomy. In young obese patients, a hip spica cast is a more appropriate postoperative means of temporary immobilization and protection of the osteotomy. The spica cast is changed to a long-leg cast following pin removal at 6 weeks as noted above.

As the patient resumes standing and walking, the corrected extremity will appear to be in a slight valgus alignment. Radiographic verification of correction of the varus deformity is best shown with standing radiographs of the lower extremity. If utilized, the KAFOs are gradually discontinued in the ensuing 4 to 6 months. Follow-up, including both clinical exams and x-rays, is essential to ensure that the correction has been maintained (Fig. 27-4). Despite initial satisfactory growth of the proximal medial tibia, recurrence can occur early; in the authors' experience, this can occur even several years later, in childhood or adolescence.

Complications to Avoid

In the past, a tibial osteotomy was considered one of the most complicated elective operations in pediatric orthopaedics.[10] Neurovascular injuries can occur both directly and indirectly. Direct nerve injuries can occur either during the dissection necessary to obtain circumferential exposure of the tibia and the fibula during the osteotomy or during manipulation of the osteotomy. In performing the osteotomy, one must be cautious to avoid penetrating the soft tissues deep to the osteotomy. Particularly when performing a fibular osteotomy, the more distal motor branches of the peroneal nerve and peroneal vein are at risk, as they course along the fibula's medial shaft. Placing small retractors subperiosteally around the fibula will help minimize penetrating beyond the osteotomy with either a saw or an osteotome.

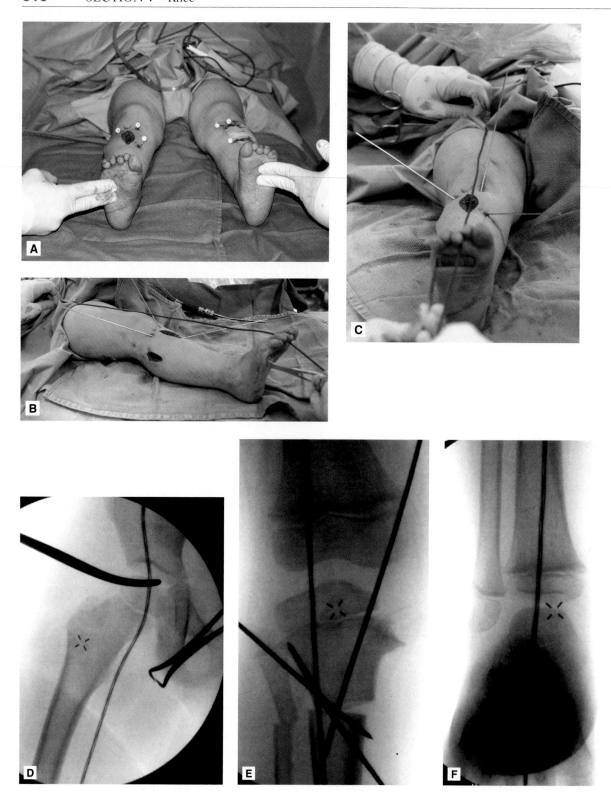

FIGURE 27-3   A. Appearance of both lower extremities after proximal tibial and fibular valgus osteotomy. **B, C.** The electrocautery cord is positioned from the center of the femoral head to the center of the ankle joint. **D.** Fluoroscopic view of the electrocautery cord position over the center of the femoral head. **E.** Fluoroscopic view of the electrocautery cord position over the distal tibia at the ankle joint. **F.** Fluoroscopic view of the electrocautery cord passing over the knee joint, demonstrating that the tibia vara has been overcorrected into slight valgus.

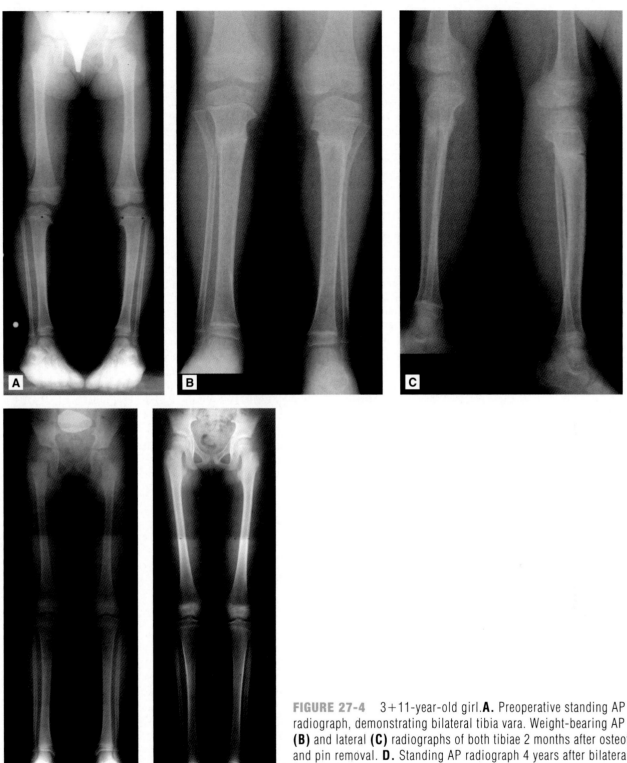

FIGURE 27-4   3+11-year-old girl.**A.** Preoperative standing AP radiograph, demonstrating bilateral tibia vara. Weight-bearing AP **(B)** and lateral **(C)** radiographs of both tibiae 2 months after osteotomy and pin removal. **D.** Standing AP radiograph 4 years after bilateral proximal tibial osteotomies.**E.** Standing long radiograph 6 years after bilateral proximal tibial osteotomies without recurrence of tibia vara.

   With the correction of tibial varus, indirect nerve injuries (uncommon) can occur where the peroneal nerve is tethered as it penetrates the crural fascia. (This usually occurs in older patients, >8–9 years, undergoing acute correction.[10]) If postoperative tethering of the peroneal nerve is suspected, the nerve should be surgically decompressed as it enters proximally into the anterolateral crural fascia. The risk of compartment syndrome (particularly the anterior compartment) can be minimized by leaving all fascial incisions open and using suction drainage. In addition, utilizing only K-wires to stabilize the osteotomies in smaller children helps avoid the additional bulk of a plate and screws, which can be an indirect cause of vascular insufficiency in the anterolateral compartments of the leg.

LATE-ONSET TIBIA VARA

Indications/Contraindications

In contrast to early-onset infantile tibia vara, patients with late-onset tibia vara are typically 8 or 9 years of age or older before a varus deformity of the leg and knee is noted. Late-onset tibia vara frequently occurs in association with distal femoral varus, proximal tibial procurvatum, internal tibial torsion, distal tibial valgus, and lateral collateral ligament laxity.[1,4,7,12] When diagnosed, late-onset tibia vara should be surgically treated. Patients with open physes should first be considered for correction by hemiepiphyseal stapling to correct the varus deformity.[7] Patients who are skeletally mature or who have inadequate growth to allow correction with hemiepiphyseal stapling should be treated by varus-correcting osteotomy of the proximal tibia, as well as a concomitant varus-correcting osteotomy of the distal femur.[1,11]

Preoperative Planning

Preoperative planning for children and adolescents with late-onset tibia vara is more demanding than it is for younger children. Older children with tibia vara are frequently obese and can have obesity-related complications, such as obstructive sleep apnea.[2] After appropriate medical workup, a standing anteroposterior radiograph of both lower extremities should be obtained on a 36- or 51-in.-long radiographic cassette. A lateral radiograph of the knee showing the tibial shaft should also be obtained. If there is concern of possible distal tibial valgus, an additional standing anteroposterior radiograph of both ankles extending to the tibial shaft should be obtained. These radiographs should be analyzed to determine the presence of distal femoral varus or valgus, proximal tibial varus and procurvatum, distal tibial valgus, and lateral collateral ligament laxity. The exact bone location of the deformities should also be assessed.[4,5,6] The authors have utilized the methods of Paley and Tetsworth[5,6] (Fig. 27-5A) in evaluating these deformities by measuring the mechanical axis deviation (MAD), the lateral distal femoral angle (LDFA), the medial proximal tibial angle (MPTA), and the lateral distal tibial angle (LDTA). Proximal tibial sagittal-plane deformity (Fig. 27-5B) should be evaluated by measuring the posterior proximal tibial angle (PPTA).

Based on the analysis, an overall surgical strategy should be planned for single-stage correction of all deformities. The most common distal femoral deformity in patients with late-onset tibia vara is distal femoral varus. Although distal femoral valgus is uncommon, it may be seen in older patients

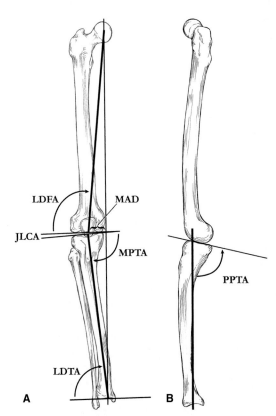

FIGURE 27-5

A. Coronal-plane illustration of the lower extremity, demonstrating the mechanical axis deviation (MAD), the lateral distal femoral angle (LDFA), the joint-line congruency angle (JLCA), the medial proximal tibial angle (MPTA), and the lateral distal tibial angle (LDTA). **B.** Sagittal-plane illustration of the proximal part of the tibia and the distal part of the femur, demonstrating the posterior proximal tibial angle (PPTA).

Gordon JE, Heidenrich FP, Carpenter CJ, Kelly-Hahnj, Schoenecker PL. Comprehensive treatment of late-onset tibia vara. J Bone Joint Surg 8/A, 2005:1561–70.

with untreated, severe, early-onset tibia vara.[4] The authors' threshold for correction of the femoral deformity has been more than 5 degrees of deformity from normal. Thus, patients with distal femoral varus and an LDFA of 92 degrees or greater or with distal femoral valgus and an LDFA of 82 degrees or less should be corrected. This level of femoral deformity can be corrected by osteotomy with blade-plate fixation or, in the case of patients with open physes, by hemiepiphysiodesis using either Blount staples (Zimmer, Warsaw, Indiana) or an eight plate (Orthofix, McKinney, Texas). The tibial deformities can be corrected by proximal and, if needed, distal tibial osteotomies, followed by gradual correction with a circular external fixator.[1,11] Lateral collateral ligament laxity can be corrected by distal transport of the proximal fibula, resulting in tightening of the lateral collateral ligament.

Surgical Procedure

Children older than 8 years should be positioned supine on a radiolucent table, with a bump placed under the hip. If, a distal femoral osteotomy is required, and it is performed through a lateral incision under tourniquet control. The opening-wedge femoral osteotomy is stabilized by a 95-degree condylar blade plate. If, a fibular osteotomy is required, and it is completed before closing the incision for the femoral osteotomy. The fibular osteotomy is performed through a 4-cm posterolateral longitudinal incision over the junction of the proximal and middle thirds of the fibula. (If lateral collateral ligament laxity is present, the fibula will require distal transport, and no fibular osteotomy is performed.)

The posterolateral intermuscular interval is developed between the posterior and lateral muscle compartments. The peroneal musculature is retracted anteriorly, exposing the periosteum of the fibula. The periosteum is sharply opened, and with careful dissection approximately 2 to 3 cm, the fibula is exposed both subperiosteally and circumferentially. An oscillating saw is used to carefully remove a 1-cm section of fibula. As with younger patients, care should be taken to minimize any injury to the neurovascular structures lying just medial to the fibula. The fibular section is placed into the femoral opening-wedge osteotomy site as bone graft, and both the femoral and the fibular wounds are closed in layers, leaving the fascia open over the fibular osteotomy. A drain (e.g., Hemovac) is placed beneath the fascia lata at the femoral osteotomy site. The tourniquet is then deflated but left in place.

Planning for the proximal and, if needed, distal tibial osteotomy should be completed preoperatively. A circular external fixator is preconstructed prior to surgery to allow gradual correction of the deformities. The authors' preference has been to use a Taylor Spatial Frame (Smith-Nephew, Memphis, TN). To predictably obtain a satisfactory outcome when utilizing this method, attention to the details of preoperative planning is imperative. The tibia deformity is carefully analyzed to identify both its plane and its degree of severity. Once the desired correction is selected, the software program determines the location and sequence of correction for closing fixation application. If the patient is skeletally immature, a single-proximal full ring is used to stabilize the proximal fragment (Fig. 27-6). If the patient is skeletally mature, a ring block of two 2/3 rings separated by two-hole Rancho cubes

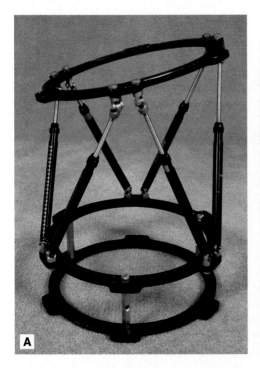

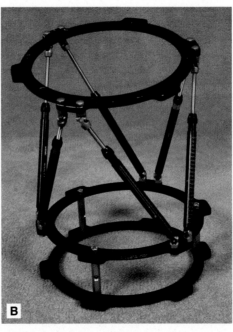

FIGURE 27-6

A, B. Single-proximal full-ring frame for stabilization of the proximal fragment in skeletally immature patients.

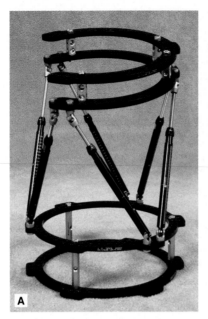

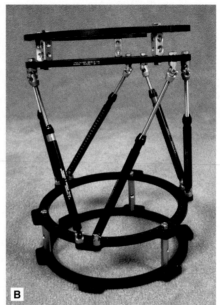

FIGURE 27-7

A, B. Double-proximal 2/3-ring frame for stabilization of the proximal fragment in skeletally mature patients.

can be used to stabilize the proximal fragment (Fig. 27-7). This preconstructed external fixator is then placed over the leg and suspended from the leg using suction tubing (Fig. 27-8).

With the tourniquet deflated, a proximal olive wire is placed from lateral to medial under fluoroscopic guidance approximately 5 mm distal to the physis in skeletally immature patients or 5 mm distal to the joint in skeletally mature patients. The wire is then tensioned and secured to the proximal ring, leaving at least a 2-cm gap between the ring and the anterior leg and a 4-cm gap between the ring and the posterior leg. A distal transverse lateral-to-medial olive wire is then placed within 5 mm of the ankle joint if a distal tibial osteotomy is planned or within 5 cm of the joint if no distal osteotomy is required. This wire is then tensioned and secured to the distal ring. The smooth proximal and distal transfibular wires are placed and secured. However, if distal transport of the fibula is needed to tighten the lateral collateral ligament, no proximal transfibular wire is placed. One or two additional proximal transverse wires are placed and secured. If a distal tibial osteotomy is required, an additional medial-to-lateral transverse wire is added distally. Titanium half-pins are then added proximally, one anteromedially and one anterolaterally. Two or three anteromedial half-pins are placed into the distal shaft of the tibia and secured to the middle or distal rings. The authors prefer 5- or 6-mm titanium half-pins.

After the external fixator has been secured, the anterior two struts are removed to allow access to the anterior leg and to destabilize the fixator. Next, the proximal tibial osteotomy is performed. The tourniquet is once again elevated, and an anterior 4-cm longitudinal incision is made over the proximal anteromedial tibia, just distal to the proximal transfixing wires. Sharp dissection is used to obtain direct exposure of the periosteum of the tibia; the periosteum is then incised (Fig. 27-9). The tibia is circumferentially exposed subperiosteally, taking care to avoid the anterior tibial artery laterally and the neurovascular bundle posteriorly (Fig. 27-10). A 4.8-mm drill bit is used to create multiple transverse bicortical drill holes in the tibia, approximately 1 cm distal to the proximal fixation (Fig. 27-11). With subperiosteal retractors protecting the soft tissues, an Ilizarov osteotome

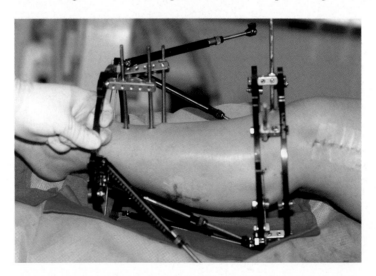

FIGURE 27-8

Intraoperative application of preconstructed double-proximal 2/3-ring frame. (A femoral osteotomy with plate fixation was also done.)

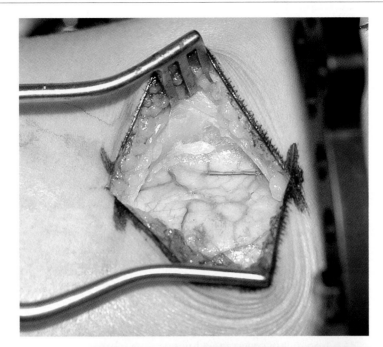

FIGURE 27-9

Exposure of the proximal anterior medial tibia through a 4-cm longitudinal incision.

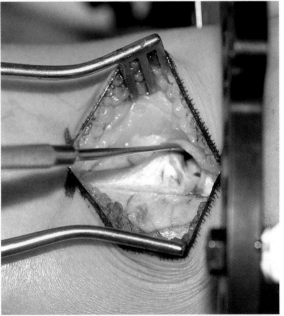

FIGURE 27-10

Subperiosteal circumferential exposure of the tibia is carried out, taking care to avoid the anterior tibial artery laterally and the neurovascular bundle posteriorly.

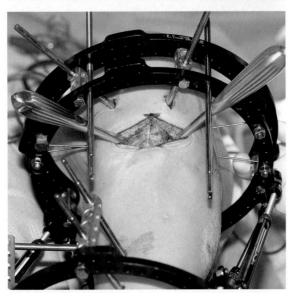

FIGURE 27-11

Crego elevators protect the soft tissues after exposure of the proximal tibia. Long half-pins through holes on the frame hold the retractors in place.

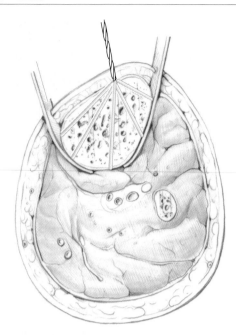

FIGURE 27-12

Anatomical transverse cut through the lower extremity, showing the multiple bicortical drill holes in the tibia. This is done approximately 1 cm distal to the proximal fixation.

is used to carefully connect the drill holes, thereby completing the osteotomy (Fig. 27-12). This is confirmed with the image intensifier (Fig. 27-13). The periosteum is approximated using absorbable sutures, and the wound is closed in layers. The tourniquet is again deflated and dressings applied.

Postoperative Management

The patient is mobilized with crutches on postoperative day 1, at which time weight bearing is encouraged and physical therapy begins. Gradual deformity correction is begun with the spatial frame on postoperative day 2 to 4. Dressings are left in place and changed on postoperative day 5 to 7. The patient then begins taking daily showers, cleaning the pin sites with soap and water.[3] Weekly radiographs are obtained to monitor bone formation and deformity correction. As the progress of daily strut turning is completed, the deformity should correct. Definitive assessment of deformity correction is determined with a standing anteroposterior radiograph of both lower extremities and a lateral radiograph of the knee showing the tibial shaft. Correction of any residual deformity can be performed at any point during this time.

After the deformity is completely corrected, the rings should be locked in place using three threaded rods with removal of the struts. Radiographs of the tibia should be obtained monthly during

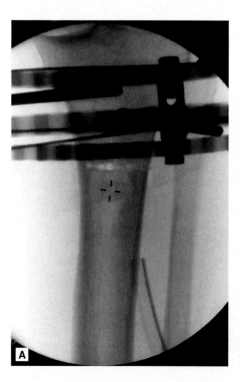
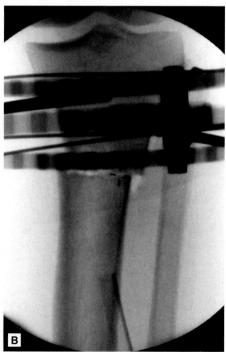

FIGURE 27-13

A, B. Intraoperative radiographs, demonstrating completion of the proximal tibial osteotomy after multiple drill holes have been made in the proximal tibia.

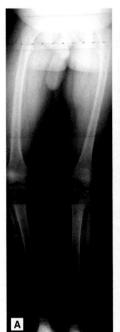
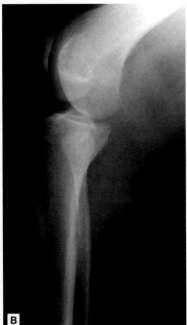
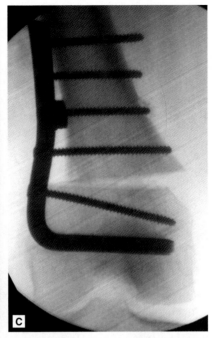
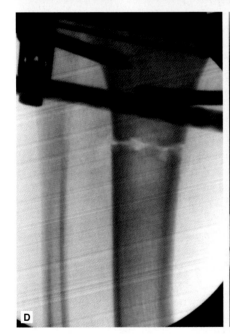
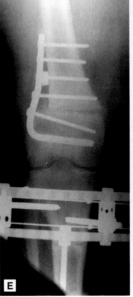
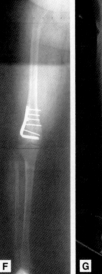
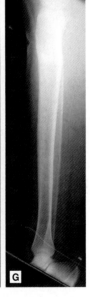

FIGURE 27-14

This 15-year-old boy had progressive bowing of the right lower extremity. **A.** Preoperative standing AP radiograph with a lateral distal femoral angle of 102 degrees, a medial proximal tibial angle of 82 degrees, and a lateral distal tibial angle of 89 degrees. **B.** A posterior proximal tibial angle of 77 degrees and medial mechanical axis deviation. **C.** Intraoperative fluoroscopic AP view, showing the completed varus-correcting distal femoral osteotomy stabilized with a 95-degree condylar blade plate. **D.** The completed proximal tibial osteotomy is stabilized with circular frame fixation. **E.** AP radiograph of the distal femur and proximal tibia taken 3 months postoperatively shows consolidation of both osteotomies, with correction of both distal femoral varus deformity and proximal tibial varus deformity. **F.** Standing AP radiograph of right lower extremity taken 6 months postoperatively shows normal alignment and joint orientation. **G.** The lateral standing radiograph demonstrates correction of proximal tibial procurvatum.

this consolidation period to monitor healing. Dynamization should be performed by sequentially removing the three threaded rods as bone consolidation and healing progress.

When the patient has been full weight bearing for 2 weeks with only a single threaded rod spanning the osteotomy site, the external fixator can be removed under general anesthesia. Typically, no additional immobilization is required, and the patient is encouraged to progressively increase his or her activity (Fig. 27-14).

Complications to Avoid

As with any external-fixator application, transfixing wires must be placed with the utmost knowledge and awareness of the leg's neurovascular anatomy. Precise wire placement is essential in both achieving external fixator stability and avoiding nerve and/or arterial injury. Often even in obese patients, the peroneal nerve is palpable passing from proximal to distal around the fibular neck. When placing a transfibular wire in this area, the nerve should be palpated; when the wire is introduced, it should be repositioned if the nerve is irritated.

Similarly, the tibial osteotomy is carefully performed with drills and an osteotomy. It is essential to take great care to avoid injuring neurovascular structures deep to the osteotomy site with either the drills or the osteotome.

PEARLS AND PITFALLS

Infantile Tibia Vara

- Waiting too long to perform the varus-correcting osteotomy in the treatment of infantile Blount disease—delay beyond 4 to 5 years of age potentiates progressive growth-plate pathology.
- Follow-up assessment is essential, as recurrence can occur.
- In performing a varus-correcting osteotomy in the treatment of infantile Blount disease:
  - Utilize a simple transverse osteotomy technique with K-wire fixation to facilitate intraoperative adjustment of the osteotomy.
  - Because varus deformity is often both bony and ligamentous, confirm both visually and fluoroscopically that full correction of the varus deformity has been achieved.
  - Do not close the fascial incision into the anterolateral compartments.
  - Adequate cast immobilization is essential with this technique. Most extremities can be satisfactorily protected with a long-leg cast. Occasionally, however, for the obese and relatively short extremity, a spica cast is necessary to ensure adequate immobilization.

Infantile or Late-Onset Tibia Vara

- Approach the fibula posterior to the peroneal musculature along the lateral intramuscular septum to minimize trauma to the lateral muscular compartment.

Varus Deformity in Late-Onset Tibia Vara

- Typically there is pathologic varus of both the proximal tibia and the distal femur. In planning deformity correction, it is imperative not to ignore the distal femoral varus in late-onset tibia vara. Overcorrection of the tibia to compensate for existing femoral varus leads to an oblique frontal plane knee-joint deformity. Even a normal-appearing distal femur may have a varus deformity, as the relative hip abduction that occurs with a genu varum deformity allows the knee joint line to remain horizontal. Distal femoral varus should be corrected if the LDFA is more than 92 degrees.
- Remember to evaluate the contralateral limb. Often patients with seemingly unilateral tibia vara will, in actuality, have bilateral deformity. The severity of the deformity in one limb frequently obscures the fact that a mild deformity is present in the contralateral limb.
- Careful attention should be paid to any laxity in the lateral collateral ligament. The inclination is to ignore the laxity, which can lead to uncorrected residual varus, or to overcorrect the tibial varus, compensating for the varus with valgus in the tibia. This can lead to pathologic genu valgum, which is particularly noticeable in obese patients.
- Hemiepiphysiodesis treatment with staples or eight-plates can be effective in treating late-onset tibia vara. If used with sufficient growth remaining, hemiepiphysiodesis may be definitive in correcting all aspects of the varus deformity, without the need for osteotomy.

REFERENCES

1. Gordon JE, Heidenreich F, Carpenter CJ, et al. Comprehensive treatment of late-onset tibia vara. *J Bone Joint Surg Am.* 2005;87:1561–1570.
2. Gordon JE, Hughes MS, Shepherd K, et al. Obstructive sleep apnea syndrome in morbidly obese children with tibia vara. *J Bone Joint Surg Br.* 2006;88:100–103.
3. Gordon JE, Kelly-Hahn J, Carpenter C, et al. Pin site care during external fixation in children: results of a nihilistic approach. *J Pediatr Orthop.* 2000;20:163–165.
4. Gordon JE, King DJ, Luhmann SJ, et al. Femoral deformity in tibia vara. *J Bone Joint Surg Am.* 2006;87:1561–1569.
5. Paley D, Tetsworth K. Mechanical axis deviation of the lower limbs: preoperative planning of multiapical frontal plane angular and bowing deformities of the femur and tibia. *Clin Orthop.* 1992;280:65–71.
6. Paley D, Tetsworth K. Mechanical axis deviation of the lower limbs: preoperative planning of uniapical angular deformities of the tibia or femur. *Clin Orthop.* 1992;280:48–64.
7. Park SS, Gordon JE, Luhmann SJ, et al. Outcome of hemiepiphyseal stapling for late-onset tibia vara. *J Bone Joint Surg Am.* 2005;87:2259–2266.
8. Schoenecker PL, Meade WC, Pierron RL, et al. Blount's disease: a retrospective review and recommendations for treatment. *J Pediatr Orthop.* 1985;5:181.
9. Schoenecker PL, Rich MM. The Lower Extremity. In: Morrissy RT, Weinstein SL, ed. Lovell and Winters Pediatric orthopaedics, 6th ed, vol II. Philadphia: Lippincott Williams & Wilkins: 1165–1184, 2006.
10. Slawski DP, Schoenecker PL. Peroneal nerve injury as a complication of pediatric tibial osteotomies: a review of 255 osteotomies. *J Pediatr Orthop.* 1994;14:166–172.
11. Stanitski DF, Dahl M, Louie K, et al. Management of late-onset tibia vara in the obese patient by using circular external fixation. *J Pediatr Orthop.* 1997;17:691–694.
12. Thompson GH, Carter JR, Smith CW. Late-onset tibia vara: a comparative analysis. *J Pediatr Orthop.* 1984;4:185–194.

28 Congenital Knee Dislocation

Charles E. Johnston, II

Few congenital anomalies present with such an obvious and dramatic clinical abnormality as congenital dislocation of the knee (CDK) (Fig. 28-1). Consultation from the newborn nursery may request an evaluation for "the knee is on backward," an appearance produced by the combination of unstable excessive hyperextension and angular deformity. The deformity is rare, being only about 1/100 as common as congenital hip dislocation, and may in fact be concomitantly present with congenital dysplasia of the hip (CDH) and a foot deformity in the ipsilateral extremity (Fig. 28-2).

Evaluation for associated chromosome anomalies and syndromes, especially those associated with congenital laxity, such as Larsen, Beals, or Ehlers-Danlos syndrome, is mandatory. Underlying neurologic conditions, such as arthrogryposis or spinal dysraphism, can be seen with CDK, implicating a lack of movement due to muscular paralysis or fibrosis as an etiologic agent for CDK. Quadriceps fibrosis and atrophy, the major obstacles to obtaining a well-functioning knee, are characteristic findings. In the absence of an obvious neuromuscular condition, these are attributed to the *in utero* position of the extremity, where the hip is usually hyperflexed and the foot immobilized at the baby's face or shoulder, with the knee hyperextended and unable to flex (Fig. 28-3).

Although the knee may seem stiff and unable to be flexed, ligamentous laxity has long been known, somewhat paradoxically, as a feature accompanying CDK and probably is responsible for the long-term instability and disability from this condition, though it is frequently downplayed. Insufficiency of the anterior cruciate ligament (ACL), due to elongation or congenital absence, is typical of bilateral syndromic CDK and probably should be addressed as part of the comprehensive surgical management (below).

Isolated or unilateral CDK (with or without ipsilateral hip dislocation) is frequently stable following reduction, with an ACL that is present and functional, leading to the designation of "stiff" CDK for the unilateral, teratologic variety, as opposed to the "lax" bilateral syndromic variety.

INDICATIONS/CONTRAINDICATIONS

Surgical treatment—open reduction of the knee with femoral shortening—is indicated for cases that do not respond to nonoperative techniques. Previously advocated for infants as early as 6 months of age, it is now recommended that surgery be delayed until such time as the surgeon feels the femur is robust enough to achieve meaningful internal fixation of a shortening osteotomy. In bilateral cases, the procedures should probably be staged for reasons of anesthesia time and blood loss in young children and infants.

Knees responding to conservative measures as described above are contraindicated for surgery.

PREOPERATIVE PLANNING

At presentation, the degree of passive flexion of the knee should be determined. It may be immediately apparent that the deformity is relatively mild when the knee will flex and reduce with gentle stretching of the quadriceps. Quadriceps contracture is assessed by applying gentle traction to the

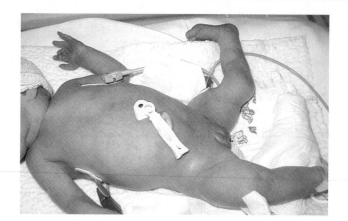

FIGURE 28-1

Left CDK in a newborn. The femoral condyles are easily palpated in the popliteal fossa.

tibia and attempting to flex the knee. If the tibia can be reduced, it will engage the distal femur and translate posteriorly with traction and flexion, and a stable articulation can be palpated. In a simple hyperextension deformity (grade 1), flexion may be increased by gentle manipulation, with maintenance of the reduction by a long-leg cast or anterior plaster slab. Conversely, an unstable articulation prevents any flexion of the knee; the tibia will subluxate laterally and proximally on the distal femur as more vigorous flexion is attempted, indicating an irreducible grade 3 dislocation. The fibrosis and shortening of the quadriceps mechanism are easily palpated in the irreducible deformity (Figs. 28-4A–4B). Other findings in irreducible CDK include obliteration of the suprapatellar pouch and contracture and fixation of the iliotibial (IT) band and hamstring tendons, which are anteriorly subluxated and bowstrung at the level of the femoral condyles.

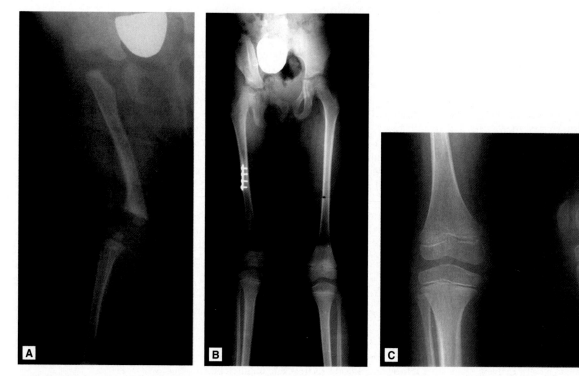

FIGURE 28-2 **A.** A 6-month-old child with an ipsilateral teratologic CDH and irreducible grade 3 CDK. No other orthopaedic abnormalities were noted at the time. **B.** The patient underwent simultaneous medial open reduction of the CDH and open reduction and femoral shortening of the CDK. At 7 years follow-up, there is slight shortening of the right lower extremity and excellent hip function, though there is residual acetabular dysplasia. (The patient eventually underwent periacetabular osteotomy.) **C.** Knee radiographs at age 8, revealing mild hypoplasia of the lateral femoral condyle and attenuation of the tibial spine. Range of motion was from 0 to 75 degrees flexion, with normal extensor strength and minimal anterior drawer instability.

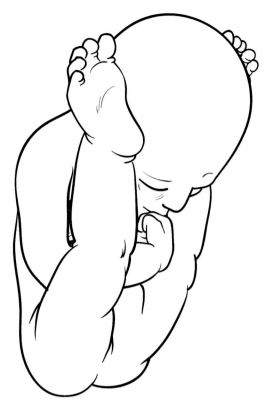

FIGURE 28-3

Typical intrauterine position associated with CDK. The hips are hyperflexed with hyperextended knees, leading to extensor fibrosis and contracture. (Redrawn after Niebauer JJ, King D. Congenital dislocation of the knee. *J Bone Joint Surg Am.* 1960;42A:207.)

The resting relationship between the distal femur and the proximal tibia should be determined on a true lateral radiograph of the knee. The degree of disturbance of the femorotibial articulation is defined as hyperextended, subluxated, or dislocated (Fig. 28-5). This relationship must be accurately visualized during treatment to document reduction of the deformity (Fig. 28-6).

The traditional approach to an irreducible CDK includes an extensive V-Y quadricepsplasty (Fig. 28-7) to overcome the shortened extensor mechanism, thus allowing the knee to flex and reduce. Although this procedure has undoubtedly produced a few satisfactory outcomes, a more likely outcome is a knee with inadequate flexion and possible redislocation due to fibrosis and scarring of the quadriceps and with inadequate quadriceps strength due to significant musculotendinous lengthening—both resulting from the extensive dissection of the quadriceps (Anterior Cruciate Ligament Reconstruction). In addition, wound healing over the anterior knee surface may be compromised due to the

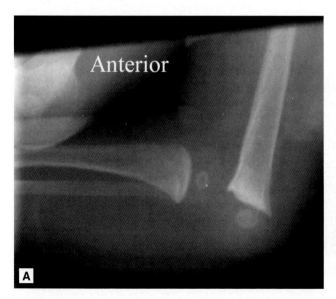

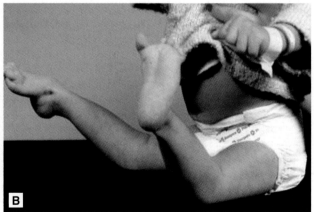

FIGURE 28-4   A–B. Radiograph and clinical appearance of a grade 3 irreducible dislocation of the knee.

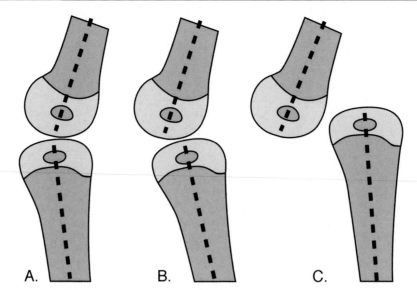

FIGURE 28-5

Radiographic classification of CDK. **A.** Grade 1: Hyperextension. **B.** Grade 2: Subluxation. **C.** Grade 3: Dislocation.

ischemia and tension produced by the flexion stretching of the contracted anterior skin (Fig. 28-7D). Serious consideration for a procedure in which there is much less intramuscular dissection and weakening is therefore appropriate. Femoral shortening is an effective method to avoid the many problems of the V-Y quadricepsplasty.

Arthrotomy must be performed to mobilize the anteriorly subluxated medial and lateral periarticular structures and allow them to relocate to their normal anatomic position posterior to the femoral condyles and the axis of rotation of the knee (Fig. 28-8). In previous surgical techniques, once the knee is reduced in flexion, the redundant posterior capsule resulting from this maneuver was generally ignored. However, failure to obliterate the redundant posterior capsule following open reduction is an invitation for a redislocation into the same incompetent posterior capsular space. The failure to perform a posterior knee capsulorrhaphy may be considered analogous to the performance of an open reduction of a congenital hip dislocation; one would never fail to perform a capsulorrhaphy to obliterate the potential space into which the femoral head could redislocate. If the ACL is also congenitally absent in a CDK reduced without capsulorrhaphy, chronic instability of the knee, or perhaps frank redislocation due to hyperlaxity, would not be an unexpected outcome. Thus the traditional extensive V-Y quadricepsplasty should be abandoned in favor of femoral shortening to minimize the extent of quadriceps dissection and subsequent weakening. Acute femoral shortening also decompresses the anterior skin, allowing knee flexion without tension/ischemia to wound edges.

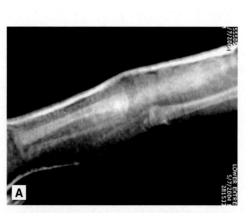
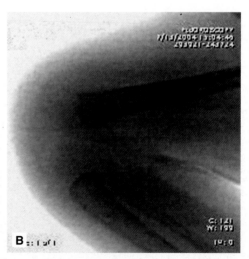

FIGURE 28-6 **A.** Failed closed reduction of the right knee in a 2-month-old child with trisomy 9 and bilateral CDK and teratologic CDH. **B.** Botox injection of the quadriceps was performed twice, at 1-month intervals, with daily physical therapy manipulations carried out by both the PT department and the parents. Two months later, full flexion and reduction were achieved.

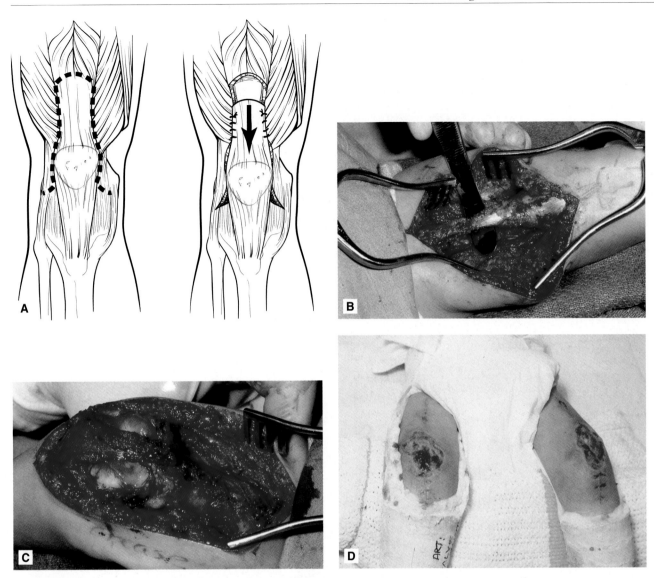

FIGURE 28-7   **A.** Traditional V-Y quadricepsplasty. (Redrawn after Curtis B, Fisher R. Congenital hyperextension with anterior subluxation of the knee; surgical treatment and long-term observations. *J Bone Joint Surg Am.* 1969;41:255.) **B.** Contracted quadriceps tendon in preparation for V-Y lengthening during open reduction. **C.** Repaired extensor mechanism following V-Y lengthening. Tenuous repair of the musculotendinous junction in the supracondylar region follows the extensive dissection, often with poor results. This procedure is no longer recommended. **D.** Dehiscence of anterior incisions following V-Y quadricepsplasty without femoral shortening. The tibiae subsequently resubluxated due to inadequate flexion.

NONOPERATIVE TREATMENT

Nonoperative treatment should begin as soon as possible in infancy and is appropriate for infants up to 12 months of age. Once the radiographic position (Fig. 28-5), the degree of initial flexibility of the quadriceps contracture, and the amount of reduction possible are determined, a manipulative technique that combines manual traction on the tibia with gentle flexion of the knee is begun, with the position maintained by an anterior plaster slab from the groin to the dorsum of the foot. Such a slab is actually easier to apply and maintain with good coaptation than is a long-leg cast in a new-born infant. Forceful manipulation is contraindicated due to risk of pressure necrosis or fracture separation of cartilaginous epiphyses. If trained physical therapists are available, serial manipulations with splinting in increasing flexion are performed daily until the knee will flex beyond 90 degrees. Radiographic confirmation of the reduction is mandatory (Fig. 28-6). Once the knee is flexed

FIGURE 28-8

Anterior subluxation of the medial and lateral periarticular structures. The patella is reflected distally *(P)*. The medial hamstrings seen under the elevator *(arrow)* are anterior to the medial femoral condyle. The iliotibial (IT) band and lateral retinaculum are anterior to the lateral femoral condyle *(double arrows)*. The distal femoral epiphysis and physis are visualized.

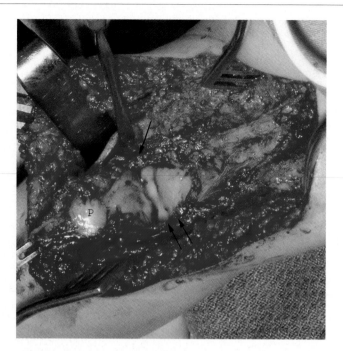

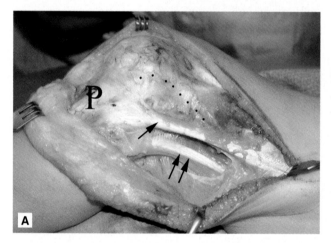

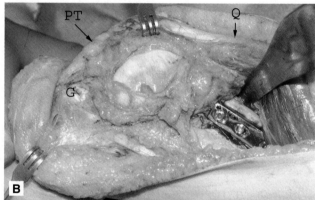

FIGURE 28-9   **A.** Extended lateral parapatellar incision. The patellar tendon *(P)*, IT band *(arrow)*, and biceps femoris posterior to the IT band *(double arrow)* are identified. The arthrotomy to mobilize the extensor mechanism, release the vastus lateralis, and expose the supracondylar region of the femur is outlined *(dots)*. **B.** Femoral shortening has been performed in the supracondylar region fixed with a four-hole plate, and the extensor mechanism has been skeletonized. Note that the extensor mechanism is intact from proximal (vastus lateralis–quadriceps tendon junction *[Q]*) to the patellar tendon *(PT)*. The IT band has been sharply released from the Gerdy tubercle *(G)*. **C.** The extensor mechanism has been skeletonized and retracted laterally (to the right). The patellar tendon is held in the forceps, and the joint is inspected via a medial arthrotomy. The ACL is congenitally absent. **D.** The extensor mechanism has been centralized with lateral advancement and imbrication of the vastus medialis, following reduction of the knee. **E.** Lateral view of the centralized extensor mechanism. No attempt has been made to close the lateral arthrotomy. The vastus lateralis has been repaired to cover the internal fixation. The IT band *(arrow)* has been reattached to the posterior capsule behind the lateral femoral condyle. Posterolateral capsulorrhaphy has already been performed deep to the reattached IT band. The knee was felt to be stable following capsulorrhaphies, so no ACL reconstruction was necessary. With the knee reduced in 90-degree flexion, a segment of the patulous posterior capsule is resected **(F)** and the femoral edge advanced to the remaining tibial segment **(G)**. **H.** Preoperative radiograph of grade 3 CDK in a boy with Larsen syndrome. **I.** Intraoperative radiograph, demonstrating reduction with femoral shortening. **J.** Three years postoperative open reduction, femoral shortening, and posterior knee capsulorrhaphies. The knee is stable in extension, and the boy is asymptomatic. *(Continued)*

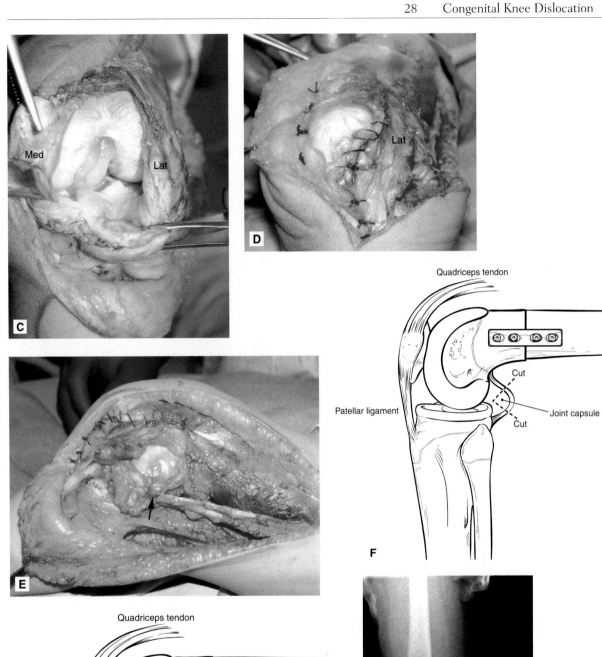

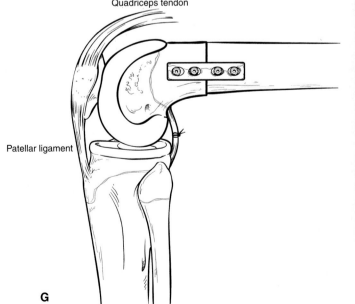

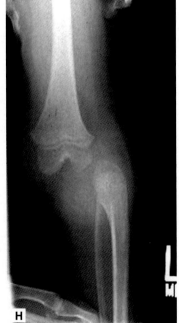

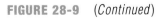

FIGURE 28-9   *(Continued)*

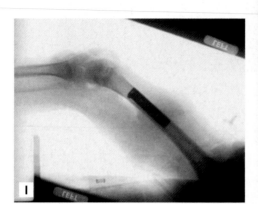

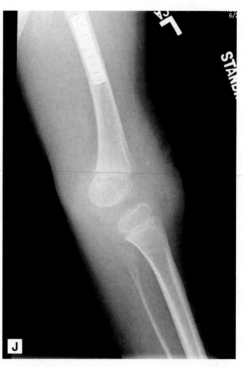

FIGURE 28-9
(*Continued*)

beyond 90 degrees, a plastic splint can be used to maintain this position and can be removed to perform range-of-motion exercises. In a patient who has ipsilateral CDH, once the knee can be reduced to such a position, a Pavlik harness can be applied to attempt to treat the hip dislocation while simultaneously maintaining the knee reduction.

In knees with irreducible deformity and a more severe quadriceps contracture, thus preventing manipulative closed reduction, the addition of botulinum toxin (Botox) to the quadriceps has been effective. The temporary paralysis of the quadriceps seems to allow gradual stretching, even when the initial flexibility seemed unfavorable for nonoperative reduction (Fig. 28-6A). The physical therapy concepts developed in Europe for clubfoot manipulation can easily be applied to manipulation of CDK. Once the Botox effect has been achieved on the quadriceps, daily serial manipulations to stretch and mobilize the fibrosed muscle can be effective and, in fact, have produced a reduction where serial manipulation without Botox was failing (Fig. 28-6B).

SURGICAL PROCEDURE

Two incisions are used—an extended lateral parapatellar arthrotomy incision and a posteromedial incision. The lateral parapatellar incision is extended proximally along the lateral femur to allow mobilization of the periarticular contracted lateral tissues (iliotibial band released from its distal insertion and vastus lateralis released from the intramuscular septum) and to provide subperiosteal access to the supracondylar region for acute shortening (Fig. 28-9A–9B). The quadriceps tendon, patella, and patellar tendon are mobilized as a continuous longitudinal structure via medial and lateral arthrotomies, which allow sharp dissection/elevation of the medial periarticular structures (pes tendons) subluxated anteriorly (Fig. 28-8). The skeletonized extensor mechanism can be retracted medially and laterally as necessary to inspect the joint and confirm reduction (Fig. 28-9B–9C). The intercondylar notch is inspected for the presence of the ACL. The femur is acutely shortened, usually around 2 to 2.5 cm, and plated (Fig. 28-9B). Following mobilization of the anteriorly subluxated periarticular structures, the knee will reduce with simple flexion, and the only repair necessary is to stabilize the extensor mechanism in the intercondylar groove, usually by a medial imbrication of the vastus medialis retinaculum (Fig. 28-9D). The lateral release is repaired only to the extent of covering the internal fixation.

Posterolateral capsulorrhaphy is now performed by bluntly dissecting the capsule from the more superficial posterior structures with the knee flexed. The dissection is simplified once the IT band and the vastus lateralis have been mobilized, as described earlier. With the knee flexed, the redundant posterior capsule can be imbricated following excision of an appropriate segment of the patulous capsule (Figs. 28-9E–9G). The imbrication is usually performed using nonabsorbable sutures, with the knee in no less than 60 degrees of flexion.

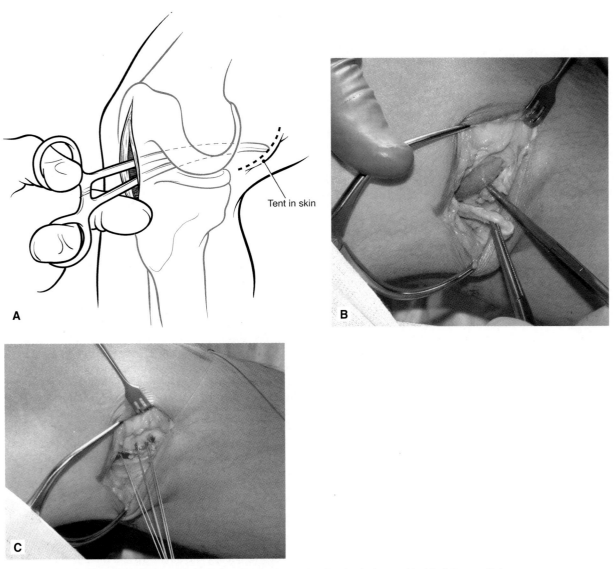

FIGURE 28-10 **A.** The incision for posteromedial capsulorrhaphy is located behind the medial femoral condyle at the joint line. **B.** In posteromedial capsulorrhaphy, a segment of redundant capsule (held in a Kocher clamp) is excised with the knee reduced and flexed. **C.** Imbrication of the remaining capsule.

Posteromedial capsulorrhaphy is performed through a separate 4-cm incision just behind the medial femoral condyle (Fig. 28-10A). This incision can best be placed by pushing a blunt instrument from inside the joint via the existing arthrotomy to the posteromedial corner of the knee and then cutting down on the instrument tenting the skin. The redundant capsule is dissected free of the superficial tissues with the knee flexed, and a segment is excised and the imbrication performed, similar to what was performed on the posterolateral side (Fig. 28-10B and 28-9C). Hamstring tendon shortening may be done in conjunction with the capsulorrhaphies, but should not be considered as a replacement for it. Following the medial and lateral capsulorrhaphies, the knee should have at least a 30-degree flexion contracture, which will stretch in 4 to 6 months following discontinuation of the immobilization.

At this point, the knee must be assessed for ligamentous instability, especially when the ACL is congenitally absent. The posterior capsulorrhaphies should prevent significant anterior drawer in maximum minus 30 degrees extension. Thus, determination of the amount of anterior drawer with the knee flexed becomes the intraoperative decision. If the anterior drawer is unacceptable, the ACL should be reconstructed—if not during the same procedure, then as a staged procedure later. ACL reconstruction in an infant under 1 year should probably be delayed until gross instability with walking is apparent. If ACL competence is satisfactory, the wounds are closed and the knee is casted in 60 degrees of flexion for 8 to 12 weeks, followed by gradual active range-of-motion exercises.

POSTOPERATIVE MANAGEMENT

A postoperative brace with varying degrees of full-extension blockage may be substituted for earlier discontinuance of cast immobilization. Follow-up evaluation focuses on ACL competence or insufficiency (Figs. 28-9H–9J).

Anterior Cruciate Ligament Reconstruction

Historically there has been a reluctance to attempt intra-articular ACL reconstruction in children due to the fear of physeal injury producing deformity and growth arrest from transphyseal procedures. These concerns are relenting, however, as both clinical and experimental studies have shown that this risk may be overstated. Both transphyseal and physeal-sparing techniques have been described. The drilling of an anchoring hole across any physis potentially risks injury. However, a smooth, centrally placed hole across a physis that is filled with a nonosseous material (e.g., a tendon) is no more likely to produce growth disturbance than is temporary smooth pin fixation, which is frequently utilized in the management of other physeal injuries. Use of interposition materials to prevent the re-formation of physeal bars is also well-established, and both animal and clinical studies using tendon material as transphyseal ligament reconstruction are providing reassurance that limb length or angular deformity complications from such procedures are less likely than previously believed.

Unpublished data from 22 congenitally dislocated knees has documented that all nine knees that had reduction by V-Y quadricepsplasty and *no* ligament reconstruction were uniformly unstable at follow-up, with poor quadriceps strength. All nine required full-time bracing or assistive devices for community ambulation. Eight of nine unsatisfactory knees (up to 15-year follow-up) were in patients with laxity syndromes, predominantly Larsen syndrome. As a result of this review, an attempt to reconstruct the ACL-deficient knee in the laxity syndrome group seemed not only justified but also mandatory if the uniformly unacceptable results in the earlier cases were to be improved.

In children under the age of 5, use of the IT band rerouted over the top of the lateral femoral condyle and through the intercondylar notch, as described by Insall, has been performed successfully concomitantly with the open reduction–capsulorrhaphy procedure. The IT band is detached from the Gerdy tubercle as part of the initial lateral parapatellar dissection that was previously described for open reduction of the knee. Following reduction of the knee and the capsulorrhaphies, the IT band is mobilized proximally in the thigh, rolled into a tubular structure, and passed antegrade over the top of the lateral femoral condyle and through the intercondylar notch (Fig. 28-11). The tubed tendon is then anchored to the proximal tibia through a tunnel that is usually kept within the epiphysis in order to perform a physeal-sparing procedure. The transferred tendon is tensioned with the tibia in maximum posterior drawer, with the suture tied over a suture anchor or a button placed on the skin of the anterior leg. The drill hole should be placed with radiographic control to minimize the possibility of an oblique transphyseal placement; ideally the tunnel should include the ossification center of the proximal tibia to provide tendon-to-bone anchorage (Figs. 28-11B–11D). Alternative transphyseal placement through a more vertical, centrally placed tunnel can also be utilized if enough tendon length is available. The author has not specifically attempted this latter alternative, however, finding that the physeal-sparing tunnel has been adequate.

Postoperative care for the knee undergoing simultaneous ACL reconstruction is the same as for the knee reduction procedure.

PEARLS AND PITFALLS

The rationale of the Insall technique, compared with other ACL substitution procedures, is that the transferred IT band is less likely to attenuate because it is an active transfer in which only the insertion of the tendon is being rerouted. Arguably, the IT band is also a deforming force, involved in the production of the CDK from the outset, and so its rerouting should be beneficial to the overall treatment and maintenance of reduction. The IT band is dissected and mobilized as part of the open reduction–shortening procedure and thus can be easily rerouted and anchored in the proximal tibia simultaneously with the reduction-capsulorrhaphy procedure.

The disadvantage of the Insall transfer—indeed with any transfer in proximity to the proximal tibial physis—remains the possibility of growth injury. In four knees in children under age 5, one physeal arrest has occurred (Fig. 28-12)—in a child with Larsen syndrome who was operated on at age 18 months. The child underwent the identical procedure on the second knee at age 3, with no physeal injury apparent at 9 years follow-up. A varus-flexion deformity occurred in the first knee, eventually corrected by a simple opening-wedge proximal tibial osteotomy at age 12. Currently at age 15, both knees are pain-free and stable, with 0 to 130 degrees range of motion and normal quadriceps strength (Fig. 28-12). A third knee operated on a child under the age of 5 with fibular hemimelia

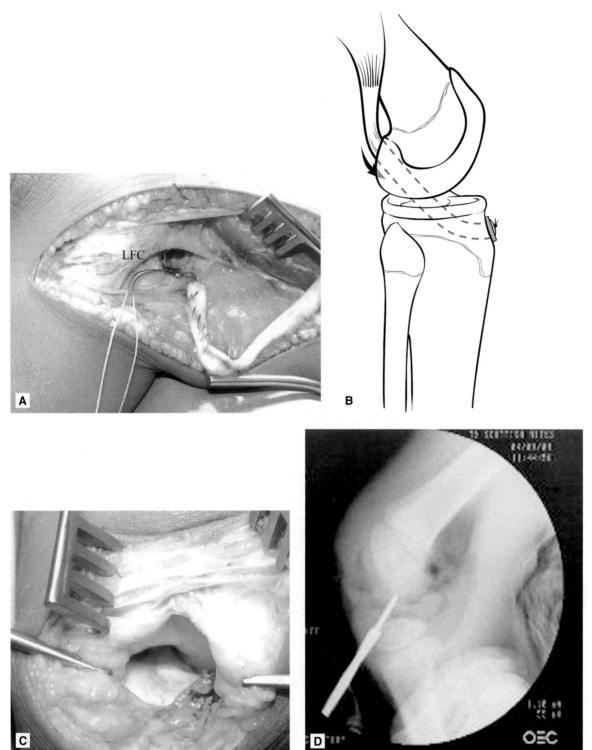

FIGURE 28-11   A. Lateral view of the knee during Insall ACL reconstruction. The IT band has been released from the Gerdy tubercle, mobilized proximally, and tubed with a running suture. A hemostat has been placed from a medial arthrotomy through the intercondylar notch over the top of the lateral femoral condyle *(LFC)* and is grasping the suture in preparation for passing the IT band antegrade through the notch to the tibial attachment site. **B.** Physeal-sparing transfer of the IT band to reconstruct the ACL. **C.** Medial arthrotomy demonstrating congenital absence of the ACL. **D.** Intraoperative fluoroscopy of placement of the tunnel in tibial epiphysis. A guide pin has been placed in the anterior portion of the ossific nucleus and a cannulated drill placed over the guide pin to create the tunnel. **E, F.** Diagram and intraoperative view of transferred IT band anchored in the tunnel in the proximal tibial epiphysis (physeal-sparing). (*Continued*)

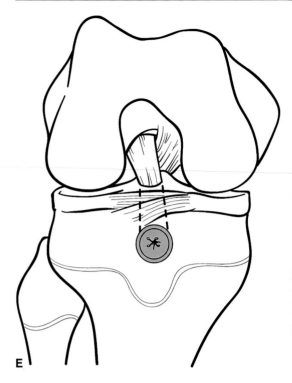

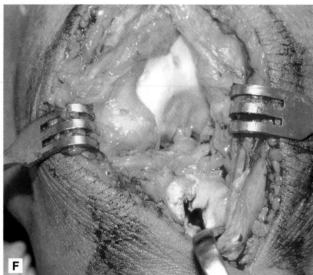

FIGURE 28-11   (*Continued*)

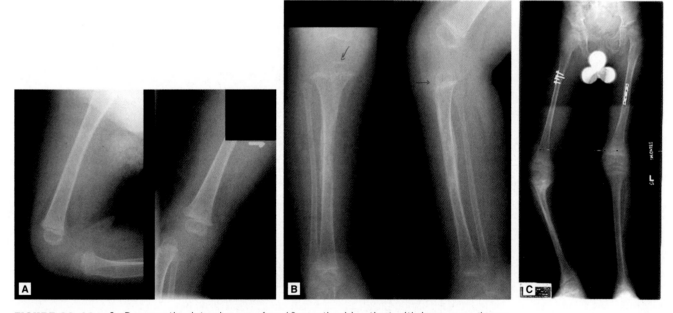

FIGURE 28-12   **A.** Preoperative lateral x-ray of an 18-month-old patient with Larsen syndrome and persistent bilateral dislocations in extension. Physeal-sparing ACL reconstruction with the transferred IT band on the right knee was performed. **B.** Radiographs of the right tibia 6 months following ACL reconstruction. A bone graft was harvested from this tibia during performance of a posterior cervical fusion 8 weeks prior to this radiograph. The tunnel for the ACL reconstruction can be seen in the proximal tibial epiphysis *(arrows)*. **C.** At age 12, a varus-flexion deformity of the right proximal tibia is noted, indicating that a physeal growth disturbance has occurred. This deformity of the right knee was corrected by a medial opening-wedge valgus-producing osteotomy. Interestingly the left knee was treated by the identical procedure at age 3, with no physeal disturbance noted.

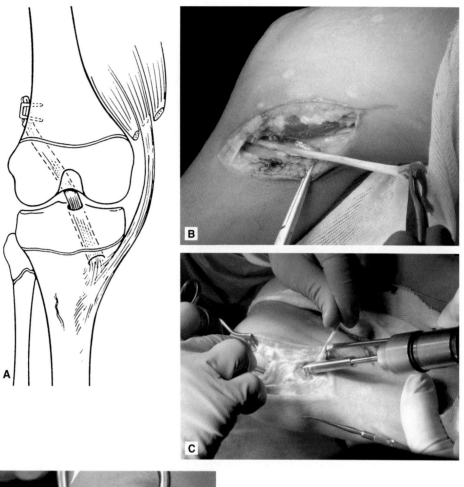

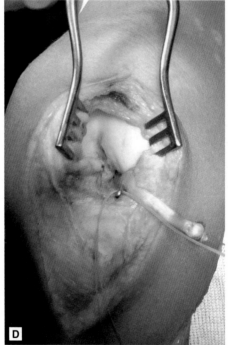

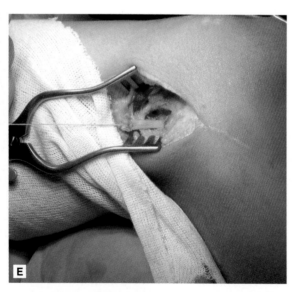

FIGURE 28-13 **A.** Transphyseal ACL reconstruction using semitendinosus (ST) rerouted through the intercondylar notch, which is then stapled to the femur for proximal fixation. **B.** Harvesting the ST using a tendon stripper via a posteromedial incision over the pes anserine insertions. **C.** Drill hole using hollow reamer to pass the ST into the knee joint traversing the proximal physis centrally. **D.** The ST has been delivered into the knee joint and is now about to be passed over the top of the lateral femoral condyle using a tendon passer inserted from a distal lateral femoral incision. **E.** The ST is tensioned in the distal lateral femoral incision before stapling to the distal femur.

and a dislocated knee has gradually become less stable with attenuation of the Insall transfer. The child has been actively running using a Syme amputation prosthesis, which may have contributed to additional stress during activity. A fourth case, also Larsen disease, has had instability in extension recur, requiring repeat reconstruction.

Like other investigators expanding the indications for transphyseal ACL reconstructions in children with traumatic deficiency of the ACL, the Insall approach has been replaced by the transphyseal procedures in syndromic knees. It is the author's opinion that the benefit of the improved stability imparted by such an ACL reconstruction in a young child outweighs the risk of the physeal injury, which, in the overall context of an extremity with CDK, can always be managed by appropriate osteotomy and/or lengthening or by contralateral epiphysiodesis (Fig. 28-12). Thus transphyseal reconstructions using semitendinosus (Fig. 28-13) have been attempted in three children under age 6 to provide better ACL stability. Follow-up is currently too short (fewer than 3 years) to comment on possible physeal injury. However, because the transfer is placed through a centrally located 6-mm hole in the tibial physis and the tendon is in fact an interposition material that would prevent a central bony bridge, the risk of serious growth disturbance is deemed minimal. Because the provision of stability by an early ACL reconstruction is invaluable to the function of such syndromic patients who otherwise would be left with disabling bilateral instability of both knees, the transphyseal reconstructions continue to be investigated with optimism.

REFERENCES

1. Curtis B, Fisher R. Congenital hyperextension with anterior subluxation of the knee; surgical treatment and long-term observations. *J Bone Joint Surg Am.* 1969;41:255.
2. Johnston CE II; Congenital Deformities of the knee. In: Scott WN, ed. *Surgery of the Knee.* 4th ed. Philadelphia: Churchill Livingstone Elsevier; 2006. p. 1191–1222.
3. Kocher MS, Garg S, Micheli LJ. Physeal sparing reconstruction of the anterior cruciate ligament in skeletally immature prepubescent children and adolescents. *J Bone Joint Surg Am.* 2005;87:2371.
4. Lo IK, Bell DM, Fowler PJ. Anterior cruciate ligament injuries in the skeletally immature patient. *Instr Course Lect.* 1998;47:35.
5. Niebauer JJ, King D. Congenital dislocation of the knee. *J Bone Joint Surg Am.* 1960;42:207.
6. Parker AW, Drez D Jr, Cooper J. Anterior cruciate ligament injuries in patients with open physes. *Am J Sports Med.* 1994;22:44.
7. Windsor RE, Insall JN. Bone-block iliotibial band reconstruction for anterior cruciate insufficiency. Follow-up note and minimum five-year follow-up period. *Clin Orthop.* 1990;250:197.

SECTION VI
SPINE

29 Posterior Spinal Fusion with Pedicle Screws

Michael D. Daubs, Yongjung J. Kim, and Lawrence G. Lenke

INDICATIONS/CONTRAINDICATIONS

The indications for the use of pedicle screw fixation are broad and cover most cases where a spinal fusion is indicated. The indications and contraindications are dictated more by surgeon experience than by anatomical or instrumentation restrictions. As surgeon experience with pedicle screw insertion increases, so do the indications. Pedicles increase in size with age; by 6 years of age, the lumbar pedicles average 5 to 8 mm in width, and the thoracic pedicles range from 3.5 to 6 mm, all of which are large enough for pedicle screw fixation. Pedicles in the pediatric age group are viscoelastic and can be gradually expanded with probing and tapping to up to 200% of their original size before fracturing.

The main contraindication for pedicle screw fixation is the complete absence of a pedicle (i.e., sometimes seen in neurofibromatosis) or the lack of an adequately sized pedicle that would allow for safe insertion based on the surgeon's experience.

PREOPERATIVE PLANNING

Prior to surgery, radiographs should be evaluated to assess the size and orientation of the pedicles in the area of the spine to be instrumented. Although not essential, computed tomography (CT) scans can be helpful in evaluating pedicle size as well as adjacent visceral structures at risk. Areas of the spine where the pedicle diameters are smaller should be noted in anticipation of a more technically demanding placement. The authors have morphologically defined four types of pedicles to

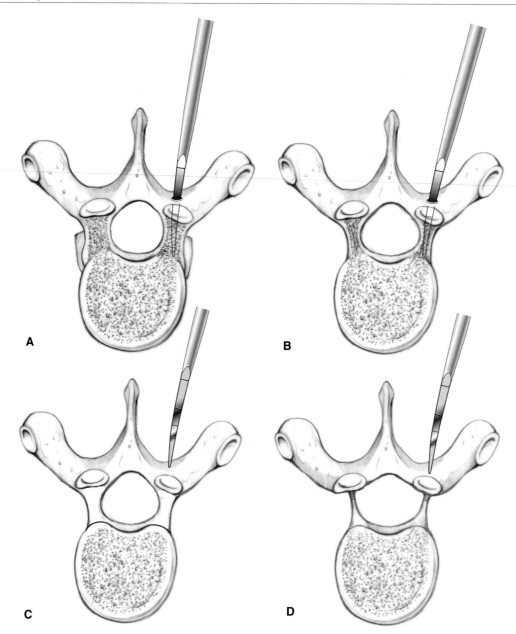

FIGURE 29-1

The morphologic pedicle classification. **A.** Type A: Large cancellous channel. **B.** Type B: Small cancellous channel. **C.** Type C: Cortical channel. **D.** Type D: Absent pedicle channel.

help with this task (Fig. 29-1). The level of difficulty of pedicle screw placement increases from type A to type D. A type A pedicle has a large, cancellous channel into which the pedicle probe is inserted smoothly without difficulty. A type B pedicle has a small cancellous channel into which the probe is inserted snugly with increased force. A type C pedicle has a cortical channel into which the probe should not be manually placed; instead the probe must be tapped with a mallet into the body. A type D pedicle has an absent channel (slit pedicle), necessitating a "juxtapedicular" pedicle probe insertion (Fig. 29-2). Pedicles in the midthoracic spine T4 through T6 have the smallest width in all age groups. In scoliosis cases, the pedicles on the concavity of the curve are typically smaller (types B and C) than those on the convex side. Taking time to think about the three-dimensional, rotational aspects of the curve and how it will affect the orientation and direction of pedicle probing and screw insertion is extremely important. The anatomical orientation of the pedicles in relation to each vertebral body does not change, but the plane of insertion and hand positioning in relation to the floor does. In more severe curves, the proper plane of insertion for the apical, concave pedicles can be nearly parallel to the floor. In these instances, it may seem that the trajectory is incorrect, but the anatomical position of the pedicle and the rotation of the spine dictate the angle of insertion should be relied upon. When first beginning, frequent reference to a spine model is encouraged, and especially in the thoracic spine, where there is less experience with pedicle screw placement.

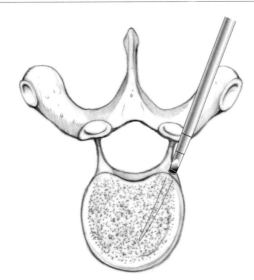

SURGICAL PROCEDURE

The patient is positioned prone on a radiolucent operating table. After positioning, 36-in. long-cassette anteroposterior (AP) and short lateral radiographs of the spine are taken to give an accurate, on-table position of the spine in both the coronal and sagittal planes to aid screw placement.

A meticulous, subperiosteal bloodless exposure is one of the most important first steps of pedicle screw insertion. It is imperative that the bony anatomy of the posterior spine be fully exposed, including the lamina, facets, and tips of the transverse processes. Accurate pedicle screw placement depends on correctly identifying the topographic landmarks and using them to obtain the correct spatial orientation and trajectory for probing and screw insertion.

Following exposure, preparation is made for pedicle screw insertion. In the thoracic spine, the facets are cleared of soft tissue, and a 1/2-in. osteotome is used to remove the inferior 5 mm of the inferior facet (Fig. 29-3). A curette is used to scrape the cartilage from the superior facet surface. At the most cephalad level of instrumentation, the facet joint is avoided and kept intact to prevent proximal junctional instability.

After the facets are prepared, the starting point for pedicle screw insertion is identified. The starting points vary slightly with each level of the spine (Fig. 29-4). In general, the starting point of insertion in the thoracic spine in the medial/lateral plane is just lateral to the midpoint of the facet joint. If the starting point is medial to this line, there is a risk of penetrating the ventral lamina and the spinal canal. In the cephalad-caudad plane, the point of entry moves from the midpoint of the transverse process in the upper thoracic spine to the upper transverse process in the midthoracic spine and back to the midpoint, of the TP at T12. In the lumbar spine, the pedicle is located at the junction of the pars interarticularis and the midpoint of the transverse process. The trajectory of insertion in the transverse plane, starting in the upper thoracic spine (T1–T3), is 15 to 25 degrees, rapidly decreasing to around 10 degrees in the midthoracic (T4–T9) region and down to 0 degrees in the lower thoracic region (T10–T12). In the lumbar spine, the transverse angle of insertion ranges from 10 degrees at L1 and gradually increases to 30 degrees at L5. In the upper levels (T1–T3), starting further

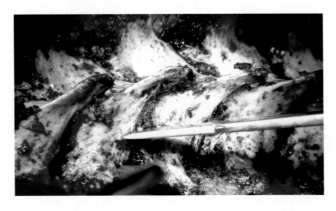

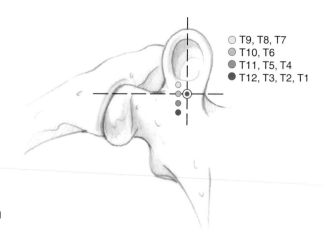

FIGURE 29-4

The various starting points of entry for pedicle screw insertion in the thoracic spine.

○ T9, T8, T7
◑ T10, T6
◑ T11, T5, T4
● T12, T3, T2, T1

lateral to the midpoint of the facet is necessary to allow for the increased angle of trajectory (20–30 degrees) in the transverse plane.

After the starting point has been correctly identified, the freehand technique of pedicle screw insertion is used. This technique requires no special equipment or imaging and utilizes the instruments routinely used in spinal surgery.

Freehand Technique

Step 1. A high-speed cortical burr is used to develop the starting point of insertion by penetrating the cortical surface 5 mm (Fig. 29-5).

Step 2. A gear-shift pedicle probe is used to palpate the cancellous "soft spot" of the pedicle entrance. In smaller-diameter pedicles, there may not be a cancellous entry point, in which case the narrow probe tip is gently used to develop the entry point. Palpation of the ventral surface of the lamina, which is solid cortical bone, is very helpful in locating the pedicle entrance. By gently palpating the ventral lamina from a medial to lateral direction, the probe will slide into the pedicle entrance of softer cancellous bone in a funnel-type fashion.

Step 3. Once the entrance is palpated, the curvilinear probe is inserted, with the tip pointed laterally to a depth of 20 mm (Fig. 29-6A) which is just beyond the medial border of the spinal canal. The curve is pointed laterally at this point to avoid inadvertent entrance into the spinal canal. The probe is then removed and pointed medially to probe the depth of the pedicle into the vertebral

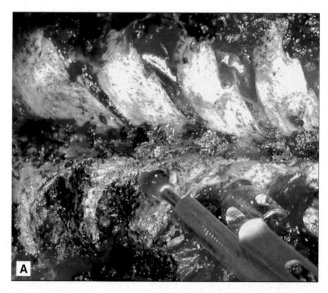
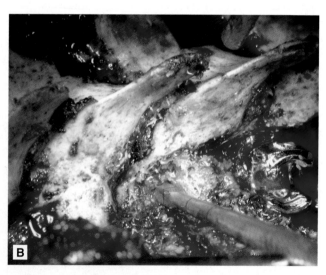

FIGURE 29-5   A. A high-speed burr is used to penetrate the posterior cortical surface at the point of entry. **B.** The pedicle probe is then inserted into the soft cancellous channel of the pedicle.

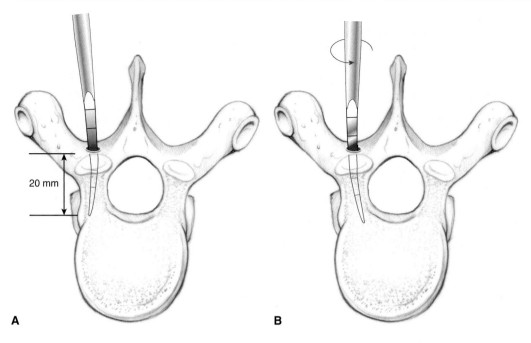

FIGURE 29-6

A) The pedicle probe is initially inserted with the curvilinear tip pointed lateral for the first 20 mm; **B)** then it is rotated medially.

body (Fig. 29-6B). The probe is aimed medially to avoid penetration laterally of the vertebral body into the great vessels or other structures. The typical depth is 30 to 35 mm in the upper thoracic spine, 35 to 40 mm in the midthoracic, and 40 to 45 mm in the lower thoracic in adolescents. The probing should be smooth and with consistent pressure. The pressure is greater than what is typically needed in the lumbar spine due to the smaller-diameter pedicles. Any sudden advancement may indicate a breach of the pedicle.

Step 4. A sounding probe is used to palpate the pedicle channel (Fig. 29-7). The medial, lateral, superior, and inferior walls, as well as the floor, are palpated for possible breaches. The upper 20 mm of the pedicle are the most common areas of medial perforation and, thus, should be carefully palpated. Because of the concerns over possible neurologic injury with medial placement of a pedicle screw, the most common area of breach is usually lateral when first performing this technique. This is also because the lateral wall is thinner than the medial wall in most pedicles. If a breach is detected laterally, the gear-shift probe can be redirected medially to form a new channel. The new channel should again be palpated with the sounding probe.

Step 5. The pedicle is tapped with a tap that is undersized by 1.0 mm from the planned screw diameter.

Step 6. The sounding probe is used to determine the depth of the pedicle channel and the corresponding screw length. A hemostat is placed on the sounding probe at the entry point of the pedicle, and the length is measured. The length of the marked probe is compared with the length of the screw to ensure it is the correct length. The screw length varies with the age and size of the patient and the anatomical level of insertion.

In pediatric deformity cases, screws are typically placed bilaterally at every level. Multiaxial screws are commonly used at the most proximal and distal levels of instrumentation. This allows motion through the mobile screw head during initial rod placement and maneuvering, instead of through the fixed screw-bone interface, which could cause loosening. Following screw insertion, radiographs or fluoroscopic images are obtained to check screw position.

Triggered electromyography (EMG) through the pedicle screws is also used to confirm correct screw position. Real-time monitoring of the thoracic nerve roots (T6–T12) with recording from the rectus abdominus is performed along with the lumbar roots—L2 through L4 (vastus medialis), L5 (tibialis anterior), and S1 (medial gastrocnemius). If the EMG threshold is less than 6 mA (thoracic) or 4 mA (lumbar), then the screw is removed, and the pedicle tract is repalpated to ensure that there are no cortical breaches. The EMG results are considered along with the radiographs, pedicle tract palpation, and intraosseous feel during placement to confirm correct screw position. Once the pedicle screws are confirmed to be in proper position, the deformity correction is performed.

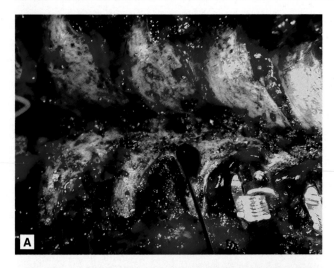

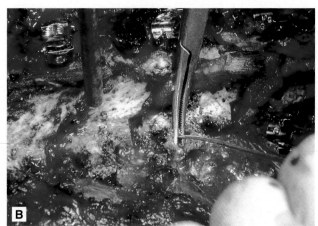

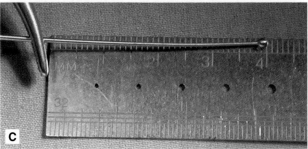

FIGURE 29-7 **A.** The sounding probe is used to palpate the four walls and the floor of the pedicle channel to check for breeches. **B, C.** With the sounding probe at the floor of the pedicle in the vertebral body, a clamp is placed at the entry point, and the depth of the pedicle (and the corresponding screw length) is measured.

Deformity Correction

Deformity correction is performed with a conventional (nonderotation) or bilateral apical vertebral derotation (BAVD) maneuver. For both techniques, the rods are first contoured to the intended sagittal and coronal planes of correction. Two clamps are used at each end of the rod, and the rod is bent over the wound to allow visualization of the deformity while contouring.

Conventional Maneuver

In the hyperkyphotic patient, the convex rod is placed first to allow for lordosing during correction. In the normokyphotic or hypokyphotic patient, the concave rod is placed first. Once the rod has been bent into the planned coronal and sagittal alignment, it is rotated 90 to 180 degrees, and the ends are inserted into the most proximal and distal multiaxial screws. The set screws are placed and left loose at one end to allow motion but are locked at the other end to avoid rod twisting. The rod is gradually translated while capturing each screw, working from proximal and distal toward the apex of the curve. The set screws are inserted and left loose at each level to allow free rotation of the rod. This is not a derotation maneuver; rather it is a method of engaging the screws and translating the spine into the corrected position. With the set screws loose (but locked at one end), coronal rod benders are used to further obtain correction. The *in situ* rod bending is a gentle, gradual maneuver that is done in small increments at each segment, with several passes to allow for viscoelastic relaxation (Fig. 29-8). Segmental compression on the convexity and distraction on the concavity of the curve are performed with the apical screws locked. During rod bending and the distraction and compression maneuvers, it is important to visually monitor the screw-bone interface for plowing of the screw through bone. Overaggressive correction maneuvers can lead to screw fixation failure through the screw-bone interface.

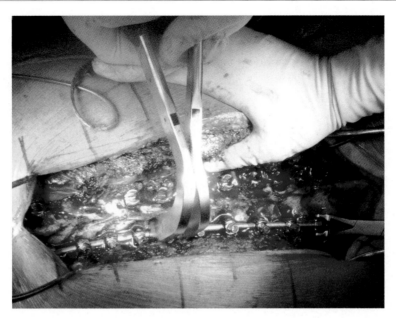

FIGURE 29-8
The coronal in situ benders are used to obtain further correction. The bending is performed with gentle force at each segment and repeated multiple times, gradually obtaining the desired correction.

Derotation Maneuver

The goal of apical derotation is to improve correction and obviate the need for thoracoplasty. BAVD maneuvers are performed only when there is adequate screw purchase. In cases where severe thoracic kyphosis or osteoporosis is present, careful consideration should be made prior to attempting BAVD, as it can cause significant strain on the apical screws and lead to fixation failure. The BAVD maneuver consists of five steps.

Step 1. Correction posts are placed over the four screws located at the curve apex, with two posts on the concave and convex sides and one open screw between them (Fig. 29-9). Some spine implant systems allow for the correction posts to be attached to each other (Fig. 29-10), which evenly distributes the force of rotation over all the attached screws. This increases safety by decreasing the chance of an individual screw plowing through bone.

Step 2. Using the posts, as well as manual pressure on the rib prominence, the apical segments are derotated (Fig. 29-10). The amount of derotational correction is dictated by curve flexibility and the strength of the screw-bone interface. As is true for all correction maneuvers, aggressive force can cause fixation failure; therefore, a constant, gentle force is required. The screw-bone interface must be monitored while the derotation is held.

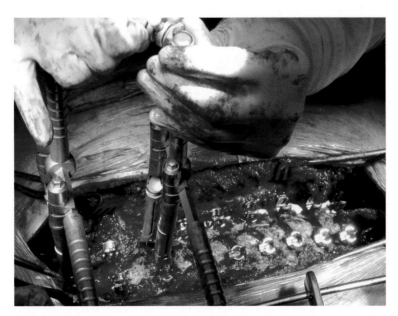

FIGURE 29-9
The correction posts have been attached to the pedicle screws at the apex of the curve. One screw is left open at the middle to allow adequate room for the connectors.

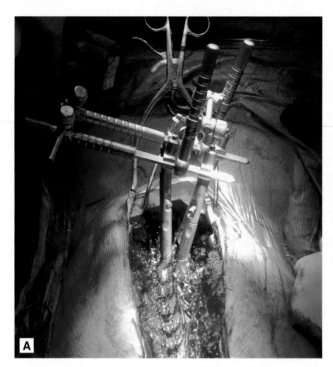
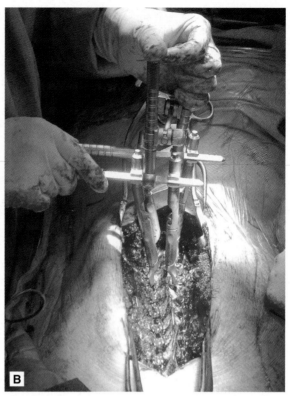

FIGURE 29-10 **A.** An intraoperative photograph taken from the head of the patient (bottom of picture), showing the BAVD device attached at the apex of the curve. **B.** The assistant is shown holding the device after the BAVD has been performed.

Step 3. While holding the correction, the previously contoured rod is placed on the concave side, and the set screws are placed. The set screws are tightened at each level, except for the three located at the apex of the curve.

Step 4. A second BAVD is performed with all but the apical set screws tightened. Following the final derotation, the apical set screws are tightened through the posts on the concavity. Standard compression/distraction and *in situ* rod bending are then used to fine-tune the correction (Fig. 29-11).

Step 5. The second rod is placed, and appropriate compression/distraction forces are once again used to enhance correction.

Derotation in a Double Major Curve

The lumbar convex curve is derotated first. It is held in position with a short rod placed on the concave side. The thoracic BAVD is then performed as described above while the assistant holds the lumbar curve on the convex side.

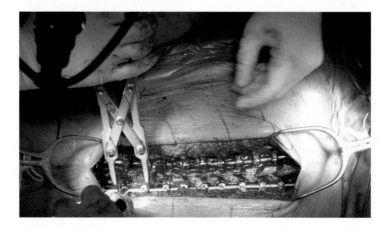

FIGURE 29-11

Compression is being placed along the convexity of the curve.

Closure

Cross-links may be placed following decortication and bone grafting. The deep fascia is closed tightly with interrupted 1-0 absorbable sutures. The superficial fascia is closed with interrupted 2-0 absorbable sutures, and the skin is typically closed with a 3-0 monofilament absorbable suture. Deep and superficial drains are placed prior to closure.

POSTOPERATIVE MANAGEMENT

Patients are mobilized on postoperative day 1, and activity is advanced as tolerated. Bracing is rarely used. Deep and superficial drains are kept in until drainage is less than 30 cc in 8 hours. Typically drains are in for 48 to 72 hours. Standing 36-in. AP and lateral radiographs are taken prior to patient discharge to check spinal alignment and to recheck instrumentation position.

COMPLICATIONS TO AVOID

The most important complication to avoid is pedicle screw malposition, as surrounding visceral structures are at risk in the thoracic and lumbar spine. The best way to avoid the complications of pedicle screw malposition is to have a thorough knowledge of the three-dimensional anatomy of the spine and its surrounding structures, as well as of internal and external pedicle bony anatomy. It is very important to know that the angle-of-insertion trajectory in relation to each vertebral segment does not change in the scoliotic spine. Thus if the proper angles of insertion are known, achieving correct placement is a matter of adjusting hand position in relation to the rotation of each vertebral segment. Carefully and repeatedly palpating all four walls and the floor of the pedicle channel with the sounding probe can help avoid a misplaced screw. If there is doubt about a screw being in the correct position, it should be removed and replaced with a hook, or this level should be skipped altogether. Spinal cord monitoring is also helpful in detecting major pedicle breeches that have caused spinal cord impingement.

Another complication to avoid is fixation failure. This most commonly occurs through the screw-bone interface and can be avoided by paying strict attention to the screw-bone interface during rod placement, derotation, compression, and distraction. If fixation failure occurs, further correction maneuvers should be halted.

In summary, the complications of pedicle screw fixation can be reduced by knowing the bony anatomy, the proper starting point and angle of insertion, and the spinal deformity in three dimensions, by learning the feel of pedicle probing and sounding, and by maintaining an awareness of the surrounding visceral structures at risk.

ILLUSTRATIVE CASE

A 15-year-old girl, Risser 4, presented with a 40-degree upper thoracic, 74-degree main thoracic, and a 42-degree lumbar Lenke type 1AN curve (Fig. 29-12A to 12J). On bending radiographs, the proximal thoracic curve corrected to 3 degrees, the main thoracic curve to 49 degrees, and the lumbar to 2 degrees. Pedicle screws were placed bilaterally from T3 to L2. A BAVD was performed, as described above, along with appropriate *in situ* bending, distraction, and compression maneuvers. The patient is doing well at 3 years postoperative.

PEARLS AND PITFALLS

- Carefully review the radiographs and know the unique characteristics of each deformity and the location of the most challenging pedicles to be probed.
- Perform a meticulous, bloodless exposure of the bony anatomy.
- Develop the feel of a correctly probed pedicle. Learn to recognize a breach.
- Avoid the tendency to place screws laterally; the medial pedicle wall is the thickest.
- If correct screw position is in doubt, remove the screw and recheck bony walls and floor.
- Verify correct location of screws by EMG screw stimulation (at T6 and below) and by intraoperative imaging.
- If a pedicle screw does not feel right, use another form of fixation.
- Pay particular attention to maintaining correct sagittal contour, particularly thoracic kyphosis. Verify this with intraoperative radiographs after all correction is completed.

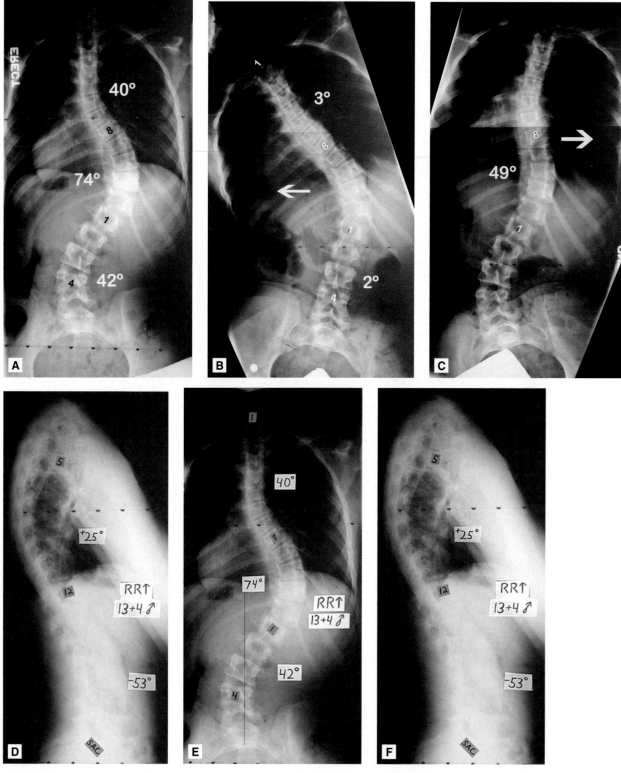

FIGURE 29-12 Standing PA **(A)**, left bending **(B)**, right bending **(C)**, and standing lateral **(D)** radiographs showing a Lenke 1AN curve. The proximal thoracic and lumbar curves are nonstructural. The main thoracic curve is a low overhanging curve with an apex at T11 that corrects to 49 degrees on bending. Preoperative **(E, F)** and 3-year postoperative **(G, H)** comparative radiographs. The patient was instrumented from T3 to L2 with pedicle screws. The proximal thoracic corrected to 1 degree, the main thoracic to 4 degrees, and the lumbar to 3 degrees. **(I)** Preoperative clinical photograph showing the prominent right rib hump and skin crease at the waist. **(J)** Three-year postoperative clinical photographs showing a well-balanced spine, loss of the skin crease at the waist, and the effect of the BAVD in reducing the rib hump without thoracoplasty. (*Continued*)

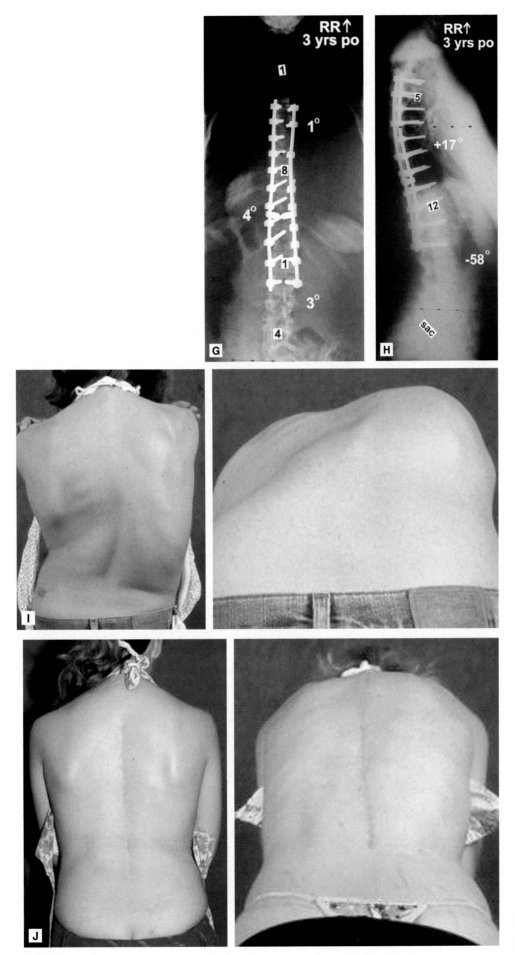

FIGURE 29-12

(*Continued*)

349

REFERENCES

1. Kim YJ, Lenke LG, Bridwell KH, et al. Free hand pedicle screw placement in the thoracic spine: is it safe? *Spine.* 2004;29:333–342.
2. Kim YJ, Lenke LG, Cho SK, et al. Comparative analysis of pedicle screw versus hook instrumentation in posterior spinal fusion of adolescent idiopathic scoliosis. *Spine.* 2004;29:2040–2048.
3. Suk SI, Lee CK, Kim WJ, et al. Segmental pedicle screw fixation in the treatment of thoracic idiopathic scoliosis. *Spine.* 1995;20:1399–1405.
4. Zindrick MR, Knight GW, Sartori MJ, et al. Pedicle morphology of the immature spine. *Spine.* 2000;25:2726–2735.

30 Posterior Spinal Fusion with Hybrid Construct Using Sublaminar Wires

David L. Skaggs

Sublaminar wires were popularized by Eduardo Luque in the treatment of neuromuscular scoliosis. Their use has since expanded to treat spinal deformity of many etiologies. An advantage of sublaminar wires over many other anchors is that gradual correction of a deformity can be achieved by tightening the wires in small steps over time. This gradual tightening takes advantage of the spine's viscoelasticity and allows stress to dissipate over time, which helps prevent anchor pull-out. This technique of gradual correction can be used at the apex of a scoliosis or at the ends of a kyphosis construct, as two examples. Reduction pedicle screws may also provide similar gradual correction but at many times the cost.

INDICATION/CONTRAINDICATIONS

The general indications for a spinal fusion for adolescent idiopathic scoliosis include a thoracic curve ≥50 degrees, a lumbar or thoracolumbar curve ≥45 degrees, or severe decompensation or cosmetic deformity. Hybrid constructs utilize a variety of anchors to attach rods to the spine, most commonly with sublaminar wires at the apex. The base of the construct is usually at least four pedicle screws, whereas the top may be hooks or four pedicle screws. The author's standard construct for idiopathic scoliosis is all pedicle screws, because of the ability to correct the rotational deformity without rib osteotomies as well as the very low risk of implant pull-out. However, direct comparison of curve correction between all pedicle screw constructs and apical sublaminar wires have shown similar results. Hybrid constructs, and sublaminar wires in particular, remain useful tools in the armamentarium of spinal deformity surgeons.

Indications for the use of a hybrid construct include scoliosis with frank thoracic lordosis, inability to safely place pedicle screws with certainty (especially at the apex of a large curve), cost considerations, and surgeon experience and training. Sublaminar wires may be used in the cervical spine. In very young children, sublaminar wires can be used even when other forms of fixation are challenging. In patients with weak bone, such as nonambulators with neuromuscular disease, full engagement of the dual cortices of the lamina with sublaminar wires often provides better fixation than do hooks or, at times, screws. Sublaminar wires may be used in combination with other anchors, such as screws or hooks, on a single vertebra in cases of very weak bone.

Contraindications include incomplete posterior elements, such as in congenital scoliosis, spina bifida, and postlaminectomy. Some have suggested that sublaminar wires should not be attempted in the setting of a syrinx or dural ectasia, though the author has used sublaminar wires in those situations safely and effectively many times with no instances of neurologic problems. Sublaminar wires may lead to intracanal adhesions, which make them more problematic to remove than other spinal anchors. Therefore a relative contraindication for sublaminar wires is a case in which a significant chance of implant removal could be anticipated.

PREOPERATIVE PLANNING

Preoperative planning is no different from planning for any other posterior spinal fusion. A detailed history and physical examination in search of any underlying cause of scoliosis is essential. In particular, the surgeon should note whether the left shoulder is higher than the right when the patient is standing, as this means the upper left thoracic curve should most likely be included in the fusion. In addition, areas of significant rotation in the Adams forward-bending test should be noted. In cases of thoracic and lumbar curves, if there is a very significant left lumbar rotatory asymmetry, serious consideration should be given to fusing the lumbar curve. Although a complete review of criteria for choosing fusion levels is beyond the scope of this chapter, the importance of level selection cannot be overstated. One avoidable pitfall in level selection is to never end a construct at the apex of kyphosis or scoliosis. Radiographs include a standing anteroposterior (AP) and lateral radiograph on a 36-in. cassette, as well as supine bending films. Magnetic resonance imaging, computed tomography, pulmonary evaluation, and nutritional optimization should also be considered when appropriate.

SURGICAL PROCEDURE

The room should be warm to prevent loss of the patient's temperature during an extended anesthesia time, when the patient is often undressed. The author's choice of preoperative antibiotics are vancomycin and ceftazidime, to include *Staphylococcus epidermidis* coverage, as this is the most common infecting organism in many series of posterior spine fusions. The patient is positioned prone over two longitudinal gel bolsters or other specialized table, with the breasts and abdomen hanging free. The shoulders should be abducted no more than 90 degrees, though with neuromonitoring of the upper extremities, this is not critical. Neuromonitoring consists of somatosensory-evoked potentials (SSEPs) and motor-evoked potentials (MEPs) of the upper and lower extremities, as well as electromyography (EMG) for pedicle screw stimulation. It is the author's preference to use aprotinin or similar agents on major spine fusions to minimize blood loss.

Subperiosteal dissection is carried out over the area to be fused, making sure not to cut the interspinous ligament above the top end fused levels in an effort to prevent kyphosis at the top or bottom of the construct. The placement of anchors may begin in a caudal-to-cephalad direction. Although this is somewhat arbitrary, it allows one to appreciate the harmonious change in rotation of the vertebral bodies while placing pedicle screws.

The spinous processes are removed in the thoracic region where the spinous process overlaps the interlaminar region, but removal may not always be needed in the lumbar region (Fig. 30-1). A Kerrison rongeur is then used to remove the ligamentum flavum (Fig. 30-2). *With two hands,* the Kerrison is placed in the midline between the ligamentum flavum into the epidural space and brought toward the surgeon's body. It is vitally important that once in the canal, the Kerrison is always pulled upward against the ligamentum and is never pushed downward into the spinal cord. An inadvertent push into the canal could lead to permanent paralysis. Assistants who believe their surgical skills are superior enough to warrant one-handed surgery at this stage are not invited back.

The Kerrison should remain against the anterior side of the ligamentum flavum at all times to sweep epidural vessels from the flavum and prevent their laceration. If epidural bleeding is encountered, it is usually venous and easily controlled with various hemostatic products; however, one must remember not to stuff these products into the canal, as doing so could cause neurologic injury from mass effect. Epidural bleeding may also be controlled by bipolar cautery. Suction is done safely and effectively by dragging the sucker tip across the ligamentum—not plunging into the canal. Wide release and/or osteotomies may be done at this time if needed.

Steel sublaminar wires may be used with steel rods. Titanium or cobalt chrome wires may be used interchangeably with titanium and cobalt chrome rods. Wires are often manufactured with a bend at one end and a ball at the other end (Fig. 30-3). In general, avoid cutting and making you own wires, as sharp edges may catch dura or epidural veins during the sublaminar passage. Sublaminar wires may be single or multiple strands; both types display equivalent mechanical behavior as part of a construct. The multistrand wires have less canal encroachment in the final construct but are probably equal at time of placement. Multistrand wires are also more pliable and seem easier to remove if necessary to do so at a future date. However, they are more cumbersome to tighten and retighten during the initial surgery.

A needle holder is used to bend the wires so that the radius of the bend is between one and two times the cephalad-caudad length of the lamina under which it will be passed. Thus, lumbar wires generally require larger bends than do thoracic wires. Because of the shingling of the cephalad

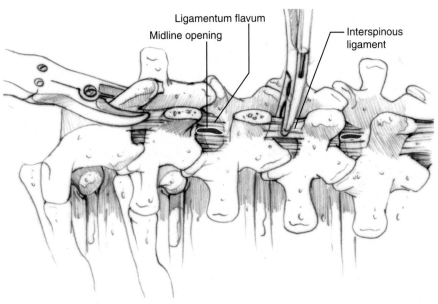

FIGURE 30-1   Spinous processes are removed almost down to the lamina. A large rongeur is used to remove the interspinous ligament down to the ligamentum flavum. In the thoracic region, and especially in cases of relative lordosis, a small rongeur may be needed to get to this point, as the large rongeur often cannot fit. A useful landmark is the midline space between the ligamentum flavum, in which a small amount of epidural fat can be seen.

lamina over the caudad lamina, particularly in the thoracic spine, the wires are passed midline under the lamina, in a caudal-to-cephalad direction. The surgeon should aim to maintain contact between the end of the wire and the anterior portion of the lamina *at all times* to prevent undue entrance into the canal (Fig. 30-4). The motion of wire passage is a combination of rotation and gliding. As in the proper technique for passing a suture with a curved needle, rotation of the curved wire should occur about the center of the radius of the curve, as if every part of the wire were passing through the point where the tip of the wire started. A small amount of gliding the tip of the wire along the anterior surface of the lamina is also done in a caudad to cephalad direction.

The end of the wire may then become visible emerging at the superior interspace. This point in the surgery may require a bit of patience and persistence. At no time should significant force be used. The author's preference is to pass the ball end (Fig. 30-4), which may then be grasped with a needle holder (Fig. 30-5). Others prefer passing a looped end, which may then be retrieved with a hook designed for this purpose (Fig. 30-6).

Once the wire has been successfully passed, it should be pulled up at both ends to prevent inadvertent canal entrance. The wire is slid until the lamina is in its center. Each wire is then bent over the lamina (Fig. 30-7). This prevents the wires from entering into the spinal canal, as at some point during surgery the wires may be inadvertently bumped.

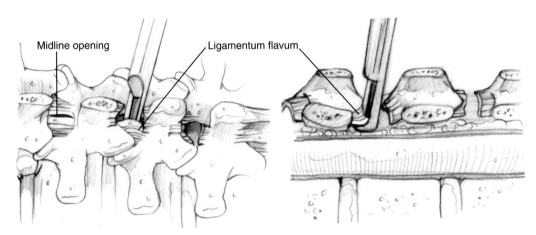

FIGURE 30-2

A Kerrison rongeur carefully enters the midline cleft between the ligamentum flavum.

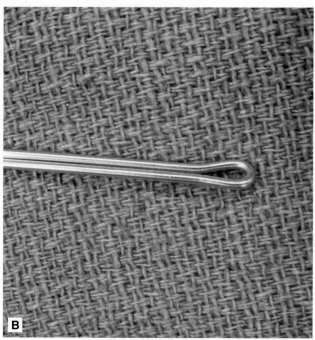

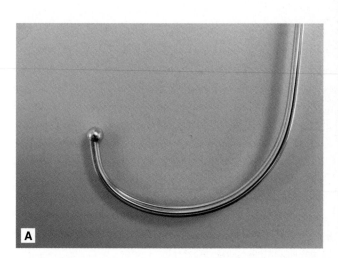

FIGURE 30-3 Solid wires are manufactured with a ball at one end **(A)** and a loop at the other end **(B).**

FIGURE 30-4

Wire is rotated with the tip touching the anterior undersurface of the lamina to guard against unneeded penetration into the canal.

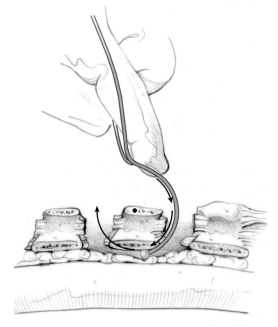

FIGURE 30-5

Ball tip of wire is grasped with a needle holder and pulled upward.

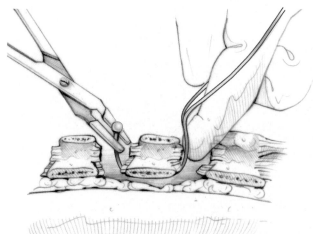

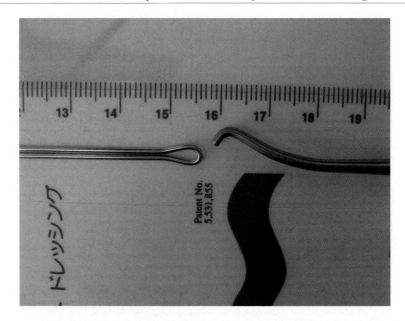

FIGURE 30-6
Loop end with hook to grasp it.

The end anchors are placed in standard fashion—usually a minimum of four pedicle screws at the bottom and four pedicle screws or hooks at the top. Wires may be at every intervening level, though some surgeons prefer to place the wires only at the apex of the curve. In a standard scoliosis case, double wires may be passed and kept together toward the concavity of the curve. Keeping the wires doubled is done more to increase the force possible before pulling through a lamina than to prevent breaking the wire.

The rod is cut, erring on the side of too long rather than too short, with the final desired contour bent into the rod. For correction mechanics, let us assume a right thoracic curve, with the left concave rod being placed first. The rod is threaded through wires and placed into the upper and lower anchors. The author's preference at this point is to allow the rod to rotate 90 degrees so the physiologic kyphosis bent into the rod is horizontal and against the scoliotic vertebrae. If ribs are to be osteotomized, that procedure may be done before inserting the first rod to aid in spine mobility and correction. The wires are tightened in an iterative process with the rod brought against the lamina at every level. Jet wire tighteners (Fig. 30-8A) or needle holders may be used. Overtightening will lead to wire breakage. Two signs that the wires should not be tightened further at a particular time are (a) the wires lose their shine, or (b) the wires begin to twist at a 90-degree angle. Ultimately, some wires break; they can be replaced using the same technique as described above.

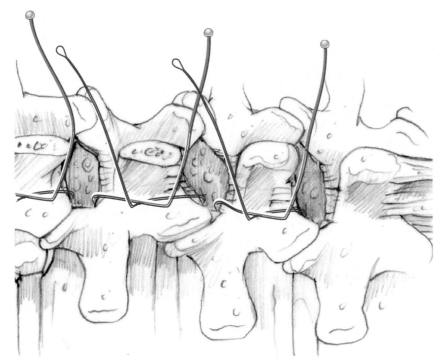

FIGURE 30-7
Wires are bent over the lamina to prevent them from being accidentally pushed into the canal later in the case.

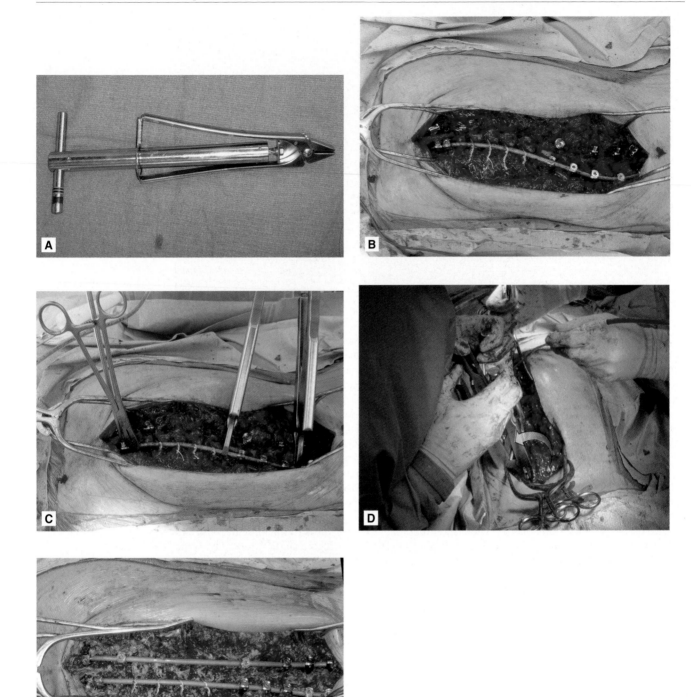

FIGURE 30-8   A. One of a number of commercially available instruments designed to aid in wire tightening. **B.** Rod against lamina after screw caps are placed in most anchors and wires are tightened. **C.** Two vice-grip rod holders are placed on the rod and maximally tilted to the patient's right. Holders can be attached to hooks if used. **D.** The rods are slowly rotated from right to left 90 degrees, turning the right thoracic scoliosis into kyphosis and the left lumbar scoliosis into lordosis. **E.** Rods appear straight from the back, confirming significant frontal plane correction.

The rod is then rotated 90 degrees, turning the scoliosis into kyphosis in a right thoracic curve. The anchors are then tightened to hold the rod in its correct position (Fig. 30-8C). In an average-size preadolescent or in a stiff curve rods smaller than 1/4 in. in diameter are likely to bend at this point, sacrificing the amount of kyphosis and scoliosis correction that could have been achieved. Distraction and compression can be done on the screws and hooks, though not on the wires. *In situ* bending of the rod may be done in the sagittal and frontal planes as needed. The convex right rod may now be placed (Fig. 30-8E). The rod may be bent with slightly less kyphosis to help derotate the apical vertebrae by pushing down on its high side. Compression and/or distraction of the top and bottom anchors may be done as needed.

Intraoperative imaging is used to confirm correct placement of implants, good correction of the spinal deformity in two planes, and good coronal alignment of the end vertebrae. Wires are cut about 2 cm in length. Decortication of all exposed bone is performed. The author uses about 3 L of jet lavage irrigation, being careful not to shoot into open interspinous spaces, as this can make the legs jump, potentially injuring the cord. Interspace openings where wires were placed are covered with sterile collagen sponges (e.g., Gelfoam or equivalent) to prevent entrance of bone graft into the spinal canal. The author uses cortical cancellous crushed allograft, in addition to the morselized spinous processes, for bone graft, being careful to place the graft under the rod and directly against bone. If rib osteotomies were performed, the space is filled with warm saline solution, and the anesthesiologist applies a Valsalva test to look for a pleural leak. If one is present, a hemovac may be placed through the leak to function as a chest tube. If no leak is present, a drain may be placed along the pleura to minimize local fluid collection and sympathetic effusions. Standard closure is then performed.

POSTOPERATIVE MANAGEMENT

Assuming solid fixation, patients are encouraged to sit up on postoperative day 1 and walk by postoperative day 2. Diet is advanced as tolerated. No brace is used unless fixation is a concern. Patients may be discharged from the hospital when they can eat, void, and no longer require intravenous pain medicines. Return to sports is between 3 and 6 months.

COMPLICATIONS TO AVOID

- When the Kerrison rongeur is in the canal, it should be gently pulled posteriorly against the ligamentum flavum at all times to avoid plunging into the cord.
- The wire should be bent at 90 degrees over the lamina to avoid inadvertently pushing the wire into the spinal cord after it is in position (Fig. 30-7).
- There is an open canal at levels where the ligamentum has been removed for wire passage; to prevent bone graft from entering the canal, Gelfoam or equivalent should be placed overlying the space.

ILLUSTRATIVE CASE

This 12-year-old boy has a mild unknown neuromuscular condition. He is community ambulatory and attends school. He has no focal neurologic signs or symptoms, and an MRI of his spine is negative. His scoliosis is troubling, as there is frank lordosis in the thoracic region (Fig. 30-9A–9J). Figures 30-8B through 30-8E are intraoperative photographs of this patient.

PEARLS & PITFALLS

- While passing the wire under the lamina, maintain contact between the end of the wire and the anterior portion of the lamina *at all times* to prevent undue entrance into the canal.
- During the course of correction, the spine usually lengthens. Plan for this by cutting the rod a little long, as it is easier to remove extra rod at the end than to replace a rod that is too short.
- Because this technique places large bending moments on the rod, choose a stiff rod—steel or cobalt chrome instead of titanium—and the largest-diameter rod possible for the child's anatomy.

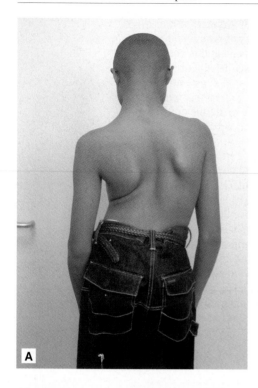

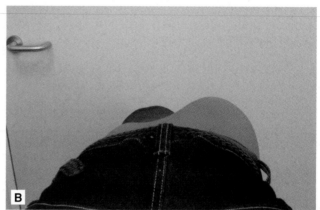

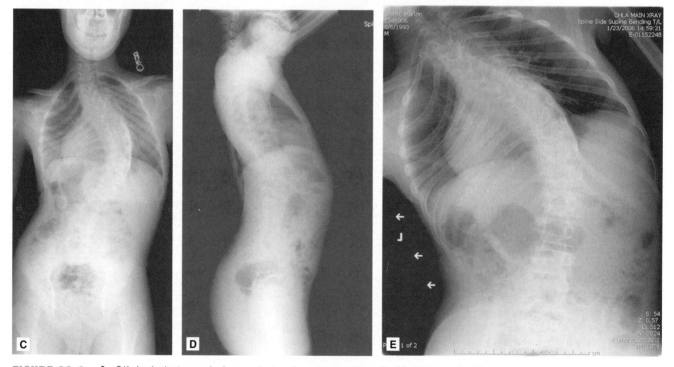

FIGURE 30-9 **A.** Clinical photograph demonstrates decompensation. **B.** Right thoracic rib hump is evident. **C.** Major curve measures 80 degrees and is longer than one would typically expect for an idiopathic curve. **D.** Lateral radiograph demonstrating sagittal alignment, notable for frank lordosis of the thoracic spine. **E, F.** Supine bending films show a moderately flexible curve. **G.** Truncal symmetry has been restored. **H.** Rib hump is gone, in part secondary to thoracoplasty of five ribs. **I.** AP radiograph demonstrates correction of the frontal plane deformity. **J.** Lateral radiograph demonstrates that thoracic lordosis has been changed to a slight amount of kyphosis. (*Continued*)

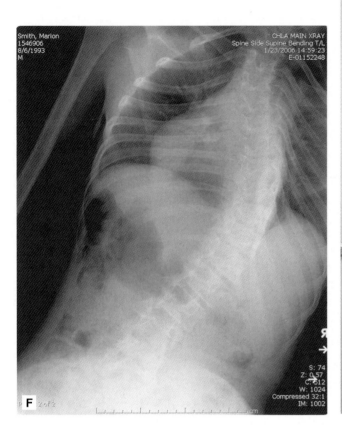

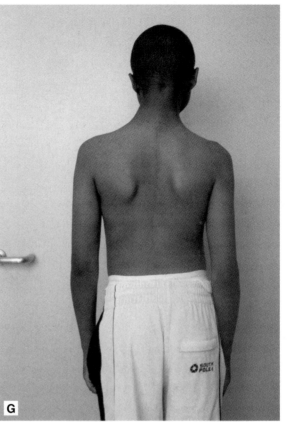

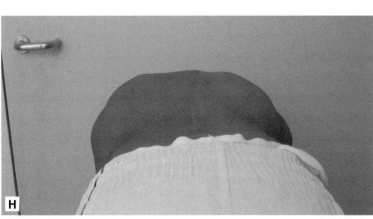

FIGURE 30-9   (*Continued*)

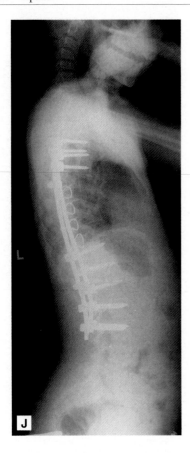

FIGURE 30-9
(*Continued*)

REFERENCES

1. Cheng I, Kim Y, Gupta MC, et al. Apical sublaminar wires versus pedicle screws: which provides better results for surgical correction of adolescent idiopathic scoliosis? *Spine.* 2005;30(18):2104–2112.
2. Cluck MW, Skaggs DL. Cobalt chromium sublaminar wires for spinal deformity surgery. *Spine.* 2006;31(19):2209–2212.
3. Girardi FP, Boachie-Adjei O, Rawlins BA. Safety of sublaminar wires with Isola instrumentation for the treatment of idiopathic scoliosis. *Spine.* 2000;25(6):691–695.
4. Parsons JR, Chokshi BV, Lee CK, et al. The biomechanical analysis of sublaminar wires and cables using Luque segmental spinal instrumentation. *Spine.* 1997;22(3):267–273.
5. Schrader WC, Bethem D, Scerbin V. The chronic local effects of sublaminar wires: an animal model. *Spine.* 1988;13(5):499–502.
6. Songer MN, Spencer DL, Meyer PR Jr, et al. The use of sublaminar cables to replace Luque wires. *Spine.* 1991;16 (8 Suppl):S418–S421.

31 Posterior Spinal Instrumentation of Neuromuscular Scoliosis to Pelvis

Vernon T. Tolo

There are many different neuromuscular disorders in which scoliosis commonly develops, among the most common being cerebral palsy, muscular dystrophy, and spina bifida. Although scoliosis may develop in children and adolescents who are ambulatory despite their neuromuscular disorder, clearly the majority of neuromuscular patients with scoliosis are nonambulatory, which is the main risk factor in the development of a progressive scoliosis in these patients. Typically, regardless of the specific neuromuscular disease, the scoliosis that results in these nonambulatory patients is nearly always a long, C-shaped scoliosis, with the apex in the thoracolumbar area and an associated pelvic obliquity. In children who have never walked, such as those with spastic quadriplegia cerebral palsy or spina bifida, this scoliosis usually begins to develop in late childhood, before the onset of puberty. In children who once walked but then stopped walking, as seen in muscular dystrophy, scoliosis typically begins to develop within 3 or 4 years of the time walking was no longer possible.

Because children with early neuromuscular scoliosis are young, with substantial growth remaining, attempts are generally made in the early stages of the scoliosis to slow the curve progression with the use of a thoracolumbar-sacral orthosis (TLSO). However, even though TLSO usage sometimes appears to be effective in delaying the curve progression, it does not obtain correction. In addition, because of the multiple medical concerns children with these neuromuscular conditions have, fulltime use of the TLSO is rarely achieved. Coexisting medical conditions, such as a seizure disorder, gastroesophageal reflux, use of a gastrostomy feeding tube, and pulmonary compromise make snug application of the TLSO difficult, if not impossible, in neuromuscular scoliosis management.

Because bracing is seldom an effective means to prevent scoliosis progression with growth, most of these curves continue to worsen year by year. If the scoliosis becomes marked at a very young age, consideration can be given to spinal instrumentation without fusion ("growing instrumentation"). If posterior spinal instrumentation and fusion are done with 5 years or more growth remaining, there will be an increased risk of the "crankshaft phenomenon," resulting from continued anterior spinal growth with a posterior fusion tether that is not growing. Once the first signs of early puberty are seen, definitive posterior spinal instrumentation and fusion can be done with substantially less risk of the crankshaft effect.

There has been controversy as to what the lower level of instrumentation should be in the surgical treatment of these neuromuscular curves—specifically whether the fusion should stop at L5 or S1. For all nonambulating patients with neuromuscular disorders, the author prefers instrumentation to the pelvis, with fusion to S1, to prevent later curve progression at the lumbosacral level and to allow for improved correction of the pelvic obliquity. In patients with neuromuscular disorders who are ambulatory, spinal instrumentation and fusion should be stopped at L4 or L5, without extension of instrumentation and fusion to the sacrum; it has been reported that ambulatory neuromuscular patients, especially those with polio, have sometimes lost the ability to walk after scoliosis treatment that included fusion to the sacrum and pelvis. This chapter addresses surgical treatment of neuromuscular scoliosis that utilizes fusion to the sacrum and instrumentation to the pelvis.

INDICATIONS/CONTRAINDICATIONS

The primary indication for this surgery is the radiographic measurement of a scoliosis greater than 50 degrees with the child in a sitting position, though there are many secondary factors to consider. Because the scoliosis in nonambulatory patients usually starts in early childhood and is a collapsible type that can be partially corrected relatively easily, it is often feasible to wait a few years after the curve has measured 50 degrees. A hard or soft TLSO is used for temporary sitting support and to allow spinal growth prior to the surgical fusion, with the plan to perform the surgery at about 70 degrees. If the scoliosis progresses to more than 100 degrees and/or if the curve becomes stiffer, surgery becomes more difficult and may require anterior discectomy and fusion in addition to the posterior instrumentation and fusion.

The primary functional improvement obtained from neuromuscular scoliosis correction is the ability to sit more evenly, with correction of the pelvic obliquity. As the pelvic obliquity worsens with the progressive scoliosis, the child has to use a forearm or hand to keep the trunk from leaning off the wheelchair. In those children with neuromuscular scoliosis who are cognitively intact and have good upper extremity function, such as those with spinal bifida or spinal cord injuries, the ability to provide a stable sitting base with a level pelvis is a prime indication for this spinal surgery as it allows improved bimanual activity functioning. For those children and teenagers who are totally dependent, the caretakers have reported improved ease of caring for the child after stabilization and correction of a marked neuromuscular scoliosis. In addition to obtaining significant correction of the deformity, another advantage of this spinal surgery is that it can halt further progression of the scoliosis.

Because the apex of most neuromuscular scoliosis is just below the thorax, the scoliosis itself probably does not interfere much with pulmonary function. However, as the curve becomes increasingly severe, the collapsing feature of this type of scoliosis may play a role in pulmonary function in some children. In Duchenne muscular dystrophy, some reports have indicated that there is a slower decline in pulmonary function if posterior spinal instrumentation and fusion are done at lesser degrees of scoliosis, with the recommendation to do this spinal surgery at any point after the scoliosis measures more than 30 degrees.

The primary contraindication for posterior spinal instrumentation and fusion is related to the coexisting medical problems these patients have. In those with muscular dystrophy, the patient's cardiomyopathy, as evaluated by echocardiography, may be severe enough to make the risks of anesthesia and surgery prohibitive. All patients with neuromuscular disease should have pulmonary evaluation prior to spinal surgery. If the patient's vital capacity is less than 20% predicted, there is a substantial risk that prolonged postoperative ventilation support (and possibly a permanent tracheostomy) will be needed after surgery—a possibility that some parents will not want to accept. Very low bone density associated with vertebral compression fractures is not common but could be a relative contraindication for surgery due to expected difficulty with spinal instrumentation placement.

PREOPERATIVE PLANNING

Preoperative imaging studies include full-length anteroposterior (AP) and lateral spine radiographs, done in both the supine and the erect positions if possible. In addition, AP supine radiographs of the spine, with the child bent first to the right and then to the left to ascertain the amount of correction expected, or an AP supine radiograph of the spine with longitudinal traction applied will help determine the stiffness of the curve and the levels of instrumentation and fusion needed for the best correction. If pedicle screw implants are to be used at the time of surgery, evaluation of the pedicle size is carried out to ascertain which levels of pedicle screws can be readily used and which may be difficult to place. Magnetic resonance imaging (MRI) is used in patients with spina bifida or with a changing neurologic examination prior to surgery; however, most patients with cerebral palsy or muscle disease do not need an MRI. Computed axial tomography (CT) is rarely employed prior to surgery in this group of patients. An AP pelvis x-ray is obtained to evaluate the hip position bilaterally, as pelvic obliquity from the scoliosis may be associated with a windswept position of the hips, particularly in cerebral palsy.

Several medical problems commonly associated with neuromuscular scoliosis need to be evaluated prior to anesthesia and surgery. Pulmonary evaluation is important. In patients who can cooperate with pulmonary function tests (PFTs), the results will allow for the measurement of vital capacity and lung volumes and will also detect any obstructive or restrictive problems with the patient's pulmonary function. A sleep study can be considered if the child is unable to cooperate with or perform the PFTs. At times, pulmonary treatment prior to surgery is needed to decrease the operative risks.

Cardiac evaluation should be done, including use of an echocardiogram. In patients with Duchenne muscular dystrophy, electrocardiograms are often abnormal, thus determination of the shortening fraction on the echocardiogram becomes the most important value in determining anesthesia risk for surgery. In addition to those with muscle diseases, patients with Friedreich ataxia commonly have echocardiographic evidence of cardiomyopathy and require preoperative evaluation.

Patients with seizure disorders should be evaluated by their neurologist, with appropriate medications used to control seizures preoperatively. Spina bifida and spinal cord injury patients may have frequent urinary tract infections; a preoperative urine culture should be obtained and necessary antibiotic treatment carried out to ensure that active urinary infection is not present on the day of surgery.

Blood transfusion is commonly needed at some point during or after the spinal fusion surgery. Although it is unusual to have a child with neuromuscular scoliosis donate autologous blood for intraoperative transfusion, the family should be provided with the information and time needed to donate donor-designated blood for the child. Usually 4 units of blood are requested, though it is common to require less than this in the perioperative period. Arrangements are also made to have a cell salvage machine in the operating room during surgery to potentially save some of the blood lost for retransfusion to the patient.

Appropriate equipment needs to be available in the operating room prior to anesthetizing the patient. A more-than-adequate supply of spinal implants and all the necessary instruments to place these implants are mandatory before starting the case. If there will be a need for ongoing or future spinal cord MRIs, titanium implants are used; if it is thought that later MRIs will not be needed, stainless steel implants are usually employed. Spinal cord monitoring equipment and technicians to record intraoperative motor-evoked potentials (MEPs) and somatosensory-evoked potentials (SSEPs) throughout the entire case need to be present. In all patients with spina bifida and spinal cord injury, latex-free operating room products are used as protection against anaphylaxis from latex allergy. Fluoroscopy availability is required. Reservation for a postoperative bed in the intensive care unit (ICU) should have been done prior to surgery.

SURGICAL PROCEDURE

Prophylactic intravenous antibiotics, including vancomycin, are started in the preoperative holding area and should be infused by the time the patient enters the operating room. General anesthesia with endotracheal intubation is completed. An arterial line is inserted to monitor blood pressure and blood gases. At least two venous lines are placed, as is a Foley urinary catheter. Electrodes for spinal cord monitoring are applied on both the upper and lower extremities and on the head and neck.

The patient is positioned prone on either large gel rolls or a spinal frame, taking care to pad all possible pressure areas. Due to the hip contractures commonly present in these nonambulatory patients, particular care needs to be used to accommodate the stiff leg position. The shoulders are abducted 90 degrees or less. Sterile prepping and draping is carried out to include the entire spine from the base of the neck (C7) to the intergluteal cleft at the level of the lower sacrum in the operative field. A surgical "time out" is completed to confirm the patient's identification and the appropriate surgical procedure.

Instrumentation and fusion are usually done from the upper thoracic spine to the sacrum, so the incision courses in the midline from approximately T1 to the sacrum. The midline fascia and the tips of the spinous processes are identified. The cartilage caps of the spinous processes are split, and subperiosteal exposure of all vertebrae to be fused is carried out to the tips of the transverse processes. One or two vertebral levels above the most cephalad implant site are also exposed, with care being taken to preserve the interspinous ligament at this level, to facilitate instrumentation of this uppermost level. At the caudal end, the posterior sacrum is exposed subperiosteally (Fig. 31-1).

Using the same midline skin incision, the posterior iliac spine (PIS) is located on one side, and an incision is made in the fascia just lateral to the PIS. Subperiosteal clearing of the lateral iliac wing down to the sciatic notch is done, using Taylor or Sofield retractors to facilitate this exposure. The author prefers to directly visualize the sciatic notch, not just palpate it. A rongeur is used to remove the fibrocartilaginous tissue at the PIS to expose bone at this site. Using progressively larger probes, a channel is created from the PIS to the lateral ilium, passing just superior to the sciatic notch. The

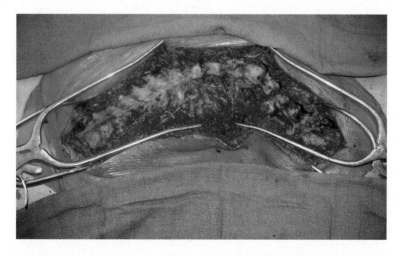

FIGURE 31-1

The spine is cleared subperiosteally to the tip of the transverse processes. Care is taken to preserve the interspinous ligament above the upper level of instrumentation.

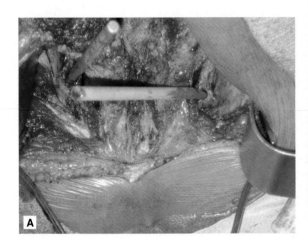

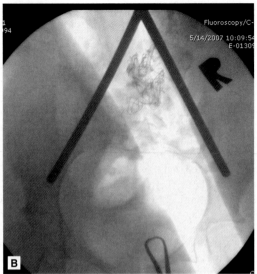

FIGURE 31-2 **A.** Temporary 1/4-in. rods are placed into the iliac wing through the posterior iliac spine, running just superior to the sciatic notch. **B.** Intraoperative fluoroscopic view of the pelvis confirms the trial iliac rod position, just superior to the sciatic notch.

final channel is completed with insertion of either a 5.5-mm (smaller children) or 1/4-in. (usually used in most patients) rod to a depth of 6 or 7 cm (Fig. 31-2). This trial rod is removed, and the channel is probed to ensure that the bony channel walls are intact and to measure the depth of the channel for later Galveston rod placement. Bone wax is used to plug the hole at the PIS to prevent blood from oozing before final rod placement. Subperiosteal dissection needs to be carried out far enough laterally at the lumbosacral level to allow a retractor to lift the paraspinous muscles dorsally to allow for visualization of the PIS through the midline wound for later Galveston rod placement. Preparation of the contralateral iliac channel is done in the same manner. (Exposure of the PIS bilaterally and the sacrum can be accomplished by detaching the entire paraspinous muscle mass from the sacrum and allowing this to move cephalad, rather than using separate fascial incisions as described above. However, it is difficult or impossible to reattach the cut distal end of this paraspinous muscle mass to the sacral region to cover the spinal instrumentation once the scoliosis correction is complete.) Although Galveston pelvic fixation has a lower profile of implant than do the iliac screws, the channel preparation for insertion is the same for both, and either form of pelvic fixation can be used (Fig. 31-3).

FIGURE 31-3

A. Galveston rods for iliac fixation are lower profile. **B.** Iliac screws can also be used.

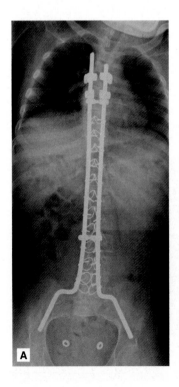

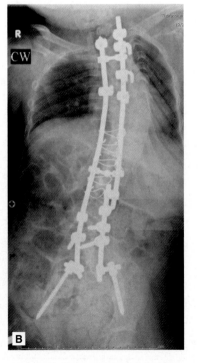

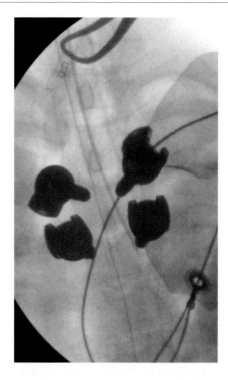

FIGURE 31-4
Fluoroscopic view of upper end of instrumentation demonstrates placement of pedicle screws.

Facets are removed with a rongeur, beginning at the L5-S1 articulation and proceeding cephalad to T12. A window of ligamentum flavum is removed at each interspinous region for later wire passage. Sterile compressed sponge (e.g., Gelfoam) is used as needed to control local bleeding. If the spinal deformity is very stiff, it may be necessary to also do foraminotomies at each intervertebral level to allow for improved scoliosis correction. Above T11, it is usually necessary to use either a power burr or bone gouges to remove the inferior articular facet at each level to be fused. All levels to be fused need to have a window of ligamentum flavum removed to allow for later instrumentation if sublaminar wires are used.

The upper spinal implants are placed next. It is preferable to use two pedicle screws at each of the upper two thoracic levels that are to be instrumented and fused (total of four pedicle screws). Pedicle screws are placed with the help of fluoroscopy as needed (Fig. 31-4). If pedicle screws cannot be adequately placed, the use of a double-level claw hook configuration is acceptable, with the lower hook in each claw placed in a cephalad direction under the inferior lamina of one thoracic vertebra and the upper hook placed in a caudal direction over the transverse process or superior lamina of the vertebra one level higher.

Once the proximal implants have been placed, 16-gauge double wires are placed in a sublaminar position, beginning at L5. These wires are passed at each level up to the proximal implants. The sublaminar wires are then separated, with a single wire on each side of the spine. Care needs to be taken to not manipulate or bump these wires too much, as they lie within the spinal canal (Fig. 31-5).

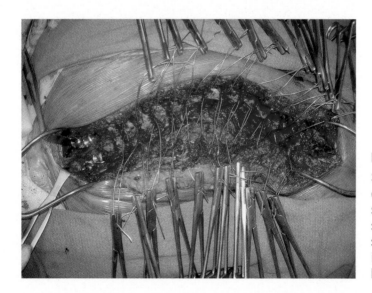

FIGURE 31-5
Sublaminar 16-gauge double wires are separated so that a single wire is on each side of the spine at all instrumented levels, beginning at L5.

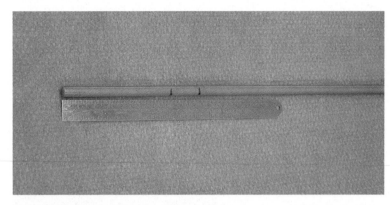

FIGURE 31-6   In this example, a mark has been made 7 cm from the end of the rod for the length to be inserted into the iliac wing, and another mark is made 1.5 cm longer to account for the offset from the iliac spine to the L5 laminar region.

The rods are then prepared for insertion. The depth of the iliac crest channel (usually 6 to 7 cm) and the offset distance from the PIS to the midpoint of the L5 lamina (usually about 2 cm or less) is added, and a mark is made at this distance from the end of the straight rod (Fig. 31-6). Hand rod benders are use to bend the rod at 90 degrees at the marked location (Fig. 31-7). The short end of the rod is placed in the slot at the end of the Galveston rod benders. While the assistant holds the long end of the rod parallel to the operating room table top and the rod plate bender is held vertical to this plane, a rod bender is placed on the short end of the rod to bend the end 90 degrees to a position perpendicular to the operating room table (Fig. 31-8). This completes the Galveston rod bend. Lordosis is then bent into the lower rod and kyphosis into the upper rod for appropriate sagittal plane alignment (Fig. 31-9). The second rod is bent in the same fashion so that the two rods are mirror images of one another (Fig. 31-10).

The initial rod can be inserted from either the concave or the convex side of the scoliosis. On the initial side, each sublaminar wire is spread apart, usually with the distal wire limb passing laterally. A surgical towel can be used to temporarily cover the wires on the second side to prevent confusion over wire identification. Once the wires have been spread, the initial Galveston rod is inserted into the iliac wing and tamped into place at the PIS. The lateral iliac wall is examined to ensure that the rod did not penetrate laterally during rod insertion. Sublaminar wire tightening is then begun at L5, followed by sequential tightening of the wires on this side to about L1 or L2. Downward pressure with a rod pusher should be placed on the rod as a counterforce to the wire tightening to minimize the chance of wire pull-through. Except in the case of milder curves, wire tightening on the initial side is stopped at this point. If the concave side wires are tightened too proximally at this stage, it will not be possible to move the rod laterally enough to engage the proximal implants. (If the curve is mild or very flexible and the initial rod can be slotted into the upper pedicle screws quite easily, however, it is appropriate to continue segmental sublaminar wire tightening above the L1 level at this time.)

FIGURE 31-7

A right-angle bend is made in the rod at the point measured to be the sum of the portion of the rod to be inserted into the iliac wing and the offset from posterior iliac spine to the L5 lamina.

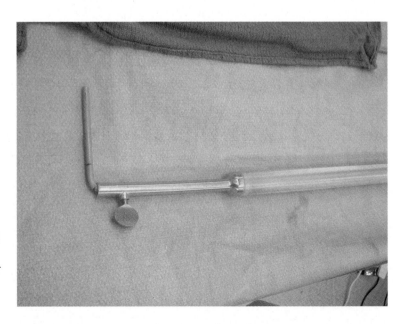

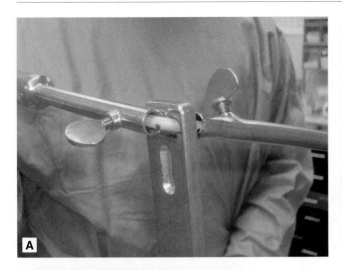

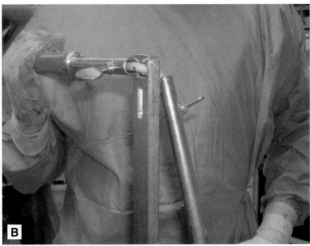

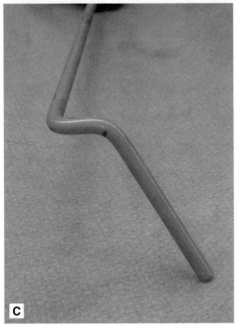

FIGURE 31-8   **A.** The bent rod is placed in the horizontal slot in the rod benders and is bent at the measurement mark for the portion to be inserted into the iliac wing. **B.** The Galveston limb is made by bending the distal rod 90 degrees to the remainder of the rod. **C.** The position of the final bend for the Galveston limb.

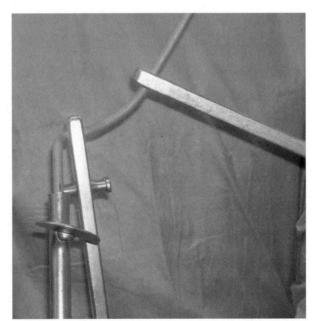

FIGURE 31-9

Using the round hole in the end of the plate benders, the rod is contoured into lordosis in the sagittal plane.

FIGURE 31-10
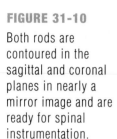
Both rods are contoured in the sagittal and coronal planes in nearly a mirror image and are ready for spinal instrumentation.

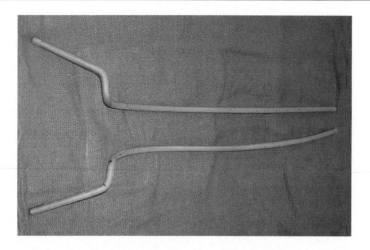

After the wires on the second side have been spread apart, the second Galveston rod is placed in the same manner as the first. Tightening of the sublaminar wires is done at L5 and continued proximally to about L1. The convex-side wires can be tightened more snugly at this point than were the concave apical wires. Cross-link devices are placed at least at one level approximately at L2 or L3 and possibly at the L5 level as well. These cross-links allow for rod separation at this level and help stabilize the lower end of the instrumentation in the pelvis as correction is taking place. The upper end of each rod is then cut with a bolt cutter to the final estimated length, based on placing the upper end of the rods near the proximal implants. It is important that the upper end of the rod be contoured into a kyphotic position to minimize the risk of pull-out of the upper implants through the bone. The upper end of the convex rod is slotted into the pedicle screws or hooks on that side and held manually in place with a rod pusher while the two most-cephalad sublaminar wires are tightened. The caps for the proximal screws or hooks are then placed to capture the rod. The remaining sublaminar wires on the convex side are then tightened. The concave-side rod is inserted into the upper spinal implants and is held in place while the upper two sublaminar wires on this side are tightened. After the implant caps have been placed to capture the rod, the remaining sublaminar wires on the concave side are tightened. Once all wires have been tightened, the twisted wire is cut at a level that leaves them about 1 to 1.5 cm in length. One additional cross-link is placed to stabilize the upper end of the instrumentation at the midthoracic level, after distraction forces have been placed across the concave-side proximal implants and compressive forces have been placed across the convex-side implants. All set screws are torqued to final tightness (Fig. 31-11).

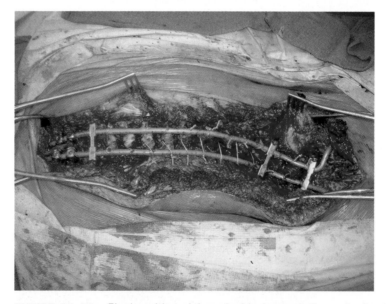

FIGURE 31-11 Final position of the spinal instrumentation, prior to placement of bone graft. The cross-links in the lumbar spine stabilize the lower portion of the instrumentation prior to placement of the rods into the pedicle screws and final wire tightening. The upper cross-link stabilizes the proximal pedicle screw or hook implants at the completion of the instrumentation.

Decortication of the midline and the lateral gutters of the instrumented spine is then done with rongeurs and a power burr. Jet lavage irrigation is done throughout the entire wound. Fusion, using local autograft from the spinous processes and crushed cancellous allograft, is completed by placing copious bone graft in the midline and over the transverse processes lateral to the rods. After the midline graft is placed, the wire ends are bent over and tamped down to prevent dorsal protrusion. Care is taken to ensure that bone graft is present deep to the cross-link implants. Prior to closure, fluoroscopic images of the pelvis are obtained to confirm appropriate placement of the Galveston rod limbs and of the upper end to ensure that shoulder balance is present.

Closure begins with suture of the fascial incisions adjacent to both iliac crests. If midline closure is done first, it is not possible to close these lateral fascial incisions. Care needs to be taken not to inadvertently pull the midline paraspinous muscles too far laterally when completing this lateral fascial closure. The midline wound is then closed in two layers, using large absorbable running sutures. A deep suction drain is usually used and is placed mainly in the lumbar region. The fascial closure is ideally closed in a watertight fashion. Subcutaneous and subcuticular closure are completed over a suction drain placed in the region of the iliac crests. Reinforcing nylon interrupted simple sutures are usually placed at the lower 4 to 6 in. of this incision to guard against wound dehiscence, as there are tensile stresses placed on this lower wound when the child sits postoperatively. Catheters for postoperative analgesia may be used to facilitate pain management after surgery. Sterile dressing is placed, and the drains are attached to suction reservoirs. The patient is then placed on the hospital bed for transport to the ICU.

If the child is communicative and has voluntary movement of any part of the lower extremities, the patient is kept in the operating room until lower extremity movement has been confirmed, even if intraoperative spinal cord monitoring was normal. Once the child has awakened sufficiently from anesthesia to voluntarily move the lower extremities to command, the child is considered to have the same neurologic function as preoperatively. The decision of whether to extubate the patient at the end of the surgical case is the anesthesiologist's responsibility. The patient is then moved to the ICU for postoperative care.

POSTOPERATIVE MANAGEMENT

Postoperative management provided by the pediatric intensivists, including fluid management, pain control, cardiac care, and pulmonary issues, is beyond the scope of this chapter. The orthopaedist needs to be involved enough to be aware of the medical issues being addressed, but is usually not the one providing the hour-to-hour care for the first day or two following surgery.

Because the segmental spinal instrumentation described in this chapter is very strong fixation, a brace or cast following surgery is not necessary. If medically stable, the child is started with sitting a day or two after surgery. Progressively longer periods of time for sitting are used each day. The criteria for hospital discharge include satisfactory wound healing, absence of pulmonary or gastrointestinal problems, ability to tolerate adequate oral or gastrostomy-tube intake, and adequate pain control with oral pain medications. Hospital stays are usually 6 to 7 days, with longer stays if postoperative ventilator assistance is needed.

After hospital discharge, there are no special precautions needed for lifting or moving the child. Sitting is allowed as much as the child can tolerate. A wound check is done about 1 week after hospital discharge. The child is seen 1 month, 3 months, and 6 months postoperatively, with spinal radiographs obtained at each office visit. These children are usually not too physically active due to their neuromuscular disease, but no specific physical activity restrictions are recommended once wound healing is complete.

COMPLICATIONS TO AVOID

The principal concern intraoperatively is a possible iatrogenic neurologic injury resulting from the spinal instrumentation and fusion. The continual intraoperative recording of a combination of MEPs and SSEPs is preferred to detect an emerging neurologic problem. However, if the child has a history of seizures, it is sometimes not wise to use MEPs, due to the cranial stimulation. If there is a change in the MEPs or SSEPs during surgery, mean arterial blood pressure is raised initially. If the signals return to normal, surgery is continued. If the signals remain abnormal, the spinal correction is reversed, and the implants may be removed. If the MEPs and SSEPs return to normal baseline, the surgical instrumentation and correction are resumed, perhaps with a somewhat lesser amount of correction. If the signals remain abnormal after correction has been released and the implants removed, the child is wakened, with an attempt to have him or her move the lower extremities to command. If there is voluntary movement in the upper extremities and not in the lower extremities, methylprednisolone protocol is begun. No further attempts at instrumentation are done, bone graft is placed over the spine, and wound closure is carried out.

Medical complications in the perioperative period will occur less often if thorough preoperative pulmonary and cardiac evaluations are done to proactively deal with potential medical complications.

Wound infection rates are higher in patients with neuromuscular scoliosis than in other patients undergoing scoliosis surgery. Preoperative nutritional status can be assessed with a serum albumin and immunocompetence screened with a total lymphocyte count. If either or both of these are below normal, nutritional supplements prior to surgery can decrease the rate of postoperative complications, including wound infection. In patients with spina bifida, ensuring healthy skin through which the scoliosis surgery incision is made may require plastic surgery before the spine surgery to minimize the postoperative wound complication rate. For the best effect, preoperative antibiotics, usually vancomycin and a cephalosporin, should have been given completely by the time of the initial skin incision for the spinal surgery.

Although the use of allograft in neuromuscular scoliosis surgery has been implicated as leading to higher wound infection rates, thorough jet lavage irrigation of the wound prior to bone graft placement may minimize infection risk.

The spine's bone density is generally lower in nonambulatory children and teenagers with neuromuscular scoliosis than in children who are able to walk. In addition, many children with cerebral palsy have lower bone density as a result of seizure medications. Therefore, implant cutout is possible at any of the sites where the implants are placed. At the proximal end, the implant failure rate is higher with hooks than with pedicle screws. To avoid excessive stress on the proximal end implants, the rod should be contoured into sufficient kyphosis and be held firmly in the implants with a rod pusher while the upper two or three sublaminar wires are tightened; this will relieve some of the stress on the upper instrumented vertebrae. As the sublaminar wires are tightened, a secondary twist in the wire usually indicates that further twisting may break the wire. When sublaminar wire tightening is done, a rod pusher is used to set the rod against the posterior lamina and to act as a counterforce to prevent the wire from cutting through the lamina. At the iliac crest sites for the limbs of the Galveston rod, care needs to be taken to ensure that the bend and contour of the rod are satisfactory to prevent the iliac limb from punching through the lateral iliac crest. If this happens, redirection and reinsertion of the rod under direct vision may work; however, if it is not possible to insert the Galveston limb, a fallback position is to use an iliac screw with a side connector attached to the rod (Fig. 31-12).

Most patients with neuromuscular scoliosis have C-shaped thoracolumbar curves; however, some have a double thoracic-lumbar scoliosis. In this instance, the technique described above for spinal

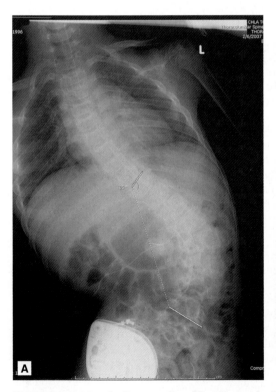
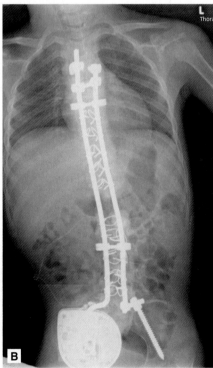
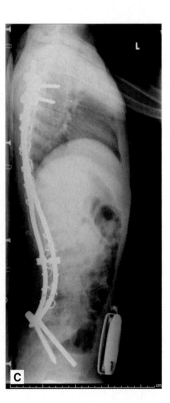

FIGURE 31-12   A. Preoperative AP radiograph of a 10-year-old boy with spastic cerebral palsy demonstrates an 85-degree scoliosis. AP **(B)** and lateral **(C)** radiographs demonstrate the postoperative correction. Because of initial Galveston rod cutout in the left iliac wing, an iliac screw was used for pelvic fixation.

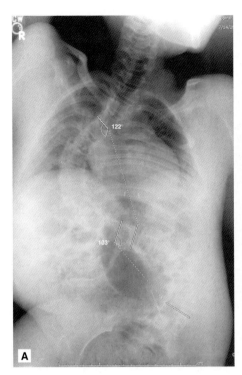
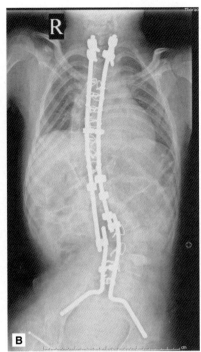
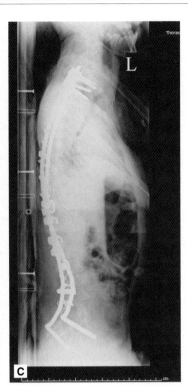

FIGURE 31-13   A. Preoperative AP radiograph of this 14-year-old boy with CP demonstrates double curves of greater than 100 degrees. Postoperative AP **(B)** and lateral **(C)** radiographs demonstrate the technique of linking rods together with pelvic fixation for severe double curve instrumentation.

instrumentation should be modified, unless the double curves are relatively mild. For more severe double curves, the spinal instrumentation to the pelvis is facilitated by initially instrumenting the lower lumbar curve with Galveston pelvic fixation, instrumenting the upper thoracic curve with proximal implants as described above, and then attaching the rods with dual rod connectors to complete the instrumentation and spinal correction. Attempting to treat a large double curve with the same construct used for the C-shaped single curve makes instrumentation technically more difficult. It also makes it harder to achieve a well-balanced spine at the end of the surgery (Fig. 31-13).

If marked thoracic kyphosis is present, the instrumentation must be modified to address this deformity. The lower half of the spinal instrumentation is placed as described above to treat the lumbar curve and pelvic obliquity. The thoracic kyphosis will then require segmental osteotomies to remove the facets and allow for improved kyphosis correction; this usually involves the use of pedicle screws at multiple levels. If instrumentation is not modified in this way, there is a high likelihood of proximal implant cutout at the proximal end of the kyphotic deformity. Once the upper thoracic kyphotic segment is instrumented, the rods are attached in the thoracolumbar area to complete the instrumentation (Fig. 31-14).

After segmental spinal instrumentation in children with spastic cerebral palsy, the muscle tone in the lower extremities is usually increased for several months postoperatively. The use of diazepam is helpful to decrease this muscle hypertonicity.

ILLUSTRATIVE CASES

A 13-year-old boy with spastic quadriplegia cerebral palsy (CP) developed a progressive right thoracic, left lumbar scoliosis, with each curve measuring about 90 degrees (Fig. 31-15A). Posterior spinal instrumentation with Galveston pelvic fixation and posterior spinal fusion from T2 to the sacrum was utilized. A cross-link stabilized the pelvic fixation at L5 and the proximal implants at T4. Pedicle screw fixation is preferred proximally if the vertebral anatomy allows it (Figs. 31-15B–15C).

A 12-year-old girl with CP presented with a 100-degree left thoracolumbar scoliosis with marked pelvic obliquity (Fig. 31-16A). Posterior spinal instrumentation from T2 to the pelvis, with fusion from T2 to the sacrum, was used to correct the deformity and the pelvic obliquity. A double-level claw hook pattern was used proximally due to the small vertebral size, which precluded pedicle screw placement (Figs. 31-16B–16C).

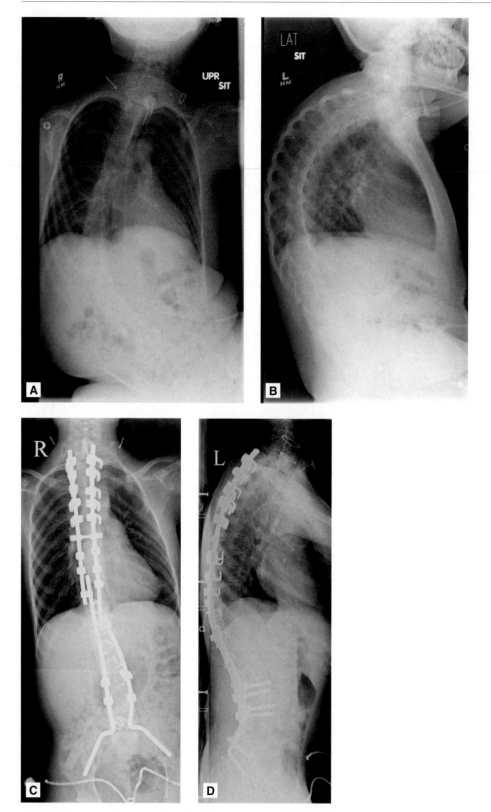

FIGURE 31-14 Preoperative AP **(A)** and lateral **(B)** radiographs of a 15-year-old boy show scoliosis and hyperkyphosis associated with CP. Postoperative AP **(C)** and lateral **(D)** radiographs demonstrate the technique of using linked rods with pelvic fixation in patients with hyperkyphosis.

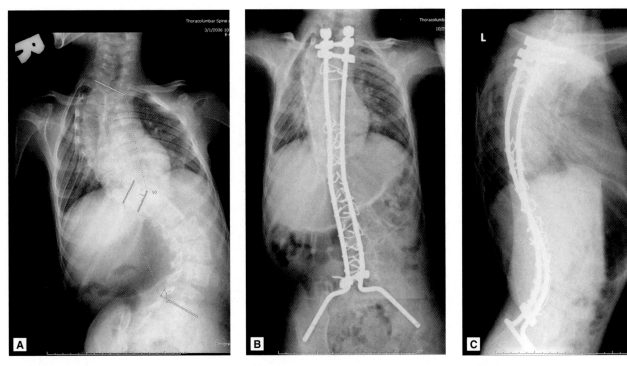

FIGURE 31-15   A. Preoperative AP radiograph with severe right thoracic, left lumbar scoliosis associated with cerebral palsy. Postoperative AP **(B)** and lateral **(C)** radiographs with Galveston pelvic fixation and pedicle screw proximal fixation.

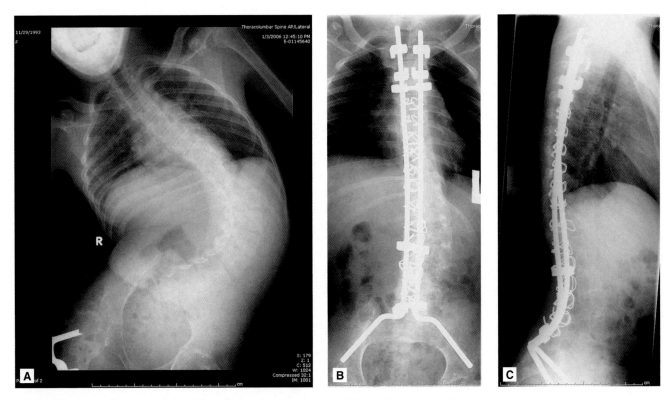

FIGURE 31-16   A. Preoperative AP radiograph with severe left thoracolumbar scoliosis associated with CP. Postoperative AP **(B)** and lateral **(C)** radiographs with Galveston pelvic fixation distally and double-level claw hook fixation proximally.

PEARLS AND PITFALLS

- Because patients with neuromuscular scoliosis have multiple associated medical problems, make sure that these problems are thoroughly evaluated *prior* to surgery.
- If there is more than 5 years of growth remaining at the time of spinal fusion, the definitive posterior spinal instrumentation and fusion should be delayed until the first signs of puberty, if possible, to prevent later crankshaft phenomenon.
- In nonambulatory patients with neuromuscular scoliosis, fuse to the sacrum, not to L5.
- If a child with neuromuscular scoliosis is walking, avoid fusion to the sacrum.
- Either Galveston rod instrumentation or iliac screws provide strong pelvic anchors for correction of the pelvic obliquity.
- Proximal spinal instrumentation with pedicle screws is preferred over the use of hooks.
- Segmental spinal instrumentation provides very stable postoperative fixation.
- Wound infection rates are higher with neuromuscular scoliosis than with other spine deformity operations.

REFERENCES

1. Benson ER, Thomson JD, Smith BG, et al. Results and morbidity in a consecutive series of patients undergoing spinal fusion for neuromuscular scoliosis. *Spine.* 1998;23:2308–2317.
2. Ecker ML, Dormans JP, Schwartz DM, et al. Efficacy of spinal cord monitoring in scoliosis surgery in patients with cerebral palsy. *J Spinal Disord.* 1996;9:159–164.
3. Jevsevar DS, Karlin LI. The relationship between preoperative nutritional status and complications after an operation for scoliosis in patients who have cerebral palsy. *J Bone Joint Surg.* 1993;75:880–884.
4. Lipton GE, Miller F, Dabney KW, et al. Factors predicting postoperative complications following spinal fusions in children with cerebral palsy. *J Spinal Disord.* 1999;112:197–205.
5. Lonstein JE. The Galveston technique using Luque or Cotrel-Dubousset rods. *Orthop Clin North Am.* 1994;25:311–320.
6. Peelle MW, Lenke LG, Bridwell KH, et al. Comparison of pelvic fixation techniques in neuromuscular spinal deformity correction: Galveston rod versus iliac and lumbosacral screws. *Spine.* 2006;31:2392–2398.
7. Sponseller PD, LaPorte DM, Hungerford MW, et al. Deep wound infections after neuromuscular scoliosis surgery: a multicenter study of risk factors and treatment outcomes. *Spine.* 2000;25:2461–2466.
8. Tolo VT. Clinical evaluation for neuromuscular scoliosis and kyphosis. In: DeWald RL, ed. *Spinal Deformities: The Comprehensive Text.* New York: Thieme Medical Publishers; 2003:272–283.

32 Posterior Occiput-C2 and C1-C2 Cervical Fusion

Purushottam A. Gholve and John P. Dormans

The craniovertebral junction and upper cervical spine are structurally a composite of bones and ligamentous structures. The geometry of the articular surfaces provides mobility, and the muscular and ligamentous attachments that span the skull and upper cervical spine provide stability. On the one hand, this versatile construct provides complex mobility to the region. But on the other hand, it makes this anatomical region more vulnerable to instability from a wide variety of causes, such as congenital abnormalities, trauma, tumors, and inflammatory and degenerative conditions. Progressive instability in this region may result in myelopathy from spinal cord compression. Major upper cervical instability is usually treated by occipitocervical or C1-C2 arthrodesis.

A number of innovative arthrodesis techniques have been described subsequent to the initial surgical description in 1972 by Foerster, who described an onlay bone graft technique using fibular autograft to stabilize progressive atlantoaxial instability secondary to an odontoid fracture. This chapter presents the general principles of occipitocervical and C1-C2 arthrodesis and elaborates on the techniques developed and published by the senior author (JPD) for posterior occipitocervical fusion.

INDICATIONS/CONTRAINDICATIONS

Documented significant instability at the atlanto-occipital or atlantoaxial joint is an indication for posterior arthrodesis of either occiput-C2 or C1-C2, respectively. Atlanto-occipital instability is determined by complex measurements on radiographs as described by the Powers ratio, the Kaufmann method, the Harris method, or a translation of more than 2 mm at the atlanto-occipital articulation (measured from the anterior surface of the occipital condyles to the posterior surface of the anterior arch of the atlas), as observed on flexion-extension lateral cervical spine radiographs. Dynamic magnetic resonance imaging (MRI), with sagittal views in both flexion and extension, may also demonstrate an associated compression of the upper cervical spinal cord.

Atlantoaxial instability is diagnosed on the basis of an increased atlantodental interval (ADI). In children over 8 years old and in adults, the ADI should be 3 mm or less, whereas in younger children, the ADI should be 4 mm or less (some consider 5 mm acceptable). Thus, in children, an ADI of 4 mm or more is considered by the authors to be atlantoaxial instability. Advanced imaging in the form of dynamic sagittal-plane flexion-extension MRI and computed tomographic (CT) scans can provide more information regarding the degree of instability and the presence of spinal cord compression. The causes of upper cervical instability that require arthrodesis of the upper cervical spine are described in Table 32-1.

PREOPERATIVE PLANNING

Preoperative MRI or CT scans help identify an abnormal course of the vertebral artery or the presence of an open posterior arch of C1 or C2. Multimodality neurologic monitoring, in the form of transcortical motor-evoked potentials (TcMEPs), somatosensory-evoked potentials (SSEPs), and

TABLE 32-1   Conditions with Upper Cervical Instability that Can Require Occipitocervical or Atlantoaxial Arthrodesis

Congenital/Developmental
Down syndrome
Occipitalization with atlantoaxial instability
Os odontoideum
Absent occipital condyles
Congenital basilar invagination

Traumatic
Atlanto-occipital dislocation
Odontoid fracture
C1 ring fracture (Jefferson fracture)
C2 fracture with spondylolisthesis (Hangman's fracture)

Infective
Grisel syndrome (upper respiratory infection with rotatory subluxation of C1-C2)
Bacterial/fungal osteomyelitis
Tuberculosis

Inflammatory
Rheumatoid arthritis
Seronegative spondyloarthropathies, such as Reiter syndrome or psoriasis
Atlantoaxial rotatory subluxation or fixation

Tumors (instability following removal of tumor)
Primary
Chordoma of clivus and occipital bone
Langerhans cell histiocytosis (surgical intervention rarely needed)
Aneurysmal bone cyst

Metastatic
Leukemia/lymphoma (surgical intervention rarely needed)

Iatrogenic
Following extensive decompressive laminectomy for tumor, trauma, or Chiari malformation

electromyography (EMG), is recommended for use during surgery. If difficult intubation is anticipated because of associated cervical instability or spinal canal stenosis, preoperative anesthesiology consult for use of in-line fiber optic intubation should be considered.

SURGICAL PROCEDURE

Posterior Occipitocervical Arthrodesis

Several techniques of posterior occipitocervical arthrodesis are described by Wertheim and Bohlman, Koop et al., Hamblen, Cone and Turner, Paquis, and Gonzalez. This chapter describes two techniques developed at the authors' institution: One using autogenous iliac bone graft and the other using autogenous rib bone graft. Both procedures are performed under general anesthesia.

After intubation in the supine position, a halo ring is applied. The patient is then carefully placed in the prone position, and the halo ring is fixed to the operating table, using the Mayfield positioning frame (Integra Corporation) (Fig. 32-1). The desired alignment of the occiput and the upper cervical spine is confirmed with an intraoperative lateral cervical spine radiograph or fluoroscopic image. Either the posterior thorax is included in the surgical field (for the rib graft technique), or the iliac graft site is prepared (for the iliac graft technique). A posterior cervical spine midline exposure extends from the external occipital protuberance to the second cervical vertebra spinous process or to the intended level of arthrodesis. The skin and subcutaneous tissue are incised in the midline, and the paraspinous muscles are subperiosteally retracted laterally. The dissection is limited laterally, to avoid injury to the vertebral arteries, and distally, to avoid unintentional distal extension of the fusion mass. In the case of an open posterior C1 or C2 arch, careful dissection is necessary to avoid direct injury to the dura or spinal cord.

Headlamps and magnifying surgical loupes are recommended for this procedure. A high-speed diamond drill is used to make four transverse burr holes at the base of the occiput, two on each side of the midline with a minimum 1-cm bone bridge between the two holes of each pair (Fig. 32-2).

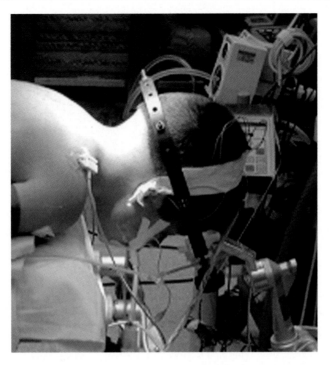

FIGURE 32-1

The child is in the prone position, with the halo attached to the Mayfield positioning frame (Integra Corporation).

The holes are below the transverse sinus and traverse both cortical tables. The transverse sinus is situated at the level of the external occipital protuberance. A high-speed diamond burr is used to create a trough below the transverse holes to accept the superior end of the bone graft.

Iliac Graft Technique   A unicortical-cancellous graft is obtained from the iliac crest. An oblique incision is made over the posterior iliac crest, and dissection is carried to the posterior iliac crest. The iliac crest apophyseal cap is sharply divided with a scalpel, and a Cobb elevator is used to expose the lateral iliac wing subperiosteally. A 3 cm by 4 cm rectangular unicortical-cancellous iliac crest graft is obtained. A notch is created in the inferior base of the graft to fit around the base of the C2 spinous process (Fig. 32-3). The graft is usually secured distally at C2, but the lower extent of

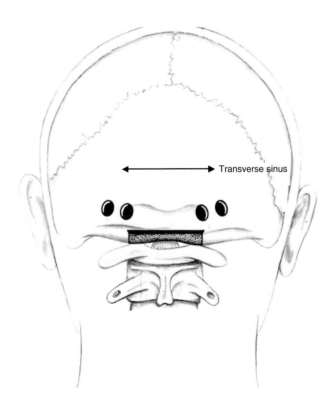

Transverse sinus

FIGURE 32-2

The occipital burr holes and rectangular trough are demonstrated. (Redrawn after Dormans JP, Drummond DS, Sutton LN, et al. Occipitocervical arthrodesis in children. *J Bone Joint Surg.* 1995;77(8):1234–1240, with permission.)

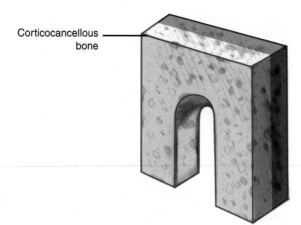

Corticocancellous bone

FIGURE 32-3

Corticocancellous graft with a notch at the base of the graft is contoured for occiput-C2 fusion.

the fusion depends on the level of instability. On each side of the midline, looped 16- or 18-gauge Luque wire is passed through the occipital burr holes and looped on itself. Wires are then passed either under the lamina of C2 (preferred) or through the base of the spinous process of C2 (or whichever is the most caudal vertebra). The left end of this wire is passed through the left arm of the graft and, similarly, the right end of the wire through the right arm of the graft (Fig. 32-4). The graft is precisely fashioned to fit securely between the trough in the base of the skull and at the base of the spinous process distally. The wires are crossed in a figure-eight fashion and are subsequently twisted with the occipital wires and then cut (Fig. 32-5). An intraoperative lateral cervical spine radiograph is obtained to check the position of the graft wire construct and the alignment of the occiput and cervical spine. Adjustments are made prior to final wire tightening by flexion or extension of the halo frame and minor refashioning of the graft. Another radiograph is necessary to confirm the correct positioning after each adjustment. The wound is closed in layers.

Rib Graft Technique The rib harvest depends on the specific topographic anatomy of the occipitocervical arthrodesis site. An oblique incision is made over the posterior rib, and the chest wall muscles are split in the line of the incision down onto the rib. Subperiosteal dissection is carried around the donor rib. The graft is obtained by cutting the rib both medially and laterally with a rib cutter. Adequate rib harvest is necessary so that enough is available for both structural and morcelized grafts. The exposed pleura is then checked for integrity, and the wound is flooded with sterile normal saline while the lungs are hyperinflated to check for any air leaks. In the case of a minor leak, the air may be suctioned from the chest cavity using a red rubber tube attached to a suction machine. The pleura is then sewn closed. With a major leak, the pleura is repaired, and placement of a chest drain tube is considered.

FIGURE 32-4

Posterior view showing each occipital wire looped on itself and the wire passed through the base of the C2 spinous process. (Redrawn after Dormans JP, Drummond DS, Sutton LN, et al. Occipitocervical arthrodesis in children. *J Bone Joint Surg.* 1995;77(8):1234–1240, with permission.)

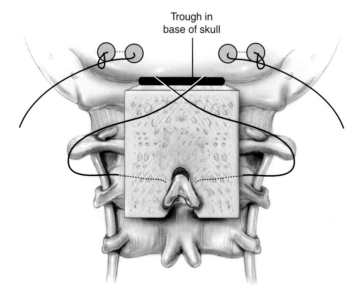

Trough in base of skull

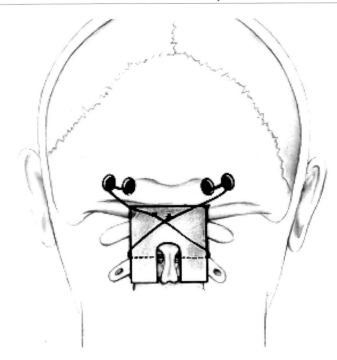

FIGURE 32-5

Schematic drawing demonstrating the final graft placement. (Redrawn after Dormans JP, Drummond DS, Sutton LN, et al. Occipitocervical arthrodesis in children. *J Bone Joint Surg.* 1995;77(8):1234–1240, with permission.)

Two full-thickness structural grafts are fashioned from the harvested rib graft, and the grafts are contoured to fit the arthrodesis site. Because the rib grafts are more elastic than are iliac grafts, they can be nicely contoured to fit very small children or infants or those with skull abnormalities. On each side of the midline, a 16- or 18-gauge wire is passed through the occipital burr holes. A braided cable or 5-0 Mersilene suture can also be used in place of wire. Distally, two sublaminar wires are passed on each side of the midline of the most caudal vertebra. Similar passage of wires under the lamina of other vertebrae in a long fusion helps increase the fixation strength. The structural grafts are placed in the arthrodesis site, and the grafts are secured under radiographic guidance by subsequently twisting and cutting the previously placed wires (Figs. 32-6 and 32-7). Flexion or extension of the halo frame, improved contouring of the graft, and appropriate tightening of the wires can allow adjustments in reduction and alignment. After satisfactory alignment has been radiographically confirmed, morcelized bone graft is packed into the central area of the arthrodesis site, and the wound is closed in layers.

Postoperative care for both techniques includes immediate application of a halo vest (measured and made prior to the surgery) and continued halo immobilization for 8 to 12 weeks postoperatively. With the rib graft technique, a chest radiograph is taken in the recovery room to rule out a pneumothorax.

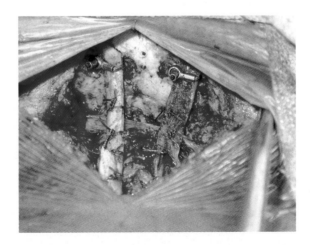

FIGURE 32-6

Rib graft in long fusion fixed with braided cables and 5-0 Mersilene suture.

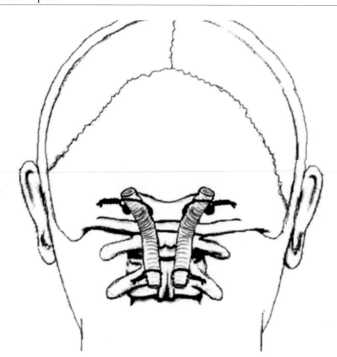

FIGURE 32-7

Schematic drawing of rib graft fixed with wire. (Redrawn after Cohen MW, Drummond DS, Flynn JM, et al. A technique of occipitocervical arthrodesis in children using autologous rib grafts. *Spine.* 2001;26(7):825–829, with permission.)

Posterior C1-C2 Arthrodesis

Several techniques are described for posterior C1-C2 fusion. The three commonly used techniques are the Gallie technique, the Mah-modified Gallie technique, and the Brooks sublaminar wire technique. Preoperative planning and positioning, including halo application and neurologic monitoring, are similar to that for the occipitocervical arthrodesis described above.

A posterior midline incision is made between the occiput and C3. The subperiosteal dissection is carried down onto C2, proceeding laterally and avoiding injury to the vertebral vessels. Too caudal an exposure may lead to an unwanted fusion at the next distal adjacent vertebral level. The posterior arch of the atlas and the bifid spinous process of the axis are identified. A horizontal incision is made through the periosteum, just above the superior margin of the posterior arch of atlas, no more than 1 cm from the midline. This helps avoid inadvertent injury to the vertebral artery and the greater occipital nerves.

Gallie Technique   A 16- or 18-gauge wire is made into a U shape, and the free ends are passed in a caudal-to-cephalad direction below the posterior arch of the atlas. An appropriately sized corticocancellous graft is obtained from the posterior iliac crest. The graft is trimmed and fashioned to conform to the posterior arch of C1 and the spinous process of C2. The graft is laid posteriorly over C1 and C2, and the looped central part of the wire is passed from superior to inferior over the graft. The looped wire is snugly fit around the spinous process of C2. The free ends of the wire are twisted in the midline (Fig. 32-8A). Additional cancellous bone graft is packed deep to the corticocancellous graft, and the wound is closed in layers. An intraoperative lateral cervical spine radiograph is used to confirm satisfactory alignment of C1-C2.

Mah-Modified Gallie Technique   This is a similar procedure to that described for the Gallie technique that includes exposure, graft harvest, and wire passage. Instead of bringing the wire loop around the base of the C2 spinous process, however, a stout threaded K-wire is passed transversely across the base of the spinous process. The K-wire is cut so that it extends 1 cm on each side of the spinous process. Following this modification, the wire loop is brought down over the ends of the K-wire, and the free ends are twisted in the midline (Fig. 32-8B).

Brooks Technique   After subperiosteal exposure, the posterior arch of the atlas and the lamina of the axis are identified. Two 18-gauge wires or braided cables are passed in a sublaminar position for both the posterior arch of C1 and the lamina of C2, with one wire or cable on each side of the midline. Care is

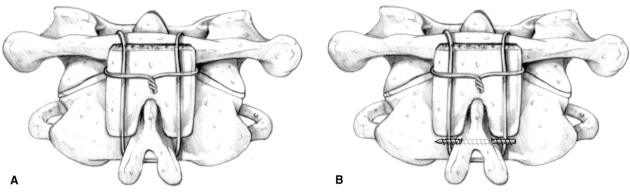

FIGURE 32-8   A. Gallie technique for atlantoaxial arthrodesis. (Redrawn after Vender JR. The evolution of posterior cervical and occipitocervical fusion and instrumentation. *Neurosurg Focus.* 2004;16(1):E9, with permission.) **B.** Mah-modified Gallie technique for atlantoaxial arthrodesis. (Adapted and modified from Vender JR. The evolution of posterior cervical and occipitocervical fusion and instrumentation. *Neurosurg Focus.* 2004;16(1):E9, with permission.)

taken to preserve the C2-C3 interspinous ligament. Two corticocancellous iliac crest grafts are harvested. Alternatively, a single rectangular iliac crest graft can be obtained. The graft is fashioned to fit between the interval of C1 and C2 lateral to the spinous process. With the bone grafts held firmly in place, the wire or cable is secured and tightened under radiographic monitoring (Fig. 32-9).

The authors' clinical experience has found the Gallie technique to be particularly applicable to older children with fully intact spinous processes. Hyperextension and posterior translation of C1

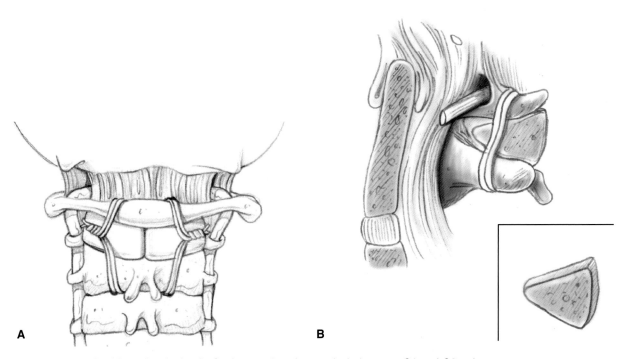

FIGURE 32-9   Brooks arthrodesis. A. Grafts are placed posteriorly between C1 and C2 spinous process and secured by tightening the sublaminar wires. (Redrawn after Drummond DS. Congenital anomalies of the pediatric cervical spine. In: Bridwell KH, Dewald RL, eds. *The Textbook of Spinal Surgery: Volume 1.* 2nd ed. Philadelphia: Lippincott-Raven; 1997:915, with permission.) **B.** Lateral view demonstrating the wedged graft between the spinous process to prevent hyperextension. The graft is shaped triangularly to achieve a good fit.

over C2 interoperatively is less of a problem with the Gallie technique when compared with the Brooks technique. In addition, it is unnecessary in the Gallie technique to pass a wire or cable beneath the lamina of C2. The main disadvantage of the Gallie technique is that the spinous process of C2 in young children is cartilaginous, which may increase the risk for wire cutout and loss of reduction; thus, in this situation, the Brooks technique is preferred.

POSTOPERATIVE MANAGEMENT

Posterior occiput-C2 and C1-C2 arthrodesis patients are immobilized postoperatively in a halo vest for 8 to 12 weeks. Oral antibiotics are prescribed for 2 or 3 days if any inflammation is noted at the pin site. Radiographic examination of the cervical spine helps check the satisfactory position of the graft and visualize early callus maturation by 5 to 8 weeks. The halo is then removed by 8 to 12 weeks. Appropriate activities are gradually increased.

COMPLICATIONS TO AVOID

The senior author (JPD) has reported complications of occipitocervical arthrodesis, including graft breakage and nonunion, fusion of an additional level caudad to the intended level, and pin tract infections. All eventually had successful occipitocervical fusion.

The following precautionary measures are necessary to prevent complications:

- Avoid too lateral of a surgical dissection, as this may injure the vertebral vessels and the greater occipital nerve.
- To prevent unintentional extension of the fusion mass, avoid too caudal an exposure.
- Identify posterior arch defects prior to surgery to prevent dural tear and/or a cerebrospinal leak.
- Pass the sublaminar wire carefully to prevent neurologic injury. Use intraoperative multimodality spinal cord monitoring.
- Less halo pin tract care is good pin tract care.
- Use titanium wires if follow-up MRIs are required (especially in postvertebral tumor excision surveillance).

ILLUSTRATIVE CASE

A 4-year-old boy was referred for orthopaedic evaluation as a part of VATER syndrome (vertebral/ vascular anomalies, anal atresia, tracheoesophageal fistula, esophageal atresia, and renal agenesis). He was born with multiple congenital anomalies, including bicuspid aortic valve, ventricular septal defect, patent ductus arteriosus, and hypospadias. He was asymptomatic, and physical exam was normal, with no neurologic changes. The lateral radiographs of his cervical spine demonstrated C1-C2 instability and a fusion of C2-C3 (Figs. 32-10A–10B). Three-dimensional reformatted CT scan confirmed occipitalization of the anterior arch and the lateral masses of the atlas. Flexion-extension MRI of his cervical spine revealed compression of the spinal cord, which was maximal in flexion (Figs. 32-10C–10D). In view of the demonstrated C1-C2 instability and occipitalization associated with a congenital C2-C3 fusion, as well as MRI evidence of anterior cord compression, a posterior occiput-C2 arthrodesis was performed (Figs. 32-10E–10F). He had an uneventful postoperative recovery. At latest follow-up, 2 years after surgery, he was asymptomatic, and the flexion-extension radiographs of his cervical spine revealed solid fusion with no movement at C1-C2 (Figs. 32-10G–10I).

FIGURE 32-10   Lateral cervical spine radiographs demonstrating C1-C2 instability: Flexion view **(A)** and extension view **(B)**. MRIs of cervical spine showing instability: Flexion of the neck **(C)**, demonstrating anterior cord compression at upper cervical spine, and extension of the neck **(D)**, demonstrating less compression. Immediate postoperative AP **(E)** and lateral **(F)** radiographs of the cervical spine. Lateral radiographs of the cervical spine 2 years postoperatively, demonstrating good posterior fusion in neutral **(G)**, flexed **(H)**, and extended **(I)** neck positions.

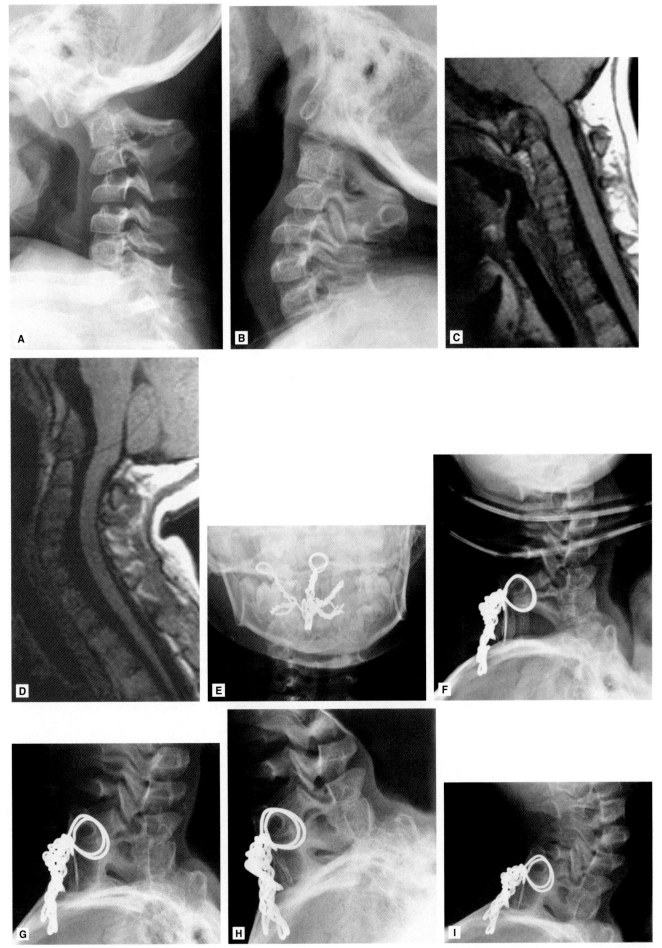

REFERENCES

1. Brooks AL, Jenkins EB. Atlanto-axial arthrodesis by the wedge compression method. *J Bone Joint Surg.* 1978;60:279–284.
2. Cohen MW, Drummond DS, Flynn JM, et al. A technique of occipitocervical arthrodesis in children using autologous rib grafts. *Spine.* 2001;26(7):825–829.
3. Copley LA, Dormans JP. Cervical spine disorders in infants and children. *J Am Acad Orthop Surg.* 1998;6:204–214.
4. Copley LA, Dormans JP, Pepe MD, et al. Accuracy and reliability of torque wrenches used for halo application in children. *J Bone Joint Surg.* 1993;85(11):2199–2204.
5. Copley LA, Pepe MD, Tan V, et al. A comparative evaluation of halo pin designs in an immature skull model. *Clin Orthop Relat Res.* 1998;357:212–218.
6. Copley LA, Pepe MD, Tan V, et al. A comparison of various angles of halo pin insertion in an immature skull model. *Spine.* 1999;24(17):1777–1780.
7. Dormans JP, Drummond DS, Sutton LN, et al. Occipitocervical arthrodesis in children. *J Bone Joint Surg.* 1995;77(8):1234–1240.
8. Drummond DS. Congenital anomalies of the pediatric cervical spine. In: Bridwell KH, Dewald RL, eds. *The Textbook of Spinal Surgery: Volume 1.* 2nd ed. Philadelphia: Lippincott-Raven; 1997:915s.
9. Gallie WE. Fractures and dislocations of the cervical spine. *Am J Surg.* 1939;46:495–499.
10. Hosalkar HS, Cain EL, Horn D, et al. Traumatic atlanto-occipital dislocation in children. *J Bone Joint Surg.* 2005;87(11):2480–2488.
11. Kaufman RA, Dunbar JS, Botsford JA, et al. Traumatic longitudinal atlanto-occipital distraction injuries in children. *Am J Neuroradiol.* 1982;3:415–419.
12. Koop SE, Winter RB, Lonstein JE. The surgical treatment of instability of the upper part of the cervical spine in children and adolescents. *J Bone Joint Surg.* 1984;66:403–411.
13. Mah J, Thometz J, Emmans J, et al. Threaded K-wire spinous process fixation of the axis for the modified Gallie fusion in children and adolescents. *J Pediatr Orthop.* 1989;9:675–679.
14. McAfee P, Cassidy J, Davis R, et al. Fusion of the occiput to the upper cervical spine: a review of 37 cases. *Spine.* 1991;18(suppl):490.
15. Powers B, Miller MD, Kramer RS, et al. Traumatic anterior atlanto-occipital dislocation. *Neurosurgery.* 1979;4:12–17.
16. Steel HH. Anatomical and mechanical considerations of the atlanto-axial articulation. *J Bone Joint Surg.* 1968;50:1481–1482.
17. Sullivan JA. Fractures of the spine in children. In: Green NE, Swiontkowski MF, eds. *Skeletal Trauma in Children: Volume 3.* Philadelphia: WB Saunders; 1994:283–306.
18. Vender JR. The evolution of posterior cervical and occipitocervical fusion and instrumentation. *Neurosurg Focus.* 2004;16(1):E9.
19. Wertheim SB, Bohlman HH. Occipitocervical fusion: indications, technique, and long-term results in thirteen patients. *J Bone Joint Surg.* 1987;69(6):833–836.
20. Willis BP, Dormans JP. Nontraumatic upper cervical spine instability in children. *J Am Acad Orthop Surg.* 2006;14(4):233–245.

33 Anterior Spinal Fusion for Thoracolumbar Idiopathic Scoliosis

Daniel J. Sucato

INDICATIONS/CONTRAINDICATIONS

The anterior approach for thoracolumbar/lumbar curves in adolescent idiopathic scoliosis (AIS) is an extremely effective and safe method for treating these curve patterns. The indications include thoracolumbar/lumbar curves greater than 40 to 45 degrees in the adolescent age group. It may also be applied to patients in the juvenile age group. Contraindications to the anterior approach for these curves are relatively few and may include patients who have had previous intra-abdominal surgery. In these patients, significant scar formation would be present, making access to the spine more challenging. It may also include patients who have an associated structural thoracic curve.[12,14]

PREOPERATIVE PLANNING

Patients who plan to undergo an anterior spinal fusion and instrumentation (ASFI) for thoracolumbar/lumbar curves should be evaluated both clinically and radiographically. The clinical examination should focus on the patient's trunk balance, spinal deformity, waistline asymmetry, and neurologic status. Assessment of trunk balance should determine both whether a truncal imbalance is present and its direction. If a thoracic curve clinically appears to have some structural characteristics, as evidenced by a significant thoracic rib on the Adams forward-bending test, then a selective ASFI of a thoracolumbar/lumbar curve would have poor cosmetic results.[14] The typical patient with a thoracolumbar/lumbar curve who would require surgery will have a trunk shift to the convexity of that curve (usually left side) that can be quantified by measuring the deviation from a plumb bob to the center of the sacrum. This type of curve is also associated with significant waistline asymmetry. Neurologic examination and history are important to ensure that there is no indication for obtaining an MRI to assess for neural axis abnormalities.[6] Abdominal reflexes, which are especially important in assessing patients with presumed idiopathic scoliosis, should be symmetric (bilaterally absent or present). Otherwise, an MRI of the spine should be obtained prior to surgery.

Radiographic assessment should include anteroposterior (AP) and lateral radiographs. The AP radiograph is used to measure the coronal measurements of the upper thoracic, main thoracic, and thoracolumbar/lumbar curves. It should also be used to assess apical vertebral translation and rotation to ensure that this is truly a structural thoracolumbar/lumbar curve without a structural thoracic curve. The patient's skeletal maturity can be assessed by evaluating the status of the triradiate cartilage and the Risser sign. The lateral radiographs should be used to measure the amount of lumbar lordosis. Junctional kyphosis between the main thoracic and thoracolumbar/lumbar curve is a relative contraindication to isolated fusion and instrumentation of the thoracolumbar/lumbar curve. Supine-bend AP radiographs can be used to assess the flexibility of the curve.

The AP radiograph is the main imaging study for planning surgical levels (Fig. 33-1). The most commonly accepted fusion level planning is to include all vertebrae within the Cobb angle of the thoracolumbar/lumbar curve (from proximal to distal end vertebrae of the two most-tilted vertebra).

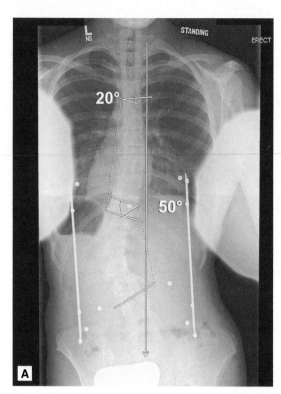
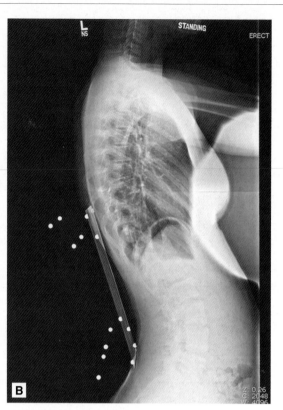

FIGURE 33-1   A. AP radiograph of a patient with a left thoracolumbar/lumbar (T/L) idiopathic scoliosis. The left T/L curve is measured from T11 to L3 to be 50 degrees. The planned fusion levels would be from T11 to L3 (the Cobb end vertebrae). The right thoracic compensatory curve does not cross the midline and measures 20 degrees. **B.** Lateral radiograph reveals normal sagittal contour.

The most common thoracolumbar/lumbar curve is measured from T11 to L3, and these are the most common fusion levels. Although supine bending radiographs do not generally assist in choosing fusion levels, they are utilized to ensure that the thoracic curve is not structural.

Hall Curve popularized the concept of a short anterior fusion. The criteria for this technique includes less than 60 degrees, which is relatively flexible. Fusion levels for this approach depend on whether the apex is at the disc or at a vertebral body. If the apex is at a vertebral body, then a three-level fusion—including the apex and one segment above and one segment below—would yield a satisfactory correction. When the apical segment is a disc, fusion and instrumentation would occur two segments above and two segments below this apical disc. It is important to understand that overcorrection of the curve is often necessary to achieve good results with this strategy and significant disc wedging below the fusion is expected.[2]

SURGICAL PROCEDURE

The anterior approach for instrumentation and fusion of a thoracolumbar/lumbar curve is performed with the patient in the lateral decubitus position. The convexity of the curve is positioned up so that access is achieved onto the convexity of the spine. In general, the rib just proximal to the proximally instrumented vertebra is utilized. For example, fusion from T11 to L3 would require an incision over the 10th rib. After the patient is positioned in the lateral decubitus position and an axillary roll is placed, the patient is secured with a bean bag with or without body positioners. The table can be flexed to provide greater access to the spine. The patient's flank and back are then prepped in the normal sterile fashion, with the umbilicus visualized to maintain anatomic perspective.

The incision is directly over the rib and extends distally in line with the rib to the costochondral junction. It is then extended just lateral to the midline and extends caudad, depending on the length of fusion. Posteriorly it is extended back, close to where the rib inserts at the transverse process. The incision is carried through the various muscle layers down to the rib periosteum, which is incised. Subperiosteal dissection around the rib is then performed circumferentially. Placing a finger in the subperiosteal layer around the rib and pulling distally as well as upward ruptures the costochondral junction with only moderate force, thus freeing the rib from all attachments except the spine (Fig. 33-2).

Posterior

Cephalad

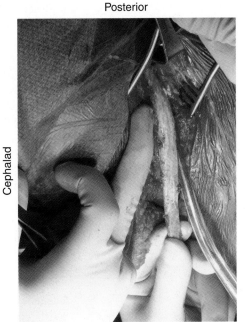

FIGURE 33-2

Following dissection down to the rib and subperiosteal dissection of the rib, the rib is free to be cut at its posterior margin (to the right), having already been disarticulated from the costochondral junction.

Usually the 10th rib is harvested, as direct access into the pleural cavity can then be achieved through the incision. (If the incision were made through the 12th rib, only the posterior portion of the incision would be above the diaphragm in the pleural cavity.) The rib is harvested by cutting it as posteriorly as possible with the rib cutter. The distal cartilage is then incised in a longitudinal fashion, with each side of the cartilage tagged with heavy suture for later closure. At this point, the retroperitoneal space can be identified by the retroperitoneal fat—a critical landmark (Fig. 33-3). The peritoneum is then bluntly dissected off the abdominal wall and the diaphragm with fingers, a sponge, or a sponge on a stick (Fig. 33-4). As this is done, the diaphragm is incised, leaving a 1- to 2-cm cuff of diaphragm along with the thoracic wall (Fig. 33-5). Marking stitches should be placed to allow for reapproximation of the diaphragm at the end of the procedure, with alternative color pairs being helpful.

As one dissects down toward the spine, the parietal pleura is identified. The peritoneum continues to be dissected off the abdominal wall, and the psoas comes into view. The psoas inserts at L1 and should be partially dissected off the spine and retracted posteriorly to provide good access to the spine (Fig. 33-6). The psoas muscle is rather easily dissected off the disks with cautery. The segmental vessels lie along the midportion of the vertebral body immediately adjacent to the psoas muscle. Thus, when dissecting the psoas muscle from the vertebral bodies, it is important to avoid inadvertent injury to the segmental vessels. Once the diaphragm is dissected down to the parietal pleura, the parietal pleura is incised, and the segmental vessels can be identified (Fig. 33-7). At this point, a chest spreader and/or Balfour retractor is placed to give good visualization within the chest and abdomen, respectively (Fig. 33-8).

The segmental vessels should be ligated. Segmental vessels may be isolated using a right-angle hemostat, which can then be used to pass a nylon suture. The sutures are then tied, and the vessel is

Posterior

Cephalad

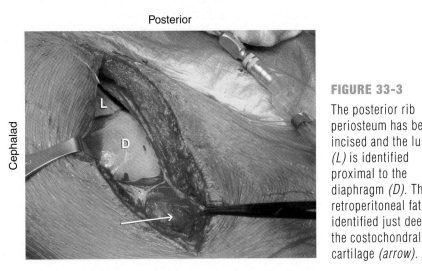

FIGURE 33-3

The posterior rib periosteum has been incised and the lung (L) is identified proximal to the diaphragm (D). The retroperitoneal fat is identified just deep to the costochondral cartilage (arrow).

Posterior

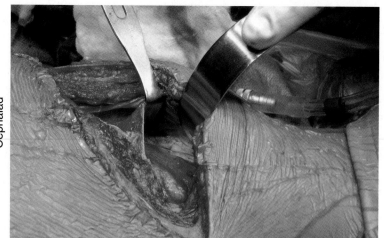

FIGURE 33-4

The peritoneal contents are bluntly dissected off the abdominal wall. The diaphragm is being retracted proximally/ posteriorly.

Anterior

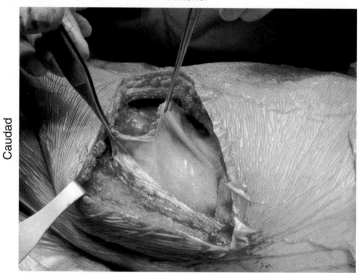

FIGURE 33-5

Incision of the diaphragm, leaving a distal cuff of diaphragm to maintain its innervation and function. Marking sutures are placed to align the diaphragm at the completion of the procedure.

Anterior

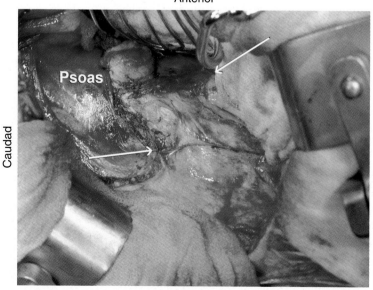

Psoas

FIGURE 33-6

Following incision of the diaphragm down to the spine. The last marking suture is noted *(arrows)*. Distal to it is the psoas muscle, and proximal is the intact parietal pleura. The spine is outlined with dotted lines.

Anterior

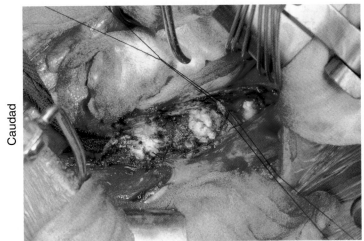

FIGURE 33-7

Ligation of the segmental blood vessels. Two silk sutures have been passed and tied to ligate the vessel. The vessels distally have already been tied off.

incised (Fig. 33-7). The cut segmental vessels are retracted anteriorly and posteriorly with blunt dissection, sharply freeing any soft-tissue attachments to the vessels.

Complete removal of the disc material is the most important aspect of the procedure to ensure a solid arthrodesis. This requires complete exposure of the disc to its posterior edge as well as all the way anterior and around to the contralateral side of the spine. One should be able to palpate to the opposite annulus. The disc can be incised with a sharp scalpel blade from anterior to posterior in a box-type cut (Fig. 33-9). This is then incised midway so that the annulus is easier to remove with the rongeur. Incision of the adjacent endplate should be performed at the junction between the vertebral body and the endplate. The periosteum is incised as far circumferentially as possible, going past the midline in the anterior aspect. The incised annulus fibrosis and nucleus pulposus are then removed with a Lexel rongeur (Fig. 33-10). The endplate is then separated from the vertebral body using a Cobb elevator (Fig. 33-11). The elevator is then turned so that it slides down the endplate, as this provides a nice clean plane for complete, efficient removal of the endplate. Each endplate can be removed with a rongeur after it is completely freed with a large Cobb. Additional endplate and annulus can be removed using ring curettes, regular curettes, pituitary rongeurs, or Kerrison rongeurs. In severe deformities, the posterior annulus is completely removed, allowing for access to the posterior longitudinal ligament (PLL). This ligament can be removed by initially penetrating it with an angled nerve hook and then removing it with a Kerrison rongeur. The author reserves the removal of the PLL for large (>60 degrees), stiff (less than 50% flexibility index) curves; it is usually not necessary in the more typical smaller, flexible curves to achieve fusion and carries some increased neurologic risk. (The editors (DLS and VTT) do not remove the PLL or the posterior annulus, as it seems unnecessary for correction. Leaving these intact provides some protection against neural injury and bleeding.)

Anterior

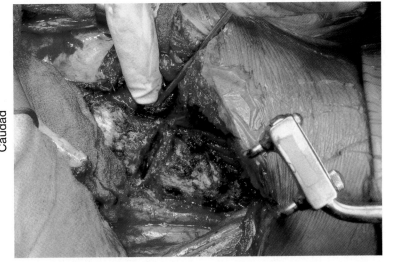

FIGURE 33-8

Following segmental vessel ligation, the spine is fully exposed from the anterior edge of the vertebral body to the posterior edge. The Balfour retractor (right) is retracting the abdominal contents anteriorly and the psoas muscle posteriorly. The proximal retractor keeps the ribs spread apart. The anterior vertebral body is being palpated.

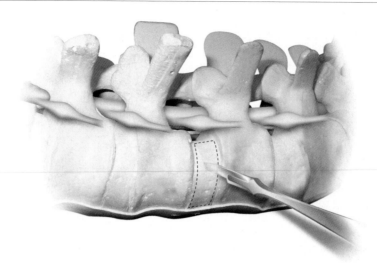

FIGURE 33-9

Incision of the annulus fibrosis in a rectangular fashion.

Following completion of a discectomy, a hemostatic agent should be placed (Gelfoam or Surgicel) in the disc space to prevent continued endplate bleeding while work is being completed elsewhere. Disc excision usually begins at the apex of the deformity, as this allows for some collapse of the spine and greater access to the proximal and distal discs.

After completion of all the discectomies, the implants can be placed. Implants can be placed using either a single screw–single rod system or a double screw–double rod system. It is important to understand the biomechanics for each system. In general, when using a single rod–single screw system, the rod diameter should be 1/4 in. (6.35 mm), with large-diameter (6.5–7.5 mm) screws. Biomechanical studies demonstrate that a single screw–single rod system is deficient in sagittal plane stiffness with flexion and extension, especially when compared with the double screw–double rod systems.[4,9,10,15] Adding anterior structural support in the form of titanium cages, femoral allograft rings, and so forth, significantly improves that sagittal plane stiffness and is equal to the double rod–double screw systems. The advantages of the single screw–single rod system include decreased cost, decreased bulk, and safety of placing a single screw compared with the double screw system. The advantage of the double screw–double rod system is greater overall stiffness, especially in the sagittal plane. The double rod system may also decrease the incidence of pseudoarthrosis, especially at the distal motion segment. Anterior structural support may not be completely necessary when a double screw–double rod system is used, possibly obviating the cost advantage of a single screw–single rod system.

When screws are placed, it is important to fully visualize the endplates of the vertebra to allow for parallel placement of screws to the endplates. In addition, the anterior and posterior margins of the vertebral body should be identified as the single screw is placed in the midposterior aspect of the vertebral body (Fig. 33-12). Because the screw should be directed in the midaxial plane, it is important to understand the rotational deformity of each vertebra. For example, at the apex, the screw will start in the posterior third of the vertebral body, and the trajectory will be anterior relative to the patient. Thus it is usually best to begin placing screws at the apex of the deformity to correctly orient oneself and then move away from the apex (proximally and distally); allowing for less rotational deformity of the spine. Placing the screw heads toward the posterior portion of the vertebral body is

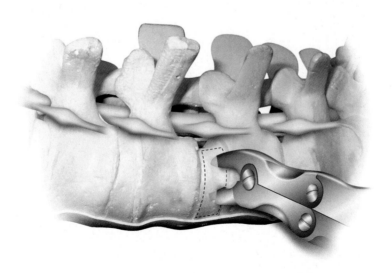

FIGURE 33-10

Initial removal of the nucleus pulposus with a Lexel rongeur.

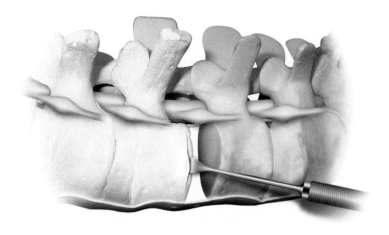

FIGURE 33-11

Dissection along the endplate of the vertebral body.

desirable to avoid creating kyphosis during compression. The awl/staple is initially introduced into the vertebral body, and then the awl is removed (Figs. 33-12A and 33-12B). A large-diameter (6.5–7.5 mm) screw is then placed in the same direction as the awl (Figs. 33-12C and 33-12D).

When placing double screws, a similar technique is used with respect to placing screws in the correct trajectory. A staple/plate is used to orient both screws, and awls are placed prior to screw insertion.

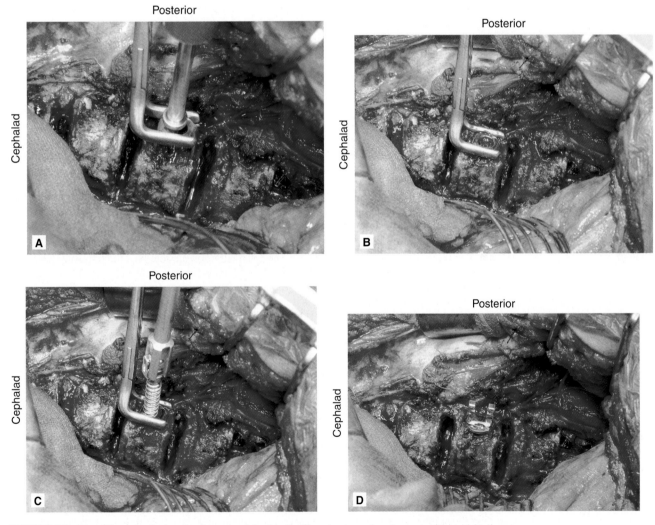

FIGURE 33-12   Placement of a single screw/staple. **A.** The staple and awl are positioned in the midvertebral body in the coronal plane and slightly posterior in the sagittal plane. **B.** The awl is advanced with the staple until the staple is flush with the cortex. **C.** The screws are advanced either with or without tapping the lateral convex cortex. **D.** Following final seating of the screw: Note the complete discectomy, allowing full visualization for safe screw placement.

Posterior

Cephalad

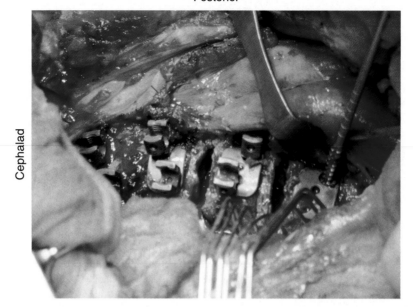

FIGURE 33-13   In the dual rod system, the plate is centered on the vertebral body and advanced into place. The screws are then placed parallel to the endplates in the frontal plane. Note that the posterior screw is directed parallel to the coronal plane or slightly anteriorly to avoid the spinal canal, whereas the anterior screw is directed slightly posteriorly. Again, complete discectomy allows for full visualization of the endplate and the anterior and posterior margins of the vertebra.

In general, the posterior screw is placed initially, followed by the anterior screw. These two screws, which are usually placed in a convergent method, increase the pull-out strength (Fig. 33-13).

It is especially important to place the most proximal and distal screws parallel to the endplates, as some mild screw plow may occur (particularly in a single rod system) during the correction maneuver. It is best to err on directing the screws slightly toward the apex of the deformity to account for this screw plow.

During screw placement, the screw length should be appropriate to allow for bicortical purchase without being excessively long. Palpation on the opposite cortex can be performed to adjust the screw length accordingly. When large screws are used in these generally healthy patients with good bone density, the screw purchase should be outstanding; screw loosening is relatively rare. If a tap is used, which the author does not find necessary, it must not penetrate past the opposite cortex, as this may injure segmental vessels in a place that would be difficult to control.

Following screw placement, the rib harvested during the initial exposure is divided into small segments and placed into the disc spaces. It is important to place these fragments as posterior and as lateral onto the concave side as possible. Usually, when a good discectomy is performed, the rib that is harvested is not enough bone to fully fill the disc space. In this case, allograft bone or some other bone graft substitute should be utilized.

Once the posterior and concave sides of the discs have been filled, the next step is to correct the spine. Rod rotation is usually performed as the primary corrective maneuver and has been traditionally performed with a single rod system (Fig. 33-14). This works exceptionally well in correcting the coronal plane deformity, as well as maintaining sagittal plane lordosis. If the table was flexed at the initial stage of the surgery. it should be leveled so that maximal deformity correction can be achieved. Following rod rotation, assessment of the deformity correction is made; minor adjustments can be made with further rotation of the rod or *in situ* bending. Compression is an additional maneuver for correcting the coronal plane deformity; however, this step should wait until anterior structural support is placed to avoid losing lordosis or creating kyphosis.

A similar correction maneuver can be performed with a double screw–double rod system (Fig. 33-15). Alternatively, several screwdrivers can be placed in the anterior screws and then be used to push down on the spine to correct the coronal and sagittal plane. The posterior rod can then be seated and fully tightened. The anterior rod, which is added after the correction has been performed, is used to increase the construct's overall stiffness.

An AP radiograph can be obtained to ensure that overall correction is achieved. A true lateral radiograph can ensure that screws are not in the vertebral canal. If complete correction is the goal, it

Posterior

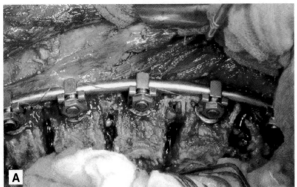

Posterior

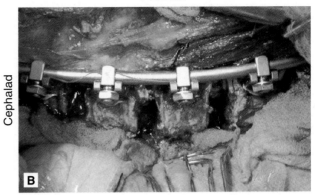

Posterior

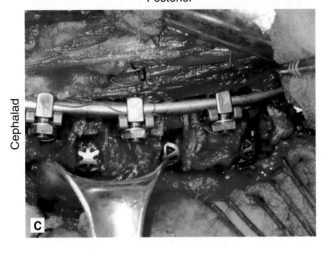

FIGURE 33-14   Spine deformity correction with a single rod. **A.** The single 1/4-in. rod is placed with the coronal plane deformity contoured into the rod and seated. **B.** Following rod rotation, the coronal plane deformity is corrected, and lordosis is restored to the spine. **C.** Anterior structural support (titanium mesh cages filled with autograft) is placed into the anterior-concave aspect of the spine.

is easy to assess on a radiograph. Likewise, if proximal end vertebra tilt is necessary to avoid over-correction in the presence of a right thoracic curve, this can also be assessed on the radiographs.

Anterior structural support can be placed before or after rod rotation and correction of the spine deformity. The author places anterior structural support following rod rotation, primarily because of the concern of stiffening the intervertebral segments, thus preventing complete deformity correction. The anterior structural support is usually placed in the levels distal to T12 to maintain lordosis, to correct the coronal plane deformity by placing the anterior structural support into the concavity of the curve, as well as increasing the overall sagittal plane stiffness of the construct (Fig. 33-14C). At each segment, distraction can be performed to seat the anterior structural support. Compression is then performed to secure the support. Compression is done in sequential levels, from proximal to distal. Additional bone graft is then placed to completely fill the disc space.

Closure of the patient is performed by initially closing the parietal pleura over the implant, using a running Vicryl suture (Fig. 33-16). The diaphragm is then closed with interrupted sutures, using pop-off needles so that the all stitches can be placed and cut at the end (Fig. 33-17). A large (24 French) chest tube can be used to avoid clotting over time.

Following completion of closure of the diaphragm and placement of chest tube, the chest is reapproximated with the rib approximator and multiple large 1-0 Vicryl sutures (Fig. 33-18). The periosteum of the rib is then oversewn with a 2-0 stitch. The muscle layers are closed sequentially, followed by skin closure. An x-ray is usually taken to ensure that the lung is completely inflated and that the implants are in a good position, with overall good correction of the spine.

In general, the results from an open ASFI of a thoracolumbar/lumbar curve are very satisfying, with excellent coronal, sagittal, and axial plane correction (Fig. 33-19).

POSTOPERATIVE MANAGEMENT

Immediately postoperatively, clear liquids are utilized until adequate bowel sounds are audible. A soft diet is then initiated and advanced as tolerated. In general, the patient's appetite is significantly diminished for a few days postoperatively, and hydration is achieved with intravenous fluids during the first 24

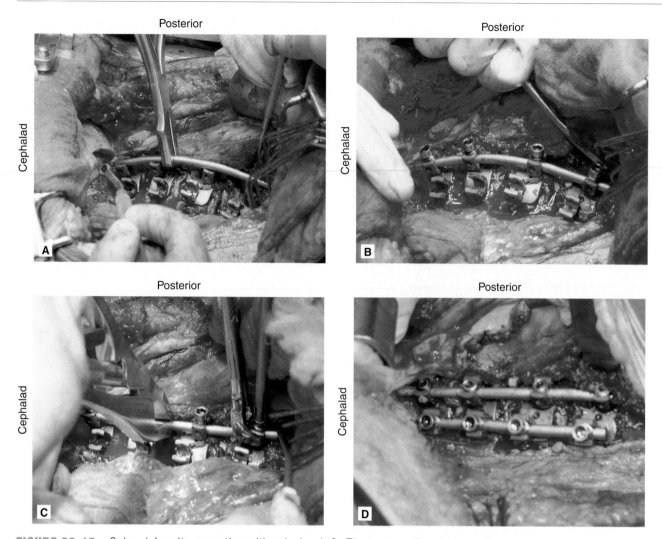

FIGURE 33-15   Spine deformity correction with a dual rod. **A.** The contoured posterior rod is initially placed in-line with the coronal plane deformity. **B.** The posterior rod is provisionally secured with the set screws. **C.** Following rod rotation, coronal plane correction has occurred. Restoration of the sagittal plane is achieved, and the set screws are fully tightened. **D.** Because complete correction of the spine has been achieved with the posterior rod, the anterior rod is laid in and secured with little or no deformity correction.

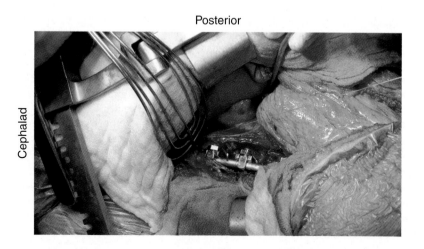

FIGURE 33-16

Closure of the parietal pleura over the implant.

Posterior

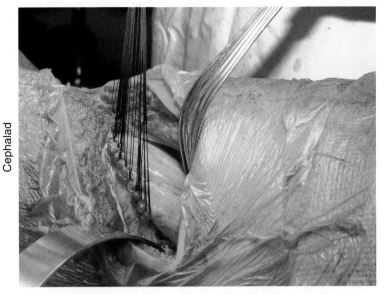

FIGURE 33-17
Closure of the diaphragm using neurolon stitches. The chest is to the right on the photograph, and the abdominal contents are to the left.

to 48 hours. Antibiotics are generally continued for 24 to 48 hours postoperatively. Stool softeners and other bowel regimens, including suppositories and enemas, may be used to facilitate bowel function.

Patients are usually mobilized on the first day to sit in the chair. On the second postoperative day, they are allowed to ambulate if and when the chest tube has been discontinued. Aggressive pulmonary toilet is necessary during the initial postoperative period to prevent atelectasis, subsequent fevers, and potential pneumonias. Postoperative ventilatory support is extremely rare at the author's institution due to aggressive pulmonary treatments with incentive spirometer, intermittent positive pressure ventilation if necessary, and chest physiotherapy. The chest tube is maintained on wall suction until there is a significant decline in the volume as well as a change to a more serous-colored fluid. The chest tube is usually removed when there is less than 80 cc per shift. A chest x-ray is obtained about 1 hour after chest tube removal.

Following discharge from the hospital, the patient usually does not require immobilization if dual rods or a single rod with anterior column support were used. However, if a single rod construct without anterior structural support was used, it is generally recommended to wear a brace for 3 months during activities (walking and standing) to prevent significant sagittal plane motion, especially flexion. (Single rod constructs without anterior structural support can allow for excessive sagittal plane motion.)

When single 6.35-mm diameter rods with anterior structural support or a double rod system are utilized, patients are allowed to do limited activities for the initial 6 weeks. Following the 6 weeks, patients are generally feeling more vigorous, and more activities are allowed at this point. Once solid fusion is visualized radiographically, especially on the lateral radiograph, full activities, including

Posterior

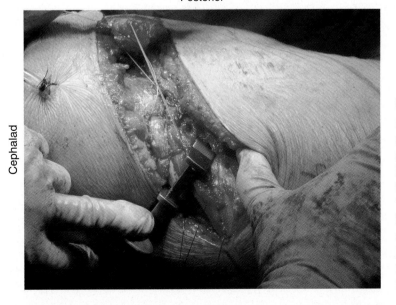

FIGURE 33-18
Closure of the chest/abdomen. A rib approximator is used to bring the ribs close together, while a large Vicryl suture secures the ribs together. A chest tube was placed just prior to reapproximating the ribs.

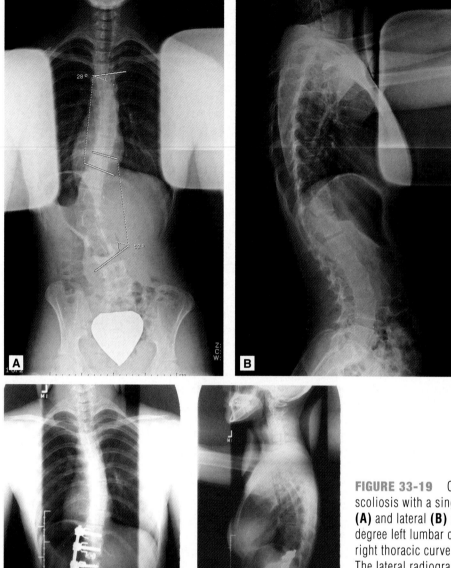

FIGURE 33-19 Correction of thoracolumbar/lumbar scoliosis with a single 6.35-mm rod. Preoperative AP **(A)** and lateral **(B)** radiographs, demonstrating a 52-degree left lumbar curve measured from T10 to L3 and a right thoracic curve measuring 28 degrees from T5 to T10. The lateral radiograph demonstrates some kyphosis at the apex of the lumbar curve (T11–T12). AP **(C)** radiograph following an anterior instrumentation and fusion from T11 to L3, with anterior structural support at each level below T12. A nice coronal plane correction is achieved without overcorrection to allow an adequate response of the thoracic curve. The proximal fusion level of T11 is chosen (one distal to the preoperative proximal end vertebra) to provide as many mobile thoracic segments for the thoracic curve response. **(D)** The lateral radiograph demonstrates nice restoration of the lumbar lordosis.

athletic activities, are then allowed. The time patient is allowed to return to contact sports is controversial and varies from one surgeon to another.

COMPLICATIONS TO AVOID

The number of complications of anterior surgery are low and fall into three main categories—intraoperative, immediate postoperative, and long-term postoperative complications. Intraoperative complications are extremely rare. One needs to be careful with segmental blood vessel ligation to avoid excessive bleeding. Retraction of the ureters are important to avoid injury. The great vessels are usually retracted adequately following dissection. Neurologic injury from ligation of the segmental blood vessels, leading to compromised spinal cord perfusion, is exceedingly rare in the lumbar spine; however, hypotensive anesthesia should be avoided during anterior surgery in the thoracic spine.[18] A cautious approach is to temporarily ligate the segmental vessels with a vessel clip, which can be removed if changes in the spinal cord monitoring occur. Neuro monitoring following ligation of the vessel with the vessel clip should be performed for 5 to 10 minutes, at which point it is generally accepted that neurologic injury will not subsequently occur.[1]

Neurologic injury from screw penetration into the canal can be avoided with an understanding of the anatomy of the vertebra, as well as dissection during discectomy back to identify the posterior annulus and/or posterior longitudinal ligament, in addition to a lateral x-ray to define screw placement.

Patients will postoperatively feel temperature asymmetry in the lower extremities. The ipsilateral legs will feel warmer following surgery secondary to dissection of the sympathetic chain in the thoracolumbar spine. This often resolves over a 6- to 12-month period. However, it may be permanent. Appropriate patient counseling preoperatively is important.

Immediate postoperative complications include atelectasis secondary to the thoracoabdominal approach with entrance into the chest, which may be exacerbated by postoperative splinting due to pain. This complication may contribute to fever within the first 48 hours and is treated with aggressive pulmonary toilet and an increase in physical activity. Postoperative ileus can occur and is treated with bowel rest. Total parental nutrition is usually unnecessary in the otherwise healthy patient.

The most common long-term complication with this surgical approach is pseudarthrosis (Fig. 33-20), with early studies demonstrating an incidence between 10 and 40%.[5,7,17] However, the pseudarthrosis

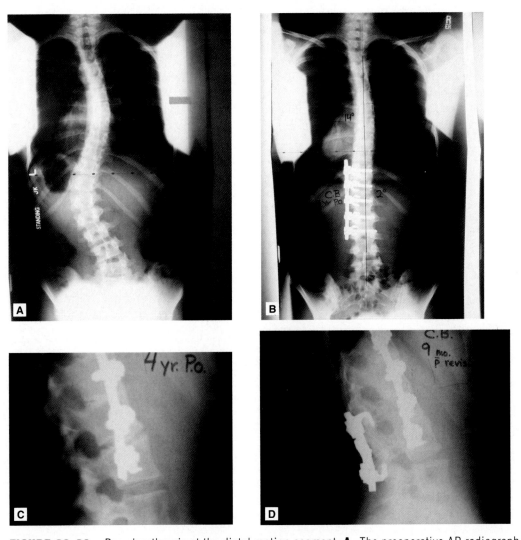

FIGURE 33-20   Pseudoarthrosis at the distal motion segment. **A.** The preoperative AP radiograph of a patient with a TL/L curve measuring 52 degrees from T11 to L3. **B.** The 1-year postoperative radiograph, following an AFI from T11 to L3, with very nice coronal plane correction. **C.** The lateral radiographs 4 years after the original surgery, demonstrating a pseudoarthrosis at the L2–L3 level without obvious implant failure. **D.** The lateral radiograph 9 months following successful revision with posterior spinal fusion of only the L2–L3 level. The anterior aspect of the spine went on to a solid fusion, as seen on this radiograph, secondary to the rigid fixation of the posterior construct.

rate has recently improved due to a better understanding of the anatomy of the thoracolumbar spine, a more complete and aggressive discectomy, aggressive bone grafting, the use of autologous bone supplemented with allograft bone and/or other bone graft substitutes, the use of stiffer constructs, and the use of anterior structural support.[3,8,11,16] The most common site for pseudarthrosis has been the distal segment, perhaps because of the rotational flexibility of the single screw with the single rod. However, use of anterior interbody structural support has significantly reduced or eliminated this problem. Treatment of pseudoarthrosis at a single level is treated with posterior instrumentation and fusion of the levels that have pseudoarthrosis (Fig. 33-20D).

Hip flexion in the short postoperative period may be affected secondary to the surgical dissection with psoas retraction posterolaterally, though this is generally unrecognized by the patient. As time goes on, relative hip flexion weakness may be perceived by the patient, especially when performing strenuous athletic activities. This is usually not a significant issue and resolves with a good strengthening exercise program.

The long-term prognosis for disc wedging below the instrumented segments is not understood. It is relatively common to see disc wedging below the instrumented segments, especially when the preoperative radiographs demonstrate a parallel disc below the intended instrumented levels or when fusion stops short of the lowest-end vertebra of the Cobb angle.[13]

PEARLS AND PITFALLS

- An accompanying structural thoracic curve with significant rib hump on clinical examination is generally considered a contraindication to this technique
- Planned fusion levels may include the proximal end to distal end vertebra of the Cobb angle, though good results have been reported with the Hall criteria.
- Anterior structural support should be considered to prevent kyphosis, particularly when using a single rod construct.
- Risk of pseudarthrosis can be minimized by bone grafting of the entire disc area, which usually requires the addition of allograft.

REFERENCES

1. Apel DM, Marrero G, King J, et al. Avoiding paraplegia during anterior spinal surgery: the role of somatosensory evoked potential monitoring with temporary occlusion of segmental spinal arteries. *Spine.* 1991;16(8 Suppl):S365–S370.
2. Bernstein RM, Hall JE. Solid rod short segment anterior fusion in thoracolumbar scoliosis. *J Pediatr Orthop B.* 1998;7(2):124–131.
3. Bullmann V, Fallenberg EM, Meier N, et al. Anterior dual rod instrumentation in idiopathic thoracic scoliosis: a computed tomography analysis of screw placement relative to the aorta and the spinal canal [elec.]. *Spine.* 2005;30(18): 2078–2083(elec.).
4. Fricka KB, Mahar AT, Newton PO. Biomechanical analysis of anterior scoliosis instrumentation: differences between single and dual rod systems with and without interbody structural support. *Spine.* 2002;27(7):702–706.
5. Hsu LC, Zucherman J, Tang SC, et al. Dwyer instrumentation in the treatment of adolescent idiopathic scoliosis. *J Bone Joint Surg Br.* 1982;64:536–541.
6. Inoue M, Minami S, Nakata Y, et al. Preoperative MRI analysis of patients with idiopathic scoliosis: a prospective study [elec.]. *Spine.* 2005;30(1):108–114(elec.).
7. Kamimura M, Ebara S, Kinoshita T, et al. Anterior surgery with short fusion using the Zielke procedure for thoracic scoliosis: focus on the correction of compensatory curves. *J Spinal Disord.* 1999;12:451–460.
8. Kaneda K, Shono Y, Satoh S, et al. New anterior instrumentation for the management of thoracolumbar and lumbar scoliosis: application of the Kaneda two-rod system. *Spine.* 1996;21(10):1250.
9. Lowe TG, Enguidanos ST, Smith DAB, et al. Single-rod versus dual-rod anterior instrumentation for idiopathic scoliosis: a biomechanical study [elec.]. *Spine.* 2005;30(3):311–317(elec.).
10. Oda I, Cunningham BW, Lee GA, et al. Biomechanical properties of anterior thoracolumbar multisegmental fixation: an analysis of construct stiffness and screw-rod strain. *Spine.* 2000;25(18):2303–2311.
11. Ouellet JA, Johnston CE II. Effect of grafting technique on the maintenance of coronal and sagittal correction in anterior treatment of scoliosis [elec.]. *Spine.* 2002;27(19):2129(elec.).
12. Sanders AE, Baumann R, Brown H, et al. Selective anterior fusion of thoracolumbar/lumbar curves in adolescents: when can the associated thoracic curve be left unfused? *Spine.* 2003;28(7):706.
13. Satake K, Lenke LG, Kim YJ, et al. Analysis of the lowest instrumented vertebra following anterior spinal fusion of thoracolumbar/lumbar adolescent idiopathic scoliosis: can we predict postoperative disc wedging?[elec.]. *Spine.* 2005;30(4):418–426(elec.).
14. Schulte TL, Liljenqvist U, Hierholzer E, et al. Spontaneous correction and derotation of secondary curves after selective anterior fusion of idiopathic scoliosis [elec.]. *Spine.* 2006;31(3):315–321(elec.).
15. Spiegel DA, Drummond DS, Cunningham BW, et al. Augmentation of an anterior solid rod construct with threaded cortical bone dowels: a biomechanical study. *Spine.* 1999;24(22):2300.
16. Sweet FA, Lenke LG, Bridwell KH, et al. Maintaining lumbar lordosis with anterior single solid-rod instrumentation in thoracolumbar and lumbar adolescent idiopathic scoliosis. *Spine.* 1999;24:1655–1662.
17. Turi M, Johnston CE, Richards BS. Anterior correction of idiopathic scoliosis using TSRH instrumentation. *Spine.* 1993;18(4):417–422.
18. Winter RB, Lonstein JE, Denis F, et al. Paraplegia resulting from vessel ligation. *Spine.* 1996;21(10):1232–1233.

34 Thoracoscopic Release, Fusion, and Instrumentation

Peter O. Newton and Andrew Perry

T he first report of thoracoscopic surgery was in 1910, after Jacobaeus used it to lyse tuberculous lung adhesions. However, it was not until the early 1990s that this minimally invasive approach was reintroduced. Thoracoscopy, also know as video-assisted thoracic surgery (VATS), was at first limited by the available technology. Due to the significant improvement in optical technology and instrumentation over the past 10 years, however, VATS has gradually gained more uses.

Because thoracoscopic procedures utilize a limited chest wall dissection to the anterior spine, there is usually less postoperative pain, reduced pulmonary impairment, and improved cosmesis. The technique, however, requires special attention to detail and is considered by some surgeons to be too demanding and/or tedious for routine use. The learning curve for the procedure is substantial, but dedicated training and cautious adoption can result in excellent outcomes with reduced patient morbidity.

INDICATIONS/CONTRAINDICATIONS

Indications

The indications for thoracoscopic anterior release and fusion are essentially the same as those for any open anterior thoracic spinal procedure. The three main indications include scoliosis, kyphosis, and congenital deformity (Table 34-1). The thoracoscopic approach is appropriate for release and fusion between the T4 and T12 vertebral levels in patients with spinal deformity. As additional experience is gained, the procedure may be extended both proximally to T2 and distally to L1.

Scoliosis   In patients with scoliosis, anterior release and fusion has traditionally been indicated for the treatment of large or rigid curves with Cobb angles more than 70 to 75 degrees that do not bend below 45 to 50 degrees. However, new techniques, such as pedicle screws and temporary rods, may be changing these indications. The degree to which flexibility can be increased is dependent on the complete removal of both the annulus fibrosis and the internal disc material. Discectomy increases curve flexibility and may provide greater coronal and sagittal plane correction than would be obtained with posterior implant systems alone. In the most severe cases of scoliosis, resection of the rib head and/or the costovertebral joint may also be required to optimize mobility. Thoracoscopic instrumentation is generally limited to patients with primary single thoracic curves, with instrumentation levels planned no higher than T4 and no lower than T12.

Prevention of crankshaft deformity is another situation that may require an anterior release and fusion procedure. This deformity may occur in skeletally immature patients, who have not yet reached their peak growth rate, following an isolated posterior instrumentation. In skeletally immature children with neuromuscular scoliosis due to cerebral palsy, however, an anterior release and fusion procedure may be unnecessary. In such cases, a posterior procedure alone may be adequate in preventing crankshaft deformity. In most patients, however, a skeletal age of 10 years or younger suggests a high probability of development of crankshaft deformity. The status of the triradiate cartilage may be a reasonable marker to identify patients who would benefit from an anterior procedure. Thus, patients with

TABLE 34-1   **Indications and Contraindications of Thoracoscopic Release and Fusion Surgery**

INDICATIONS

- Scoliosis
  - Primary thoracic curve, with planned implants no higher than T4 or lower than T12
  - Large curves >70–75 degrees
  - Stiff curves, bend >50 degrees
  - Prevention of crankshaft deformity in the immature
  - Pseudoarthrosis risk (e.g., Marfan syndrome, neurofibromatosis, or prior spinal irradiation)
- Kyphosis
- Congenital scoliosis
  - In situ fusion
  - Hemiepiphysiodesis

CONTRAINDICATIONS

- Pulmonary insufficiency/intrathoracic adhesions
- Reduced distance from chest wall to spine
- Small children
- Large curves
- Large, stiff, high thoracic curves

an open triradiate cartilage who are Risser 0 could be treated with an anterior release and fusion in an effort to limit future anterior growth. The use of pedicle screw constructs may negate prevention of crankshaft as an indication for anterior fusion, though this remains controversial.

Lastly, in patients with increased risk for pseudoarthrosis formation (e.g., patients diagnosed with neurofibromatosis, Marfan syndrome, or prior irradiation), an anterior release and fusion procedure can be beneficial. Adequate anterior discectomy provides a large area of cancellous bony surface, increasing the likelihood of solid fusion as compared with arthrodesis attempted by posterior methods alone.

Kyphosis   The question of anterior release or straight posterior fusion has become more of an actuality with the advent of powerful, third-generation stiff segmental instrumentation. A recent study comparing traditional anterior/posterior fusion with posterior-only surgery for adolescent hyperkyphosis reported no additional improvement in radiographic outcome with the former. Preliminary anterior release and fusion is considered no longer necessary when correcting kyphosis with a posterior column-shortening procedure and pedicle screw instrumentation. However, it is the opinion of the authors that very rigid or large curves (>120 degrees) may still require an anterior release. For these curves, thoracoscopic anterior release prior to a posterior instrumentation and fusion can potentially result in better correction of kyphosis.

Congenital Deformity   The majority of patients undergoing treatment for congenital deformities of the spine are less than 5 years of age and may require anterior release and fusion over several levels. The technical challenges of thoracoscopy increase as the size of the child decreases, so endoscopic procedures can be difficult in this segment of the pediatric population. Nevertheless, the anterior portion of either a circumferential fusion or hemiepiphysiodesis is endoscopically possible. In addition, excision of lower thoracic-level hemivertebrae has been reportedly done thoracoscopically in these patients.

Contraindications

Thoracoscopic release and fusion is not indicated in those patients who would not be candidates for a similar open approach. The following contraindications to the procedure are listed in Table 34-1. Many surgeons consider thoracoscopic instrumentation contraindicated in patients with high left thoracic curves (>20–25 degrees), as this curve cannot be controlled with thoracoscopic instrumentation and may result in an elevated left shoulder postoperatively.

VATS requires an adequate space in the chest cavity for manipulation of both the endoscope and the working instruments. This space generally requires collapse of the lung on the side of the chest cavity being operated on. As such, the patient's pulmonary status must allow single-lung ventilation. Pleural adhesions between the lung and the chest wall limit the ability to deflate this organ. Although minor adhesions can be divided, a nearly complete pleural symphysis between the chest and lung can make adequate lung collapse extremely challenging. Prior medical history of compromised pulmonary function, a history of previous thoracotomy, or pulmonary infection (which may have resulted in intrathoracic pleural adhesion formation) should all be considered relative contraindications. In patients with severe pulmonary insufficiency and poor preoperative lung function, from whatever cause, VATS is contraindicated.

In patients with severe curves (>100 to 120 degrees) in which the spine has become closely approximated to the rib cage, the field of vision and maneuverability of the working instruments can be compromised. Preoperatively, a working distance of 2 to 3 cm on radiographs should be considered the minimum before attempting a VATS procedure.

Achieving single-lung ventilation and obtaining adequate working space in children weighing less than 30 kg can be challenging. Although children weighing less than 30 kg have been safely treated with the anterior thoracoscopic approach, the relative benefit of this minimally invasive technique seems to be reduced in very small patients. In larger patients, visualization is often limited by excessive bleeding or inconsistent lung deflation. At any point during the endoscopic procedure, conversion to an open approach must be considered if visualization is inadequate.

PREOPERATIVE PLANNING

Preoperative planning begins with proper patient selection. Patient lung function must be assessed, with specific attention to asthma or severe restrictive or other cardiopulmonary diseases. Careful evaluation of standing and bending radiographs is essential to decide on the levels to be released and/or instrumented. Patients must also be counseled on the possibility of conversion to an open procedure should the need arise.

SURGICAL PROCEDURE

Surgical Equipment

Thoracoscopic surgery requires high-quality endoscopes and a three-chip video system to ensure good visualization. Endoscopes with angled viewing (0 to 45 degrees) are essential to view all aspects of the spine and the implants. Endoscopic retractors for the lung, peanut dissectors, a suction/irrigation device, and harmonic scalpel are all required. For disc excision, surgical tools typical to open spine surgery, including rongeurs, curettes, and modified mechanical endplate shavers, are required. In addition, conventional tools for harvesting iliac crest bone graft, including a bone mill for morcelizing graft, are required if autogenous bone grafting is planned. Somatosensory-evoked potential monitoring in the upper and lower extremities can also be valuable.

Patient Positioning

The patient is positioned on a radiolucent table in the lateral position, with an axillary roll in place. The legs should be scissored to prevent excessive pressure on the down-side leg. Positioning the patient in the lateral position allows for anterior placement of ports on the chest wall, which in turn enables greater circumferential visualization and access to the vertebral bodies and disc. In the prone position, it is difficult to place ports on the anterior chest wall, making circumferential (anterior and far-side) disc exposure more difficult. Having the surgeon or assistant stand anterior to the patient and placing the video display monitor behind the patient helps with spatial orientation of the operative field and allows for a better "mind's eye view" of the procedure. The harmonic scalpel generator, electrocautery generator, suction/irrigation, and cell saver are positioned at the head of the table on either side of the anesthetist.

Port Location

Typically the number of ports is dictated mainly by the deformity and the number of levels that require surgery. Four ports are usually sufficient for a six- to eight-level release and fusion. Port spacing is also dependent on the working distance from the chest wall to the spine and on angulations of the endoscopic viewing optics. The higher the viewing angles of the endoscope, the greater the possible spacing of the ports while maintaining an in-line view of the disc space. Typically the instrument for discectomy is placed in the port that is parallel to the discs, and the endoscope is placed either one port proximal or distal to this level. Port placement along the anterior axillary line optimizes exposure and visualization of the anterior spine while also affording a larger field of view with the scope and an increased working distance for the instruments.

When anterior instrumentation is planned, three ports along the posterior axillary line are combined with two ports on the anterior axillary line. Skin marking helps with proper placement of the thoracoscopic portals and is a crucial initial step for this procedure (Fig. 34-1). With the patient in the direct lateral position on the operating table, the image intensifier is used to mark a longitudinal line on the patient that corresponds to the sagittal alignment of the spine. The midlateral position of the vertebra to be instrumented is marked on the lateral chest wall and usually approximates the posterior axillary line. With the image intensifier in the anteroposterior plane, the orientation of each vertebra to be instrumented in the frontal plane is also marked on the posterior aspect of the patient. The intersection of a line marking the frontal plane orientation and the midlateral portion of that vertebral body demarcates the ideal chest wall entry site for appropriate screw trajectory.

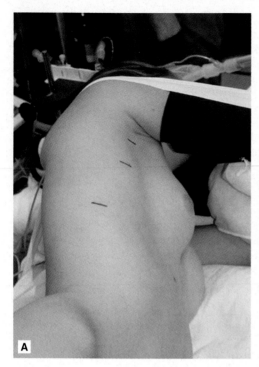
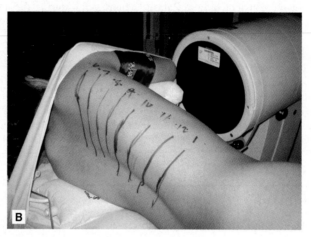

FIGURE 34-1   A. On-table surface markings for planned placement of anterior ports for thoracoscopic release procedure. **B.** The planned positions for the posterior ports used for placing anterior vertebral body screws thoracoscopically.

Skin incisions (1.5 cm in length) are made, and with blunt dissection through the musculature, the chest cavity is entered with Mayo scissors. The rigid tubular ports are then placed between the ribs along the anterior axillary line. Care should be taken in placing the portals, particularly when placing them distally, to avoid penetrating the diaphragm.

Spine Exposure

The first step to ensure optimal visualization is to achieve complete lung deflation. An 11.5-mm diameter trocar (Thoracoport) is placed through 1.5-cm long skin incisions located along the anterior axillary line. The ipsilateral lung is deflated and confirmed via direct visualization through the port. Deflation is best performed with a double-lumen endotracheal tube.

With three portals in place, exposure of the spine can be increased with a fan retractor placed on the lung. The levels to be released and/or instrumented are determined by counting from the head of the first rib. This is sometimes difficult to visualize and often requires palpation with a peanut dissector.

The spine is exposed by longitudinal incision of the pleura, approximately 5 mm anterior to the rib heads. Exposure of the discs is accomplished by retracting the pleura and segmental vessels off the anterior aspect of the spine. The harmonic scalpel is used to coagulate and divide these vessels, which allows excellent hemostasis during circumferential exposure of the spine (Figs. 34-2 and 34-3). Once the loose areolar tissue is divided, the pleura, azygos vein, esophagus, and aorta are reflected anteriorly off the spine. Sponges are packed between the anterior longitudinal ligament and these structures to provide protection during the discectomy and instrumentation. The packing of sponges also improves circumferential visualization of the discs from the right to left rib heads (Fig. 34-4). Distal exposure to the T12 through L1 disc space requires division of the diaphragm insertion by extending the longitudinal incision of the pleura onto the inferiorly retracted diaphragm and by blunt stripping of the diaphragm from the anterior aspect of the spine.

Discectomy and Bone Grafting

Disc excision is initiated with incision of the annulus and anterior longitudinal ligament with the harmonic scalpel. An up-biting rongeur is used to remove the most anterior and concave aspect of the annulus of the disc first (Fig. 34-5). Clear identification of the direction and path of discectomy is required to avoid removing excessive bone, as this may result in heavier bleeding and will interfere with visualization. The discectomy then moves toward the convex side to the level of the rib head. The deep aspects of the disc should only be removed under direct visualization. In addition, the posterior longitudinal

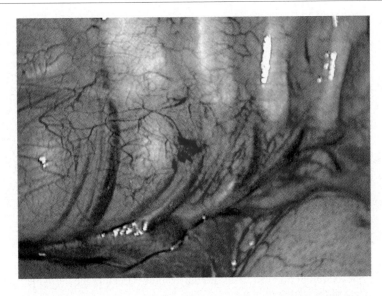

FIGURE 34-2
Proximal aspect of the spine with the lung retracted.

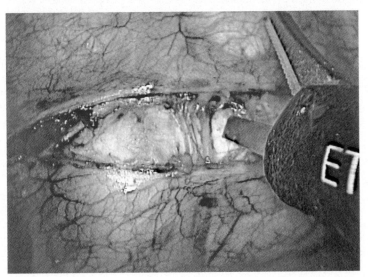

FIGURE 34-3
The segmental vessels coagulated prior to division with the harmonic scalpel. Division of these vessels allows wide exposure of the concave side of the spine.

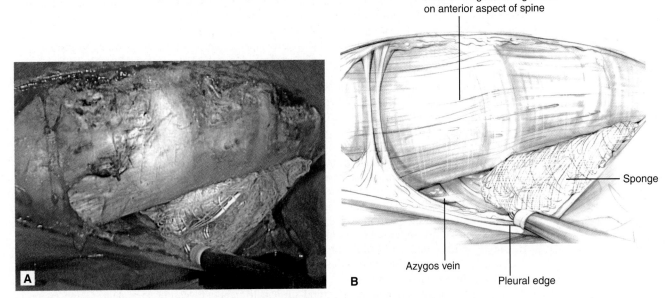

FIGURE 34-4   A. Packing sponges used to retract the great vessels and expose the circumference of the spine. **B.** Line drawing depicting the relationships of the above structures

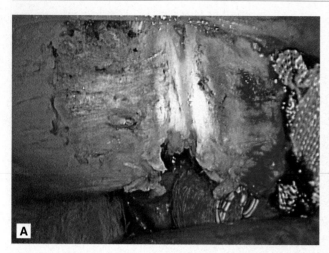
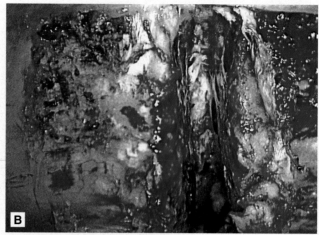

FIGURE 34-5   **A.** Discectomy is initiated at the most anterior and concave aspect of the disc with an up-biting rongeur. **B.** Deep excision of the disc is followed by removal of endplate cartilage from the superior and inferior aspects of the vertebral body.

ligament should not be breached to prevent injury to the neural elements. (Many surgeons, including the editors, leave the posterior annulus intact as added protection against injury to the spinal cord.)

An angled curette or rongeur is useful in removing the endplate cartilage. Once this is excised, hemostasis can be aided by immediate cancellous bone grafting or by placement of hemostatic agents (e.g., Surgicel; Ethicon, Somerville, NJ). The endoscopic retractor and working instruments are varied from port to port to maintain ideal visualization and access to the different levels of the spine.

Cancellous grafting of each evacuated disc space is recommended because arthrodesis is the ultimate goal of surgically treating spinal deformities. This graft may be autologous from the patient's ribs or ilium, allogenic (freeze-dried or frozen), or an artificial bone graft substitute. Enough morcelized graft to fill the disc space is delivered through a tubular plunger device. A critical look at the postoperative radiographs will often demonstrate the extent of discectomy and grafting that was performed. In cases in which an anterior release is combined with posterior instrumentation, the anterior portion of the surgery is now complete, unless the surgeon chooses to close the pleura, as described below.

Instrumentation

Insertion of the vertebral body screws requires at least three posterior axillary line ports, the position of which would have already been planned with the image intensifier. However, before making a skin incision, the port location can be confirmed by placing a K-wire through the chest wall at each proposed site. An anteroposterior view is used to ensure the orientation of the K-wire with the vertebra. A rigid 15-mm Thoracoport is used to place instrumentation.

The starting point for the screw is in the mid to superior aspect of the vertebral body just anterior to where the rib head articulates. An awl is used to initiate the hole, followed by a tap. The screw path is tapped through the far cortex. A ball-tipped calibrated probe is used to determine the exact length of the screw. Screws are available in 2.5-mm increments to accommodate the variety of vertebral body dimensions. Visualizing directly through the anterior and posterior portals, as well as with the endoscope and image intensifier, ensures proper screw placement. Subsequent screws are placed in similar fashion, moving the portal one rib space distally. Care should be taken to appropriately align each screw to make later rod insertion as straightforward as possible (Fig. 34-6). Each screw should be placed with bicortical purchase. However, given the location of the aorta on the left side of the vertebral bodies, excessive screw penetration should be avoided. Typically, two or three screws can be placed through each skin incision.

A malleable calibrated template is inserted through the distal port to determine rod length. The rod is contoured to the desired shape, anticipating a 1- to 1.5-cm shortening of the spine due to compression. A hex-end holder is then used to maintain the orientation of the contoured rod while it is being placed onto the head of the vertebral body screws (Fig. 34-7).

As each screw cap is captured on the rod, morcelized autogenous bone graft is added prior to compression of the construct. An interbody device or cortical allograft is used at the more distal levels, where the interspace may require structural support to maintain sagittal alignment. Compression is achieved with an endoscopic compressor (Fig. 34-8). Deformity correction is accomplished by cantilevering a rod into position, beginning by engaging the proximal screws first. This combination of rod

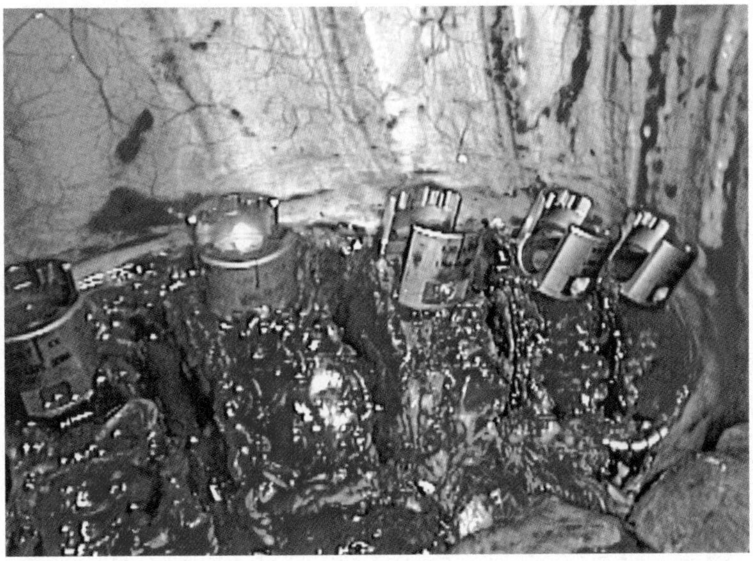

FIGURE 34-6

Vertebral body screw insertion. Appropriate screw alignment is required to facilitate rod insertion and ensure deformity correction.

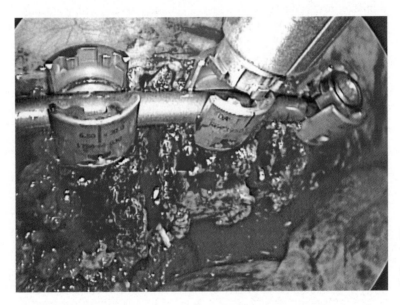

FIGURE 34-7

The rod is sequentially engaged, beginning with the proximal screw.

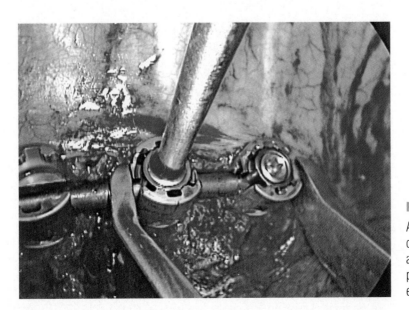

FIGURE 34-8

As each screw is captured, bone grafting and compression are performed with an endoscopic compressor.

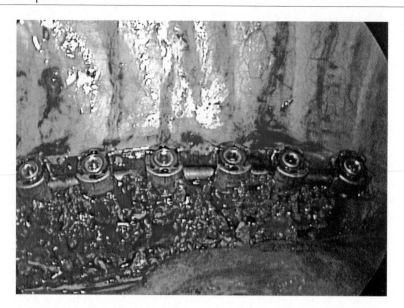

FIGURE 34-9

Entire construct with morcelized bone graft in place between each vertebra.

cantilevering, facilitated with an approximating device, and segmental vertebral body compression provides coronal plane correction of the scoliosis, sagittal restoration of kyphosis, and axial plane derotation of the spine (Fig. 34-9).

Pleural Closure

Pleural closure completes the procedure and is accomplished with an endoscopic stitching device (Figs. 34-10 and 34-11). The advantages of the pleural closure are debated, but may include limiting bleeding, maintaining the bone graft in position, and decreasing pleural scarring. A chest tube is inserted through an inferior portal after removal of debris and irrigation of the ipsilateral hemithorax. Lung reinflation is confirmed, and bronchial suctioning of the dependent lung is done to reduce the likelihood of developing postoperative atelectasis.

POSTOPERATIVE MANAGEMENT

Patients who undergo thoracoscopic surgery have a slightly shorter time to discharge and recover than those who have the open thoracotomy procedure. The chest tube is removed when the output slows to 50 to 75 ml per 8-hour period, which usually correlates to day 4 postoperatively.

Once the chest tube is removed, a postoperative thoracolumbar-sacral orthosis (TLSO) is prescribed for 3 months (worn when the patient is out of bed) if a single anterior rod system was utilized. Posterior instrumentation cases generally do not require postoperative external immobilization.

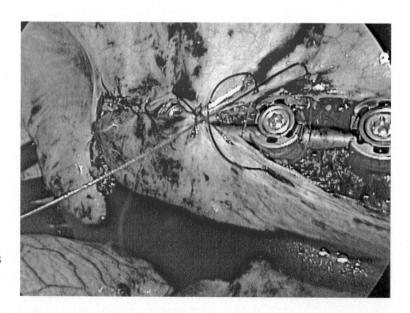

FIGURE 34-10

An EndoStitch device is used to reapproximate the pleura.

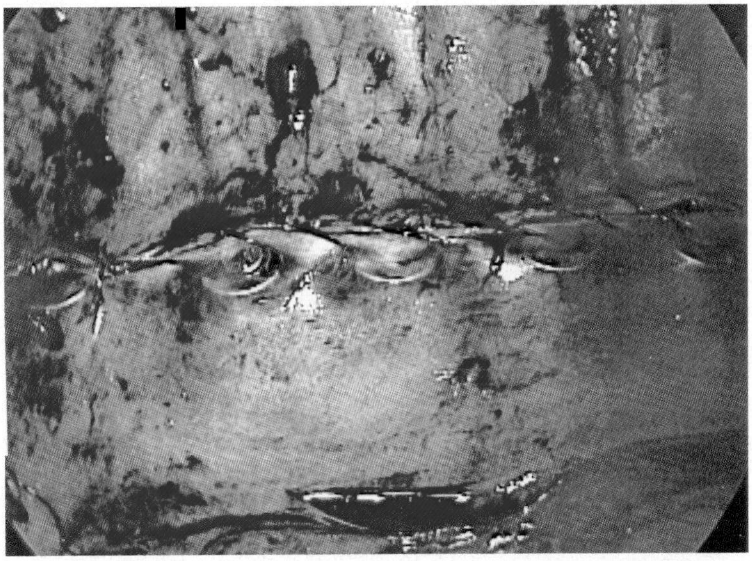

FIGURE 34-11
Following closure of the pleura, irrigation of the chest cavity is performed.

COMPLICATIONS TO AVOID

The complications of thoracoscopic release and fusion are essentially the same as those of open anterior spinal surgery. Intraoperatively, complications that may occur with either procedure include injury to the heart, great vessels, lung, diaphragm, spinal cord, or thoracic duct. However, with the endoscopic approach, these complications may be more challenging to deal with.

The greatest likelihood for iatrogenic injuries occurs when visualization is suboptimal. As such, maintaining adequate visualization is the most important aspect of the procedure. The most common hindrance to visualization is excessive bleeding, which can come from the segmental vessels during spinal exposure, from epidural veins, or from exposed bone. Before continuing dissection in another area, each source of bleeding must be minimized as much as possible through the appropriate use of electrocautery, ultrasonic coagulation, bone waxing, and early disc space bone grafting.

The likelihood of lung injury occurs when there is inadequate deflation or retraction of the structure. A lung that has significant pleural adhesions is at risk of injury during placement of the initial thoracoscopic portal. Directly sighting down the portal from outside to inside the chest is one way to ensure that no lung tissue is in the path of the instruments. After establishing a portal, an endoscope can be used to confirm that a clear path exists from the portal to the spine.

Injury to the thoracic duct that is recognized during surgery by the presence of cloudy fluid may be repaired by sutures or clips. If a chylous effusion develops postoperatively, a nonfat diet and/or thoracic duct ligation may help.

Spinal cord injury during thoracoscopic release and fusion surgery may result from either direct trauma during disc excision or from vascular insufficiency secondary to segmental vessel ligation. Appropriate visualization, especially into the depth of the disc space, can help reduce the occurrence of this complication. An attempt to maintain the segmental vessels during exposure of the spine should be considered in high-risk patients. Monitoring of spinal cord function after placing an endoscopic vessel clip may be useful in revision cases, congenital deformity, and kyphosis.

ILLUSTRATIVE CASE

A 14-year-old girl who was otherwise healthy presented with a 45-degree right thoracic, 29-degree left upper thoracic, and 23-degree lumbar scoliosis (Fig. 34-12). The thoracic kyphosis between T5 and T12 was 3 degrees, and the Lenke classification of this curve was considered to be 1A–. The end vertebrae of the thoracic curve were T5 proximally and T11 distally. These were chosen as the levels for anterior instrumentation and fusion. The patient underwent a thoracoscopic anterior release and fusion, with Frontier titanium single-rod instrumentation placed between T5 and T12. Two structural fibular allografts were placed between T10–T11 and T11–T12 disc spaces. All levels received morcelized iliac crest bone. The operative time was 5 hours, with an estimated blood loss of 300 ml. The chest tube was removed on the day of discharge (postoperative day 4). The patient wore a TLSO for 3 months postoperatively. Her radiographs and clinical appearance 6 months postoperatively suggested satisfactory correction and demonstrated radiographic evidence of arthrodesis (Fig. 34-13).

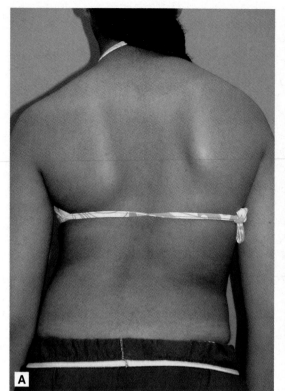
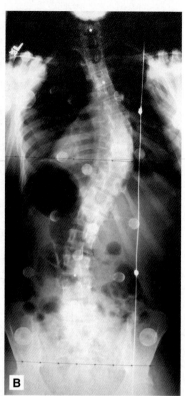

FIGURE 34-12

Clinical appearance **(A)** and preoperative anteroposterior (AP) radiograph **(B)** of a 14-year-old girl with a 45-degree Lenke 1A–curve.

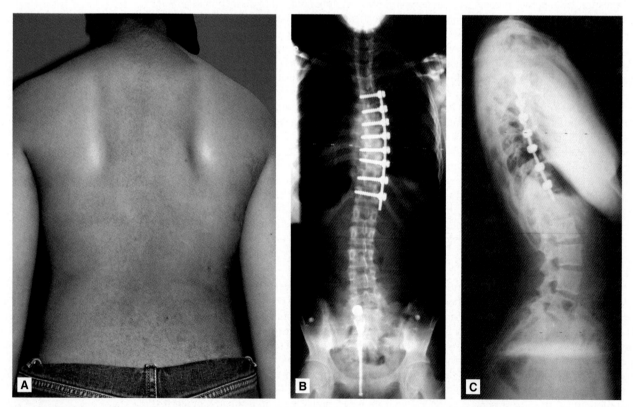

FIGURE 34-13   A, B, C. Postoperative radiographic views and the clinical appearance of the patient 6 months after the procedure.

PEARLS AND PITFALLS

- Thoracoscopic surgery provides a safe and effective alternative to open thoracotomy.
- Proper patient selection and preoperative planning of surgery are essential.
- Complications can be reduced by adequate intraoperative visualization.
- Potential advantages compared to an open procedure include the following:
  - Better cosmesis
  - Decreased blood loss
  - Less postoperative pain
  - Decreased wound care
  - Shorter length of hospitalization
  - Earlier return to prehospital activities
- Disadvantages include:
  - Specialized equipment and imaging technology
  - Cost
  - Steeper learning curve
  - Longer surgical time
  - Inability to control upper thoracic spine, with possible results of a high left shoulder

REFERENCES

1. Al-Sayyad MJ, Crawford AH, Wolf RK. Early experiences with video-assisted thoracoscopic surgery: our first 70 cases. *Spine.* 2004;29(17):1945–1951, 1952 (disc.).
2. Arlet V. Anterior thoracoscopic spine release in deformity surgery: a meta-analysis and review. *Eur Spine J.* 2000;9(Suppl 1):S17–S23.
3. Faro FD, Marks MC, Newton PO, et al. Perioperative changes in pulmonary function after anterior scoliosis instrumentation: thoracoscopic versus open approaches. *Spine.* 2005; 30(9):1058–1063.
4. Grewal H, Betz RR, D'Andrea LP. A prospective comparison of thoracoscopic vs. open anterior instrumentation and spinal fusion for idiopathic thoracic scoliosis in children. *Pediatr Surg.* 2005;40(1):153–156, 156–157 (disc.).
5. Newton PO, Parent S, Marks M, et al. Prospective evaluation of 50 consecutive scoliosis patients surgically treated with thoracoscopic anterior instrumentation. *Spine.* 2005;30(17 Suppl):S100–S109.
6. Newton PO, Shea KG, Granlund KF. Defining the pediatric spinal thoracoscopy learning curve: sixty-five consecutive cases. *Spine.* 2000;25(8):1028–1035.
7. Newton PO, White KK, Faro F, et al. The success of thoracoscopic anterior fusion in a consecutive series of 112 pediatric spinal deformity cases. *Spine.* 2005;30(4):392–398.
8. Picetti GD III, Ertl JP, Bueff HU. Endoscopic instrumentation, correction, and fusion of idiopathic scoliosis. *Spine.* 2001;1(3):190–197.
9. Sucato DJ. Thoracoscopic anterior instrumentation and fusion for idiopathic scoliosis. *J Am Acad Orthop Surg.* 2003;11(4):221–227.
10. Wong HK, Hee HT, Yu Z, et al. Results of thoracoscopic instrumented fusion versus conventional posterior instrumented fusion in adolescent idiopathic scoliosis undergoing selective thoracic fusion. *Spine.* 2004;29(18):2031–2038.

35 Thoracoplasty

Christopher W. Reilly

Thoracoplasty is a technique used mainly to improve the cosmetic appearance of the posterior chest wall. Many surgeons have utilized this technique in a variety of ways. It has been combined with anterior and posterior surgical spinal procedures, including thoracoscopic surgeries. The rationale for thoracoplasty evolved from the limited correction of the rib hump deformity achieved with posterior spinal instrumentation and fusion. Although recent advances in instrumentation constructs may have reduced the indications for thoracoplasty, it remains a useful technique.

INDICATIONS/CONTRAINDICATIONS

Thoracoplasty is usually done on the convex side of the scoliotic curve, with the goal of reducing the rib hump deformity. It has also been used on the concave side of the scoliosis, potentially allowing the rib cage and spine to move posteriorly, which is an advantage in severely hypokyphotic idiopathic spinal deformities. Thoracoplasty can dramatically improve the cosmetic result of a scoliosis procedure, especially if correction of the rib deformity is limited during spinal instrumentation alone. This may be advantageous in stiff idiopathic or congenital deformities in older adolescents. Thoracoplasty can also be performed in isolation. Patients with a solid fusion who are unhappy with their posterior chest wall contour may, in some cases, be managed with a thoracoplasty, avoiding the need for spinal osteotomy. The popularity of thoracoplasty has declined as surgeons have achieved more rotational correction with pedicle screw constructs during the initial spinal instrumentation. However, thoracoplasty can still be a powerful tool if applied with the appropriate indications.

As well as providing for correction of the chest wall deformity, thoracoplasty will also improve correction of the primary spinal deformity. Some thoracoplasty techniques, both anterior and posterior, can release the costovertebral junction. The rib head has a stout ligamentous attachment to its vertebral body, the annulus, and the superior body. Resection of the rib head may lead to increased mobility, which is an advantage in the correction of hypokyphotic deformities that are typical in idiopathic patients. Improvement in correction of the apex of a stiff deformity may be significant, approaching that provided by an anterior spinal release. Concern regarding the negative effects of thoracoplasty on pulmonary function has led some surgeons to explore more aggressive posterior osteotomy techniques to achieve improved correction.

A final indication for thoracoplasty is the excellent autogenous bone graft that it provides. This is most commonly an issue in young patients. Rib graft can provide an autogenous bone graft for fusion in cervical spine deformities in very young patients or in patients with poor pelvic bone quality. Rib bone quality is maintained, even in nonambulatory patients, because of the continuous work of respiration. The ribs are also relatively bigger than the pelvis in young patients, often providing the best source of autograft. The same technique used for reduction of a rib hump deformity can be used to harvest a long rib segment through the primary incision or through an additional small incision. The rib bed heals well in young children, quickly forming a new rib. The extrapleural technique minimizes any negative effect on pulmonary function. The rib can be split longitudinally, providing a structural graft that can span the occipitocervical and cervicothoracic junctions.

411

The major contraindication to thoracoplasty is reduced pulmonary function. Concern regarding pulmonary function has reduced the incidence of anterior spinal surgery and the use of thoracoplasty. Unfortunately, the patients with the most severe chest wall deformities, who will cosmetically gain the most from thoracoplasty, also frequently already have reduced pulmonary function. In addition, patient-based outcome studies indicate that patient satisfaction does not correlate well with deformity correction or posterior trunk surface contour. It appears that thoracoplasty leads to a measurable reduction in pulmonary function immediately postoperatively, which is slow to return to preoperative values. Once recovery from surgery for idiopathic scoliosis, which included thoracoplasty, is complete, the change in pulmonary function is small. The long-term changes in pulmonary function and the effect of thoracoplasty in later life have not been defined.

Thoracoplasty is associated with greater blood loss and should be avoided in patients with a bleeding diathesis or in patients who are very concerned about the risk of transfusion. A previous thoracotomy should be considered a relative contraindication to a thoracoplasty. Significant pleural scarring makes the technique more challenging, leading to greater blood loss and possible pleural rents.

PREOPERATIVE PLANNING

Thoracoplasty is most efficiently carried out when a preoperative decision is made to proceed with the technique. The decision to use the technique may be made after the spinal deformity has been instrumented, allowing the surgeon to evaluate the residual chest wall contour. However, the procedure is more difficult to do with instrumentation in place, and the secondary gain of greater primary curve correction is lost.

In deformity procedures, the thoracoplasty should be planned at the apex of the deformity, addressing the area of greatest rib prominence. In general, resection of small sections of the apical five ribs leads to a dramatic improvement in chest wall contour. Usually the lowest rib resected will be the 10th rib. There is little point in performing a thoracoplasty on the 11th or 12th rib because of their mobility. If the thoracoplasty stops at the 9th rib, the 10th rib will stand out and may end up being a painful prominence in teenagers who sit in hard-backed school chairs.

The surgeon should plan for, and warn the family about, the possibility of a chest tube. Even if the resection remains extrapleural, the local posterior hematoma can transudate through the pleura and may lead to a significant effusion that requires chest tube placement a few days postoperatively. Delayed chest tube placement delays the patient's discharge and is a major disappointment for the family and surgeon.

SURGICAL TECHNIQUE

Thoracoplasty is usually combined with a primary spinal procedure, though it can be performed in isolation. A number of variations of thoracoplasty techniques have been described. The traditional midposterior rib resection was described by Steel. Posterior thoracoplasties also include paramedian concave and convex techniques. A thoracoplasty can also be performed as part of a thoracoscopic spine procedure.

A Steel thoracoplasty is designed to remove the apex of the rib prominence posteriorly (Fig. 35-1). The procedure is most easily done after exposure of the spine has been completed. The surgeon should center the rib resection on the apex of the deformity, usually resecting segments from five ribs. The interval between the latissimus dorsi muscle and the paraspinal muscles is opened. The latissimus dorsi is lifted up, exposing the posterior aspects of the ribs while leaving the paraspinal muscles in their normal location. Cutaneous nerves cross this plane and should be protected. The posterior aspects of the ribs are then directly visible. Cautery can be used to split the periosteum overlying the rib over a span of 3 to 4 cm. The periosteal sleeve can then be elevated off the rib, taking care to protect the intercostal bundle and keep it with the periosteal sleeve. Howarth and Key elevators are useful initially, and a laminar finder allows the rib to be freed circumferentially. The pleural layer is robust, and the laminar finder can usually be slid along the rib to elevate the periosteum over a 3- to 4-cm length. A segment of rib can then be removed with a rib cutter. A larger segment (about 3 cm) should be removed at the apex, with subsequent resections made slightly smaller, effectively tapering toward the intact rib. Care must be taken to avoid leaving excessive rib medially, which, if left prominent, can create a paraspinal ridge, like a razorback.

At this point, the spinal instrumentation can be undertaken. Local oozing can be controlled with packing or Gelfoam. Grafting of the rib bed is not required. Some surgeons elect to stabilize and close the gap by placing a heavy suture through drill holes in the cut end of each rib. The suture is then tied tight, closing the gap. *However, this technique should be avoided.* The correction of the surface contour achieved with a thoracoplasty is not simply a correction of the rib shape in the axial plane. With thoracoplasty, the lateral end of the rib drops inferiorly as the patient lies in bed. This alteration in

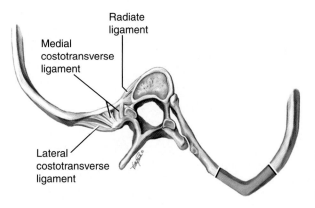

FIGURE 35-1

Posterior thoracoplasty as described by Steel.

vertical position of the rib adds to the power of the resection. The rib rotates down, hinging on the costosternal junction, thus preserving the anterior rib contour. Closing the gap has an undesired effect on the shape of the anterior chest wall, pulling back the rib, potentially exacerbating any breast asymmetry and reducing the lung volume. The inferior rotation of the posterior rib through thoracoplasty also means that significant cosmetic correction can be achieved without removing large segments of rib.

The paramedian thoracoplasty is a modification of the Steel technique. Like the Steel technique, this procedure is best performed after exposure of the spine is completed. Instead of elevating the latissimus dorsi muscle and approaching the rib lateral to the paraspinal muscles, however, in the paramedian approach the transverse process is removed, allowing for resection of a 2-cm rib segment centered on the costotransverse articulation (Fig. 35-2). The initial dissection is carried around the tip of the transverse process, which can then be resected at its base with a rongeur. This procedure provides immediate access to the rib. Initially, cautery should be used to define the superior and inferior borders of the rib. The pleura and neurovascular bundle can then be elevated off with an elevator, as in a standard approach. The resected portion of rib, again longest at the apex of the curve, is not the most prominent section of the rib. However, the paramedian resection allows the prominence to drop away effectively.

The paramedian approach has a number of advantages over the Steel technique. The exposure can be done rapidly, and a smaller additional dissection is required. It also improves visualization of the local anatomy for screw placement and facilitates placement of derotation sticks by completely freeing the lateral side of the screw head. The posterior sensory branches emerging from the midposterior portion of the rib are not at as much risk. The bone quality of the more midline portion of the rib, around the costotransverse articulation, is excellent. The paramedian approach also avoids any rib prominence, which can occur after a Steel thoracoplasty. The risk of a pleural rent or later pleural effusion appears to be the same as with the Steel technique.

Variations of the paramedian thoracoplasty have been described. Instead of completing two cuts in the rib, a single cut, just lateral to the costo-transverse joint, can be made. The medial portion of the rib can then be removed with a rongeur, which disrupts the costovertebral joint and removes the rib head (Fig. 35-3). An advantage of this approach is the potential increased mobility that disruption of the costovertebral ligament complex provides, which may specifically improve sagittal plane correction.

A concave paramedian thoracoplasty has also been described. Both rib head sparing and sacrificing variations can be used. Concave rib resection may allow the concave chest wall to spring out, improving the sagittal chest wall contour in a hypokyphotic patient. This also avoids the potential exacerbation of the deficient anterior chest wall, which can potentially occur with convex thoracoplasty. Resection of the concave apical rib heads removes an area of significant stiffness,

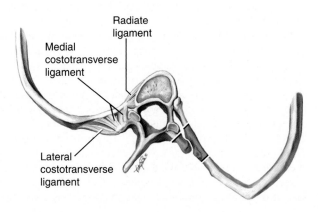

FIGURE 35-2

Paramedian thoracoplasty.

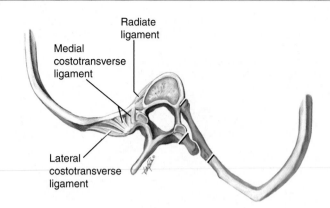

Radiate
ligament

Medial
costotransverse
ligament

Lateral
costotransverse
ligament

Modified paramedian
thoracoplasty with rib
head excision.

allowing improved correction of the primary deformity. The concave rib heads are more anteriorly placed than those on the convex side, which makes exposure a little more difficult. The approach can be bloody, and the risk of pleural rent and pneumothorax may be higher.

A thoracoplasty can also be completed as part of an open or thoracoscopic anterior spinal procedure. Rib head resection may already be required for optimum anterior screw placement. To complete the anterior thoracoplasty, the pleura overlying the medial end of the rib is divided with cautery. The subperiosteal plane can then be developed with a laminar finder. The rib is cut lateral to the costotransverse joint, resecting 3 to 4 cm of rib. In a thoracoscopic procedure, the rib can be quickly cut and removed using a large Kerrison rongeur. Pleural closure is extremely difficult after a multilevel anterior thoracoplasty and usually should not be attempted, as these patients will all require chest tubes.

POSTOPERATIVE MANAGEMENT

In most cases, routine postoperative management of patients undergoing thoracoplasty does not differ from management of other deformity patients. A postoperative anteroposterior chest x-ray is indicated to check for a pneumothorax or hemothorax. Pain management may be more challenging in these patients, and chest wall pain may limit lower lobe ventilation, necessitating more aggressive respiratory therapy. Chest wall pain can be partially controlled with an intercostal block placed after the rib resection is completed. Monitoring of the patient's postoperative respiratory status should be carefully carried out. It is possible for a very significant fluid collection to slowly develop, resulting in desaturation, usually at night. Late chest tube placement may be required.

No specific change in patient positioning or mobility is required. Although it is difficult to evaluate, the addition of a significant thoracoplasty may add a day to the patient's length of stay.

COMPLICATIONS TO AVOID

Thoracoplasty, whether performed open or thoracoscopically, is an invasive procedure that can be associated with a number of significant complications. The costovertebral junction is a transitional area, rich in neurovascular structures and complex muscular and bony anatomy. The intertransverse area is traversed by the posterior primary ramus of the intercostal nerve and an associated vascular bundle. Bleeding may be significant. Elevation of the pleura off the rib and resection of the rib itself are also associated with the potential for significant blood loss. Ongoing ooze from the thoracoplasty bed may obscure spinal anatomy during pedicle screw placement. This oozing can usually be controlled with local packing, but may slow the procedure.

Decreased sensation along the incision is common in deformity patients due to disruption of the posterior primary ramus as it runs through the paraspinals and then to the skin. Division of this neurovascular bundle is almost unavoidable when a thoracoplasty is completed. The midline numbness may be exacerbated by division of more lateral sensory branches coming off the intercostal nerve. This is a significant problem in midlateral thoracoplasties, although not in paramedian rib resections. The sensory nerves supplying the posterior chest wall are visible and should be avoided.

Flail segments can be produced with overzealous rib resections. For this reason, resections of more than five ribs should be avoided. The location of the rib resection is also very important. The 10th rib should not be left as the lowest intact rib. In addition, if a midlateral resection is going to be used, the surgeon must avoid leaving a significant residual spike of medial rib, as doing so can leave a visible razorback-like prominence. It appears that thoracoplasty may also be associated with an increased risk of developing a proximal junctional kyphosis above the spinal instrumentation.

If the rib head is preserved, the intact periosteal sleeve will lead to formation of a dysplastic-looking rib, reconnecting the floating lateral portion of the rib. If the rib head is resected, the lateral portion of the rib will be stabilized in the local scar. Hypermobility is usually not a problem. However, it is possible for a painful spinal costal pseudoarthrosis to develop. The floating lateral rib may also become incorporated in the spinal fusion mass, leading to restriction of costal motion. If this occurs over the entire exposed costal bed, a significant change in chest wall motion may develop. Fusion at a single site may lead to a single stiff prominent rib that will irritate the patient. Careful attention to the surgical technique and avoidance of excessive rib resection will minimize these problems. The value of rib head resection is unclear in this technique. Although rare, both painful pseudoarthrosis and costospinal fusion appear more likely to occur in paramedian thoracoplasties.

The most significant problem after thoracoplasty is the accumulation of pleural fluid, often necessitating chest tube placement. Careful elevation of the pleural layer off the rib prior to sectioning the rib will minimize the chance of creating a pleural rent. In most cases the pleura will be intact at all levels. Placement of a drain along the resection bed may also limit the local hematoma and minimize transudation. If a major hole in the pleura is created, a chest tube should be placed. Small rents in the pleura do not necessarily require chest tube placement.

These patients experience more pain postoperatively. They may have great difficulty with respiratory therapy and may develop atelectasis as a result. In complicated patients, thoracoplasty may have a detrimental effect on pulmonary function and may delay extubation. The long-term effect of thoracoplasty in spinal deformity patients is difficult to evaluate.

CONCLUSIONS

Thoracoplasty provides an additional tool in the management of spinal deformity patients. In carefully selected cases, it can provide a dramatic improvement in the rib hump deformity, increased correction of the primary curve, and an excellent source of bone graft. The use of thoracoplasty has declined as pedicle screw spinal instrumentation constructs have allowed surgeons to more effectively correct the chest wall deformity in smaller curves. In addition, concerns regarding pulmonary function limit the use of thoracoplasty in larger deformities. In addition, it appears that primary curve correction and rib hump correction may not correlate well with patient-based outcome measures.

ILLUSTRATIVE CASE

A paramedian rib head–preserving thoracoplasty was performed in this 16-year-old girl who had a 95-degree right thoracic scoliosis (Figs. 35-4 to 35-7. To see a bending photo pre and post see Figs. 30-9B and H). Her chest wall correction was excellent. A good amount of autograft was available from the thoracoplasty. Her postoperative radiograph demonstrates the absent medial end of the rib.

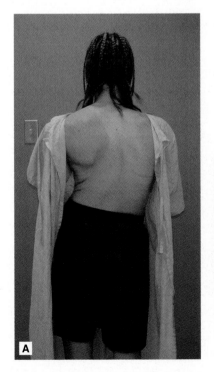

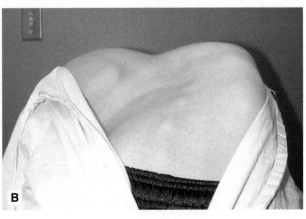

FIGURE 35-4

Clinical photographs demonstrate a significant cosmetic deformity **(A)** and a marked rib hump on the forward-bending test **(B)**.

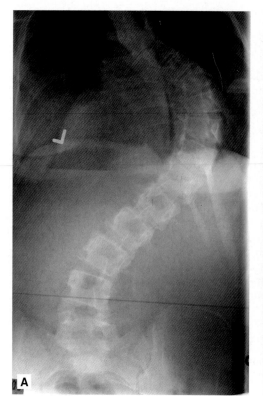
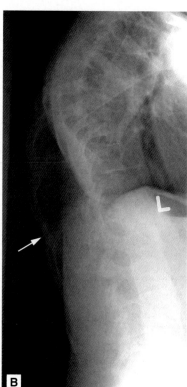

FIGURE 35-5

Preoperative AP **(A)** and lateral **(B)** radiographs demonstrate a 95-degree right thoracic curve with a severe rib hump deformity.

PEARLS AND PITFALLS

- Thoracoplasty can dramatically improve the posterior rib prominence, but underlying pulmonary function must be considered. Carefully consider pulmonary implications of this technique in patients with restricted lung function.
- Midline thoracoplasty, resecting 2 to 3 cm of rib, effectively corrects the rib hump deformity and minimizes the dissection and the potential for sensory loss.

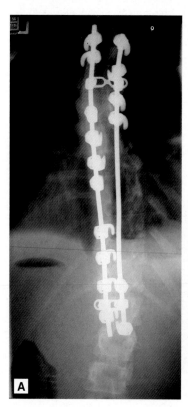
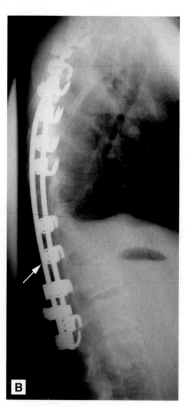

FIGURE 35-6

Postoperative AP **(A)** and lateral **(B)** radiographs demonstrate good correction of the primary spinal deformity and the rib hump deformity, which is now much less prominent on the lateral radiograph. Note the absence of the medial end of five ribs at the apex of the curve on the AP radiograph. A paramedian rib head–sparing thoracoplasty was completed during this instrumentation procedure.

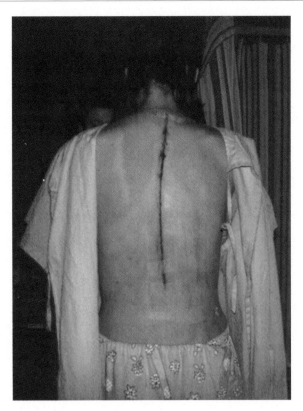

FIGURE 35-7

Standing appearance post-op day 3 is excellent, with a dramatic improvement in the clinical deformity.

- Resection of five rib segments is tolerated well. Do not leave the 10th rib intact. It may be prominent and bother the patient when sitting against a hard-backed chair.
- Do not repair the resected defect by suturing together or plating the rib. Letting the ribs float avoids reducing chest volume and allows the ribs to rotate inferiorly and to fall forward. The periosteal sleeve will reestablish the bony connection.

REFERENCES

1. Chen SH, Huang TJ, Lee YY, et al. Pulmonary function after thoracoplasty in adolescent idiopathic scoliosis. *Clin Orthop Relat Res.* 2002;399:152–161.
2. Kim Y, Bridwell J, Lenke KH, et al. Proximal junctional kyphosis in adolescent idiopathic scoliosis following segmental posterior spinal instrumentation and fusion: minimum 5-year follow-up. *Spine.* 2005;30(18):2045–2050.
3. McClellan J, Grevitt M, Webb J. Thoracoplasty. In: Weinstein SL, ed. *The Pediatric Spine: Principles and Practice.* 2nd ed. Philadelphia: Lippincott Williams & Williams; 2001:282–291.
4. Mehlman CT, Crawford AH, Wolf RK. Video-assisted thoracoscopic surgery (VATS). Endoscopic thoracoplasty technique. *Spine.* 1997;22(18):2178–2182.
5. Min K, Waelchli B, Hahn F. Primary thoracoplasty and pedicle screw instrumentation in thoracic idiopathic scoliosis. *Eur Spine J.* 2005;14(8):777–782.
6. Mummaneni PV. Sasso RC. Minimally invasive, endoscopic, internal thoracoplasty for the treatment of scoliotic rib hump deformity: technical note. *Neurosurgery.* 2005;56(2 Suppl):E444.
7. Oda I, Abumi K, Lu D, et al. Biomechanical role of the posterior elements, costovertebral joints, and rib cage in the stability of the thoracic spine. *Spine.* 1996;21:1423–1429.
8. Soultanis K, Pyrovolou N, Karamitros A, et al. The use of thoracoplasty in the surgical treatment of idiopathic scoliosis. *Stud Health Technol Inform.* 2006;123:327–333.
9. Steel HH. Rib resection and spine fusion in correction of convex deformity in scoliosis. *J Bone Joint Surg Am.* 1983;65:920–925.

36 Costotransversectomy

John T. Smith

An infinite variety of complex congenital and acquired deformities of the spine produce severe sagittal, coronal, and rotational spinal deformity. Surgical management of the most severe deformities may require complete or partial vertebral resection. Notable causes of these severe deformities include congenital kyphosis, congenital scoliosis, and acquired kyphoscoliosis resulting from extensive laminectomy. In addition, neurologic injury may occur as a result of impingement anterior to the spinal cord from various pathologies, including tumor, infection, or deformity, and may benefit from decompression anterior to the spinal cord. These challenging procedures present significant neurologic risk. Visualization of the adjacent neurologic structures is critical to minimize the risk of neurologic injury during deformity correction and/or spinal cord decompression.

A variety of surgical approaches have been recommended, depending on the age of the patient, the type of deformity, and the severity of the curve. In 1894, Menard[4] provided the first-known description of the use of a costotransversectomy for the treatment of a spinal abscess in tuberculosis. Seddon[6] published an update on this technique in the era of modern spine surgery, again noting its utility as a surgical approach to the spine. With broader indications, Ahlgren and Herkowitz[1] described a modified posterolateral approach to the thoracic spine and found it valuable for the biopsy of spinal lesions, decompression of paraspinal infections, and treatment of thoracic disc herniations.

Costotransversectomy approaches have been used extensively for a variety of conditions, including thoracic disc herniation,[2] excision of spinal neurinoma,[9] and excision of ventrally based space-occupying intraspinal lesions.[3] To improve visualization of the hemivertebra resection, Ruf and Harms[5] described a posterior-only approach for excision of the hemivertebra combined with immediate segmental pedicle screw fixation. Shono et al.[7] described a similar procedure for resection of isolated non-incarcerated hemivertebra causing kyphoscoliosis, using a posterior approach for excision followed by segmental spinal instrumentation and fusion, achieving excellent results. The author recently reported results of using the costotransversectomy approach for complex congenital and acquired kyphoscoliosis.[8] The purpose of this chapter is to describe the costotransversectomy approach to managing complex spinal deformity involving vertebral resection or osteotomy. This approach may also be used for spinal cord decompression.

INDICATIONS/CONTRAINDICATIONS

Indications

Costotransversectomy approaches have been used for a variety of purposes, including the following:

- Thoracic disc herniations
- Excision of spinal neurinomas
- Hemivertabrae resection
- Spinal osteotomy
- Space-occupying lesions anterior to the spinal cord, such as tumor or infection

Contraindications

- Any lordotic thoracic spine is a relative contraindication, as visualization is more difficult in this situation.
- In a patient with a single good lung, an ipsilateral costotransversectomy is risky but may be demanded by the pathology.

PREOPERATIVE PLANNING

Because these patients are generally at high risk for neurologic injury, a detailed neurologic examination and documentation is necessary preoperatively. Imaging studies most often include both magnetic resonance imaging (MRI) and three-dimensional computed tomography (3D CT) scan. The neural structures and three-dimensional bony deformity should both be well appreciated by the surgeon. For deformity correction, bending or hyperextension radiographs may be of assistance.

SURGICAL PROCEDURE

The patient is placed prone on the operating table and carefully padded. The author prefers the use of a radiolucent operating table that allows for 30 degrees of rotation in both directions in the central longitudinal axis. This setup offers better intraoperative visualization and the use of intraoperative fluoroscopy (Fig. 36-1). Spinal cord monitoring of somatosensory-evoked potentials (SSEPs) or motor-evoked potentials (MEPs) are established before the start of the procedure. If acceptable potentials are confirmed, they serve as confirmation of spinal cord function during correction of the deformity. If adequate potentials cannot be obtained due to established spinal cord compression or preexisting neurologic abnormalities, additional caution during correction is warranted. In such cases, a wake-up test is performed intraoperatively at the completion of the decompression and deformity correction in patients with normal motor function. Because these cases represent such a high risk for neurologic injury, the anesthesiologist should be asked to aim for normal blood pressure, not decreased, to avoid placing the spinal cord at additional risk for an ischemic event.

The back is prepped and draped widely out to the posterior axillary line. A standard midline incision is made, as required, to treat the specific deformity. A subperiosteal exposure of the spine is completed. It is important to determine preoperatively the adequacy of the posterior element by 3D CT scan, keeping in mind that in certain deformities these may be abnormal or absent.

Fluoroscopy is used to determine the level of hemivertebra excision or osteotomy. A transverse incision is then made through the paraspinous muscle at the level of the hemivertebra or the site of posterior vertebral resection or osteotomy (Fig. 36-2). The adjacent ribs are exposed subperiosteally for approximately 3 cm. Adequate visualization often demands removal of two or three ribs adjacent to the anomalous vertebra, though at times a simple osteotomy through adjacent ribs may suffice; this decision is made intraoperatively. The ribs needed for sufficient exposure of the anomalous vertebra are then resected. Attention must be paid to segmental vessels in the middle third of the vertebral body. Usually, one can dissect these away from the vertebral body, taking advantage of a

FIGURE 36-1

Preferred patient positioning on a radiolucent operating table. This table allows for 30 degrees of rotation around the axial plane for better intraoperative visualization.

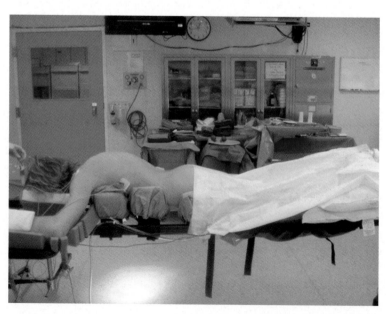

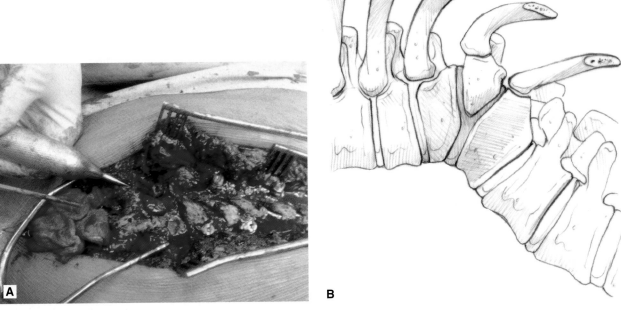

FIGURE 36-2 **A, B.** Exposure of the spine and ribs through a transverse incision in the paraspinous muscle.

natural plane. If vertebral resection is planned, the costovertebral joint should be removed. However, if exposure to the anterior canal is all that is needed (i.e., for removal of infection or tumor), this joint may be left intact and can serve as a landmark and protection. Care is taken to preserve the adjacent pleura by packing a moist sponge between the vertebra and the pleura and then placing a blunt retractor around the anterior aspect of the vertebral body. If a pleural tear occurs, repair of the defect is completed, if possible, and placement of a chest tube is mandatory.

Prior to vertebral resection, spinal instrumentation is placed a minimum of two levels above and below the vertebral resection. One may want to consider placement of pedicle screws or other anchors early in the case before bleeding occurs. If complete destabilization of the spine is anticipated, a temporary stabilizing ride may be placed on the contralateral side across the level of vertebral resection. Longer constructs may be needed, depending on the specific deformity. The author's preference is to use a pedicle screw construct, although surgeon preference may be to use a hybrid construct of pedicle screws, hooks, and/or wires in the thoracic spine. Consideration should be given to titanium implants to allow for postoperative MRIs.

Rongeurs and curettes are used to remove the lamina of the anomalous vertebra (or the vertebra directly posterior to the area of pathology) and its associated pedicle (Fig. 36-3). The laminectomy

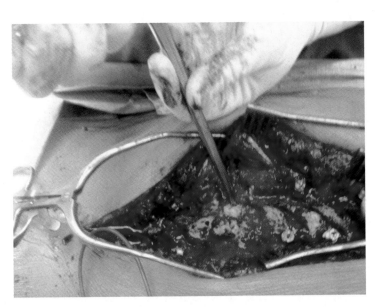

FIGURE 36-3

With pedicle screws in place to ensure stability, a laminectomy of the anomalous vertebra is completed using rongeurs and curettes. The dura and segmental nerve roots must be protected.

and pedicle excision allow for direct visualization of the dura and intraspinal contents, which are protected along with the paraspinous venous plexus. The associated segmental nerves may be visualized and protected as they exit the foramina. However, if exposure is necessary, the nerves should be sacrificed, as painful neuromas are uncommon and the dermatomal loss of sensation appears to be well tolerated. Retraction of the adjacent dura for visualization must be gentle and requires a skilled assistant. Various hemostatic agents, such as powdered Gelfoam and thrombin, are useful to minimize venous bleeding during resection. Prophylactic use of bipolar electrocautery aids in hemostasis within the spinal canal. For removal of intraspinal pathology, this may be all the exposure that is necessary.

If the goal of the surgery is to remove part or all of the vertebrae, once the pedicle is removed, the discs and endplates of the anomalous vertebra are easily visualized, providing identifiable anatomic planes for dissection. These are also relatively avascular (Fig. 36-4). There are two different approaches for removing a hemivertebra, With both techniques, sharp curettes and rongeurs are necessary for safety. In the first approach, the discs cephalad and caudad to the hemivertebra are removed first and then the vertebrae. An alternative approach is to remove the hemivertebrae first with a series of curettes going through the area where the pedicle was resected. In the latter approach, bony bleeding is controlled with bone wax or other hemostatic agents. In either case, the last portion of the vertebrae to be resected is the posterior cortex. After this is sufficiently thinned, it is pushed anteriorly away from the spinal cord. This point is critical, as the spinal cord is tethered over this region if there is any kyphosis; thus it is at significant risk of injury. The anterior longitudinal ligament is usually left intact.

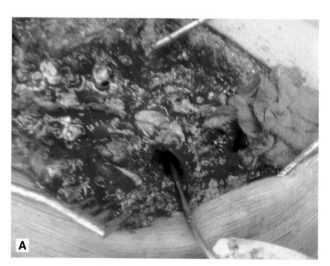

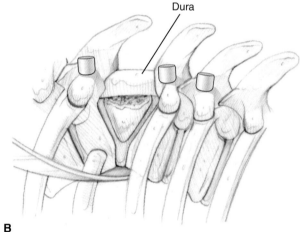

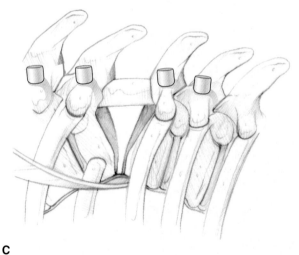

FIGURE 36-4   A–C. After removal of the rib, the hemivertebra is resected, beginning with the pedicle and working anterolaterally around the spinal cord, taking care to protect the cord.

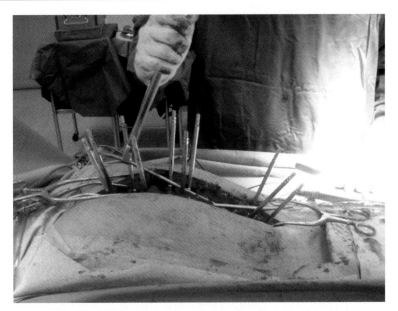

The surrounding segmental vascularity that often accompanies these deformities can make adequate hemostasis challenging. Substantial blood loss may be encountered during the resection, requiring the use of bipolar cautery, bone wax, thrombin-soaked Gelfoam, direct compression, and patience. Once the hemivertebra has been removed, the endplates of the adjacent vertebrae are decorticated to expose the underlying cancellous bone. If required for correction of the deformity, appropriately sized wedges in the vertebral bodies approximating the amount of desired correction are made. Care should be taken to preserve the anterior longitudinal ligament to act as a stabilizing restraint and to prevent translation during correction. Following adequate resection of the vertebrae, significant correction through the resected site should be possible, with manual pressure on the surrounding spine. Recall that if resection has been significant enough to cause spinal instability, a temporary rod spanning the resected area should be placed prior to resection. The resected hemivertebra may be morcelized for bone graft and packed loosely in the gap left by the vertebral resection. If required, additional anterior column support, using an appropriately sized femoral or humeral ring allograft or cage, may be added.

For patients with acquired kyphoscoliosis, bilateral costotransversectomies may be performed to facilitate vertebral resection or decancellation osteotomy under direct visualization.

Rods are then appropriately contoured. Combinations of cantilever bending and translation forces are used to obtain gradual correction of the deformity intraoperatively (Fig. 36-5). During this process, it is important to visualize the dura to determine whether there is any impingement by the superior or inferior lamina on the dural contents (Fig. 36-6). If this is seen, further resection of adjoining

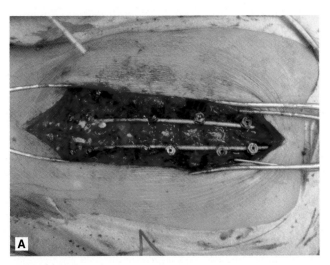

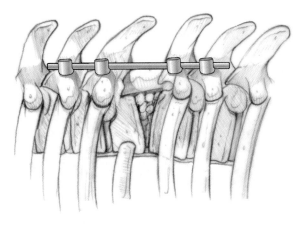

FIGURE 36-6   A, B. Final correction of the deformity with instrumentation completed.

laminae is required. Careful observation of the spinal SSEPs and MEPs is critical during this process. If there is a change in neuromonitoring, one should make certain that the blood pressure is adequate, look for and remove soft-tissue or bony impingement on the dura, and finally accept less correction with appropriate recontouring of the implants.

A standard posterior arthrodesis is performed over the instrumented levels. The author's preference is to use a combination of local autogenous bone and supplemental morcelized allograft bone for fusion. A superficial surgical drain is placed after closure of the deep fascia. If there was violation of the pleura, a chest tube is placed, and the wounds are closed in a standard fashion. The patient is awoken from general anesthesia to confirm intact motor function.

POSTOPERATIVE MANAGEMENT

It may be preferable to admit the patient to the intensive care unit for close observation, monitoring for any delayed change in neurologic or pulmonary function. Careful attention must be given to postoperative fluid management, as incipient fluid retention is expected and can result in pulmonary compromise. Suction drainage is maintained until output is less than 1 cc/kg per day. This patient population will develop a visible retropleural hematoma, which is commonly misinterpreted as a pleural effusion. This hematoma will gradually resolve over time and does not generally require placement of a chest tube. Patients with stable fixation are mobilized with standard activity restrictions as they are able. Solid fusion is expected by 6 months and should be confirmed radiographically.

COMPLICATIONS TO AVOID

Potential adverse events associated with this approach fall into two categories: Reversible and irreversible. Reversible complications include excessive intraoperative bleeding, dural tears, failure of instrumentation, pleural tears, pneumothorax, pseudoarthrosis, structural graft displacement, infection, and other routine problems associated with complex spinal deformity surgery. Potential irreversible complications are incomplete neurologic injury, paralysis, or death from excessive intraoperative bleeding resulting from inadvertent vascular injury.

RESULTS

The author recently reported results of using the costotransversectomy approach in 17 patients with complex congenital or acquired kyphosis.[8] The mean age at surgery was 11.9 years (4 to 16 years). The diagnosis was congenital kyphosis in 15 patients and complex kyphoscoliosis following failed previous surgery in 2 patients. The mean preoperative sagittal deformity was 70 degrees (range 25–160 degrees), and coronal deformity was 49 degrees (range 7–160 degrees). All but one patient was treated with vertebral resection or osteotomy through a single posterior approach and costotransversectomy, an anterior and posterior fusion, and posterior segmental spinal instrumentation. The mean kyphosis correction was 31 degrees (range 0–82 degrees) and the scoliosis correction 25 degrees (range 0–68 degrees). The average follow-up was 60.6 months (range 24–144 months). Complications included one failure of posterior fixation, requiring revision; one patient with lower extremity dysesthesias; and two patients with late-progressive pelvic obliquity below the fusion. There were no neurologic injuries. Patient outcomes were determined using simplified outcome scores based on patient satisfaction. Outcome was rated as satisfactory in 13, fair in 2, and poor in 1.

ILLUSTRATIVE CASE

A 17-year-old boy presented with a painful, progressive kyphoscoliosis. A radiograph revealed a type I congenital kyphosis secondary to a posteriorly based segmented hemivertebra at T11 (Fig. 36-7). He had no associated neurologic signs or symptoms but was having activity-related back pain. A 3D CT scan demonstrated intact laminae and provided three-dimensional visualization of the hemivertebra critical to preoperative planning (Fig. 36-8). The MRI showed mild impingement of the spinal cord at T11.

The patient underwent resection of the hemivertebra via a costotransversectomy through a posterior-only approach. Segmental spinal instrumentation was used to correct the deformity. The resected hemivertebra and a femoral ring allograft were placed prior to correction for anterior column support. A standard posterior arthrodesis was performed using morcelized allograft and local bone. The patient was slowly mobilized without bracing and discharged on the fifth hospital day. Postoperative radiographs showed excellent correction in the sagittal plane (Fig. 36-9).

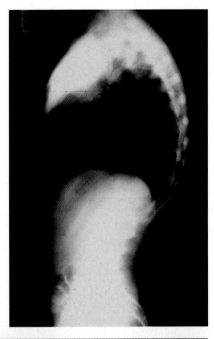

FIGURE 36-7

Standing lateral view of the spine, showing a significant kyphosis secondary to a posteriorly based hemivertebra at T11.

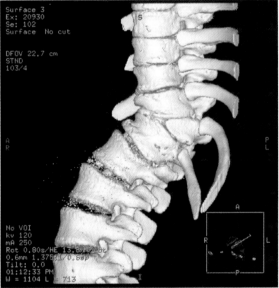

FIGURE 36-8

3D CT scan of the thoracolumbar junction, showing the posteriorly based hemivertebra. 3D CT scans are essential to adequately visualize the three-dimensional anatomy of these deformities and are critical for preoperative planning.

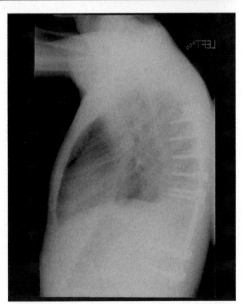

FIGURE 36-9

Postoperative lateral radiograph taken after hemivertebra resection and posterior instrumentation and fusion.

PEARLS AND PITFALLS

- Adequate exposure is critical. Do not hesitate to take out an additional rib(s) or make additional rib osteotomies.
- Meticulous attention to hemostasis, including use of bipolar cautery within the canal, bone wax on bone bleeding, and thrombin agents, is vital to visualization.
- Use of headlight and magnification loupes are helpful.
- If complete destabilization of the spine is possible, a temporary rod should be placed first.

REFERENCES

1. Ahlgren BD, Herkowitz HN. A modified posterolateral approach to the thoracic spine. *J Spinal Disord.* 8:69–75, 995.
2. Dinh DH, Tompkins J, Clark SB. Transcostovertebral approach for thoracic disc herniations. *J Neurosurg.* 2001;94(Suppl): 38–44.
3. Hamburger C. Modification of costotransversectomy to approach ventrally located intraspinal lesions. *Acta Neurochir.* 1995;136:12–15.
4. Menard V. *Etude Pratique sur le Mal du Pott.* Paris: Masson et Cie; 1900 (as cited in *Campbell's Operative Orthopedics.* 6th ed. St. Louis: CV Mosby; XXXX:2091).
5. Ruf M, Harms J. Posterior hemivertebra resection with transpedicular instrumentation: early correction in children aged 1 to 6 years. *Spine.* 2003;28(18):2132–2138.
6. Seddon HJ. In: Platt H, ed. *Modern Trends in Orthopedics.* 2nd ed. London: Butterworth and Co; 1956.
7. Shono Y, Abumi K, Kaneda K. One-stage posterior hemivertebra resection and correction using segmental posterior instrumentation. *Spine.* 2001;26:752–757.
8. Smith JT, Gollogly S, Dunn HK. Simultaneous anterior-posterior approach through a costotransversectomy for the treatment of congenital kyphosis and acquired kyphoscoliotic deformities. *J Bone Joint Surg Am.* 2005;87:2281–2289.
9. Takamura Y, Uede TK, Tatewaki K, et al. Thoracic dumbbell-shaped neurinoma treated by unilateral partial costotransversectomy: case report. *Neurol Med Chir (Tokyo).* 1997;37:354–357.

37 Convex Hemiepiphysiodesis for Treatment of Congenital Scoliosis

John F. Sarwark, Najeeb Khan, and Alfred Cook

Congenital scoliosis—a lateral curvature of the spine caused by vertebral anomalies present at birth—may result in an imbalance in the longitudinal growth of the spine. Early recognition and early treatment of congenital scoliosis is aimed at maintaining length and balance of the spine, as instrumentation and correction of congenital scoliosis at an older age may be difficult and risky. It is estimated that 75% of congenital curves are progressive, and only 5% to 10% can be treated with bracing (which treats the compensatory curve, not the congenital curve directly); thus early surgical treatment remains an effective therapeutic intervention.

Congenital scoliosis is classified as follows (Fig. 37-1):

- Failure of formation
  - Partial failure of formation (wedge vertebra)
  - Complete failure of formation (hemivertebra)
- Failure of segmentation
  - Unilateral failure of segmentation (unilateral unsegmented bar)
  - Bilateral failure of segmentation (block vertebra)
- Mixed

The natural history of congenital scoliotic curves is often one of progression, particularly if the curve is diagnosed before the age of 10. Progression of the curvature may accelerate during the adolescent growth spurt. The most progressive of all congenital spinal anomalies is a concave-side unilateral unsegmented bar with one or more contralateral convex-side hemivertebra(e), which has the potential to progress at a rate of 10 to 12 degrees per year, depending on the length of the unsegmented bar. A block vertebra, on the other hand, causes the least severe scoliosis. The rate of deterioration is usually less severe if the abnormality is in the upper thoracic region, more severe in the thoracic region, and most severe in the thoracolumbar region.

The keys to success of early operative intervention include careful selection of patients with defined progressive curves, short curves, young age at operation, solid arthrodesis at the anterior and posterior levels, and effective postoperative immobilization. In a series of 30 patients who underwent anterior and posterior convex epiphysiodesis, more than 76% showed correction; arrested or slowed progression was seen in the remaining patients.

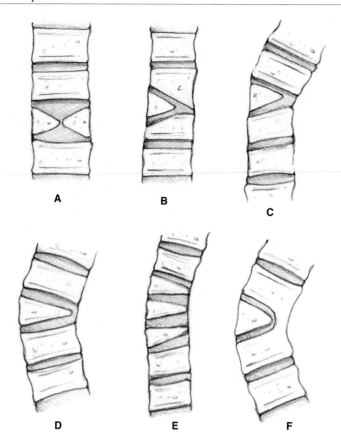

Defects of formation. **A.** Anterior central defect. **B.** Incarcerated hemivertebra. **C.** Free hemivertebra. **D.** Wedge vertebra. **E.** Multiple wedge vertebrae. **F.** Unsegmented bar with associated hemivertebra.

INDICATIONS/CONTRAINDICATIONS

The indications for anterior and posterior fusions and not only an isolated posterior fusion, are as follows:

- To correct sagittal and coronal plane imbalance
- To increase the correctability of the scoliosis by discectomy
- To eliminate growth of the anterior physis to prevent bending or torsion of the fusion mass upon further growth (crankshaft phenomenon)
- To correct curves with significantly higher potential for progression
- To improve or stabilize pulmonary function
- To help young patients who are fused at the lumbar level with a Risser sign of 0 (more than 4 to 5 years of growth remaining) and who have significant residual deformity of at least 30 degrees scoliosis and 10 degrees of rotation

For thoracic curves, the amount of crankshaft effect that can be tolerated is weighed against the inconveniences and risks of the thoracotomy necessary to perform the anterior epiphysiodesis if a single hemivertebra is being treated. A costotransversectomy approach can be considered for the anterior discectomy and fusion. The ideal candidate for convex hemiepiphysiodesis is a congenital scoliotic curve without major kyphosis or lordosis, a progressive curve with a magnitude less than 70 degrees, a curve length consisting of five segments or fewer, an age less than 5 years, no cervical spine involvement, and no unilateral unsegmented bar as the etiology of the curve.

PREOPERATIVE PLANNING

In addition to a thorough spine and neurologic examination, it is necessary to evaluate for specific associated physical findings often found in patients with congenital scoliosis. The skin of the back should be carefully examined for cutaneous abnormalities, such as hair patches, lipomata, dimples, and scars, all of which may indicate an underlying anomalous vertebra or spinal cord. Evidence of neurologic involvement, such as a clubfoot, calf atrophy, absent deep tendon reflexes, and atrophy of one lower extremity compared with the other, should also be noted. Other congenital anomalies that may coexist with congenital scoliosis should also be noted, such as genitourinary and cardiac anomalies; a Klippel-Feil syndrome with a short, stiff neck; and craniofacial malformations. Diastematomyelia occurs in approximately 5% of patients with congenital scoliosis.

Preoperative imaging includes full spine x-rays and magnetic resonance imaging (MRI). In addition to evaluating the scoliotic curve and neural structures, other anomalies, such as Klippel-Feil, cervical hemivertebra, and rib synostosis with congenital scoliosis, should be noted. A three-dimensional computer-assisted tomographic (CT) exam may be helpful in defining the congenital defect. Genitourinary anomalies, occur in about one-third of children with congenital scoliosis, therefore a preoperative renal ultrasound is recommended.

SURGICAL PROCEDURES

Plan to fuse the entire length of the scoliotic curve with subperiosteal exposure on the convex side only, to try to avoid fusion from occurring in a young spine from subperiosteal exposure on the concave side.

Fusion of congenital scoliotic curves requires addressing the curve both from the anterior and the posterior aspects. This can be done with a single-incision posterior surgical approach or with a combined anterior-posterior surgical approach. Regardless of the approach, it is important to have both a posterior and an anterior fusion to achieve adequate correction of the deformity, to decrease the likelihood of pseudarthrosis, and to avoid bending or twisting of the fusion mass over time (crankshaft effect). If the combined approach is chosen, it is usually safe to do the anterior and posterior surgical procedures under the same anesthesia.

The anterior surgical procedure consists of removing the disc, the cartilage endplates, and the bony endplates on the convex site. If a hemivertebra exists, a partial hemivertebra excision may be done with a rongeur and curette. Bone graft is also placed into the disc space for fusion. An autogenous rib graft, obtained at the time of thoracotomy exposure, can be placed within a trough created in the anterolateral portion of the vertebral bodies. No anterior instrumentation is used.

The level of the curve determines the type of anterior surgical approach, if the combined anterior and posterior technique is used, as surgical exposure is on the convex side. Depending on the location of the curve, an anterior surgical approach may be a thoracotomy for T1 through T11, a thoracoretroperitoneal approach for levels T11 and below, or a purely retroperitoneal approach for lumbar and lumbosacral curves.

After the anterior fusion has been completed, a posterior surgical procedure is carried out, with or without spinal instrumentation. The posterior approach is a standard subperiosteal exposure and fusion on the convex side only. The decision to use posterior instrumentation depends on such factors as the severity of the curve, length of fusion, and expected compliance with postoperative immobilization.

The outcome of hemiepiphysiodesis *in situ* is either (a) fusion to stop progression of the curve without improvement in the long term or (b) steady improvement of the curve. It is uncommon to see increased deformity after convex hemiepiphysiodesis when the unfused concave part of the spine grows and the convex side does not.

A challenge with convex hemiepiphysiodesis is the intraoperative determination of how much vertebral apophysis to excise. If too much is excised, a complete bilateral fusion will result without an epiphysiodesis effect and without subsequent curve correction. If too little vertebral apophysis is excised, a pseudarthrosis with continued convex-side growth may result.

SURGERY

Posterior (Combined) Approach: Transpedicular Convex Anterior Hemiepiphysiodesis Combined with Posterior Arthrodesis

This approach is an effective combined anterior and posterior hemiepiphysiodesis that is performed utilizing a single posterior surgical approach.

After general anesthesia has been accomplished, the patient is positioned prone on a radiolucent operating table with a frame or chest rolls. Preoperative prophylactic antibiotics are given. Either a portable x-ray or a fluoroscopic image with a skin marker is obtained to identify the appropriate level for the incision. After standard sterile preparation and draping, a single midline posterior incision is made. Dissection is subperiosteal to retract the paraspinous muscles on the convex side of the curve only as far lateral as the tips of the transverse processes in the thoracic spine and lateral to the facet joints in the lumbar spine.

With fluoroscopic imaging, the pedicles of the intended fusion levels are identified at the intersection of a line bisecting the transverse process and the facet joint. After entering the pedicles using a pedicle guide, the position is verified against these markers, using intraoperative fluoroscopic

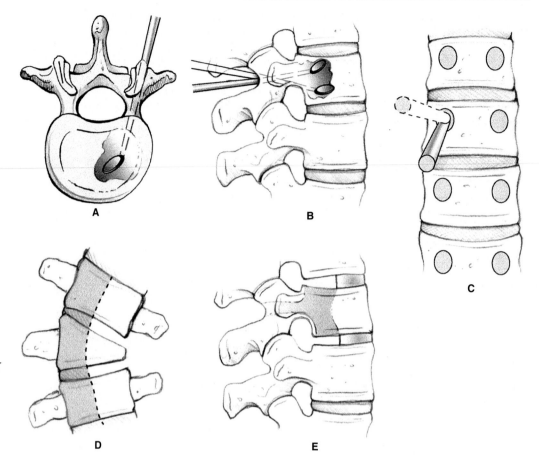

FIGURE 37-2

Transpedicular convex anterior hemiepiphysiodesis. **A.** Axial view of curette entering pedicle. **B.** Sagittal view of curette transversing the pedicle to begin the eggshelling procedure. **C.** Coronal view of the pedicle being entered and endplates being curetted. **D.** Region of the vertebral bodies that will be fused. **E.** Sagittal view demonstrating the upper and lower endplates once the intravertebral discs have been removed in preparation for fusion.

imaging. Once the correct levels have been exposed and confirmed, the convex vertebral body is approached through the pedicle with a straight curette. A decancellation (or removal of cancellous vertebral bone) of the convex half of the vertebral bodies is continued with curved curettes. Using progressively larger curettes, cancellous bone removal continues until only the cortical rim of the pedicle remains. The pedicle margins then expand into the vertebral body (Fig. 37-2). Brisk bleeding may occur during decortication.

In this approach, the surgeon will remove the vertebral body cancellous bone, the vertebral apophysis, and disc material *on the convex side only*. Communication with each pedicle hole across the vertebral apophysis and disc space should be achieved. As decortication continues via the pedicle approach, the pedicle medial cortex integrity must be maintained as the boundary adjacent to the spinal canal. The caudad and cephalad pedicle cortices border the intervertebral neural foramina.

For allograft or autogenous bone graft, a rongeur or bone cutter is used to fashion small cortico-cancellous strips small enough to be placed into the pedicle windows. The bone graft strips are packed into the decancellated portion of the vertebral bodies, with special attention given to packing across the disc spaces.

After the transpedicular bone grafting is complete, a posterior arthrodesis is performed for all vertebrae in the scoliotic curve, plus one or two levels superior and inferior to these vertebrae, in the standard fashion. The transverse processes and posterior elements on the convex side are exposed and decorticated. The facet joints are excised bilaterally at the levels that need to be fused. Bone graft fragments are placed over the posterior decorticated spine (convex side). Pedicle screw instrumentation of the convex side only may be added if the vertebral anatomy allows.

The lumbodorsal fascia and skin are closed in a standard fashion.

Combined Anterior and Posterior Convex Hemiepiphysiodesis

This combined anterior and posterior approach is used for similar indications as in the posterior (combined) transpedicular technique.

The patient is positioned on a radiolucent operating table in a straight lateral position with the convex side up. It is possible to tilt the operating table to turn for either the anterior or the posterior exposure as the case proceeds. Once the spine has been locally exposed both anteriorly and posteriorly,

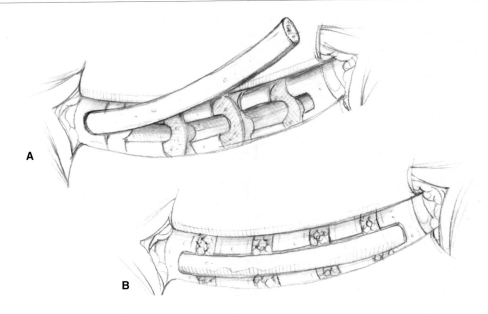

FIGURE 37-3
A. Rib graft is placed in a trough. **B.** Small autogenous cancellous bone chips are packed alongside the rib in the disc spaces to aid in fusion.

needles or other markers are inserted on both anterior and posterior aspects of the spine so that both are visible on one cross-table fluoroscopic image. After the correct level has been confirmed, the segmental vertebral vessels are ligated to improve local anterior surgical exposure. The periosteum of the anterior vertebral bodies is incised and peeled forward to the lateral edge of the anterior longitudinal ligament and backward to the base of the pedicle.

The annulus of the disc is incised at its superior and inferior margins, and the superficial portion of the nucleus pulposus is removed. The cartilaginous endplates, which are quite thick in children, are then removed. At least one-third of the vertebral apophysis (but never more than half) is removed. Following removal of the cartilaginous endplates, the cortical bony endplate is removed with a curette.

After the discs have been excised throughout the spinal region to be fused, a trough is made in the lateral side of the vertebral bodies. The autogenous rib graft is then laid in the trough (Fig. 37-3). The autogenous rib graft is augmented by packing cancellous bone graft (either iliac crest autograft, autogenous bone chips prepared from the removed rib, or allograft) into the disc spaces.

The posterior fusion procedure consists of a standard, subperiosteal exposure of the convex side only over the area to be fused. The facet joints are excised, any facet cartilage is removed, and the entire area is decorticated. A bone graft is then applied. The lumbodorsal fascia and skin are closed in a standard fashion. If the vertebral anatomy allows, pedicle screw instrumentation may be used for fixation.

A corrective Risser cast (with thigh extension for LS curves) is applied while the child is still under general anesthesia. Alternatively, the patient may be fit postoperatively with a custom thoracolumbosacral orthosis (with thigh extension for LS curves). Less immobilization is usually needed if spinal instrumentation has been used to augment the convex fusion.

POSTOPERATIVE MANAGEMENT

For both the combined anterior/posterior and posterior surgical approaches, the child is placed in a thoracolumbosacral orthosis for 4 to 6 months. Clinical follow-up is continued until the end of growth. Results may appear excellent for years but can deteriorate during the adolescent growth spurt, particularly with curve progression above or below the area of prior fusion.

COMPLICATIONS TO AVOID

- Failure to fuse the entire curve
- Failure to apply sufficient bone graft
- Failure to apply an appropriately snug cast or brace when instrumentation is not used
- Premature removal of the cast or brace
- Failure to recognize and repair pseudarthroses promptly

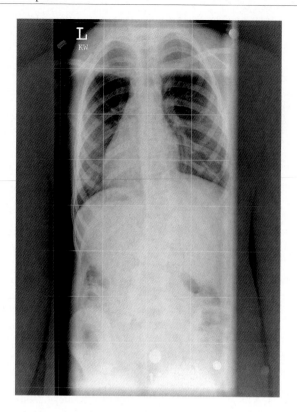

FIGURE 37-4

A preoperative radiograph revealing a L1 hemivertebra and a right thoracolumbar curve.

ILLUSTRATIVE CASE

A 3-year-old girl presented to the orthopaedic clinic with congenital scoliosis. Radiographs at the initial visit revealed an L1 hemivertebra. The right thoracolumbar curve at that time measured 26 degrees. The patient did not have any obvious neurologic deficits. The patient was observed over the next 2 years with minimal changes in her curve. At 6 years of age, shortly after the 2-year period she presented for a follow-up visit that revealed progression of her curve (Fig. 37-4). An MRI performed

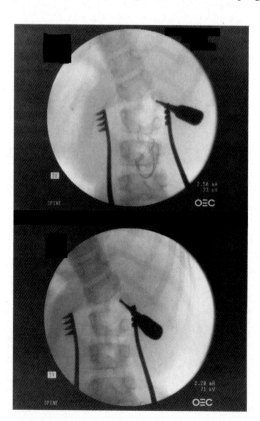

FIGURE 37-5

The pedicle was entered with a curette with fluoroscopic guidance. A trough was created from the superior endplate of L1 through to the inferior endplate of T12. A similar trough was created through the inferior endplate of L1 to the superior endplate of L2.

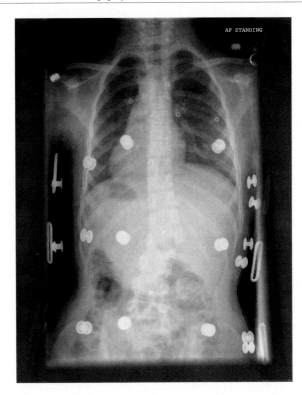

FIGURE 37-6
A postoperative radiograph of the patient in a brace after fusion.

for preoperative planning did not show any neural abnormality. Subsequently the patient underwent L1 hemivertebra partial excision with posterior *in situ* fusion and an anterior hemiepiphysiodesis of T12 through L2 through a transpedicular approach (Fig. 37-5). Once the L1 hemivertebra was identified, a portion was readily removed. A trough was created from the superior endplate of L1 through to the inferior endplate of T12. A similar trough was created through the inferior endplate of L1 to the superior endplate of L2. A mixture of bone from the hemilaminectomy and allograft was used for the fusion (Fig. 37-6). After more than 2 years of follow-up, the patient is doing well, without any complaints of back pain and with x-rays revealing a solid fusion (Fig. 37-7).

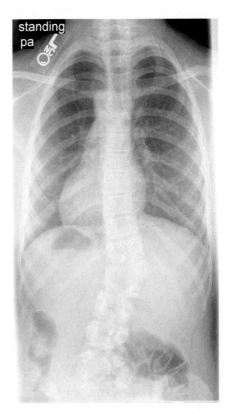

FIGURE 37-7
A 2-year follow-up radiograph reveals a solid fusion.

PEARLS AND PITFALLS

- Epiphysiodesis by fusion of the entire curve—not merely the apical segment—should be done.
- Fusion should be done both anteriorly and posteriorly on the convex side of the curve only.

REFERENCES

1. Andrew T, Piggott H. Growth arrest for progressive scoliosis: combined anterior and posterior fusion of the convexity. *J Bone Joint Surg Br.* 1985;67(2):193–197.
2. Canale ST, Campbell WC, eds. *Campbell's Operative Orthopaedics: Volume 2.* 10th ed. St. Louis: Mosby; 2003:1859–1868.
3. Deviren V, Berven S, Smith JA, et al. Excision of hemivertebrae in the management of congenital scoliosis involving the thoracic and thoracolumbar spine. *J Bone Joint Surg Br.* 2001;83(4):496–500.
4. Keller PM, Lindseth RE, DeRosa GP. Progressive congenital scoliosis treatment using a transpedicular anterior and posterior convex hemiepiphysiodesis and hemiarthrodesis: a preliminary report. *Spine.* 1994;19(17):1933–1939.
5. Thompson AG, Marks DS, Sayampanathan SR, et al. Long-term results of combined anterior and posterior convex epiphysiodesis for congenital scoliosis due to hemivertebrae. *Spine.* 1995;20:1380–1385.
6. Uzumcugil A, Cil A, Yazici M, et al. The efficacy of convex hemiepiphysiodesis in patients with iatrogenic posterior element deficiency resulting from diastematomyelia excision. *Spine.* 2003;28(8):799–805.
7. Winter RB, Lonstein JE, Denis F, et al. Convex growth arrest for progressive congenital scoliosis due to hemivertebra. *J Pediatr Orthop.* 1988;8:633–638.

38 Hemivertebra Excision

Daniel Hedequist and John B. Emans

Hemivertebra excision is a challenging operation that can lead to significant deformity correction while involving only a short section of spine. Treatments available for an isolated hemivertebra include in situ fusion, convex hemiepiphysiodesis, or hemivertebra excision. In situ fusion remains the safest treatment choice for an isolated hemivertebra, but to be successful, fusion must extend above and below the hemivertebra into normal spine and little or no correction is usually achieved. Convex hemiepiphysiodesis is easily accomplished and safe, but the results with regard to curve correction are unpredictable. Hemivertebra excision involves a short section of spine and potentially allows for complete deformity correction, but remains a demanding operation with potential for neurologic complications and extensive blood loss.

The excision of an isolated hemivertebra may be performed as a staged or simultaneous anterior-posterior procedure or as a posterior-only procedure. Posterior-only approaches are advantageous in that they avoid anterior surgery, allow for similar correction of the deformity, and may be performed with a low complication rate. The disadvantages of posterior-only surgery include the technically demanding nature of the procedure; the potential for significant blood loss, which may impair visualization and inhibit deformity correction; the need for more manipulation of the dural sac and its contents; and the reported higher reoperation rates.

Combined anterior-posterior surgery allows for the most complete visualization and control of the spine and may be performed as either a staged procedure with separate anesthetics or as a single anesthetic procedure. A single anesthetic surgery may either be a sequential anterior then posterior approach or a simultaneous approach as described in this chapter.

The advantages of a simultaneous anterior-posterior approach to hemivertebra excision are complete exposure and control of the operative site. This allows for a single anesthetic and does not require repositioning or redraping of the operative field. The authors' experience with this approach has been reliable deformity correction and a high fusion rate in the absence of neurologic complications.

The authors use both simultaneous anterior-posterior procedures as well as posterior-only approaches for hemivertebra excision. A posterior-only approach is easiest in a kyphotic deformity, particularly in the thoracolumbar or lumbar spine. For fragile patients where blood loss entails risk or for very lordotic deformities (or when doubt exists about manipulating the dura and its contents), simultaneous anterior and posterior procedures are preferred. We will describe the operative technique for simultaneous exposure and surgery in this section.

INDICATIONS/CONTRAINDICATIONS

Excision of a hemivertebra may be indicated when there is a hemivertebra causing progressive imbalance or curve progression in a growing child. In general, fully segmented hemivertebra in the thoracolumbar, lumbar, and lumbosacral regions of the spine will cause progressive deformity above and below and are an indication for early surgical treatment. However, fully incarcerated or semisegmented hemivertebra may not cause progressive deformity and may be better observed or treated differently. In general, hemivertebra resection should completely correct the patient's deformity. If the deformity involves a long section of the spine in a very young child, consideration should be given to growth-oriented treatments, such as a Vertical Expandable Prosthetic Titanium Rib (VEPTR) or growing rods.

Patients between the ages of 18 and 30 months may be the best age for hemivertebra excision. However, the procedure can be performed on younger or older children. At this ideal age, vertebral size and strength are amenable to excision as well as to spinal implant placement, as there is enough bony surface available to obtain reliable fusion. These children also represent minimal anesthetic risk. Concern has been expressed about early circumferential fusion and the creation of iatrogenic canal stenosis; operating after the age of 18 months probably makes stenosis unlikely. If supplemental fixation in the form of a body cast is needed, children of this age can tolerate periods of immobilization and can still be carried fairly easily by parents.

PREOPERATIVE PLANNING

Congenital scoliosis is frequently associated with other organ system abnormalities, especially the genitourinary, auditory, musculoskeletal, and cardiac systems. A thorough examination of the patient is warranted, as is a screening ultrasound of the genitourinary system and screening echocardiogram of the cardiac system. Because more than 30% of patients with scoliosis will have associated spinal dysraphism, a thorough neurologic exam is required, as is a screening magnetic resonance imaging (MRI) of the spinal cord and brain stem, to assess the spinal axis.

Upright preoperative anteroposterior and lateral x-rays of the spine help assess balance, while preoperative bending, supine, or push-prone radiographs assess the anatomy and flexibility of the adjacent curvatures. A computed tomography (CT) scan of the spine with three-dimensional reconstructions is indispensable in preoperative assessment and surgical planning. Radiographs often do not reveal posterior laminar fusions or bifid lamina that may be present at surgery and that can cause confusion when trying to identify levels in the operating room.

Preoperative planning should include the goal of complete correction of the deformity at that level, which may best be thought of as a wedge resection. If the deformity is kyphotic, more posterior column must be resected; if lordotic, more anterior column. The hemivertebra body must be resected, but equally important, any disc and endplate cartilage above and below must also be resected back to the endplate. The resection must continue well past the midline over to the concave annulus at that level; otherwise, complete correction will not occur or will at least be quite difficult. Excising the vertebral body in children is easy, but resecting the rubbery, resistant endplate and disc material can be much more difficult.

SURGICAL PROCEDURE: ANTERIOR/POSTERIOR RESECTION

Before entering the operating room, the surgeon should initial the anterior operative field on the convexity of the curve at the chest or flank to avoid entering on the curve concavity. Appropriate anesthesia, arterial monitoring, Foley catheter placement, and motor-evoked potential (MEP) and somatosensory-evoked potential (SSEP) monitoring are performed prior to surgical positioning.

Patients are then placed in the lateral decubitus position (convex side facing upward), centered on the break in the operating table, with the posterior aspect of the body placed all the way to the lateral edge of the table to facilitate retractor placement (Fig. 38-1). This prevents the handles of the self-retaining retractors from hitting the bed and not allowing opening and retraction. The entire posterior and anterior fields of the patient should be prepped and draped. Exposure is facilitated by accentuating the deformity

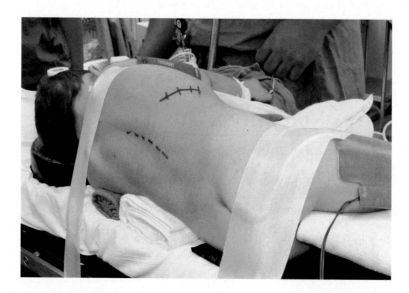

FIGURE 38-1

Lateral positioning of the patient with convexity of curvature facing upward. Notice the roll under the apex of the deformity and the patient positioned at the lateral aspect of the bed.

with the kidney bar or removable roll. Patient taping or positioning should be done in such a way to allow deformity correction after excision. Radiographic identification of the desired operative level before making the incision is helpful, as the exact location of the deformity can be confusing.

Anterior exposure of the spine may be performed in a transthoracic, transthoracic-retroperitoneal, or purely retroperitoneal manner, depending on the location of the deformity. Hemivertebrae located between T11 and L2 may be exposed through a transthoracic-retroperitoneal (thoracoabdominal) approach via 10th-rib excision. Hemivertebrae between L3 and the lumbosacral junction may be exposed via a retroperitoneal flank exposure. Exposure of the spine may be done either by a general surgeon familiar with the exposure or by the spinal surgeon if he or she is familiar and comfortable with anterior transperitoneal access. Exposure need only be enough to visualize and remove the area of wedge resection and is usually accomplished through a very limited exposure. A full thoracoabdominal approach is usually not needed, and the hemivertebra at the diaphragmatic attachment can be accessed without a full incision of the diaphragm.

The posterior region of the spine is exposed via the standard midline incision and wide exposure of the appropriate level. An exposure above or below the desired segment may result in inadvertent fusion posteriorly. As mentioned previously, there may be associated laminar fusions or bifid fusions, making clear identification of levels difficult. Once the posterior region of the spine is exposed, a radiograph should be taken for confirmation of levels. This can be aided by placing a spinal needle in the disc space anteriorly and a marker on an appropriate posterior landmark.

Once confirmed at the appropriate level, the procedure begins with either hook or screw placement, as blood loss may make this difficult when bony excision begins. Anchor placement may be either with supralaminar and infralaminar hooks at the levels above and below the hemivertebra or with pedicle screw placement at these levels. Combinations may enhance stability. If the anatomy at the levels above or below do not permit instrumentation, instrumenting, but not fusing, one level longer for implant stability may be done, with a plan to take the implants out at a later date. However, an inadvertent fusion to the additional level usually results. Regardless of hook or screw placement, there are downsized pediatric implants available; the authors recommend using titanium in case future MRIs may be warranted.

Once implant anchors are placed, attention is turned to the anterior field, where the segmental vessel is first ligated at the appropriate level. Usually the segmental vessel at the level of the hemivertebra is small or absent, and there should be no need to ligate above or below the hemivertebra. If a substantial segmental vessel is to be ligated, the vessel can be tied off, or temporarily clamped but not divided, until no change is observed in MEP and SSEP monitoring. Blunt dissection should be carried all the way to the concave margin of the disc at the level of the hemivertebra. When possible, a subperiosteal flap should be created anteriorly to allow maximum exposure and protection (Fig. 38-2). This is done by making a subperiosteal incision with electrocantery at the inferior margin of the vertebral body above and the superior margin of the vertebral body below. This is then connected by a longitudinal cut along the discs and hemivertebra. The subperiosteal flap is then created using a electrocantery and a Cobb elevator anteriorly

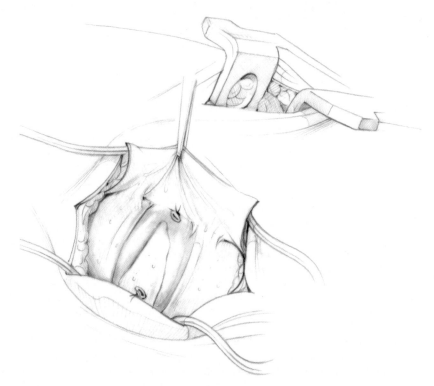

FIGURE 38-2

Anterior exposure with creation of periosteal flap anteriorly and posteriorly.

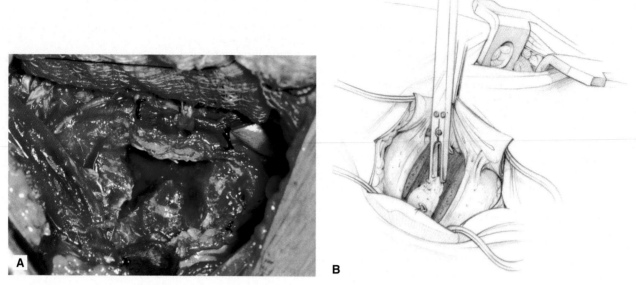

FIGURE 38-3   A, B. Resection of the anterior portion of the hemivertebra after discectomies.

past the midline to the contralteral side. Posteriorly the flap is brought back to the pedicles of the hemivertebra. The discs and endplate cartilage above and below the hemivertebra are removed with a Cobb elevator and rongeur to the posterior longitudinal ligament (PLL). The concave anterior periosteal flap acts as a protective measure against great vessel injury during discectomies, and the convex anterior flap allows the surgeon visualization to take the discs out all the way posterior to the PLL.

Removal of the anterior portion of the hemivertebra is performed with ronguers, curettes, Kerrisons, and a burr, if needed (Fig. 38-3). If used, the burr can be diamond tipped to allow for feeling the posterior vertebral cortex so that the dura is not penetrated. A large vessel is commonly centered in the middle of the posterior surface of the hemivertebra and can be controlled with bone wax, if posterior cortex is still present, or with bipolar, if the PLL or epidural veins are exposed. As mentioned, the posterior periosteal flap should allow visualization of a portion of the pedicle and of the PLL. This aids in visualization of the posterior margins and extradural space.

Resection of the posterior cortex is the last step of anterior body resection and is facilitated by resecting as much as possible of the pedicle and complete disc removal to the PLL. The wedge resection should include hemivertebra, discs, and cartilage above, below, and posterior to the hemivertebra and should extend to the concave annulus. If large sections of cartilage remain, they may inhibit complete correction or prolapse into the canal when deformity is corrected. Once complete removal has been done to the pedicle, Gelfoam is placed into the space to stop further bleeding and attention is turned to the posterior incision.

The removal of the posterior elements begins near the midline, with resection of any flavum between hemilamina and adjacent vertebral elements (Fig. 38-4). A Kerrison rongeur aids in resecting the remaining hemilamina and facet joints above and below. Resection of the transverse process is then performed, followed by resection of the pedicle; this is often done as a single piece. Resection of the pedicle must be done with visualization and protection of the nerve root (Fig. 38-5). The remaining pedicle may then be done in a piecemeal fashion. Once the pedicle is removed, complete visualization of the nerve root above and below should be obtained to allow for protection during the wedge closure. The surgeon should make sure there are no pedicle remnants that could impinge on the roots. When a rib is present at this level, the rib head and neck may be resected to avoid impingement on the roots. The residual posterior elements above and below should be shaped to correspond to their new position after correction. Any residual intervening flavum should be removed to allow bony contact and to prevent infolding with correction. The lamina may be undercut to ensure that there is not impingement on the canal when correction occurs.

Once complete resection is performed, the correction of the deformity can occur. The break in the table or a bump underneath the patient must first be removed. If possible, the table break should be bent in the opposite direction. Any large Gelfoam packing should be removed from the anterior wound. Correction can be achieved mostly by pushing on the spine, body, or vertebral elements (Fig. 38-6). Bony anchors should be reserved principally for holding, not correcting, as they are of limited strength in children this age. If correction does not occur easily, the anterior incision should be investigated to determine whether more bone should be resected and to ensure that the excision goes all the way to the concave annulus. There may also be impingement posteriorly. Closing down of the wedge with curve correction can be facilitated by placing a hand in the anterior wound and using fingers to push down on the spine to close the wedge. Placement and capturing of the rod is then performed. It is of

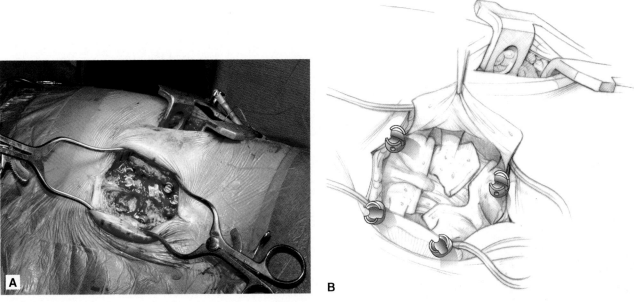

FIGURE 38-4   A, B. Posterior exposure and implant placement. In this case, three rods were used. The gold anchors are supra- and infralaminar hooks. The hooks are compressed to help close down the opening, as they seem stronger in young children than pushing against pedicle screws, which may plow a bit. Once compressed, the pedicle screws are locked down to the rod.

paramount importance that the nerve roots be visualized during correction to avoid impingement or entrapment (Fig. 38-7). Once the rod is captured, further correction is done by compression of the screws or hooks; however, the immature bone tolerates only gentle compression (Fig. 38-8). Radiographs should then be taken to confirm correction and implant position.

The incisions are closed in the appropriate manner. Younger patients should be placed in a body cast that includes one arm and/or one or both legs, depending on the level of resection and stability, for 6 to 12 weeks. Newer constructs, including pedicle screws, are stronger and may permit use of a thoracolumbar-sacral orthosis (TLSO) brace for 3 months. If there is trunk imbalance or a substantial curve above or below the resection, bracing should be extended for as long as needed until the spine seems balanced.

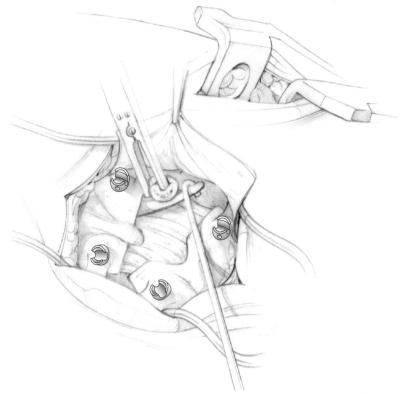

FIGURE 38-5

Pedicle resection occurs after resection of the hemilamina and transverse process. Note protection of the exiting nerve root.

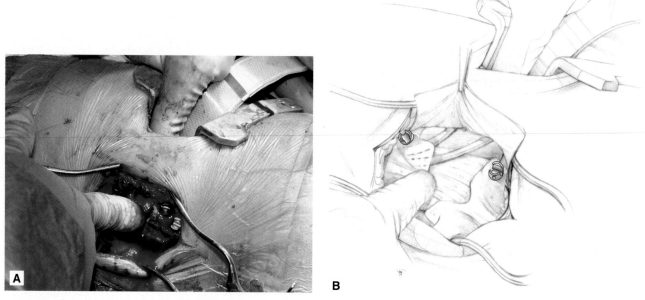

FIGURE 38-6 **A, B.** Correction of the deformity begins by unbreaking the table and placing downward force on the spine from the anterior incision. Visualization of the exiting nerve roots and dura are paramount.

RESULTS

The authors have published results on this technique in two separate papers with more than 30 patients. Correction rates were seen similar to those in other papers in the literature. The authors have had no pseudarthroses, no infections, and no neurologic complications. There was one implant failure due to set screw loosening; however, successful management was done with continued casting and no loss of correction. This technique remains a safe, reliable, and well-studied procedure for hemivertebra excision.

COMPLICATIONS TO AVOID

The most worrisome complication is one of a neorologic deficit. Risk can be minimized by appropriate neurologic screening on physical examination and with a preoperative MRI. All operations should ideally be performed with MEPs and SSEPs. One key to avoiding a nerve root injury is to have a keen awareness of the location of the nerve root above and below the pedicle being resected. Once the pedicle is resected, visualization and protection of the nerve roots needs to be done as correction of the deformity is performed.

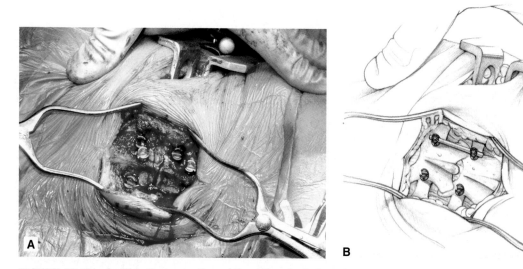

FIGURE 38-7 **A.** Note the correction of the deformity before the placement of the initial rod and B after placement of rod.

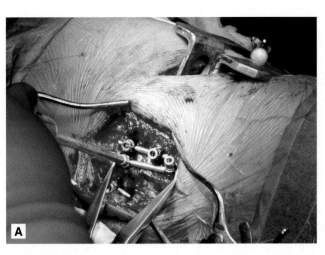
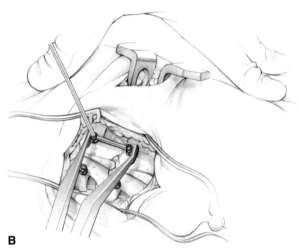

FIGURE 38-8   A, B. Further correction may be obtained by compression. This needs to be done gently, given the patient's size and implant size.

A thorough preoperative evaluation of the anatomy via plain films and CT scanning is paramount to avoid confusion at the time of surgery and to minimize the potential of not being at the correct levels on both sides of the spine. Bifid lamina or fusions seen on CT scanning will help prevent confusion and potential mistakes during the operation.

Thorough preoperative evaluation and planning, meticulous exposure, and a stepwise technique in the operating room will allow for an excellent outcome, while minimizing the chances for a complication.

ILLUSTRATIVE CASE

An 18-month-old boy presented with a progressive thoracolumbar deformity secondary to an unsegmented hemivertebra (Figs. 38-9 and 38-10). The patient underwent successful hemivertebra excision via simultaneous exposures. He was placed in a cast for 6 weeks postoperatively and healed uneventfully. His final radiographs 10 years later show a well-balanced spine, excellent fusion, and no adjacent deformity (Fig. 38-11).

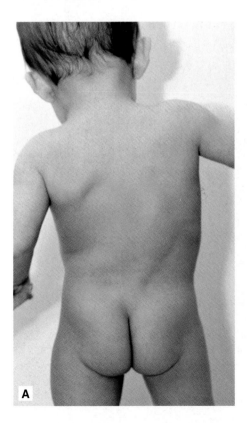
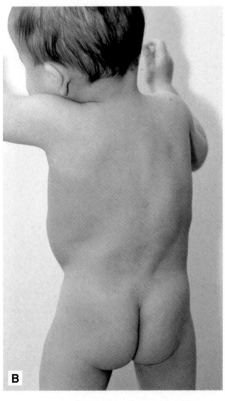

FIGURE 38-9. A, B. Clinical photos of a patient with a hemivertebra and thoracolumbar deformity.

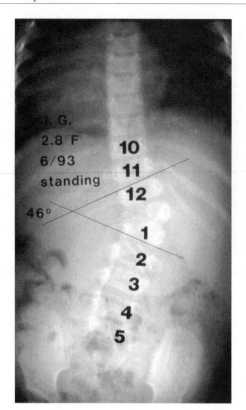

FIGURE 38-10
Radiograph showing the hemivertebra with resultant curvature of the spine.

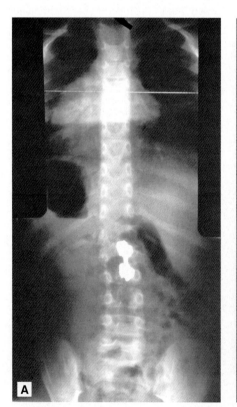

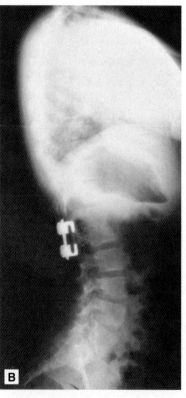

FIGURE 38-11
A, B. Final radiographs showing complete deformity correction and fusion.

PEARLS AND PITFALLS

- Examine bending films prior to surgery to ensure that there is sufficient mobility surrounding the hemivertebrae for the spine to be straight after the hemivertebra is removed. Beware that other unrecognized congenital anomalies may be present.
- Sharp curettes are essential, as they minimize the amount of force needed to remove bone.
- Bipolar cautery is useful to minimize intracanal bleeding.

EDITORS' NOTE

The editors (DLS and VTT) now perform the great majority of hemivertebrae excisions from a posterior-only approach. In a discreet hemivertebra, the spinal cord or lumbar nerve roots are toward the concavity of the curve, while the hemivertebra is toward the convexity. Thus the majority of the operation is at a distance from the neural elements. Use of loupe magnification and a headlight is helpful.

With this technique, the child is positioned prone, with good fluoroscopic imaging of the hemivertebrae verified. The hemilamina and surrounding ligamentum flavum are removed. Pedicle screws are placed in the vertebrae above and below the hemivertebra that is to be removed. The pedicle is entered with a pedicle probe, and this track is expanded with a series of curettes (Fig. 38-12). In the thoracic region, about 4 cm of the attached rib is removed as is the transverse process. The rib head may be removed or left in place and later pushed out laterally during closure of osteotomy.

Using a series of straight and downgoing currettes, the cancellous portion of the vertebral body is removed in its entirety. Frequent use of bone wax on cancellous bone limits bleeding and maximizes visualization. In young children, a layer of cartilage and/or periosteum remains intact and separates the excised vertebrae from structures anterior and lateral to the vertebral body. During this time, the pedicle is quite significantly expanded, but care is taken to leave the medial wall of the pedicle and the posterior wall of the vertebrae intact (Fig. 38-13). This is key from a safety standpoint; as long as the medial pedicle wall and posterior vertebral cortex are intact, the neural structures are protected. The discs above and below the isolated hemivertebra are then

---

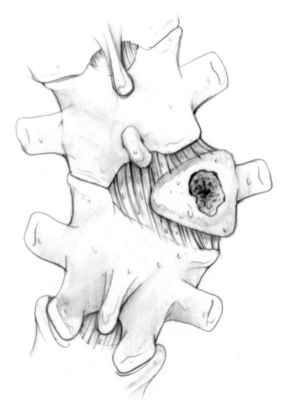

FIGURE 38-12

The pedicle is entered with a standard pedicle probe and expanded with a series of increasing sized curettes. This often creates a hole large enough to see into.

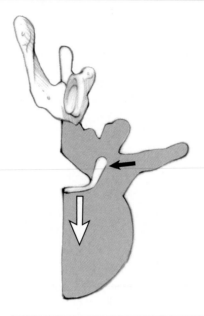

FIGURE 38-13

Cross-section of hemivertebrae. The medial wall of the pedicle (black arrow) is the second-to-last thing to be removed. The posterior wall of the vertebral body is the last thing to be removed by pushing anteriorly, away from neural elements (white arrow).

removed, including the growth plate of the vertebrae above and below the hemivertebra. At times, some bone of the above and below vertebrae may need to be removed (Fig. 38-14). At this stage, it is not unusual to encounter threads of the pedicle screw of the inferior vertebral body, confirming that more than enough tissue has been removed.

The challenge at this point is usually to dissect sufficiently medially across the midline of the spine. Intraoperative fluoroscopy with the curette in place may help confirm the medial extent of dissection. Every effort should be made to remove tissue up to, but not including, the concave annulus. During this part of the dissection, the lateral wall of the pedicle usually breaks open, allowing one to drop one's hands toward the floor and direct the currette more medially. At this point, one can see surprisingly well into the cavity with the help of a headlamp.

The penultimate part of the dissection is removal of the medial wall of the pedicle, usually with a pituitary rongeur or currette, while gently retracting nerve root and dura from this area. Bipolar cautery is helpful in this area when separating the dural sac from the bone to be removed. The final maneuver is to push the thinned-out posterior cortex of the vertebral body anteriorly, thus completing the hemivertebra excision. The open wedge should now close easily, with the surgeon having appropriate paranoia about making certain no bone or tissue buckles into the spinal canal during closure. Any gaps may be filled with bone graft.

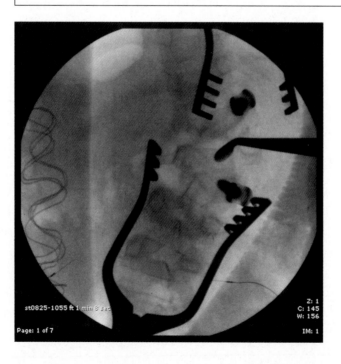

FIGURE 38-14

In this case, not only are the inferior disc and endplate removed, but also some of the vertebral body is removed to maximize correction.

> **Pearl:** In the thoracic spine in young children, pedicle screw fixation may be tenuous. Standard lumbar hooks should be placed on the rib above and below the excised hemivertebra, just lateral to the transverse process. These hooks are then attached with a rod and compressed across the ribs to achieve closure of the osteotomy while avoiding any compromise of the pedicle screws. The final rod may then be placed across the pedicle screws, and the temporary rib-to-rib rod removed.

REFERENCES

1. Belmont PJ Jr., Kuklo TR, Taylor KF, et al. Intraspinal anomalies associated with isolated congenital hemivertebra: the role of routine magnetic resonance imaging. *J Bone Joint Surg Am.* 2004;86(8):1704–1710.
2. Hedequist DJ, Emans JB. The correlation of preoperative three-dimensional computed tomography reconstructions with operative findings in congenital scoliosis. *Spine.* 2003;28(22):2531–2534.
3. Hedequist DJ, Hall JE, Emans JB. The safety and efficacy of spinal instrumentation in children with congenital spine deformities. *Spine.* 2004;29(18):2081–2086.
4. Hedequist DJ, Hall JE, Emans JB. Hemivertebra excision in children via simultaneous anterior and posterior exposures. *J Pediatr Orthop.* 2005;25(1):60–63.
5. Ruf M, Harms J. Hemivertebra resection by a posterior approach: innovative operative technique and first results. *Spine.* 2002;27(10):1116–1123.

39 Growing Spinal Instrumentation

Eric W. Hooley and Behrooz A. Akbarnia

INTRODUCTION

Managing children with progressive early-onset scoliosis (EOS) can be very challenging. Some cases, may resolve spontaneously without the need for treatment. Left untreated, however, progressive curves can produce significant thoracic deformity, leading to severe cardiopulmonary complications. Surgical treatment should be considered when nonoperative measures, including bracing and casting, are not indicated or fail to arrest progression. In this chapter we describe the principles involved in treating EOS with growing posterior spinal instrumentation.

The growing rod techniques continue to evolve and are primarily directed at the correction of the spine and thoracic deformities from a posterior approach without entering the chest cavity, while simultaneously preserving and/or stimulating spine and trunk growth. Recent studies confirm that although this method provides many challenges, it is able to promote continued spinal and chest wall growth while maintaining curve correction.

INDICATIONS/CONTRAINDICATIONS

Growing spinal instrumentation is indicated for curves that do not meet the criteria for observation or for curves that fail or do not meet the criteria for nonoperative management. These curves are generally greater than 50 degrees or are progressing rapidly (>10 degrees) between examinations. The posterior elements of the spine in these patients should be large enough to allow for appropriate spinal fixation, and patients should be young enough to have sufficient growth left. Typically patients are between 1.5 and 10 years of age. Contraindications to growing spinal instrumentation may include active infection, very stiff curves, or osteopenic bones that are too soft to withstand the corrective loads needed when this spinal instrumentation is placed.

PREOPERATIVE PLANNING

After a complete medical history and physical examination have been completed, appropriate and necessary imaging studies should be obtained and include full-length erect anteroposterior (AP) and lateral radiographs, so that the entire spine, pelvis, and thorax can be visualized. AP spine-bending radiographs of the spine or an AP radiograph while traction is applied provide helpful information as well. A computed axial tomography (CT) scan of the spine with three-dimensional reconstructions can assist in understanding the curve in cases with congenital bony abnormalities. Magnetic resonance imaging (MRI) can add information concerning neural axis anomalies and should usually be obtained preoperatively.

Consultation should be made with the patient's pediatrician to maximize the patient's medical status prior to surgery. Other specialists' input (particularly from the pulmonologist and cardiologist) should be sought as needed to assist with associated conditions or syndromes that the patient might have.

Both single and dual rod techniques are used, however, we prefer the dual rod technique which we believe provides better results. The levels that need to be incorporated into the spinal instrumentation construct are determined, and foundation sites are chosen prior to surgery. Each foundation site consists of an assembly of at least four bony anchors that are strong enough to withstand the deforming loads that will be placed on them. The anchors may be either hooks or screws. The foundations usually span at least two vertebrae in order to provide enough strength for the corrective forces that are to be applied. The cephalad foundation is often around T2 to T4, and the caudal foundation is one or two levels below the end vertebra, usually around L2 to L4.

SURGICAL PROCEDURE

The patient is given a dose of preoperative antibiotics, and anesthesia is obtained. The patient is then placed in a prone position, and all pressure points are well padded. Small children are often positioned with two longitudinal chest rolls placed on the operating table; larger children may benefit from a four-post frame setup or Jackson table setup. Intraoperative spinal cord monitoring is used at the surgeon's discretion.

After prepping and draping, a midline incision is made over the levels to be included in the construct. The exposure of the cephalad and caudal foundation sites is made subperiosteal, either through one or two incisions but care is taken to keep exposure of the spine between the foundation sites subcutaneous or subfascial to prevent premature, unwanted, spinal fusion.

At the foundation sites, hooks or screws are used to create a claw anchor. Pedicle screws provide stronger anchors and may be used if the vertebral anatomy allows. If hooks are used, downgoing hooks are placed cranially, with upgoing hooks placed caudally at each claw anchor site. A combination of

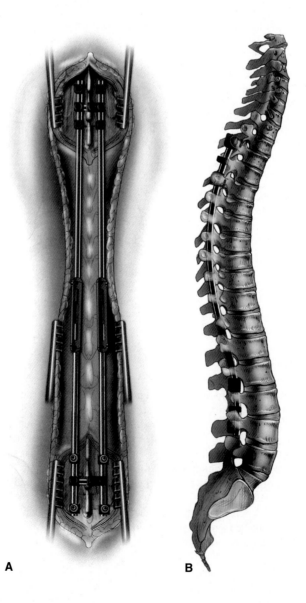

FIGURE 39-1

Coronal **(A)** and sagittal **(B)** views of a subcutaneous growing spinal instrumentation construct that uses hooks at the foundation sites.

A   **B**

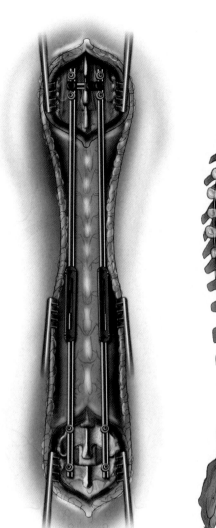

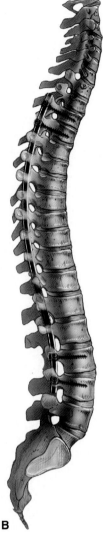

FIGURE 39-2

Coronal **(A)** and sagittal **(B)** views of a subcutaneous growing spinal instrumentation construct that uses pedicle screws at the foundation sites.

A   B

laminar, transverse process, facet, or pedicle hooks may be used, depending on the patient's vertebral anatomy and the surgeon's experience. Supralaminar hooks are less likely to dislodge as compared to transverse process hooks in the upper thoracic region. If pedicle screws are used, at least four at each foundation site are needed to create a stable anchor and a crosslink is not usually required.

Two small-diameter rods are contoured for sagittal alignment and used for each anchor site compressing the anchor levels for stability. The contoured rods are firmly attached to the foundation site anchors after being placed in a subcutaneous or subfascial position (Figs. 39-1 and 39-2). The ends of the rods from the cephalad and caudal anchors are then attached by a tandem connector on each side. The connectors are usually placed at the thoracolumbar junction, since this area has the straightest sagittal plane alignment it is also possible to use a side-to-side connector to attach the upper and lower rods if more sagittal contouring is needed or the use of a tandem connector is not possible (Fig. 39.3).

Rotation and distraction of the contoured rod is then performed, followed by locking of the tandem connector on each side. Care should be used in these maneuvers so that excessive force does not cause early failure of the anchor sites. All implants should be positioned to give the lowest profile. The foundation sites are then prepared to facilitate a posterior fusion between the vertebrae to which the claw anchor has been attached. Local bone or allograft may be used to assist in the foundation fusion process. The wound is carefully closed in routine fashion.

POSTOPERATIVE MANAGEMENT

For many patients, a brace, such as a thoracolumbar-sacral orthosis (TLSO), is used to assist in the fusion process for the first 3 to 6 months. Some patients may benefit from longer brace wear. Patients are followed at routine 6-month intervals, before and after each lengthening. Standing radiographs are obtained during these visits and are carefully assessed for implant complications and curve progression.

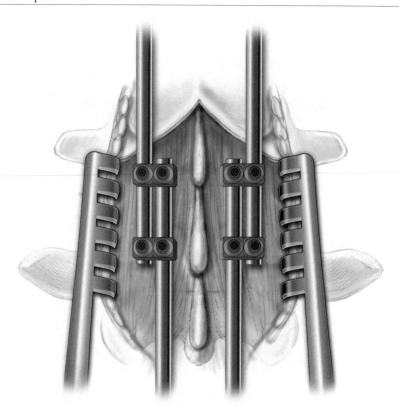

FIGURE 39-3

Side-to-side connectors attaching the cephalad and caudal rods in a subcutaneous position.

Lengthenings are scheduled every 6 months and can be performed in a variety of ways. More commonly, the tandem connectors are palpated, and a local exposure is made over them under general anesthesia. Once the connectors are uncovered, and usually one set screw loosened, the rods are distracted either from inside or outside the connector, followed by retightening of the set screw(s). The wound is closed in routine fashion.

The lengthening procedures may be accomplished in an outpatient setting or as a brief inpatient stay, depending on the patient's medical condition and needs. The patient is seen at 2 weeks following the lengthening for a routine wound check and is then scheduled as needed, with at least one visit just prior to the next lengthening in 6 months. During the interim, the patient's parent or guardian is instructed on the potential complications and is urged to keep in close contact with the surgeon should anything arise.

During the lengthenings, shorter connectors may need to be exchanged for longer connectors to accommodate the increase in length as the patient grows. If new connectors do not allow for the needed length, then the rods will need to be removed and new, longer rods inserted in much the same manner as they were placed during the index procedure.

When the lengthenings no longer result in further distraction, or when the patient has reached skeletal maturity, the patient is scheduled to undergo the final spinal instrumentation and fusion procedure. This procedure usually requires exposure of the previously instrumented levels, but may necessitate a more cephalad and/or caudal exposure if the curve has progressed outside the original curve. All growing instruments are removed, and the final spinal instrumentation construct is implanted. The final assembly consists of appropriately contoured rods attached to pedicle screws and/or hooks, based on the surgeon's preference and the patient's vertebral anatomy. Osteotomies are often incorporated into the final fusion procedure to obtain improved and acceptable balance in the coronal sagittal planes. Patients usually wear a brace for 6 months and are followed at routine intervals with radiographs. If, at maturity, the curve is not large enough to require spine infusion, it may be possible to remove the implants and leave the spine unfused.

COMPLICATIONS TO AVOID

Complications do not occur infrequently and include wound infection, skin breakdown over the implants, implant failure, curve progression, junctional kyphosis, and crankshaft phenomenon. These patients should be followed closely with routine radiographs to identify and treat these complications appropriately.

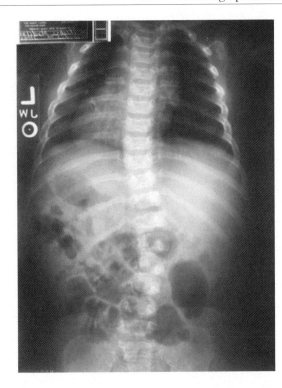

FIGURE 39-4

21-degree curve from T10 through L2 at age 8 months

ILLUSTRATIVE CASE

A 20-month-old girl presented with progressive scoliosis that was first noticed at 6 months of age. The patient had an otherwise normal medical history. She was the product of a full-term delivery with a birth weight of 8 pounds. There was no family history of scoliosis, and she was reaching her developmental milestones appropriately. Genetic counseling found no associated syndrome. An ultrasound found no renal anomalies, and an MRI revealed no intraspinal abnormalities.

On examination, the patient was 35.5 inches tall and weighed 31 pounds. She had a right thoracolumbar prominence that measured 20 degrees with the scoliometer. Her neurologic examination was normal.

Her radiographs over a 10-month period showed an increase in her curve, extending from T10 to L2 from 21 degrees to 73 degrees (Figs. 39-4 and 39-5). Her coronal plumb line was 24 mm to the

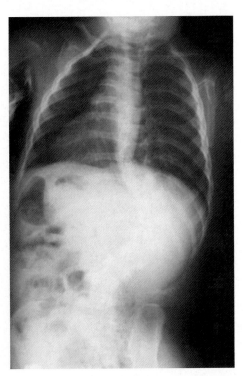

FIGURE 39-5

The curve from T10 through L2 has progressed to 73 degrees by age 20 months.

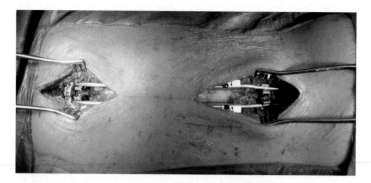

FIGURE 39-6   Intraoperative picture of the hook and rod construct, showing cephalad and caudal anchor sites. The rods have been placed subcutaneously. The caudal aspect of the tandem connectors are also seen.

right, and her sagittal balance was +71 mm. Kyphosis measured 50 degrees, and lordosis measured 53 degrees. Traction films showed that the curve corrected to –13 degrees. The length from T1 to S1 measured 255 mm.

The patient was taken to the operating room for insertion of dual growing rod instrumentation (Fig. 39-6). Hook and rod constructs were made at T3 through T4 and at L3 through L4 to serve as the cephalad and caudal foundations, respectively. After the rods were contoured and attached to their respective anchors, the cephalad and caudal rods were attached with a growing rod connector (Fig. 39-7).

Planned lengthenings have continued at 6-month intervals . The patient's latest films at 3 years show that the primary curve has decreased to 28 degrees, and the length from T1 to S1 has increased to 346 mm (Fig. 39-8). She is balanced in both the coronal and sagittal planes.

CONCLUSION

With proper patient selection and attention to details, growing rod instrumentation is a very useful technique in the treatment of these challenging cases of early-onset scoliosis. This technique obtains deformity correction but still allows the spine to grow and the thoracic cage volume to increase. Complications are as expected for a treatment that requires multiple operations over many years.

FIGURE 39-7

Initial postoperative AP **(A)** and lateral **(B)** images showing the final dual rod construct with good correction of the curve at 20 months of age.

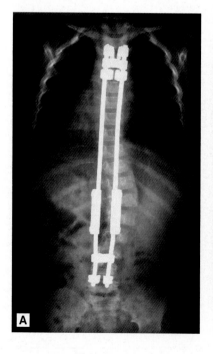

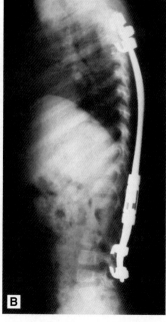

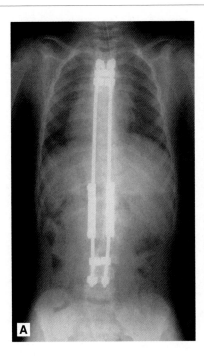
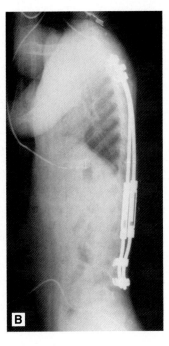

FIGURE 39-8

Latest postoperative AP **(A)** and lateral **(B)** images at age 4. The curve correction has been maintained, and coronal and sagittal balance is excellent.

PEARLS AND PITFALLS

- To prevent unwanted fusion, use subperiosteal dissection only in the areas to be fused.
- Place the tandem connectors at the thoracolumbar junction in order to affect the sagittal balance the least.
- Avoid being overly aggressive with correction at the index procedure or at the first lengthening to avoid implant failure.
- Watch especially for overcorrection in kyphotic patients.
- Keep implants in the lowest profile position.
- Make sure the curve is sufficiently flexible to benefit from this procedure and, if not, apply preoperative traction or perform an anterior annviotomy prior to surgery.
- Monitor patients closely for complications and act quickly on wound problems.
- Lengthen every 6 months or sooner to get maximal correction and growth.

REFERENCES

1. Akbarnia BA. Management themes in early onset scoliosis. *J Bone Joint Surg Am.* 2007;89:42–54.
2. Akbarnia BA, Asher MA, Bagheri R, et al. Complications of dual growing rod technique in early onset scoliosis: can we identify risk factors? Scoliosis Research Society 41st Annual Meeting. Monterey, California; 2006.
3. Akbarnia BA, Marks DS. Instrumentation with limited arthrodesis for the treatment of progressive early-onset scoliosis. *Spine.* 2000;14:181–189.
4. Akbarnia BA, Marks DS, Boachie-Adjei O, et al. Dual growing rod technique for the treatment of progressive early-onset scoliosis: a multicenter study. *Spine.* 2005;30:S46–S57.
5. Harrington PR. Treatment of scoliosis: correction and internal fixation by spine instrumentation. *J Bone Joint Surg Am.* 1962;44:591–610.
6. Klemme WR, Denis F, Winter RB, et al. Spinal instrumentation without fusion for progressive scoliosis in young children. *J Pediatr Orthop.* 1997;17:734–742.
7. Luque E, Cardosa A. Segmental spinal instrumentation in growing children. *Orthop Trans.* 1977;1:37.
8. Moe JH, Kharrat K, Winter RB, et al. Harrington instrumentation without fusion plus external orthotic support for the treatment of difficult curvature problems in young children. *Clin Orthop Relat Res.* 1984;185:35–45.
9. Thompson GH, Akbarnia BA, Kostial P, et al. Comparison of single and dual growing rod techniques followed through definitive surgery: a preliminary study. *Spine.* 2005;30:2039–2044.
10. Sponseller PL, Yazici M, Demetracopoulos C, et al. Evidence basis for management of spine and chest wall deformities in children. *Spine.* 2007;32(19 Suppl):581–590.
11. Thompson GT, Akbarnia BA, Campbell RM. Growing rod techniques in early-onset scollosis. *J Pediatr Orthop.* 2007;27(3):354–361.

40 Opening Wedge Thoracostomy and the Titanium Rib Implant in the Treatment of Congenital Scoliosis with Fused Ribs

Robert M. Campbell, Jr.

Titanium rib opening-wedge thoracostomy is a surgical procedure that attempts to correct the three-dimensional thoracic deformity of congenital scoliosis associated with fused ribs by lengthening and enlarging the constricted hemithorax (Fig. 40-1). This procedure directly aids growth of the underlying lung, while indirectly correcting scoliosis without fusion, so that thoracic spinal growth can continue to contribute to thoracic volume and further lung growth. The titanium rib (Fig. 40-2), or VEPTR (Vertical Expandable Prosthetic Titanium Rib), is made by Synthes Spine Company of Westchester, Pennsylvania. It is FDA approved, and it is available for use under the Humanitarian Device Exemption (HDE) regulations.

INDICATIONS/CONTRAINDICATIONS

Indications

The indications for use of VEPTR opening-wedge thoracostomy for fused ribs and scoliosis are as follows:

- Progressive thoracic congenital scoliosis in patients age 6 months up to skeletal maturity
- Three or more fused ribs on the concave side of the curve
- Greater than 10% reduction in the space available for the lung (the ratio of the radiographic height of the concave lung compared with the convex lung)
- Presence of thoracic insufficiency syndrome,[4] the inability of the thorax to support normal respiration or lung growth.

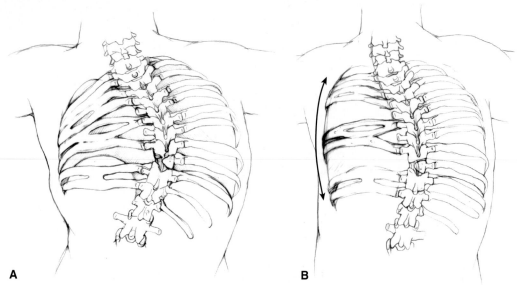

A   **B**

FIGURE 40-1   A. In fused ribs and scoliosis, the concave hemithorax compresses the underlying lung, with constriction worsening over time because of growth inhibition of the fused chest wall. This results in progressive thoracic insufficiency syndrome. **B.** The goal of thoracic reconstruction for thoracic insufficiency syndrome is to create the largest, most symmetrical thorax possible. Opening-wedge thoracostomy for fused ribs and scoliosis addresses the three-dimensional deformity of the thorax by lengthening the constrictive concave hemithorax *(arrow),* restoring potential space for growth of the concave lung, and indirectly correcting the congenital scoliosis, all without limiting growth in height of the spine through fusion. Unlike traditional spinal surgery, VEPTR instrumentation does not correct deformity; rather it serves as a means of stabilization for the acute thoracic reconstruction.

The diagnosis of thoracic insufficiency syndrome can be based either on the thoracic disability related to the biomechanical acts of respiration or on growth inhibition of the thorax. In a normal thorax, inspiration is accomplished primarily by a diaphragmatic contraction that provides expansion of the overlying lungs with assistance of anterolateral expansion of the chest wall through the intercostal muscles. Fused ribs and scoliosis is a volume depletion deformity, type II, of the thorax (Table 40-1).[2]

In fused ribs and scoliosis, thoracic insufficiency syndrome is present because the fused chest wall cannot expand to aid the diaphragm in expansion of the underlying lung. The other component of thoracic insufficiency syndrome—growth inhibition—is also present because the extensively fused chest wall constricts the growth of the underlying lung.

FIGURE 40-2   A. The 220-mm radius rib-to-rib VEPTR. **B.** The hybrid rib-to-spine VEPTR construct. **C.** The hybrid rib-to-pelvis VEPTR construct via iliac crest pedestal S-hook fixation. **D.** The 70-mm radius primary lateral expansion VEPTR. VEPTR components are made of titanium alloy and are MRI compatible. *(Continued)*

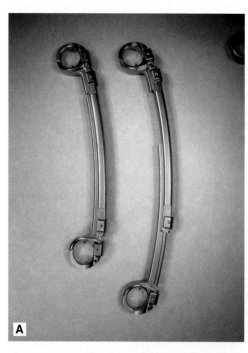

A

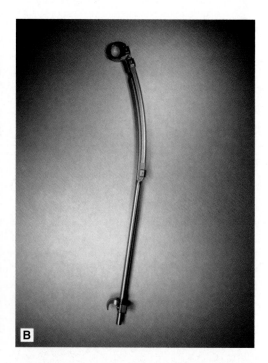

B

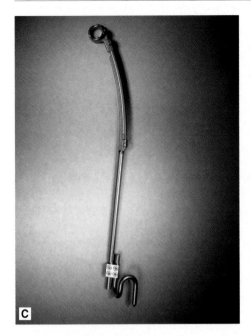

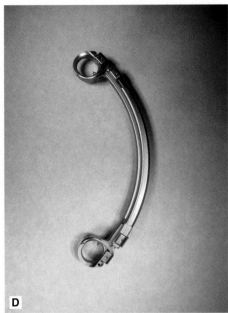

FIGURE 40-2   (*Continued*)

Contraindications

- Inadequate soft-tissue coverage for the devices
- A body weight less than 25% normal for age
- Severe, rigid kyphosis greater than 50 degrees
- Absent diaphragm function
- Inability to tolerate repetitive surgeries

Relative Contraindications

- Absence of proximal ribs for VEPTR device attachment: This situation can be corrected by the clavicle augmentation/first rib procedure. In this procedure, a rib autograft is taken from the contralateral side. The clavicle on the side of the proximal rib deficiency is osteotomized lengthwise, bringing the anterior half under the brachial plexus as a vascularized pedicle and interposing the rib autograft between the pedicle and the transverse process of T2 (Fig. 40-3). Within 3 months this forms an augmented first rib suitable for attachment of VEPTR devices posteriorly.
- A history of prior spine fusion, involving a significant portion of the thoracic spine, is not a contraindication. However, these patients do not appear to respond as favorably to VEPTR treatment compared with those who have "virgin" spines. Rigid curves within the fusion mass do not correct, spinal growth is marginal, and pulmonary outcome tends to be unfavorable.[5]

PREOPERATIVE PLANNING

The history includes an emphasis on past respiratory problems. Episodes of pneumonia; the need for oxygen, continuous positive airway pressure (CPAP), or ventilator support during episodes of pneumonia; sleep disturbances, which may suggest early cor pulmonale, are noted. Birth histories such as prematurity with sequelae of bronchopulmonary dysplasia, history of diaphragmatic hernia, tracheobronchial malacia, or other causes of intrinsic lung disease, also need to be documented. A history of past spine surgery, noting age at operation and extent of fusion, should also be determined. It should also be determined whether congenital renal abnormalities have been ruled out by prior ultrasound or magnetic resonance imaging (MRI) and whether spinal cord abnormalities have been ruled out by MRI.

TABLE 40-1 Volume Depletion Deformities of the Thorax[2]	
Unilateral Thoracic Volume Depletion Deformity	
Type I	Absent ribs and scoliosis
Type II	Fused ribs and scoliosis
Global Volume Depletion Deformity	
Type IIIa	Jarcho-Levin Syndrome
Type IIIb	Jeune Syndrome

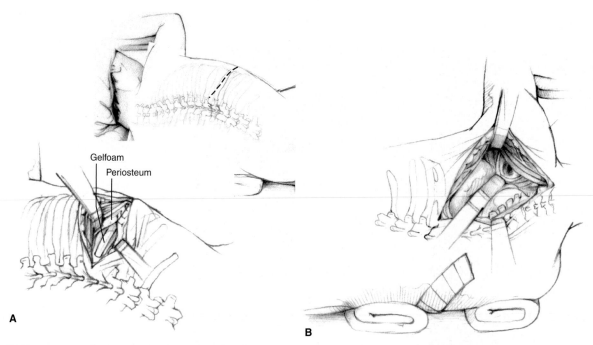

Gelfoam
Periosteum

A

B

FIGURE 40-3 **A.** For patients with proximal rib deficiency in which there is no attachment point for the VEPTR rib cradle, an osseous "first rib" for VEPTR placement can be reconstructed by the clavicle-augmentation procedure. The patient is first placed in the lateral decubitus position, with the deficiency side down. The entire ninth rib is harvested as an autograft, cut near the costochondral junction, and disarticulated from the spine. The rib periosteum is then packed with a strip of Gelfoam to maintain its cylindrical shape so it can reform the rib. The periosteum is repaired with a running Vicryl suture. A dressing is applied. **B.** The patient is transferred to a lateral decubitus position, with the deficiency side now up. The patient is draped so that both the anterior and posterior chest are accessible. A limited posterior thoracotomy is performed proximally. There is usually a vestigial rib protruding from the proximal thoracic spine; this is dissected out, along with its transverse process. Blunt dissection is used to create a tunnel beneath the brachial plexus and the vascular bundle, extending anteriorly to the clavicle. **C.** A limited anterior thoracotomy is then performed through a transverse skin incision placed just beneath the clavicle. Dissection continues through the muscle (arrow) under the clavicle, without damage to the superior vessels, until the tunnel created by the posterior approach is reached. **D.** Without stripping periosteum, the clavicle is osteotomized by first drilling holes at 5-mm intervals longitudinally, from distally to proximally, up to within 1 cm of the sternoclavicular joint. A small osteotome is then used to complete the osteotomy. **E.** The anterior clavicular half, with its intact periosteum, is carefully brought inferiorly, hinging at the intact medial side. Two holes are drilled through the distal end for passage of a 0 Prolene suture. The medial end of the clavicle half undergoes a gentle osteoclasis; that half is then directed underneath the intact posterior clavicle half to form a vascularized pedicle for the rib autograft. The ninth rib autograft has two holes drilled in each end. Two holes are also drilled in the vestigial rib/transverse process protruding from the proximal thoracic spine. A Prolene suture is threaded through the holes in the distal end of the clavicular half and then into the end of the autograft. The rib autograft is then passed through the anterior incision to extend posteriorly to the proximal thoracic spine. The suture is tied to stabilize the splice between the clavicle half and the autograft. The other end of the autograft is sutured with Prolene into the spine through the previously drilled holes into the vestigial rib/transverse processes. Bone graft, often obtained from the lateral cortex of ribs in the field, is packed around the splice between the transverse processes and the rib autograft. The reconstructed first rib is gently inclined downward at a 45-degree angle to ensure clearance for the brachial plexus. Both thoracotomies are then closed. Within 3 months, there is adequate healing to consider VEPTR implantation into the reconstructed first rib. The new proximal rib is usually wide enough to allow placement of a standard superior rib cradle, with the cradle cap placed in a burr hole inferior to the upper edge of the reconstructed rib. Care should be taken not to place VEPTRs anterior to the midaxillary of the reconstructed rib, because of the danger of brachial plexus compression. Usually a medial hybrid VEPTR can be placed without difficulty; often a rib-to-rib VEPTR can be placed closely adjacent to the hybrid. **F.** A 4-month-old patient with severe proximal rib deficiency and congenital scoliosis. **G.** 8-year follow-up after a clavicle/first rib augmentation procedure and placement of bilateral VEPTRs. (*Continued*)

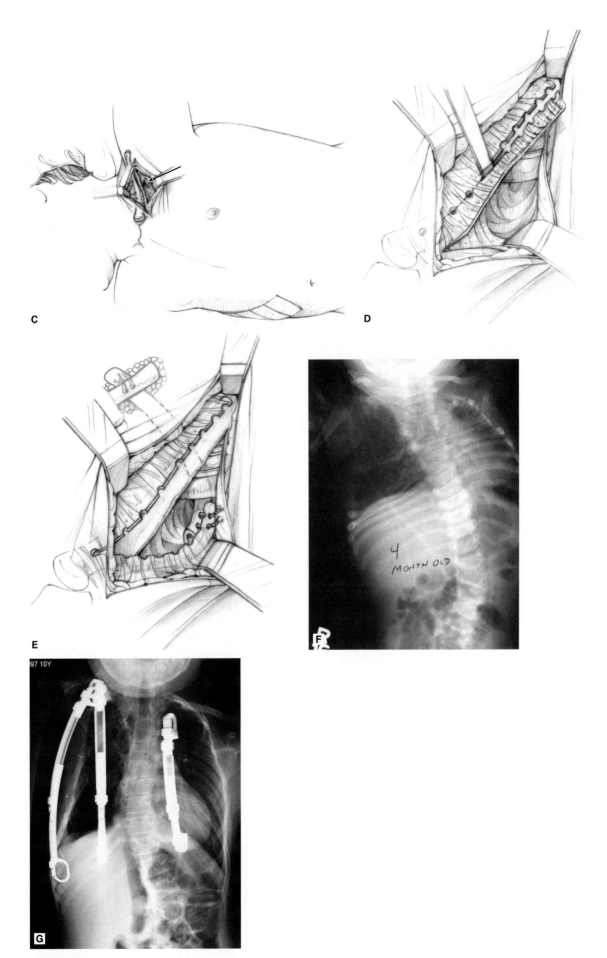

C

D

E

F

G

FIGURE 40-3 (*Continued*)

459

TABLE 40-2	Assisted Ventilation Rating
+0	No assistance, on room air
+1	Supplemental oxygen required
+2	Nighttime ventilation/CPAP
+3	Part-time ventilation/CPAP
+4	Full-time ventilation

Clinical respiratory insufficiency may be graded by the assisted ventilation rating (AVR) (Table 40-2).[2] The physical examination should include measurement of the resting respiratory rate, which is then compared with normative values to determine whether there is occult respiratory insufficiency. Fingers are examined for clubbing, which is a sign of chronic respiratory insufficiency. Standard spinal evaluation for curve flexibility, head decompensation, truncal decompensation, and trunk rotation is included.

Thoracic function through respiratory chest wall expansions is tested by the thumb excursion test.[4] The examiner's hands are placed around the base of the thorax, with the thumbs posteriorly pointing upward at equal distances from the spine. With respiration in the normal thorax, the thumbs move away from the spine symmetrically due to the anterolateral motion of the chest wall (Fig. 40-4). In fused ribs and scoliosis, however, the fused chest wall commonly has poor or absent motion. The hemithorax is disabled, because only the diaphragm is left to power respiration due to the absent intercostal muscle function. The contralateral convex hemithorax chest wall may have some ability to expand and contribute to respiration, but with increasing rotation of the spine in progressive curves and associated distortion of the rib cage, the convex chest wall will become rigid, adding to the total thoracic function disability. The thumb excursion test, a simple clinical assessment of thoracic function, is a valuable way to test for thoracic insufficiency syndrome.

Preoperative radiographs should include anteroposterior (AP) and lateral images of the spine, including the rib cage and the pelvis. Cobb angle, head and truncal decompensation, and space available for lung are determined. Supine lateral bending radiographs are used to determine flexibility and extent of hemithorax constriction on the concave side of the curve (Fig. 40-5). If kyphosis is present, a cross-table lateral radiograph with a bolster under the apex of the kyphosis is taken to determine flexibility.

Computed axial tomography (CT) scans are performed to assess the three-dimensional deformity of the thorax, and presence of intrinsic lung disease (e.g., bronchiectasis or chronic atelectasis), (Fig. 40-6) and potential bone anchor points (lamina, pedicles, ribs). The preoperative CT scan

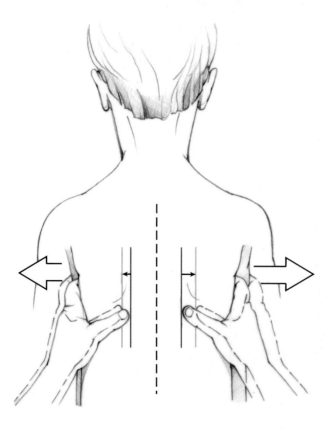

FIGURE 40-4

Thumb excursion test.

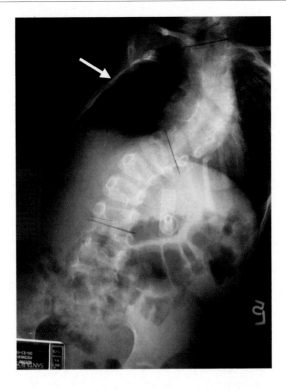

FIGURE 40-5

This 3-year-old girl shows marked thoracic constriction *(arrow)* proximal to the apex of the curve.

should also be checked carefully for areas of dysraphic spine within the area of surgical approach. In these areas, dissection should be cautious, with medial exposure only above and below the areas of dysraphism. Particularly dangerous is an area of midthoracic spine dysraphism, where the medial edge of the scapula lies within the spinal canal on the concave side of the curve (Fig. 40-9). The CT scan is performed at 5-mm intervals, unenhanced, including cervical spine, chest, and lumbar spine. A fluoroscopy of the diaphragm or dynamic MRI of the lungs may be performed to document normal function, and a screening MRI is performed to detect spinal cord abnormalities, such as tethered cord or syrinx. Cervical spine series, including flexion-extension laterals, are performed to document any abnormality or instability. An echocardiogram is performed to detect early cor pulmonale.

The author's institution routinely uses a trispecialty evaluation system in which the patient, in addition to orthopaedic evaluation, is seen by both a pediatric general surgeon and a pediatric pulmonologist. General surgery evaluation is important for in-depth understanding of the rib cage conditions, as well as associated gastrointestinal, renal, cardiac, and congenital lung malformations in some children. Pediatric pulmonary evaluation is also important to gain an understanding of the pulmonary function, including the risk of progression of respiratory insufficiency, and of intrinsic lung disease that may be complicating the patient's thoracic insufficiency syndrome. If all investigators believe that the patient has progressive thoracic insufficiency syndrome and that VEPTR opening-wedge thoracostomy is the best treatment of choice, then a surgical treatment recommendation is made. If there are any dissenting votes, an alternative recommendation is made.

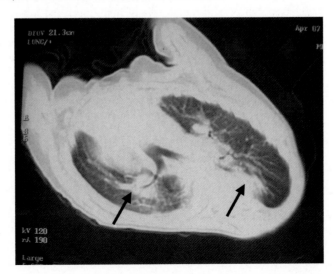

FIGURE 40-6

The CT scan of this child with scoliosis shows severe windswept deformity of the thorax in the transverse plane and bilateral chronic atelectasis *(arrows).*

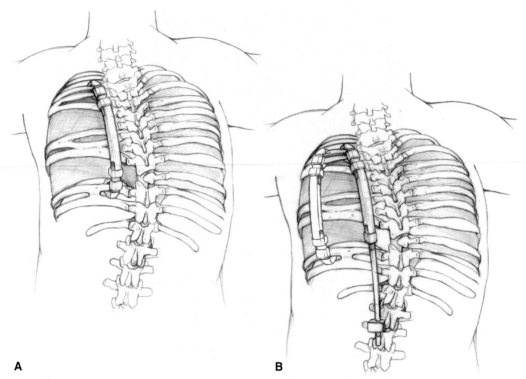

A   **B**

FIGURE 40-7   **A.** In children under 18 months, the opening-wedge thoracostomy correction is stabilized by a single rib-to-rib VEPTR placed adjacent to the spine. **B.** In children older than 18 months, the lumbar canal can accept a laminar hook, so the opening-wedge thoracostomy correction is stabilized by a rib-to-rib and a rib to spine VEPTR.

SURGICAL PROCEDURE

The Exposure

A central venous line, arterial line, and Foley catheter are placed. The patient is placed in a modified lateral decubitus position, with the chest tilted slightly anterior. An axillary roll is used, with foam padding also placed underneath the pelvis and the lower extremities. A soft bolster is also placed under the apex of the deformity. The patient is stabilized by 2-in.-wide cloth tape over a hand towel placed on top of the pelvis, taped down to each side of the operating room table. Another hand towel and cloth tape are brought across the lower extremities (Fig. 40-8). The upper arms are draped out of the field with a pulse oximeter attached to the upper hand. The shoulders are brought out at right angles to the axis of the body, with the elbows extended 90 degrees. Padding is placed between the arms and under the elbows. Spinal cord monitoring of both upper and lower extremities by somatosensory-evoked potentials (SSEPs) is performed; if practical, transcranial motor-evoked potentials (TrMEPs) are also monitored. Prophylactic antibiotics (IV Ancef, 30 mg/kg) are given prior to the procedure.

The patient is draped so that the torso is exposed from the top of the pelvis to the top of the shoulders. Anteriorally, the nipple is exposed, so that the area of breast development in females can be identified and avoided. An incision through this area may damage the breast tissue in an immature female, causing later growth disturbance of the breast by adolescence. In contrast to a usual thoracotomy incision, a curvilinear J incision is made, forming a long flap that starts proximally at T1, halfway between the medial edge of the scapula and the posterior spinous processes of the spine, and is carried longitudinally to the level of the 10th rib. (Fig. 40-9). Emans has emphasized that having this long flap aids in closure of the incision after opening-wedge thoracostomy (Emans J. Personal communication, 2000).

Exposure continues with cautery, transecting the latissimus dorsi, trapezius, and rhomboid muscles in line with the skin incision. The scapula is elevated by blunt dissection proximally, and the common insertion of the middle and posterior scalene muscle into the second rib is identified. This is an important landmark as the neurovascular bundle is immediately anterior and should be protected. An anterior flap is developed by cautery up to the costochondral junction, though the full anterior extent of this dissection is not needed in all cases. To complete the exposure, the paraspinous

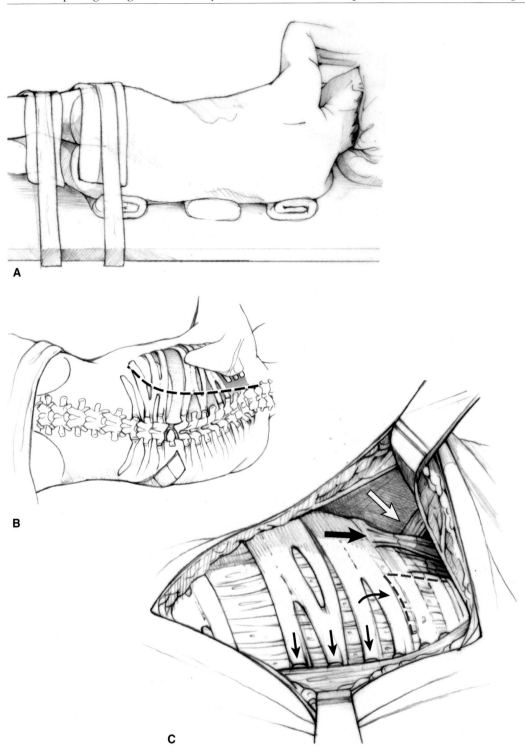

FIGURE 40-8   A. The patient is placed in lateral decubitus position. **B.** The incisions.
C. Exposure should show the common insertion of the middle and posterior scalene muscle
(straight black arrow). The neurovascular bundle lies immediately anterior to this *(white arrow).*
The safe zone for superior rib cradle insertion is posterior to the scalene muscle and on ribs two
or lower *(curved black arrow).* The paraspinal muscles are reflected from lateral to medial by
cautery up to the tips of the transverse processes. *(small black arrows).*

FIGURE 40-9

When the medial edge of the scapula is within the spinal canal through an area of dysraphism, the thoracotomy can be safely performed by retraction of the scapula posteriorly out of the canal, with resection of soft-tissue structures directly off the scapula and away from the spinal cord *(arrow)*.

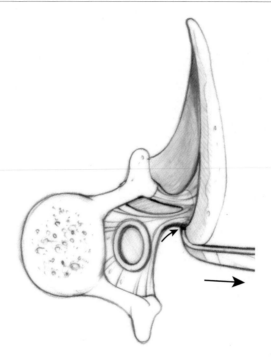

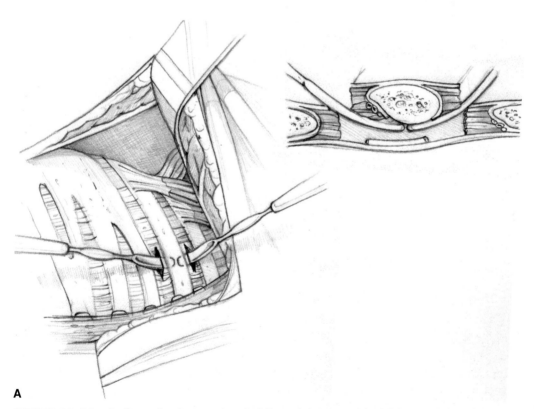

A

FIGURE 40-10 **A.** Freer elevators are inserted through intercostal incisions, separating the periosteum and the pleura anteriorly off the rib. This forms a soft-tissue tunnel for the superior rib cradle. The superior rib cradle is implanted **B.** An opening-wedge thoracostomy is begun anteriorly, close to the costochondral junction, and extended posteriorly in a groove of the fused ribs in the middle of the fused rib mass *(dotted line)* until the tip of the transverse process of the spine is encountered. **C.** The opening-wedge thoracostomy is distracted by an AO bone spreader to both lengthen the constricted hemithorax and indirectly correct the congenital scoliosis. (*Continued*)

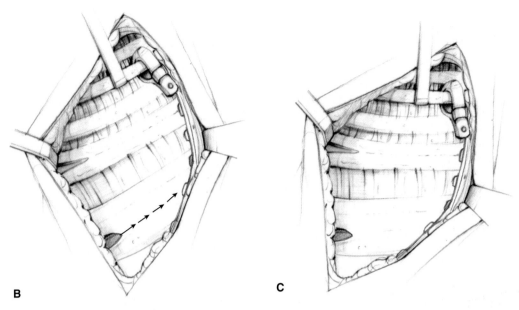

B   **C**

FIGURE 40-10
(*Continued*)

muscles are reflected by cautery from lateral to medial until the tips of the transverse processes are palpable (Fig. 40-8C). Dissection continues no further medially, because exposure of the spine may provoke inadvertent fusion. Care should be taken to leave a thin layer of soft tissue overlying the ribs to avoid damage to the periosteum, because of the risk of devascularizaiton and the subsequent inability to produce reactive bone to the stress of a rib cradle.

To identify the levels of ribs, the first rib may be palpated through the exposure and the ribs counted distally clinically. Radiographic confirmation is seldom necessary in experienced hands.

Pitfall   The usual thoracotomy approach in dysraphism (cutting through the rhomboid muscles with cautery) may result in direct spinal cord injury. To avoid this, a rake should be used to retract the scapula posteriorly to pull it out of the spinal canal. The rhomboid muscles should be sectioned directly off the bone of the scapula, away from the area of dysraphism (Fig. 40-9).

The Superior Rib Cradle

The first step in VEPTR placement is implantation of the superior rib cradle of the titanium rib. The cradle site should be located at the uppermost portion of the thoracic constriction. A 1-cm incision is made by cautery in the intercostal muscle, immediately beneath the rib of attachment. Next a Freer elevator is inserted, pushing through the intercostal muscle to the lower edge of the rib, stripping the combined pleura/periosteum layer off the anterior portion of the rib. A second portal is placed by cautery above the rib of attachment. A second Freer is inserted in this portal, pointing distally to strip off the periosteum of the rib. The two Freers should touch in the "chopstick" maneuver, confirming

FIGURE 40-11

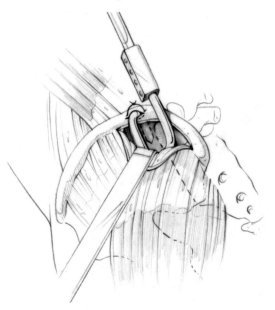

The iliac crest pedestal S-hook fixation is performed through a vertical incision over the midiliac crest. The abductor muscles are taken down by cautery and reflected. A transverse incision is made in the apophysis, and the S hook is inserted. This provides a large moment arm for correction of pelvic obliquity. The hook should be just lateral to the sacroiliac joint.

that a continuous soft-tissue tunnel has been made (Fig 40-10A.). The trial instrument is then inserted into the incisions to enlarge them superiorly and inferiorly. A 1-cm bone should be encircled by the superior rib cradle. If the rib chosen is too slender, then two ribs are encircled with an extended cradle cap that is added to the construct to encircle it.

The rib cradle cap is inserted by forceps into the superior portal, facing laterally to avoid the great vessels and the esophagus; it is then turned distally. Next the superior rib cradle is inserted into the inferior portal, mated with the cradle cap, and attached with a cradle cap lock. The superior cradle is gently distracted by forceps superiorly to test for instability. If unstable, the superior cradle can be moved another level distally to a stronger rib for attachment. The superior cradle should not be placed above the second rib, because this endangers the brachial plexus. Likewise, the superior cradle should not be placed above the rigid curve in a proximal segment of flexible spine, because the distraction power of the VEPTR will only induce a proximal compensatory curve and not correct the rigid curve.

Superior cradle insertion is similar when the attachment rib has fibrous adhesions instead of intercostal muscles linking it to the ribs above and below. When the superior cradle needs to be placed within a mass of fused ribs, however, the inferior portal for the superior cradle is created by a bone burr, creating a slot 5 mm by 1.5 mm. A 5-mm superior portal is cut by burr for placement of the cradle cap.

The Opening-Wedge Thoracostomy

The object of the opening-wedge thoracostomy is not to separate fused ribs into individual ribs, but rather to provide a cleavage point for lengthening the constricted hemithorax. Much like wedging a cast, the thorax is sectioned transversely on the concave side, and the thoracostomy is distracted apart to "straighten" the thorax (lengthening the concave rib cage), with indirect correction of the scoliosis. The chest wall constriction, *often proximal to the apex of the scoliosis,* includes not only the mass of fused ribs but also any adjacent constricted chest wall identified by persistent narrowing of the rib intercostal space as seen on the bending films.

When the constriction is primarily a fused rib mass of three or four ribs, a single opening-wedge thoracostomy will usually be adequate. The thoracostomy interval, following the groove between the two central fused ribs, is marked by cautery posteriorly. Anteriorly the fused ribs usually have separated, and the thoracostomy is easily begun at the costochondral junction. It extends posteriorly through cautery lysis of muscle or fibrous adhesions in line with the marked interval (Fig. 40-10B). The underlying pleura is protected by elevating the muscle or fibrous tissue with a clamp. When the junction of fused ribs is reached, a #4 Penfield elevator is inserted under the rib mass, pointing posteriorly along the groove, to strip away the pleura/periosteum layer. With the lung protected by the Penfield, a Kerrison rongeur is used to cut an interval along the groove in the fused ribs for a distance of 2 cm. The Penfield is inserted further, and the thoracostomy is continued posteriorly until the tips of the transverse processes are reached. An AO bone spreader is then inserted into the interval at the posterior axillary line to widen the thoracostomy (Fig. 40-10C).

Medial to the transverse processes, there is usually fibrous tissue; this is carefully lysed by a Freer elevator, with care taken not to violate the spinal canal. If, medially to the transverse process, bone is present, it is carefully resected by subperiosteal stripping with a Freer elevator and then resection under direct vision by rongeur. Care must be taken not to sacrifice any anomalous segmental vessels that may penetrate the fused rib mass. To avoid entering the spinal canal, the final 5 mm of fused rib bone is disarticulated from the vertebral column by carefully pulling it free with a curved curette. Bone wax is placed over any bleeding surfaces. The thoracostomy interval is further widened with the bone spreaders to ensure that the superior hemithorax segment is completely mobilized down to the spine.

A Kidner dissector is used to gently take down pleura proximally and distally beneath the osteotomized ribs to mobilize the pleura. Small pleural rents do not require repair. However, if an extensive pleura tear occurs, it is repaired with a patch of bioabsorbable membrane (Surgisis) that is attached by an absorbable interrupted suture. Once the thoracostomy interval is widened a distance of several centimeters, the AO bone spreader is replaced with the Synthes rib distractor, and the thoracostomy is slowly widened to its maximum extent. With successful lengthening of the constricted hemithorax, the oblique proximal ribs will also begin to assume a more horizontal position. The superior rib cradle, tilted medially at initial insertion, will also begin to align with the longitudinal axis of the body. If there are more than four fused ribs constricting the hemithorax, or if the ribs below the fused rib mass are closely adherent with fibrous tissue, then a second or even third thoracostomy will be needed to correct the deformity. At least a two-rib thickness should be present in each section of the chest that is osteotomized by the opening-wedge thoracostomies. Use soft-tissue sparing technique when performing the thoracostomy osteotomies, avoiding the stripping of rib periosteum because of the subsequent risk of devascularization of the rib.

Implantation of a Hybrid VEPTR

When patients are older than 18 months, the lumbar spine is usually spacious enough for a laminar hook. Therefore, a hybrid VEPTR from proximal ribs to lumbar spine can be used for maximum correction (Fig. 40-7B).

With the Synthes rib spreader left in place to continue lengthening the constricted chest wall through the thoracostomy, attention is turned to the lumbar spine, where the inferior end of the VEPTR lumbar hybrid extension is to be attached. A 5-cm paraspinous skin incision is made 1 cm lateral to the midline at the level of the proximal lumbar spine. A flap is elevated medially to expose the midline of the spine. Cautery is used to longitudinally section the apophysis of the two posterior spinous processes at the correct interspace. A Cobb elevator is used to strip the spine laterally, while attempting to leave the interspinous ligament intact in order to prevent development of kyphosis. The ligamentum flavum is then resected and the laminar hook inserted. Gelfoam is placed over the exposed dura if needed. Autograft, usually from rib resection, is placed from the superior lamina to the top of the hook, anchoring it with a single-level fusion. To hold the hook in place until the bone block fuses, a 1-0 Prolene suture is wrapped around the shank of the hook and around the posterior spinous process at that level. In patients with extensive congenital scoliosis, there is risk of lumbar spine dysraphism of the posterior spinal elements. Therefore, a large Cobb elevator should be used in stripping the paraspinous muscles to minimize the risk of violating the canal during exposure. It is important not to violate the cortex of the lamina of attachment, as this would weaken its ability to withstand the distraction forces. If the interspace is too small for the hook, then a superior laminotomy is performed.

The size of lumbar extension needed is determined by measuring from the bottom of the rib of attachment, encircled by the superior rib cradle, down to the endplate of T12. The T12 location can usually be estimated by palpating the 12th rib clinically. The distance in centimeters should correspond to the number inscribed on the rib sleeve and the hybrid lumbar extension. The hybrid device is assembled and locked with a distraction lock. To estimate the proper length, the device is placed into the field, with the rib sleeve engaged into the implanted superior cradle proximally and the spinal rod marked by a skin marker approximately 1.5 cm below the bottom of the spinal hook. The hybrid is removed from the field, and the rod is cut. The end of the rod is bent into slight lordosis and valgus by a French bender so that it will line up with the axis of the spine after implantation and conform to the lordosis of the lumbar spine.

A subfascial canal is created for safe passage of the sized lumbar hybrid extension. A long Kelley clamp is threaded from the proximal incision, through the paraspinal muscles, and into the distal incision, with care taken not to violate the chest wall and the pericardium. A #20 chest tube is attached to the clamp and is pulled upward into the proximal incision. The end of the rod of the hybrid is placed inside the end of the chest tube, and the device is carefully guided through the canal by the chest tube into the distal incision. The tube is removed, and the rod is threaded into the hook and then upward into the superior cradle. A distraction lock engages the superior cradle to the rib sleeve.

To perform the initial tensioning of the device, a Synthes C-ring is attached to the rod just above the hook. A distractor is then used to distract the device between the hook and C ring. The hook is then tightened to the rod. The Synthes rib distractor, which was positioned between two ribs to hold the thoracostomy open, is now removed. If there is adequate distraction from the hybrid device, then the opening-wedge thoracostomy should maintain its open position.

It is important to place the hybrid lumbar extension in the lumbar spine so that it is below any areas of junctional kyphosis seen on the lateral weight-bearing x-ray. The VEPTR hook should be placed at least two levels below any junctional kyphosis to prevent accentuating the kyphosis. If posterior elements are lacking, a Dunn-McCarthy "S" hook to the iliac crest is used (Fig. 40-11) with the hybird.

Implantation of the Second VEPTR: Rib-to-Rib Construct

A second rib-to-rib construct VEPTR device should be added laterally to assist the hybrid device in correcting deformity and to decrease load on the medial rib cradle. The second superior cradle is usually attached around the ribs encircled by the hybrid device medially. The inferior cradle site chosen for attachment should be a stable, sizeable rib that is no lower than the 10th rib and that is relatively transverse in orientation. The 11th and 12th ribs are not good as attachment points, because they are floating ribs and do not attach anteriorly to the sternum. The span of the chest wall bridged by the VEPTR should be as long as possible to maximize future device expansion potential. The portals for the inferior cradle site are prepared in the same fashion as the superior cradle site.

The length of the rib-to-rib VEPTR should be based on the *corrected* length of the constricted hemithorax. After the superior cradle is implanted, the thoracostomy interval is again opened by the Synthes distractor to maximum correction. The distance from the inferior edge of the rib cradle attachment superiorly to the superior edge of the inferior rib of attachment is measured. The distance in centimeters will correspond to the number inscribed on the rib sleeve and inferior cradle of the rib- to- rib VEPTR needed. The inferior cradle is threaded into the rib sleeve, and the combined rib sleeve/inferior rib cradle is ready for implantation.

The Synthes rib distractor is removed. The inferior cradle cap is inserted, facing laterally, into the distal portal of the inferior rib cradle site; it is then turned superiorly so that it can mate with the inferior rib cradle. If the inferior rib of attachment is somewhat oblique in orientation, an extended cradle will be needed to span the extra distance required to surround the rib. The inferior rib cradle is next placed in the superior portal of the inferior cradle site and locked to the end cradle cap with a cradle cap lock. The proximal rib sleeve is engaged into the superior cradle at an angle and is then slowly levered into place. A distraction lock is placed proximally. The rib-to-rib VEPTR is distracted 0.5 cm to tension the construct and is then locked with a distal distraction lock.

After the lateral device is distracted, the medial hybrid device is distracted again to balance the distraction force for final medial construct tensioning. The hook is tightened, and the distraction C-ring is removed.

Both the standard superior rib cradle and the inferior rib cradle of the rib-to-rib VEPTR are in neutral position. If the inferior osseous rib of attachment is oriented differently from the superior rib, then the VEPTR may not fit well around the inferior rib. In such a situation, a 30-degree right-handed or left-handed inferior VEPTR cradle may be used to better fit the inferior cradle around the rib.

The ideal age for VEPTR intervention from a pulmonary viewpoint is age 6 months to 2 years. However, VEPTR hybrid placement may not be practical for children age 18 months or younger, because there may not be adequate room in the lumbar spinal canal for a laminar hook. In these children, a medial rib-to-rib titanium rib can be used to stabilize the thoracostomy (Fig. 40-7A). Although correction with the rib-to-rib VEPTR construct may not be as great as with a VEPTR hybrid, it can keep the thoracostomy open until the child reaches age 2 years. At that time, greater correction can be obtained by replacing it with a hybrid if desired. If so, the inferior cradle and the rib sleeve are removed, a longer rib sleeve is added with a matching hybrid lumbar extension bridging to the proximal lumbar spine, and the hybrid tensioned.

Closure

To aid closure so that there is minimal tension on the suture line, the skin and muscle flaps are grasped with dry laparotomy sponges and stretched toward one another. Two deep drains (#7 and #10 Jackson Pratt) are placed. A chest tube is needed only if there is significant pleural rent or tear in the lung visceral pleura. Subcutaneous pain catheters for local anesthetic are helpful in controlling postoperative pain and are placed near implanted devices.

The musculocutaneous flap is first approximated along the apex, with several interrupted figure-of-eight sutures of 0 Vicryl. During this step, care should be taken to monitor both the pulse oximeter and the SSEPs and MEPs tracings of the upper extremities to detect signs of acute thoracic outlet syndrome. This syndrome can occur during closure, because the fused anomalous ribs are distracted superiorly by the VEPTR device into a brachial plexus that may be congenitally shortened. While pulling the soft-tissue envelope inferiorly to close the space, acute pressure may develop on the brachial plexus. If there are any signs of brachial plexus depression, especially a decrease in the ulnar nerve tracings, or loss of pulse oximeter reading, the closure is relaxed slightly, and monitoring signs usually improve. If necessary, distraction may be relaxed on the VEPTR devices. If continued alterations in pulse oximeter and/or spinal cord monitoring are encountered, even with relaxation of the closure, it may be necessary to resect the anterolateral portion of the first and second ribs, lateral to the devices, to provide clearance for the brachial plexus.

After the apex is secured, the proximal and distal muscle layers are closed with running suture of 0 Vicryl with skin closure by 4-0 Monocryl suture. Adhesive skin closures (Steri-Strips) are then placed over the wound, and a bulky dressing is applied. Surgical polyurethane foam is placed over the dressings to further pad the incisions. AP and lateral radiographs are taken in the operating room to check the position of devices, to verify correction, to check for pneumothorax, and to confirm proper position of the endotracheal tube above the carina.

POSTOPERATIVE MANAGEMENT

Patients are usually left intubated 24 to 72 hours. VEPTR thoracic reconstruction acutely alters pulmonary function mechanics to a much greater extent than does a standard thoracotomy, so immediate extubation is often not well tolerated. However, some institutions do allow patients to be extubated the next morning if they are doing well. The hematocrit is checked daily for 3 days. Although blood loss usually averages 50 cc,[5] continual oozing underneath the large flaps results in a 50% risk for postoperative transfusion. In general, a hematocrit of 30% or greater is optimal for oxygen- carrying capacity for these patients. Fluid management should be on the restrictive side to prevent acute pulmonary edema, as emphasized by Smith (Smith J. Personal communication, 2000).

Once weaned off the ventilator, the patient can be transferred to the surgical ward. Jackson Pratt drains are removed when their individual drainage decreases to 20 cc or less over a 24-hour period. Chest tubes are removed once their drainage equals 1 cc/kg of patient weight over 24 hours. If the patient goes into respiratory distress after drains and chest tubes are removed, the surgeon may consider reaccumulation of the pleural effusion with compression of the lung. In which case, temporary chest tube drainage will be helpful.

Vigorous pulmonary toilet, including percussion, is needed postoperatively. The patients are mobilized as soon as possible. No bracing is used because of the constrictive effect on the thorax.

VEPTR Outpatient Expansion

The VEPTR devices are first expanded 6 months after implantation in outpatient surgery under general anesthesia. No spinal cord monitoring is necessary unless changes were encountered in the initial implantation. Positioning is similar to the implantation procedure. The distraction locks of the devices are exposed through 3-cm incisions, either through the thoracostomy incision, if it is adjacent to a distraction lock, or through a new incision paralleling the device, if the distraction lock is distal from a previous incision. The distraction locks are removed, the devices are expanded by the expansion forceps until a maximum reactive force is encountered, and new distraction locks are placed (Fig. 40-12).

Thick muscle flaps should be maintained over the devices by meticulous soft-tissue technique to minimize the risk of skin slough. If the distraction lock is exposed through the thoracostomy incision, a Freer elevator is inserted proximally along the top of the device and used to elevate the overlying muscle. Cautery is inserted into the soft-tissue tunnel created by the Freer elevator and is used to release the muscle deeply on each side of the device to mobilize a thick muscle flap with the free edge at the skin incision. The same approach is used distally. When device expansion is complete, the mobilized muscle flaps are closed without tension over the locks. When the skin incision parallels the device, the muscle incision is made by cautery along the side of the device to the mid-rib sleeve. The cautery is then turned sideways to release the muscle flap off the device. The full-thickness muscle flap is reflected by a Freer elevator, the expansion procedure performed, and the full-thickness flap brought back over the device for closure.

Postoperatively AP and lateral standing spine x-rays are performed. Patients are usually able to be discharged within 24 hours of surgery, though at some centers this is done on an outpatient basis for particularly stable children. All devices are expanded on schedule every 6 months. Pulmonary function tests are performed yearly once the patients are old enough to cooperate.

VEPTR Replacement Procedure

Once the devices have been maximally expanded, a replacement procedure is performed to replace the rib sleeve and the inferior cradle/hybrid lumbar extension portion of the devices, while retaining the superior cradles/spinal hooks/Dunn-McCarthy pelvis hooks. This can usually be accomplished through limited incisions over the end and middle portion of the hybrid devices and the upper and distal portion of the rib-to-rib construct VEPTRs.

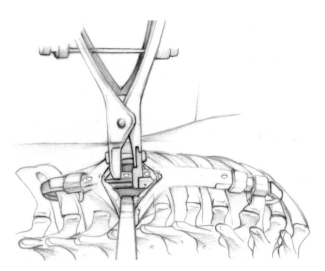

FIGURE 40-12

Once unlocked, the VEPTR is slowly expanded by expansion forceps until the reactive force is too great to continue. The VEPTR is then locked in its expanded position.

Endpoint of VEPTR Treatment

Because lung growth by either alveolar cell multiplication or hypertrophy continues to the age of skeletal maturity, continued VEPTR treatment is recommended until the time of skeletal maturity, as assessed by the Risser sign. Definitive posterior spine fusion can be considered at that time, with removal of hybrid VEPTR devices, but the more lateral VEPTR devices can be left in the patient if they are asymptomatic. These devices do not require any further expansion. Yearly follow-up post-fusion is advised, with radiographs and pulmonary function testing.

COMPLICATIONS TO AVOID

The most common complication is the slow, asymptomatic, superior migration of the superior rib cradle through the rib of attachment. Several months after implantation, the rib of attachment undergoes hypertrophy, and in most cases, the rib cradle is filled with new bone. Some of the new bone can also form below the cradle, so that the device appears to be migrating into the hypertrophied rib. However, it actually remains in its original position. Complete migration through the rib of attachment occurs an average of 3 years after implantation, though this is also usually asymptomatic. This migration is treated by accessing the superior cradle at the time of expansion surgery through a limited incision and reimplanting it into the rib of attachment, which is usually reformed. A CT scan may help define the position of the cradle relative to the rib. Curved curettes are extremely useful for shaving the hypertrophied rib down to an acceptable size for reimplantation of the cradle.

Another common complication is skin slough or infection. This is treated with debridement without removal of devices and irrigation with dilute microbicide (Betadine) irrigation. The skin edges are loosely approximated with Prolene sutures, leaving a 5-mm gap in the wound and allowing it to close by secondary intention. The patient is maintained on 4 to 6 weeks of intravenous antibiotics, with culture results determining the specific antibiotic. Sometimes it is helpful to add a wound vacuum-assisted closure (VAC) overlying the device to help with healing.

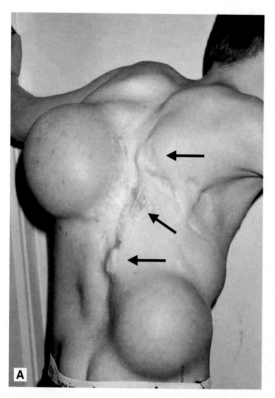
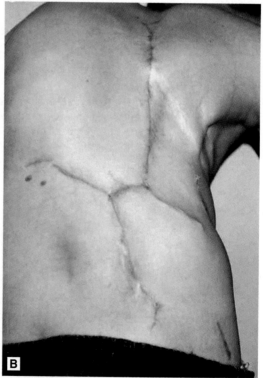

FIGURE 40-13   A. A child with poor skin coverage over the VEPTR *(arrows)* following repeated lengthenings. Soft-tissue expanders have been inserted to provide adequate soft tissue for rotational flap coverage. **B.** The thinned skin has been resected, and the skin mobilized by the soft-tissue expanders has been used as rotational flaps to cover the VEPTR. (Courtesy Mr. Tristian de Chalain, plastic surgeon, and Stewart Walsh, M.D., pediatric orthopaedist; Starship Children's Hospital; Auckland, New Zealand.)

TABLE 40-3 San Antonio VEPTR Complications, 1989–2004[2]	
n = 201 pt(1,412 procedures)	
Mean proc/pt	7.02/pt
Mean f/u	6 yr
Infection rate/proc	3.3%
Skin slough % pt	8.5%
Migration Index (Risk of migration/patient/year) 0.09	
Mean time to mig	3.2 yr
% pt with mig	27%
Pt device breakage %	6%

Recurrent infections require removal of the rib sleeve and the lumbar hybrid extension or the inferior rib cradle. The patient is maintained on 6 weeks of antibiotics. When sedimentation rate/C-reactive protein has normalized and the wound is healed, reinsertion of the device can be considered.

Skin slough is treated by debridement and mobilization of flaps. In patients with long-standing VEPTR devices, dense soft-tissue scarring sometimes occurs over devices, and recurrent skin slough becomes a problem. For these patients, soft-tissue expanders are placed laterally to mobilize the skin. The skin is then transferred posteriorly over the devices with the assistance of a plastic surgeon (Fig. 40-13).

Table 40-3 provides a review of complications over a 15-year period at the author's institution.

ILLUSTRATIVE CASE

A 3-year-old girl with severe congenital scoliosis and fused ribs (Fig. 40-14A) was treated with VEPTR opening-wedge thoracostomy. At 11-year follow-up, the scoliosis has been stabilized with growth of the thorax (Fig. 40-14B). Vital capacity is 58% normal. The patient is now skeletally mature and will undergo a posterior spine fusion with removal of the hybrid VEPTR and retention of the lateral VEPTR to maintain the expansion of the hemithorax.

PEARLS AND PITFALLS

- VEPTR may be performed in cases of previous fusions, though these patients do not appear to respond as favorably to VEPTR treatment as compared with those who have "virgin" spines.

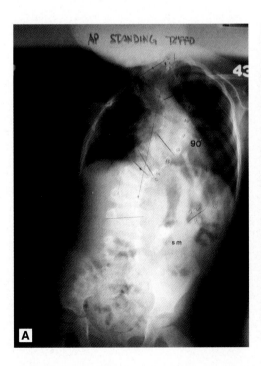
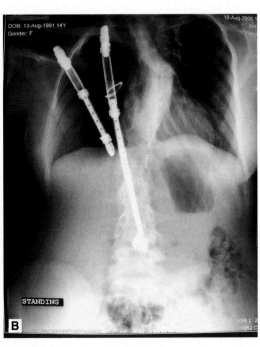

FIGURE 40-14

A. A 3-year-old girl with severe congenital scoliosis and fused ribs. **B.** At 11-year follow-up, the scoliosis has been stabilized with growth of the thorax.

- The thumb excursion test is a simple clinical assessment technique of thoracic function and is a valuable way to test for thoracic insufficiency syndrome.
- The preoperative CT scan should be checked carefully for areas of dysraphic spine within the area of surgical approach. In these areas, dissection should be cautious, with medial exposure only above and below the areas of dysraphism. Particularly dangerous is an area of midthoracic spine dysraphism, where the medial edge of the scapula lies within the spinal canal on the concave side of the curve.
- If the patient goes into respiratory distress after drains and chest tubes are removed, reaccumulation of the pleural effusion with compression of the lung should be considered. In which case temporary chest tube drainage will be helpful.
- A 1-cm bone should be encircled by the superior rib cradle. If the rib chosen is too slender, then two ribs are encircled with an extended cradle cap added to the construct to encircle it.
- If possible, avoid placing the superior cradle above the second rib as this will endanger the brachial plexus.
- Do not place the superior cradle above the rigid curve in a proximal segment of flexible spine, because the distraction power of the VEPTR will only induce a proximal compensatory curve and will not correct the rigid curve.
- It is important to place the hybrid lumbar extension in the lumbar spine below any areas of junctional kyphosis seen on the lateral weight-bearing x-ray. The VEPTR hook should be placed at least two levels below any junctional kyphosis to prevent accentuating the kyphosis.

REFERENCES

1. Campbell RM Jr, Hell-Vocke AK. Growth of the thoracic spine in congenital scoliosis after expansion thoracoplasty. *J Bone Joint Surg Am.* 2003;85:409–420.
2. Campbell RM Jr, Smith MD. Thoracic insufficiency syndrome and exotic scoliosis. *J Bone Joint Surg Am* . vol 89A: supp(1), 108–122.
3. Campbell RM Jr, Smith MD, Hell-Vocke AK. Expansion thoracoplasty: the surgical technique of opening-wedge thoracostomy. Surgical technique. *J Bone Joint Surg Am.* 2004;86(Suppl 1):51–64.
4. Campbell RM Jr, Smith MD, Mayes TC, et al. The characteristics of thoracic insufficiency syndrome associated with fused ribs and scoliosis. *J Bone Joint Surg Am.* 2003;85:399–408.
5. Campbell RM Jr, Smith MD, Mayes TC, et al. The effect of opening wedge thoracostomy on thoracic insufficiency syndrome associated with fused ribs and congenital scoliosis. *J Bone Joint Surg Am.* 2003;85:1615–1624.

41 Temporary Distraction Rods in the Correction of Severe Scoliosis

David L. Skaggs, Jacob M. Buchowski, and Paul Sponseller

The use of temporary distraction rods for the correction of severe scoliosis has recently gained popularity. Temporary distraction rods can be used instead of halo traction for severe spinal deformity of the thoracic and lumbar spine. With the use of temporary distraction rods, more significant corrective force may be applied directly to the spine as compared to halo traction. In addition, gradual correction of the spine may obviate the need for anterior release.

INDICATIONS/CONTRAINDICATIONS

Temporary rods may be used in most cases of severe spinal deformity of the thoracic and lumbar spine, including severe pelvic obliquity. The only requirement is that there is reasonable bone strength to anchor the rods near the top and bottom of the deformity. Anchor points may include the spine, pelvis, or ribs. In general, in most instances that halo traction is considered for a thoracic or lumbar spinal deformity, a temporary rod may be considered as well.

This technique is contraindicated if continuous neuromonitoring of the spinal cord is not possible. To date, temporary distraction rods have not been employed in the cervical spine. Temporary rods have been used to treat kyphotic deformities, but this may represent a population at increased risk for neurologic injury from traction. A relative contraindication is the inability of the patient to tolerate staged procedures due to significant medical comorbidities or poor nutritional status.

PREOPERATIVE PLANNING

Patients with severe spinal deformity often have accompanying underlying medical conditions necessitating attention to other organ systems. Pulmonary consultation is frequently required, as well as cardiac or neurosurgical consultation depending on the patient's individual needs. Children with severe pulmonary restriction are often nutritionally depleted, and this should be addressed before proceeding with staged spinal surgery, even considering placement of a gastrostomy tube.

Standard anteroposterior (AP) and lateral radiographs of the spine should be obtained. In cases of severe spinal deformity, bending films are less helpful than are traction films (Figs. 41-1B–1D). Traction films are particularly helpful in predicting the usefulness of temporary distraction rods. A general rule of thumb is that the first surgery with temporary rod will be able to achieve better correction than the correction of a spinal deformity on a supine traction film in which the surgeon is pulling very

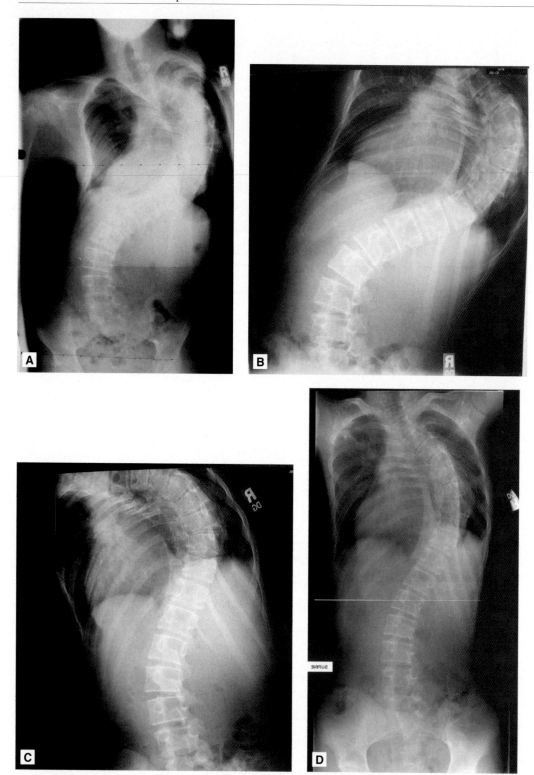

FIGURE 41-1   A. AP radiograph of a 16-year-old boy with 132 degrees of scoliosis. Vital capacity is 30% of normal. Family has asked that no anterior approach or rib osteotomies be performed. **B.** Right bend film shows correction of major curve to 107 degrees. **C.** Left bend film. **D.** Supine traction film performed by the author. Pulling very hard approximates the minimal correction that can be expected following the first surgery with placement of the temporary rod. **E.** AP radiograph following first surgical procedure, with placement of a temporary rod and osteotomies. Cobb angle is 77 degrees, improved from 132 degrees preoperatively. **F.** AP standing radiograph 1 week following second surgical procedure, with final instrumentation intact. No anterior surgery was performed. No osteotomies of ribs were performed. Curve is now 32 degrees, improved from 132 degrees preoperatively. The patient gained 5 inches in height. (*Continued*)

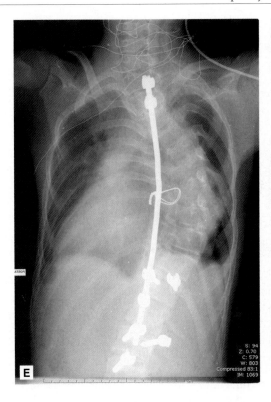

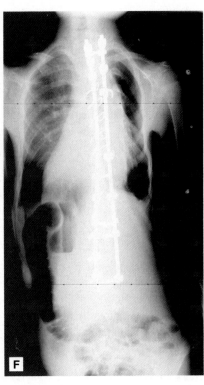

FIGURE 41-1
(Continued)

hard. As these patients have large deformities and will be undergoing distraction of the spine, an MRI of the cervical, thoracic, and lumber spine is a standard preoperative study.

A major advantage of the temporary rod technique is avoidance of an anterior spinal release, because correction through posterior surgery is generally sufficient. However, if a surgeon chooses to perform an anterior release, this would be done before placement of the temporary rod.

A total of two operative procedures about one week apart should be planned. At the first surgical procedure, the temporary rod is placed in addition to any necessary posterior spinal releases and osteotomies. At the second surgical procedure, the temporary rod is removed, the final spinal implants are placed, and fusion is performed. When the tension on the temporary rod is released at the time of the second surgery, there is no significant return of the spine to its previous deformity position. Thus having more than 7 days between these procedures would seem to add little additional correction. Additional procedures in which the temporary rods are lengthened over the course of weeks have been attempted, but have been shown not to significantly improve deformity correction. However, in some cases the amount of correction obtained at the first surgery may be sufficient. In this case, final fusion may be performed at the first surgery. (See Illustrative Case 2, Figure 41A–J).

Preoperative planning should include evaluation of the bony anchor points for the temporary rod. A basic principle in choosing anchor points for the temporary rod is to expect that these anchors will plow through bone a bit, compromising the holding power of the final anchor. Thus, the temporary anchors should not be used as permanent anchors at either end vertebra of the final instrumentation construct. For example, because pedicle screws will plow upward in the upper thoracic spine during their use in securing a temporary rod, they should not then be used as end vertebra anchor points in the final implant.

The upper portion of the rod is usually attached to the ribs or the spine. When attaching to ribs, standard spinal laminar hooks may be used; usually large sizes fit best. Anchoring to two ribs instead of one is usually best as this disperses the load; quite significant forces are being applied, and temporary rods have been known to tear through a single rib. An advantage of applying the temporary rod to the ribs rather than the spine is that it leaves the spine free; the permanent rod may then be placed on the spine while the temporary rod is still actively applying distraction to the ribs (Fig. 41-2). A disadvantage of using ribs as an anchor point is that one cannot push quite as hard on ribs compared to the spine.

If one chooses to use the spine as an upper anchor point, hooks are generally preferable over pedicle screws for two reasons. Most important, when pushing upward on thoracic pedicle screws, plowing through the bone occurs more easily than when pushing downward; thus it is easy to ruin the pedicle screw site as a permanent fixation point. In addition, upgoing infralaminar or transverse process hooks have the little bit of "sloppiness" that allows for easier alignment. Because the curves being treated with this technique are usually greater than 100 degrees, one can imagine that two pedicle screws on an adjacent tilted vertebrae are not going to point toward the bottom of the construct. A subtle point when planning the placement of the upper and lower anchor points is to go slightly above and below the most tilted vertebrae to allow these anchor points to line up with a straight distraction rod.

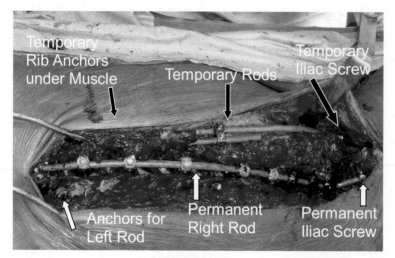

FIGURE 41-2   The temporary rod *(black arrows)* is attached to two ribs at the top and to an iliac screw in the pelvis. Following distraction and osteotomies, the pelvis is now level, the scoliosis is significantly corrected, and the permanent right rod *(white arrows)* can be placed while the temporary rod is still in place holding correction. In this particular case, the entire surgery was done at one stage, as the temporary rod led to sufficient immediate correction.

The bottom anchor points are usually in the lumbar spine or pelvis. Because the pedicles are generally stronger in the lumbar spine and the direction of force is downward, the use of two pedicle screws as a distal anchor point works well.

In cases of pelvic obliquity, or when the final fusion will be to the pelvis, the pelvis or iliac crest may be chosen as an anchor point for the temporary rod. This may be in the form of an S hook or a temporary iliac screw. When using an iliac screw, a small amount of migration is common when it is used as a distraction rod due to the significant forces applied to the rods. Therefore, a temporary iliac screw should be placed superior and lateral to where the permanent iliac screw will be placed (Figs. 41-2 and 41-3). Alternatively, an S hook may be placed over the top of the iliac crest or the sacral ala (Fig. 41-4). Regardless of which type of anchor is chosen, there is a mechanical advantage in correcting pelvic obliquity if the anchor is placed lateral to the spine. In general, the very top of the iliac crest appears to be the best place; lateral to that, the anchor point may slip further laterally. In small children, however, the top of the iliac crest may be too small to accept an iliac screw; an S hook is probably best for these patients.

FIGURE 41-3

When placing any temporary iliac screw *(thin arrow)*, the starting point should be at least 2 cm lateral to the intended starting point of the permanent iliac screw *(thick arrow)*. Some plowing of the temporary screw should be expected, though this should not affect the purchase of the permanent screw.

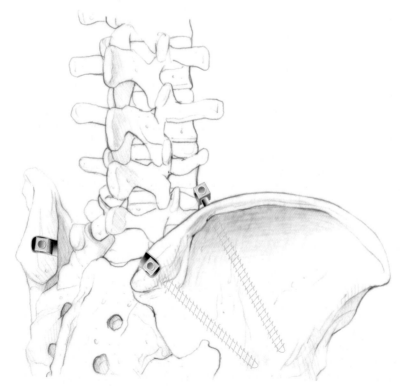

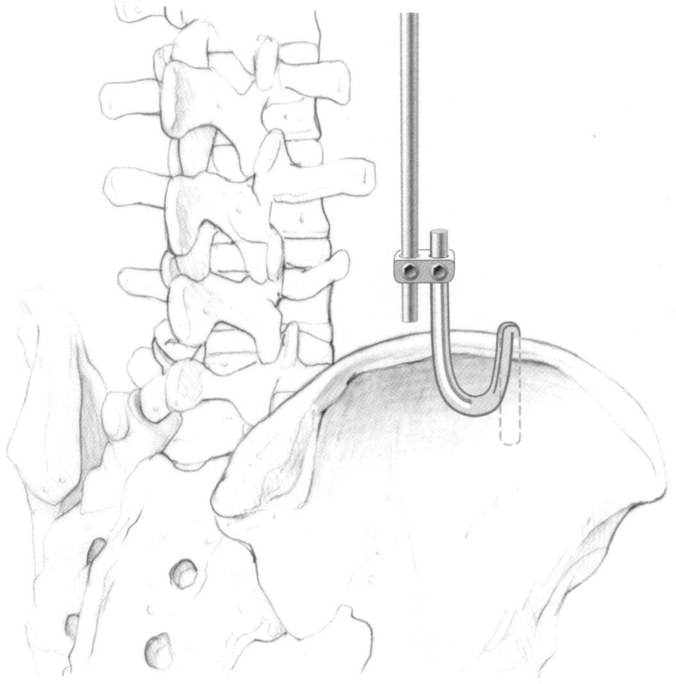

FIGURE 41-4

An S hook over the top of the iliac crest. Subperiosteal dissection is generally not needed. The anterior track can usually be started with a very small fascial incision, which is enlarged with the surgeon's finger.

SURGICAL PROCEDURE

As distraction of the spine is planned, reliable neurologic monitoring is absolutely essential, including motor-evoked potentials (MEPs) and somatosensory-evoked potentials (SSEPs) of the upper and lower extremities. Vancomycin and ceftazidime are used as antibiotic prophylaxes to cover *Staphylococcus aureus* and *Staphylococcus epidermidis,* as well as gram-negative bacteria.

The patient is placed in the prone position. The skin incision is made in a standard fashion. Dissection is carried down to the bony anchor points first, prior to dissection of the entire spine. The goal is to place the temporary rod in the spine and begin distraction *as early as possible* in the procedure. This takes advantage of the viscoelastic nature of the spine, allowing for continuous correction of the deformity during the remainder of the surgical procedure. In general, the temporary rod is placed with distraction prior to periosteal stripping of the opposite side of the spine.

Upper Anchor Points

Subperiosteal dissection is carried out through a midline incision along the lamina. Two infralaminar or pedicle hooks may be placed in standard fashion. The hooks are placed at laminae not intended to be upper-end vertebra of the final fusion, as some plowing through the bone may occur.

Ribs are often chosen as the upper anchor points. To approach the ribs, subperiosteal dissection is first carried out along the lamina, then laterally over the transverse processes, until the medial ribs are palpated. Circumferential subperiosteal dissection of the ribs is not necessary. Standard laminar hooks may be placed on the rib in an upgoing fashion. In an effort to stay out of the chest, the surgeon should try to dissect subperiosteally along the anterior surface of the ribs (Fig. 41-5). The surgeon may be subperiosteal relative to the neurovascular bundle or may include the neurovascular bundle between the hook and rib; it doesn't seem to matter either way. Prior to closing, the area surrounding the rib dissection is filled with warm saline. The anesthesiologist is asked to perform a Valsalva maneuver to assess whether the thoracic cavity has been entered. If the thorax has been entered, a small drain with a one-way valve, such as a Hemovac, may be placed to act as a chest tube for drainage.

Lower Anchor Points

Spine   Standard lumbar pedicle screws are usually used as the lower anchor points. In general, two screws are used on adjacent vertebrae, though this may be adjusted depending on the quality of the bone. Supralaminar hooks may be used as well. Although it is not as important in the lumbar spine as compared with the thoracic spine, vertebrae cephalad to the end vertebrae of the final construct should be chosen for the hooks, as some plowing through bone may be expected with the pedicle screws used with the temporary rods. One does not want to compromise the quality of the pedicle screw at the end of the final instrumentation construct.

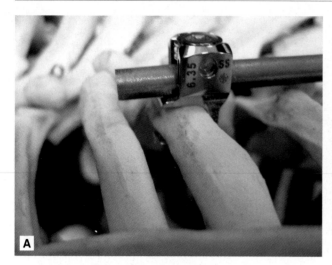

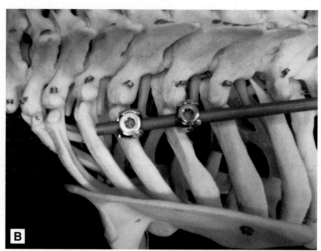

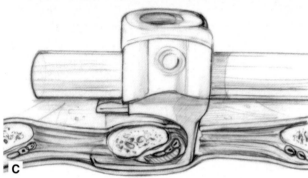

FIGURE 41-5   A. Large lumbar hook fits well on ribs of moderate- to large-size children. **B.** Hooks are placed just lateral to transverse processes, with an upward distraction force. **C.** Cross-sectional drawing of the lumbar hook incurring on a rib. The exact location of the neurovascular bundle within or outside of the hook is not important. One should aim to remain subperiosteal on the anterior surface of the rib.

Pelvis   Dissection is continued laterally to expose the iliac crest. If an iliac screw will be used for final instrumentation, the posterior-superior iliac crest is first identified; then the site is prepared for a long iliac screw going as close as possible to the sciatic notch without entering it. The screw is then inserted. For the iliac screw to be used with the temporary rod, dissection should be continued laterally along the iliac crest. The temporary screw should be placed at least 2 cm lateral and roughly parallel to the permanent screw (Fig. 41-3). This position anticipates a bit of plowing through bone but without compromising the permanent screw. The center of the iliac crest becomes thinner as one moves laterally. In small patients, a second screw may not engage adequate bone, in which case an S hook should be used.

To place an S hook, dissection is continued laterally over the iliac crest to the highest point (Fig. 41-4). In patients in which the iliac apophysis is still cartilaginous, the cartilage should be left intact, as it serves as a bumper to prevent migration of the S hook into the iliac crest. A cautery is used to dissect muscle attachments from the top of the iliac crest. Depending on the size of the bone and the S hook, the inner and outer tables of the iliac crest generally do not require significant (or any) periosteal stripping. The inner table can be palpated anteriorly by running a finger over the top of the iliac crest. This creates a tunnel for the anterior portion of the S hook. The single-rod portion of the S hook may then be slipped over the top of the iliac crest anteriorly along the tunnel created by the finger. Although this is an area of the body in which orthopaedic surgeons may have some hesitancy due to lack of experience, there are no vital structures here that are prone to injury, as long as one sticks along the iliac crest or iliacus muscle and does not venture anteriorly into the retroperitoneal space. It is easier to place an S hook more laterally than an iliac screw, and this lateral position creates a substantial moment arm that helps correct pelvic obliquity. In addition, an S hook is technically easy to connect to a longitudinal rod with a side-to-side connector.

Placement of the Temporary Rods

The simplest construct is to attach one rod to the upper anchor points and a second rod to the lower anchor points, with the two rods connected by a side-to-side connector and with a great deal of overlap of the rods present. Distraction is then applied across these rods in a serial fashion by loosening and tightening the side-to-side connector. In large curves, it may be a challenge to get the two anchor points and rods lined up straight enough for this to occur. However, a combination of distraction and rod manipulation is usually sufficient to get the rods parallel. In cases of extreme deformity, one may need to apply a very small rod to the upper anchor points and another very small rod to the lower anchor points, with these two rods connected to a third rod with multiaxial transverse connectors (Fig. 41-6; to allow soft tissue coverage during closure). This configuration can later be replaced by lower profile rods, as described above.

Releases, Osteotomies, and Additional Anchors

Once the temporary rod is in and distraction has been applied, one should proceed with subperiosteal dissection and release of the remainder of the spine. In most cases, a number of osteotomies, particularly at the apex of the concavity, are indicated for correction of these severe curves. Because significant distraction is being placed during the osteotomies, the osteotomy will occasionally complete itself with a crack and visible opening. Additional anchor points, such as pedicle screws, may be placed at this time. One shortcoming of using a temporary rod is that it is technically difficult to place pedicle screws at the apex of the deformity on the concave side of the curve. This is because the temporary rod physically limits how anterior the surgeon's hands can go to place the pedicle screw in the rotated vertebral bodies. This positioning improves over time with further distraction and vertebral derotation. Pedicle screws that could not be placed initially may be able to be placed later in the surgery following osteotomies and during further distraction or at the second-stage procedure. An effective alternative is to use sublaminar wires at the apex of the deformity. Sublaminar wires in this instance help translate the spine medially in an iterative fashion, with subsequent tightening and retightening of the wires during placement of the final rod (Fig. 41-7H; Illustrative Case 1). Sublaminar wires may be used during the temporary rod (Fig 41-E).

An essential part of this procedure is to apply multiple episodes of small amounts of distraction throughout the surgery. Patience is a virtue in this procedure. The passage of time, soft-tissue dissection, facetectomies, and osteotomies allow further correction of the spinal deformity. At the conclusion of the surgery, one should aim for deformity correction that is better than the best preoperative distraction radiograph or that has at least 50% correction of the Cobb angle.

No bone graft is used at the initial procedure, as fusion is not the goal. The author's (DLS) preference is to perform irrigation with a jet lavage and detergent prior to closure. Although the author is not aware of any infections with these staged procedures, paranoia about infection is appropriate.

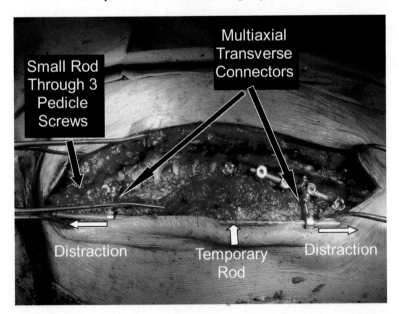

FIGURE 41-6   Small temporary rods are placed in the upper and lower anchor points and connected to a temporary rod by two multiaxial transverse connectors. This type of temporary rod configuration is generally too prominent to close soft-tissue over, but it does provide a good start at distraction and aligning the upper and lower anchors, which then allows lower-profile rods and connectors to be placed later in the case.

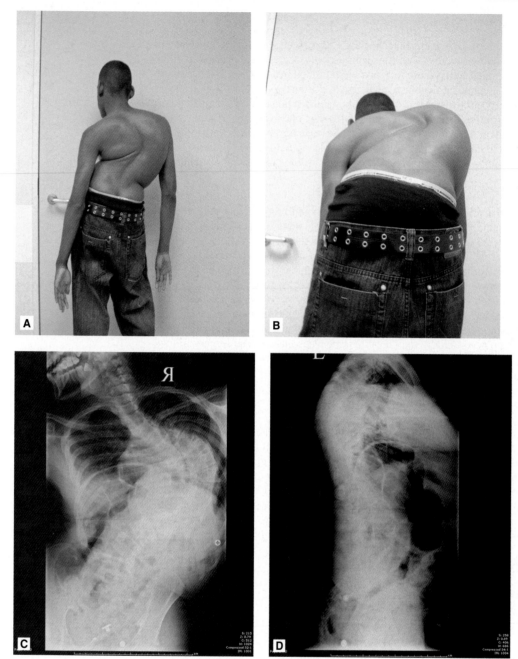

FIGURE 41-7 **A, B.** A 16-year-old boy with unknown neuromuscular disorder. He is ambulatory. AP **(C)** and lateral **(D)** radiographs of a 151-degree curve with significant elevation of the right shoulder. **E.** Traction film performed with the surgeon pulling very hard. Curve corrects to 117 degrees. Intraoperative radiograph **(F)** and photograph **(G)** of patient with a 151-degree scoliosis, shortly after applying the temporary distracting rod. Prior to doing osteotomies, the curve corrected to 89 degrees. Intraoperative skeletal traction (20 lb) was applied to the head through Mayfield tongs and through the leg on the side of the high pelvis. The upper construct *(short white arrow)* consists of a short rod through two upgoing laminar (or pedicle) hooks. The lower construct *(long white arrow)* consists of a short rod through two lumbar pedicle screws. The distracting rods are attached with a side-to-side connector to the upper and lower constructs and to each other *(black arrows).* **H.** Radiograph at the completion of the first surgery. Note that further correction of the deformity occurred following osteotomies and addition of sublaminar wires. AP **(I)** and lateral **(J)** radiograph 2 weeks after the second surgical procedure. Note that the right shoulder was higher preoperatively, and now the left shoulder is higher. Compression of the upper left screws could have improved the left shoulder position. **K, L.** 2 weeks following the second surgery the torso is greatly improved, though not perfect. The left shoulder is high. *(Continued)*

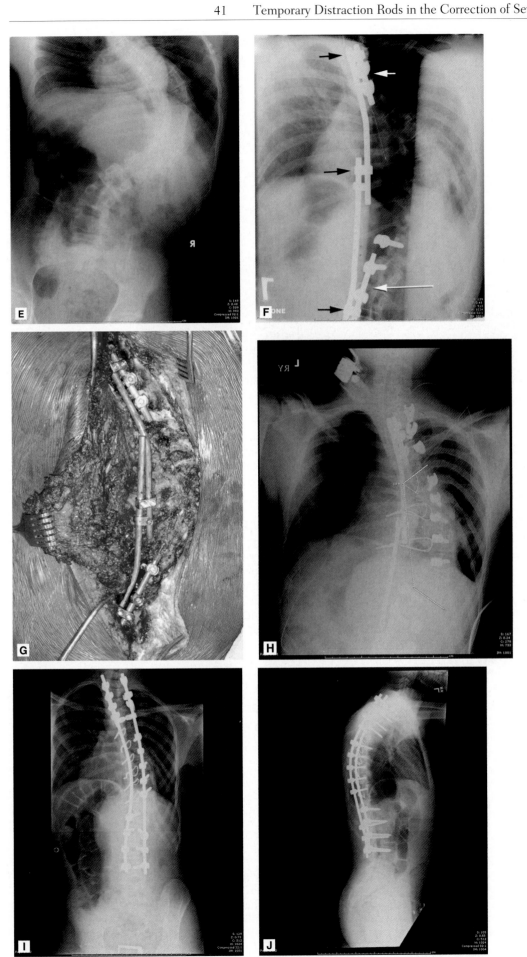

FIGURE 41-7

(Continued)

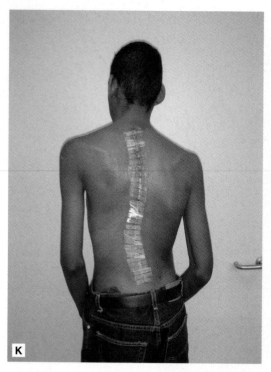
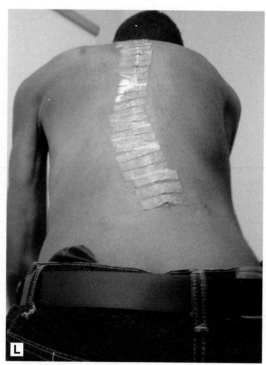

FIGURE 41-7 *(Continued)*

Closure is challenging at times, as quite significant distraction and lengthening have been placed across the soft tissues. Furthermore, the temporary rod usually remains lateral to the transverse processes. Raising thick local flaps with the paraspinal muscles is often required, including the trapezius, latissimus dorsi, and rhomboids in one thick layer. These large potential dead spaces should be drained with closed-suction drains.

POSTOPERATIVE MANAGEMENT

Nutrition is a primary concern in the postoperative period given the staged surgery and the less-than-perfect nutrition of most of these patients. Total parental nutrition is usually ordered on these patients immediately postoperatively and should continue until a regular adequate oral intake is demonstrated. Mobilization, such as sitting, standing, and walking, to help avoid pulmonary and other problems is encouraged. Keep in mind at the time of the temporary rod application that sufficient implant stability should be obtained to allow for ambulation.

COMPLICATIONS TO AVOID

- Infection
- Nutritional depletion between surgeries
- Neurologic compromise secondary to distraction
  - Careful postoperative neurologic examinations
  - Preoperative MRI

ILLUSTRATIVE CASE 1

A temporary rod used during a two-stage procedure (Fig. 41-7).

ILLUSTRATIVE CASE 2

Temporary rod used during a one-stage procedure (Fig. 41-8A–8L). This is a 12-year-old girl with adolescent idiopathic scoliosis and a Cobb angle of 112°. MRI was negative. The plan was for a two staged procedure separated by 1 week. The first planned surgery was placement of a temporary rod, followed by releases, facetectomies and osteotomies, with the second surgery planned for replacement of the temporary rod with the final implants. At the time of surgery, it was noted that there was ample correction with the temporary rod and related procedures alone (Fig. F), and thus the final

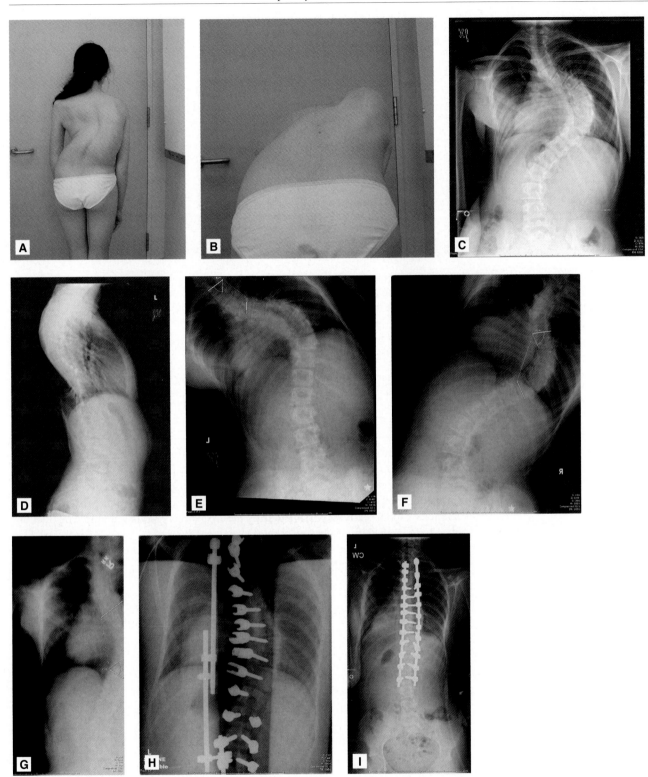

FIGURE 41-8 **A.** PA photograph. **B.** Expected rotatory asymmetry. **C.** PA radiograph demonstrating 112° Cobb angle. Left shoulder is lower. **D.** Lateral radiograph. Note rib prominence is visible. **E.** Left bending film. Note the upper left thoracic curve is 32 degrees. **F.** Right bending film demonstrating the Primary curve improves to a 73° Cobb angle. **G.** Supine traction film (pulling very hard) corrected to 67 degrees. **H.** Intraoperative radiograph demonstrating the temporary rod anchored to 2 ribs on the top left. Distraction caused some derotation of the revertebral bodies, making placement of the concave apex pedicle screws easier. **I.** Post-operative standing radiograph demonstrates correction of the 108° curve to 26°. The left shoulder is elevated immediately postoperatively, compared to being depressed pre-operatively, despite pushing down with 4 pedicle screws at the upper left portion of the construct. (*Continued*)

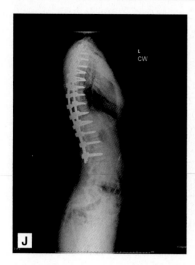
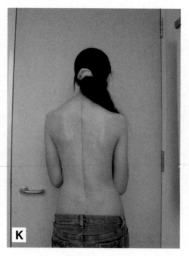
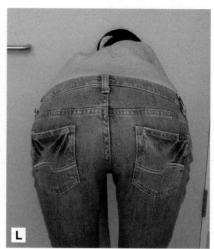

FIGURE 41-8   (*Continued*) **J.** Post-operative lateral radiograph. Note the absence of a rib prominence when compared to the pre-operative lateral, confirming rotational deformity was significantly corrected. **K.** Clinically her mild left shoulder elevation improved with time. **L.** Her rotatory asymmetry is markedly improved from pre-op, though not perfect.

implants were placed at that time. I have found that many times the second surgery is not needed as the temporary rod and related releases results in better than anticipated correction.

PEARLS AND PITFALLS

- Avoid using the most proximal and distal fusion levels as fixation points for the temporary rod, as some plowing of temporary anchors can be expected.
- Pedicle screws in the upper thoracic vertebrae tend to plow in a cephalad direction rather easily. Therefore, upgoing hooks are usually used for cephalad fixation of the temporary rod.
- Place the temporary rod as early as possible during the first surgery, so that multiple distractions can be applied to the rods during subsequent release and osteotomies.
- Beware of elevating the left shoulder with correction of the right thoracic curves.
- Neuromonitoring is essential, as the spine will be lengthened.

REFERENCE

1. Buchowski JM, Bhatnagar R, Skaggs DL, et al. Temporary internal distraction as an aid to correction of severe scoliosis. *J Bone Joint Surg Am.* 2006;88(9):2035–2041.

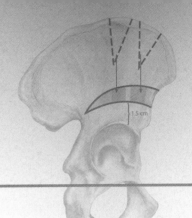

Index

Note: Page numbers followed by *f* and *t* indicate figures and tables, respectively.